Cognitive Neurology

Cognitive Neurology
A Clinical Textbook

Edited by

Stefano F. Cappa
Professor of Neuropsychology
Vita-Salute San Raffaele University
and Head of Neurology, San Raffaele
Turro Hospital

Jubin Abutalebi
Contracted Professor,
Faculty of Psychology,
University Vita-Salute
San Raffaele Milan, Italy

Jean-François Démonet
INSERM Research Director,
Inserm U825, Toulouse (France)

Paul C. Fletcher
Wellcome Trust Senior Research
Fellow in Clinical Science,
University of Cambridge

Peter Garrard
Department of Clinical Neurosciences,
University of Southampton School of Medicine,
Southampton General Hospital,
Southampton

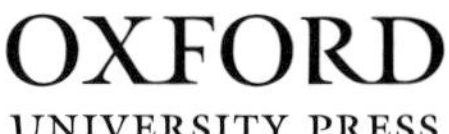

OXFORD
UNIVERSITY PRESS

Great Clarendon Street, Oxford OX2 6DP

Oxford University Press is a department of the University of Oxford.
It furthers the University's objective of excellence in research, scholarship,
and education by publishing worldwide in

Oxford New York

Auckland Cape Town Dar es Salaam Hong Kong Karachi
Kuala Lumpur Madrid Melbourne Mexico City Nairobi
New Delhi Shanghai Taipei Toronto

With offices in

Argentina Austria Brazil Chile Czech Republic France Greece
Guatemala Hungary Italy Japan Poland Portugal Singapore
South Korea Switzerland Thailand Turkey Ukraine Vietnam

Oxford is a registered trade mark of Oxford University Press
in the UK and in certain other countries

Published in the United States
by Oxford University Press Inc., New York

First published 2008

British Library Cataloguing in Publication Data

Data available

Library of Congress Cataloging-in-Publication Data

Data available

Typeset by Cepha Imaging Private Ltd., Bangalore, India
Printed in Great Britain
on acid-free paper by
Biddles Ltd., King's Lynn, Norfolk

ISBN 978–0–19–856927–5

10 9 8 7 6 5 4 3 2 1

Foreword

A clinical cognitive neurology textbook sounds a daunting read. Stefano F. Cappa and his co-editors have marshalled a group of young but experienced authors in a novel and exciting manner. The result is a manual of clinical relevance that is both readable and full of facts. More, they are often novel facts, but above all placed within the context of modern theories of cognitive function, often elaborated with the help of modern investigative techniques. The book presents cognitive neurology in its current journey along a road from psychological and neuropsychological description towards a brain based understanding of how cognitive processes come about in biological term. Further the comparatively recent appreciation of the role of compensation that occurs after injury or degeneration (at least in early stages) is accounted for explicitly in discussion of symptoms and syndromes. The capacity for plastic reorganization in the adult, even elderly brain is making a big impact on the interpretation of cognitive 'signs'. Likewise there is an ongoing impact on the understanding of how plastic mechanisms become engaged with resulting implications for cognitive manipulation for therapeutic purposes. A popular example of this is the current popularity of brain training games and devices. The serious underlying science is becoming a major issue occupying the mind of those practicing cognitive neurology.

The book is organized into an initial orienting methods section that is short and treated succinctly and effectively in three introductory chapters. There follow expositions of the clinical features of cognitive disorders associated with acute brain damage, chronic neurodegenerative disease leading to dementia, and finally other disorders leading to cognitive dysfunction. The third section of this group is especially interesting, dealing with cognitive disorders associated with psychiatric diseases and neurological disorders not traditionally associated with such problems, for example multiple sclerosis.

A book about cognitive disorders that offers principles of treatment is not common and there is real wisdom and information to be found in this concluding section.

Cognitive neurology is coming of age. The empirical behavioural approaches introduced by pioneers such as Warrington and Milner to behavioural characterization are now proving especially valuable when investigators attempt to discover the brain basis of cognitive symptoms and syndromes. Their methods, notably imaging and neurophysiology, also promise much in terms of monitoring treatment in the future. This very informative book will bring those reading it up-to-date with modern advances and modern practice. I believe the book is also admirably suited for inspiring those interested in understanding more of the effects of brain disease on higher cognitive functions.

Richard Frackowiak
Professor of Cognitive Neurology
Institute of Neurology UCL and
Director of the département d'études cognitives
Ecole Normale Supérieure
Paris

February 2008

Contents

Contributors

Jubin Abutalebi
Centre for Cognitive Neuroscience,
Faculty of Psychology,
Vita-Salute San Raffaele University,
Via Olgettina 58,
20132 Milan, Italy

Jean-Marie Annoni
Department of Neurology and Neuropsychological Unit,
Geneva University Hospitals and Medical School,
1211 Geneva, Switzerland, and
Department of Neurology,
Lausanne University Hospital,
1011 Lausanne, Switzerland

Jennifer H. Barnett
Department of Psychiatry,
University of Cambridge,
Addenbrooke's Hospital, Hills Road,
Cambridge CB2 2QQ, England

Ferdinand Binkofski
Department of Neurology and Neuroimage Nord,
University Hospital of Schleswig-Holstein,
Campus Lübeck,
Ratzeburger Allee 160,
D-23538 Lübeck, Germany

Julien Bogousslavsky
Department of Neurology,
University of Lausanne,
1011 Lausanne, Switzerland

John Bowler
Department of Neurology,
Royal Free Hospital,
London NW3 2QG, England

William S. Brooks
Prince of Wales Medical Research Institute,
Barker Street, Randwick,
New South Wales NSW 2031 and
University of New South Wales,
Sydney,
New South Wales NSW 2052, Australia

Stefano F. Cappa
Vita-Salute San Raffaele University,
DIBIT- Via Olgettina 58,
20132 Milan, and
Department of Neurology San Raffaele Turro,
Via Stamira d'Ancona 20,
20127 Milan, Italy

Lisa Cipolotti
Department of Neuropsychology,
National Hospital for Neurology and Neurosurgery,
Queen Square,
London WC1N 3BG, England

Jean-François Démonet
INSERM U825, Pole Neurosciences,
CHU Purpan, 31059 Toulouse, France

John E. Duda
Parkinson's Disease Research, Education and Clinical Center
Philadelphia VA Medical Center
3900 Woodland Avenue
Philadelphia, Pennsylvania 19104, USA

Paul C. Fletcher
Department of Psychiatry,
University of Cambridge,
Addenbrooke's Hospital, Hills Road,
Cambridge CB2 2QQ, England

Peter Garrard
Department of Clinical Neurosciences,
University of Southampton School of Medicine,
Southampton General Hospital,
Southampton SO16 6YD, England

Maria Luisa Gorno-Tempini
Memory and Aging Center,
Department of Neurology,
University of California at San Francisco,
San Francisco, California, USA

Christoph Helmstaedter
University Clinic of Epileptology Bonn,
Neuropsychology,
Sigmund Freud Str. 25,
53105 Bonn, Germany

Jürg Kesselring
Department of Neurology,
Rehabilitation Centre,
CH-7317 Valens, Switzerland

John B. J. Kwok
University of New South Wales,
Sydney, New South Wales NSW 2052 and
Garvan Institute of Medical Research,
Darlinghurst, New South Wales NSW 2010,
Australia

Andrew J. Larner
Cognitive Function Clinic,
Walton Centre for Neurology and
Neurosurgery,
Lower Lane, Fazakerley,
Liverpool L9 7LJ, England

Sandra Lehmann
Division of Rehabilitation,
Department of Clinical Neurosciences,
University Hospital,
CH-1211 Geneva 14, Switzerland

Belinda Lennox
Department of Psychiatry,
University of Cambridge,
Addenbrooke's Hospital, Hills Road,
Cambridge CB2 2QQ, England

Clement T. Loy
University of New South Wales,
Sydney, New South Wales NSW 2052 and
Garvan Institute of Medical Research,
Darlinghurst, New South Wales NSW 2010,
Australia

Angelo Maravita
Università di Milano-Bicocca,
Via dell'Innovazione 10,
20126 Milan, Italy

Ian G. McKeith
Wolfson Research Centre,
Newcastle General Hospital,
Newcastle upon Tyne, NE46BE,
England

Ulrich Müller
Department of Psychiatry,
University of Cambridge;
Cambridgeshire and Peterborough Mental
Health Partnership NHS Trust,
Downing Site Cambridge, CB2 3EB,
England; and
Behavioural and Clinical Neuroscience
Institute (BCNI)

Jared Narvid
Memory and Aging Center,
Department of Neurology,
University of California at San Francisco,
San Francisco, California, USA

Jérémie Parienté
INSERM U825, Pole Neurosciences
CHU Purpan, 31059 Toulouse, France

Kathrin Reetz
Department of Neurology and Neuroimage
Nord,
University Hospital of Schleswig-Holstein,
Campus Lübeck,
Ratzeburger Allee 160,
D-23538 Lübeck,
Germany

Armin Schnider
Division of Rehabilitation,
Department of Clinical Neurosciences,
University Hospital,
CH-1211 Geneva 14,
Switzerland

Peter R. Schofield
Prince of Wales Medical Research Institute,
Barker Street, Randwick,
New South Wales NSW 2031 and
University of New South Wales,
Sydney, New South Wales NSW 2052, and
Garvan Institute of Medical Research,
Darlinghurst, New South Wales NSW 2010,
Australia

Sean A. Spence
University of Sheffield,
Academic Clinical Psychiatry,
The Longley Centre,
Norwood Grange Drive,
Sheffield S5 7JT, England

Guillaume Thierry
School of Psychology,
University of Wales,
Bangor LL57 2AS, Wales

Daniela Wyss
Department of Neurology,
Rehabilitation Centre,
CH-7317 Valens, Switzerland

Abbreviations

ACC	anterior cingulate cortex
ACE	Addenbrooke's Cognitive Examination
AChEI	acetylcholinesterase inhibitor
ACTH	adrenocorticotrophic hormone
AD	Alzheimer's disease
ADAS-Cog	Alzheimer's Disease Assessment Scale—Cognitive Section
ADHD	attention deficit hyperactivity disorder
ADL	activities of daily living
AED	anti-epileptic drug
AIP	anterior intraparietal area
ALS	amyotrophic lateral sclerosis
ApoE	apolipoprotein E
APP	amyloid precursor protein
ARMS	at-risk mental states
ASOH	allele-specific oligonucleotide hybridization
BECTS	benign epilepsy with centrotemporal spikes
BHC	benign hereditary chorea
BIT	behavioural inattention test
BLIP	brief limited intermittent psychosis
BOLD	blood oxygen-level dependent (signal)
BPO	body part as object (error)
BPSD	behavioural and psychological symptoms of dementia
CAA	cerebral amyloid angiopathy
CADASIL	cerebral autosomal dominant arteriopathy with subcortical infarcts and leucoencephalopathy
CBD	corticobasal degeneration
CBF	cerebral blood flow
CBT	cognitive behavioural therapy
CCAS	cerebellar cognitive affective syndrome
CERAD	Consortium to Establish a Registry for Alzheimer's Disease
ChEI	cholinesterase inhibitor
CIBIC	Clinician's Interview-Based Impression of Change
CIT	constraint-induced therapy
CJD	Creutzfeldt–Jakob disease
$CMRO_2$	cerebral metabolic rate for oxygen
CNS	central nervous system
COMT	catechyl-*O*-methyltransferase
CSF	cerebrospinal fluid
CSWS	continuous spikes and waves during slow wave sleep syndrome
CT	computerized tomography
CVA	cerebrovascular accident
DAI	diffuse axonal injuries
DAT	dementia of the Alzheimer type *or* dopamine transporter
DFT	dementia of the frontal type
DLB	dementia with Lewy bodies
DLDH	dementia lacking distinctive histology
DLPFC	dorsolateral prefrontal cortex
DMS	delusional misindentification syndrome
DRPLA	dentatorubropallidoluysian atrophy
DS	Down syndrome
DTI	diffusion tensor imaging
DT-MRI	diffusion tensor magnetic resonance imaging
DUP	duration of untreated psychosis
ECT	electroconvulsive therapy
EDSS	Expanded Disability Status Scale
EEG	electroencephalography
EMF	evoked magnetic field
EOAD	early-onset Alzheimer's disease
ERP	event-related potential
ESES	electrical status epilepticus in sleep
fCJD	familial Creutzfeldt–Jakob disease
FDA	Food and Drugs Administration (US)
FDG	fluorodeoxy-glucose
FEP	first-episode psychosis
FFI	fatal familial insomnia
FFT	fast Fourier transform
FLE	frontal lobe epilepsy
fMRI	functional magnetic resonance imaging
FTD	frontotemporal dementia

FTDP-17	FTD with parkinsonism linked to chromosome 17
FTLD	frontotemporal lobar degeneration
FTLD-U	FTLD with ubiquitin-only inclusions
fvAD	frontal variant Alzheimer's disease
fvFTD	frontal variant frontotemporal dementia
GABA	gamma aminobutyric acid
GAF	Global Assessment of Functioning (scale)
GFAP	glial fibrillary acidic protein
GKS	gamma knife surgery
GOM	granular osmiophilic deposit
GSS	Gerstmann–Sträussler–Scheinker
GT	gambling task
GTCS	generalized tonic-clonic seizure
HCHWA-D	hereditary cerebral haemorrhage with amyloidosis Dutch type
HD	Huntington's disease
HIV	human immunodeficiency virus
HMPAO	TC99-hexamethylyl-propyleneamine
HPA	hippocampal–pituitary–adrenal (axis)
HRQoL	health-related quality of life
HSV	herpes simplex virus
HVLT-R	Hopkins Verbal Learning Test-Revised
IADL	instrumental activities of daily living
IEED	involuntary emotional expression disorder
IFN	interferon
IGE	idiopathic generalized epilepsy
IQCODE	Informant Questionnaire on Cognitive Decline in the Elderly
IV	intravenous
JME	juvenile myoclonus epilepsy
LB	Lewy body
LBD	Lewy body disease
LBVAD	Lewy body variant of Alzheimer's disease
LEV	levitiracetam
LI	latent inhibition
LKS	Landau-Kleffner syndrome
LN	Lewy neurite
LOAD	late-onset Alzheimer's disease
LP	Lewy pathology
LTG	lamotrigine
MAP	motor action potentials
MAPT	microtubule-associated protein tau
MBI	mild brain injury
MCI	mild cognitive impairment
MEG	magnetoencephalography
MIBG	meta-iodobenzylguanidine
MMN	mismatch negativity
MMSE	Mini-Mental State examination
MND	motor neuron disease
MRI	magnetic resonance imaging
MRS	magnetic resonance spectroscopy
MS	multiple sclerosis
MSFC	Multiple Sclerosis Functional Composite
MTL	medial temporal lobe
NAA	*N*-acetyl aspartate
NARI	noradrenaline reuptake inhibitors
NART	National Adult Reading Test
NAT	noradrenaline transporter
NBM	nucleus basalis of Meynert
NFT	neurofibrillary tangle
NMDA	*N*-methyl-D-aspartic acid
NPC	Niemann–Pick disease type C
NPI	Neuropsychiatric Inventory (test)
NSAID	nonsteroidal anti-inflammatory drug
OCD	obsessive-compulsive disorder
OER	oxygen extraction ratio
PAS	periodic acid–Schiff
PASAT	Paced Auditory Serial Addition Test
PCA	posterior cortical atrophy
PD	Parkinson's disease
PDD	Parkinson's disease with dementia
PET	positron emission tomography
PHF	paired helical filament
PiD	Pick's disease
PNFA	progressive nonfluent aphasia
PPA	primary progressive aphasia
PPI	prepulse inhibition
PrP	prion protein
PS	presenilin (PS1 and PS2)
qEEG	quantitative electroencephalography
RBD	REM sleep-behaviour disorder
rCBF	regional cerebral blood flow
RCT	randomized clinical trial
REM	rapid eye movement sleep
rINN	recommended international non-proprietary name
SC	superior colliculus

SCA	spinocerebellar ataxia
sCJD	sporadic Creutzfeldt–Jakob disease
SD	semantic dementia
SMA	supplementary motor area
SNRI	serotonin and noradrenaline re-uptake inhibitor
SP	senile (amyloid) plaques
SPECT	single-photon emission computerized tomography
sRF	somatosensory receptive field
SSPE	subacute sclerosing panencephalitis
SSRI	selective serotonin re-uptake inhibitor
T4	thyroxin
TBI	traumatic brain injury
TCS	transcranial sonography
TLE	temporal lobe epilepsy
ToM	theory of mind
TPM	topiramate
TSE	transmissible spongiform encephalopathy
TSH	thyroid stimulating hormone
UBI	ubiquitin-only inclusions
ULN	unilateral neglect
USN	unilateral spatial neglect
VaD	vascular dementia
VBM	voxel-based morphometry
VBZ	carbamazepine
VCI	vascular cognitive impairment
vCJD	variant Creutzfeldt–Jakob disease
VIP	ventral intraparietal area
VLPFC	ventrolateral prefrontal cortex
VM	ventromedial
VNS	vagal nerve (electrical) stimulation
VPA	valproic acid
vRF	visual receptive field
WAIS-R	Wechlser Adult Intelligence Scale Revised
WCST	Wisconsin Card Sorting Test

Part 1

Assessment methods

Chapter 1

Introduction and clinical examination

Jean-François Démonet

1.1 Overview of cognitive neurology

Cognitive neurology has as its aim the assessment and treatment of disorders of human behaviour and cognition while relating these disorders to dysfunctions and/or lesions of the brain. The approach is highly interdisciplinary and relies on a variety of scientific domains and methods.

The first source of knowledge is the medical sciences, in particular, the areas of neuroanatomy, neurophysiology, and clinical neurology. Evidence from the clinical neurosciences allows clinicians to suspect specific brain lesions or dysfunctions that are likely to account for a given cognitive and/or behavioural disorder. However, results from neuroimaging (X-ray computerized tomography (CT), magnetic resonance imaging (MRI)) are frequently immediately available and represent 'short cuts' that make reasoning based on indirect cues about the site of the lesion less necessary than formerly. It may even be tempting to reverse the usual approach, i.e. to predict disclosure of a symptom based on a refined neuroimaging of lesions. However, in practical terms, owing to the randomness of the anatomy of lesions and the multidimensionality of their consequences on human behaviour and performance, this type of prediction only rarely proves useful at the individual level. Nevertheless, as in every domain of medicine, priority is given to the actually observed symptoms rather than to the full set of possible consequences of a given lesion or disease.

The second source of knowledge to be invoked relates to the main theoretical and experimental conceptualizations from cognitive psychology and psycholinguistics. These allow researchers and clinicians to decipher disorders of human behaviour and cognition in a systematic way, i.e. to describe disorders and seek for specific effects on theoretical grounds. These theories lead to the construction of models of the information processing that is thought to take place in the human mind/brain. According to these conceptualizations, two types of processing can be distinguished depending on whether these operations are: (1) specific to a sensorimotor modality such as the visual identification of categories of objects; or (2) not confined to any one modality or possibly active on every modality. While the latter correspond to attentional, executive, or amodal semantic functions and representations, the former have been thought to involve highly specific processing entities such as the modules as defined by Fodor (1983).

The best known examples of functional models of cognitive functions come from the seminal works on language processing by Coltheart, Marshall, Morton, and Newcombe, which brought about the so-called 'dual routes' model of reading that distinguishes between addressing and assembly procedures in processing written inputs (e.g. see Marshall and Newcombe 1973).

In neuropsychology, this approach is based on the transparency hypothesis put forward by Caramazza (1986). In this hypothesis the pattern of performance observed in a patient with cognitive disorders allows researchers to make inferences about the underlying cognitive system in the same way as they would from patterns observed in normal subjects. The abnormal performances observed are thought to reflect dysfunction of some components of the system even though compensatory processes are likely to intervene following brain lesion that may alter earlier patterns.

These cognitive models are still unsatisfactory, are constantly revised, and are even challenged by other approaches (such as the parallel-processing computational models that questioned the validity of the earlier dual route models of reading; e.g. Ans *et al.* 1998). However, their heuristic value has been conspicuous in various domains of cognitive functions such as language, perception, and memory. These models might even be helpful to the cognitive neurologist in clinical practice in that he/she can explore cognitive performance in a patient while seeking key features suggesting a specific dysfunction of a component of the model. For example, contrasting the reading of pseudowords and irregular words would allow the clinician to assess, respectively, possible disorders of assembly and addressing procedures in reading.

Even though fruitful, this analytical approach, which implies lengthy and thorough evaluations in each patient, may not be suitable in clinical practice. The immediate aim of cognitive and behavioural assessment is often to confirm the existence of a definite disturbance in a given cognitive domain (e.g. to diagnose aphasia, deficit of episodic memory, or dysexecutive syndrome) or, even more frequently, to diagnose a dementia so that decisions on medical treatment and remediation can be taken.

1.2 Outline of Part 1

Part 1 presents the principles and main methods for assessing cognitive and behavioural disorders as well as exploring the dysfunctions and lesions of the human brain that cause these disorders.

- Chapter 1 covers the bases of the clinical examination in cognitive neurology. Clinical examination is obviously the earliest step of the assessment of cognitive and behavioural functions. It is also a crucial stage at which an informal evaluation by the clinician of the patient's attitude and behaviour, his/her demands and complaints (or the absence of such complaints!), and the medical and general context leading to neuropsychological assessment will take place. These data are of major importance and will allow the clinician, more or less efficiently depending on his/her expertise, to plan further detailed investigation of specific cognitive/behavioural domains, neurophysiological or neuroimaging investigations, or therapeutic interventions.
- Chapter 2 presents the different types and examples of neuropsychological 'tools' that allow clinicians to assess cognitive and behavioural disturbances.
- Chapter 3 covers the main neurophysiological and neuroimaging methods for exploring the lesions and the dysfunctions of the human brain. These abnormalities are very diverse in both time course (from acute to chronic) and aetiology (from developmental to degenerative), involving as well focal, acquired lesions.

1.3 Clinical examination

A crucial step in neuropsychological assessment is the interview of the patient and, if possible, his/her relative(s). This involves tactful yet systematic questions to determine disorders observed in the patient as well as his/her complaints. When possible it is important to conduct interviews of the patient and relatives separately. Discrepancies between the interview of the patient and that of carers, friends, or members of his/her family are worth noting, especially to detect anosognosia or, less frequently, overestimation of cognitive disorders in the patient.

Systematic questionnaires for the relatives will be helpful in assessing behavioural disturbances or the impact of cognitive disorders on daily activities as well as the increase of burden for relatives (e.g. Neuropsychiatric Inventory (NPI; Cummings *et al.* 1994), Caregiver Burden Inventory (Novak and Guest 1989)).

- The circumstances of disorders' occurrences, their duration, and evolution over time have to be precisely recorded as well as the conditions of daily living (alone, with family and/or friends), level of education, and type of occupation (past or present).
- The medical context will be systematically explored to list familial and personal antecedents, as well as on-going pathological conditions and treatments, especially neuropsychiatric disorders and central nervous system (CNS) drugs.
- The existence of bilingualism, incomplete mastering of written language for the language(s) spoken by the subject, as well as disorders of learning to read and write in childhood are important features that may hamper many cognitive tests.
- Manual preference will be determined by a systematic questionnaire (e.g. Edinburgh Inventory; Oldfield 1971).
- The impact of the supposed cognitive disorders on the patient's daily abilities in his/her familial, professional and social environment will be evaluated, ideally with the help of a reliable relative. This evaluation should explore domains of activity such as food preparation, drug intake, management of budget and administrative forms, use of the telephone, ability to travel alone and buy basic items (instrumental activities of daily living (IADL; Lawton and Brody 1969)). The patient's autonomy in performing basic tasks such as feeding, bathing, and sphincter functions (activities of daily living (ADL; Katz 1983)) should also be assessed.

The patient interview must be complemented by a session of informal assessment and clinical examination. The clinician will thus evaluate briefly, among other functions, temporal spatial orientation as well as ability to understand verbal instructions, to name objects and drawings, to formulate adequate sentences, and to register and retrieve new verbal information as well as features of the recent news. It is also important to evaluate the patient's ability to maintain his/her attention engaged in a given task as well as the degree of his/her motivation and participation in the proposed assessment. In patients showing important fluctuations of attention and/or fatigue, the future formal assessments will be carried out over several short sessions. The general medical context and time course of on-going acute health problems will lead the clinician to postpone non-essential aspects of cognitive evaluation.

The neurological examination will briefly assess motor functions (including voluntary ocular saccades, parkinsonian symptoms, and other movement disorders), gait, and balance as well as sensory functions, seeking especially for visual, tactile, and auditory acuity deficit as well as visual field deficit and signs of unilateral neglect. It will be useful to investigate primitive reflexes (Borroni *et al.* 2006), impairments of gesture series realization (as described by Luria 1966), and pathological imitation behaviour (Lhermitte *et al.* 1986).

Time permitting, another important stage of this first contact with the patient is to explore his/her ability to evoke the main biographical steps and milestones in personal and familial life. Not only does this part of the interview allow the clinician to evaluate informally the richness of past memories in the patient at different life periods (giving some hints of the existence of a temporal gradient in his/her remote memory) but also this part of the interview may give the patient the opportunity to reveal some omitted yet clinically relevant elements such as traumatic episodes or psychiatric treatments. While exploring autobiographical episodic memory, it seems more fruitful to rely on personally relevant milestones such as recent holidays or familial meetings rather than formal units in calendar (last month, last year). The biography will be explored according to the usual periods (school period, academic/professional training, wedding, children's births, jobs/unemployment periods, retirement). It may also be interesting to assess the ability of the patient to sketch out the structure of his/her family (e.g. ages, names, and occupations of children and grandchildren). Again, it is very important to double-check these biographical details with a reliable member of the patient's entourage. In the case of an acute medical condition, family and relatives will be of invaluable help in finding out how the patient has behaved in the recent past and, for example, the circumstances that preceded his/her admission to a hospital.

References

Ans, B., Carbonnel, S., and Valdois, S. (1998). A connectionist multiple-trace memory model for polysyllabic word reading. *Psychol. Rev.* **105**, 678–723.

Borroni, B., Broli, M., Costanzi, C., Gipponi, S., Gilberti, N., Agosti, C., and Padovani, A. (2006). Primitive reflex evaluation in the clinical assessment of extrapyramidal syndromes. *Eur. J. Neurol.* **13**, 1026–8.

Caramazza, A. (1986). On drawing inferences about the structure of normal cognitive systems from the analysis of patterns of impaired performance: the case for single-patient studies. *Brain Cogn.* **5**, 41–66.

Cummings, J.L., Mega, M., Gray, K., Rosenberg-Thompson, S., Carusi, D.A., and Gornbein, J. (1994). The Neuropsychiatric Inventory: comprehensive assessment of psychopathology in dementia. *Neurology* **44**, 2308–14.

Fodor, J. (1983). *The modularity of mind.* MIT Press, Cambridge, Massachusetts.

Katz, S. (1983). Assessing self-maintenance: activities of daily living, mobility and instrumental activities of daily living. *J. Am. Geriatr. Soc.* **31**, 721–6.

Lawton, M.P. and Brody, E.M. (1969). Assessment of older people: self-maintaining and instrumental activities of daily living. *Gerontologist* **9**, 179–86.

Lhermitte, F., Pillon, B., and Serdaru, M. (1986). Human autonomy and the frontal lobes. Part I. Imitation and utilization behavior: a neuropsychological study of 75 patients. *Ann. Neurol.* **19** (4), 326–34.

Luria, A.R. (1966). *Higher cortical functions.* Basic Books, New York.

Marshall, J.C. and Newcombe, F. (1973). Patterns of paralexia. A psycholinguistic approach. *J. Psycholinguist. Res.* **2**, 175–99.

Novak, M. and Guest, C. (1989). Application of a multidimensional caregiver burden inventory. *Gerontologist* **29**, 798–803.

Oldfield, O.D. (1971). The assessment and analysis of handedness: the Edinburgh inventory. *Neuropsychologia* **9**, 97–113.

Chapter 2

Neuropsychological testing

Jérémie Parienté and Jean-François Démonet

2.1 Introduction

Single cognitive domain tests, global cognitive 'batteries', or non-test assessment, such as questionnaires or inventories for the patient, his/her relatives, or the clinician, can be used in various situations and practices ranging from clinical medicine to theoretical neurosciences, or education and social sciences. As the field of neuropsychological assessment tends to grow, an aim in testing patients should be to reflect real-life behaviour and its disturbances.

Cognitive assessment requires from the examiner a good theoretical and practical knowledge of the tests used. Because of the broad range of the cognitive functions and the necessity of assessing subject's performance over several trials for each function, assessing the cognitive status of patients is time-consuming. Therefore, the way in which patients will be assessed has to be guided by strategic decisions involving a trade-off between the minimal list of tests deemed necessary and the risk of patient fatigue over a too prolonged session of testing (typically the duration of a session should not exceed 90 minutes including short breaks). This strategy for testing depends on the aim of the evaluation: determination of the patient's cognitive status as it contributes to diagnosis; 'baseline' evaluation before initiating a treatment; evaluation of an improvement or a deterioration of cognitive functions at follow up; forensic or research purposes.

Among the various purposes of neuropsychological assessment, clinical diagnosis remains the main reason for using cognitive and behavioural tests. This evaluation has to be adapted to its aims and the different tools chosen will vary with clinical circumstances that are as diverse as: late, progressive, or acute recent onset of a cognitive deficit; single cognitive domain impairment or behavioural disturbances; in- or outpatient clinic; etc. Facing these different situations the clinician will have to choose the appropriate tools to answer the question that motivates the neuropsychological examination.

Cognitive tests share different properties: sensibility and specificity to a specific diagnosis; either inter- or intrarater, intersession reproducibility. These data as well as norms (generally stratified for diverse parameters such as age, gender, level of education of control subjects) have to be available in publications after the tests have been validated. Therefore, quantitative scores obtained in a patient are the main outcome of the vast majority of cognitive tests and behavioural scales; these scores have to be compared to the validated norms. However, qualitative aspects of the patient's performance during a test are invaluable sources of information for the clinician. Indeed, in many cases important variations in performance can be observed even in the context of a single test, depending on the nature of the task or the type of stimuli proposed to the patient. From such qualitative observations and the identification of specific error profiles, the notions of association and dissociation between cognitive functions or processes were derived. These concepts have been historically the bases of the development of knowledge in neuropsychology and have proved to be crucial for further advances. The co-occurrences or associations of symptoms lead clinicians to identify syndromes that relate to either anatomical or functional brain impairment. For example, the association of agraphia, acalculia, finger anomia, and right/left confusion defines Gerstmann's syndrome, which is anatomically based as it results from lesions of an inferior region of the left parietal lobe, which harbours the cortical territories necessary to these functions. An example of a functional syndrome is the co-occurrence of dysexecutive and memory disorders secondary to Parkinson's disease, which indirectly induces dysfunction of functional pathways involving striato-frontal loops. Dissociations between preserved and impaired cognitive abilities have been used to delineate distinct processes within a given domain (Shallice 1988). For example, dissociations between categories (e.g. animate versus inanimate objects, or verbs versus nouns) can be found in naming performance suggesting that different underlying processes come into play during such a simple task. These observations were used to build up functional models of cognitive abilities, especially in the language domain (Coltheart *et al.* 1991). Naming can also be used for analysing the type of errors. For example, the preponderance of semantic relative to phonological errors (or vice versa) in post-stroke aphasic patients is an important feature that allows clinicians to determine the level of language disorganization according to cognitive models and possibly the site of the lesion.

In this chapter we will first describe briefly the methodology of the neuropsychological evaluation and how it has to be adapted to situations and questions. We will then give, in table format, a summary of the main neuropsychological and behavioural tests used in clinical and research assessment. This format has been chosen to be readily available to the clinician. For further details about tests listed (or not) in this chapter, the reader should refer to dedicated books (Boller and Grafman 2000; Lezak *et al.* 2004).

2.2 Methodology

As mentioned above the choice of the tests will depend on the situation in which the patient will be evaluated. Time given, expertise of the examiner regarding neuropsychology in general and the tests in particular, but also the type and severity of the cognitive deficit, behavioural problems, and, of course, the aim of the assessment will guide the examiner to select the appropriate tests to customize the evaluation to the patient's needs—either a ready-to-use battery of tests yielding a global cognitive assessment or different single cognitive domain tests to focus on the cognitive profile specific to the patient. The latter approach will enable the examiner to reveal syndrome or dissociations between altered and preserved processes, categories, or domains.

Of the vast array of neuropsychological tests, no single one could fulfil the requirements of every possible clinical situation and purpose. In practical terms, the clinician should be acquainted with a selection of validated global batteries and domain-specific tests that would bring out a first clinical appreciation. It will then be necessary to resort to more specific cognitive tests depending on the impairments found initially.

2.2.1 Methodology varies with the objectives

2.2.1.1 Clinical evaluation

During this type of assessment with a clinical purpose, the examiner will have to remain flexible and adapt to the ongoing collection of observations. While a battery of tests may be helpful in the first step of the evaluation, it is often necessary to interpret 'on-line' the results of the subtests to adapt the testing strategy and focus on the identified deficits.

- **Screening**. Brief and accurate tests are required. They need to be sensitive but less specific in order to be able to diagnose all the potential patients. Patients with scores below the cut-off at this first evaluation will then be assessed by more specific tests. For example, a Mini Mental State Examination (Folstein *et al.* 1975) could be a first step in the evaluation of a patient with a memory complaint. If it is found that none of the three words has been recalled, a Grober and Buschke test (Grober *et al.* 1988) will help the clinician to better understand the memory disturbance and its sensitivity to semantic cuing.
- **Follow-up**. In this type of assessment it is necessary to repeat the same tests over a certain period of time. In this situation there is less utility in using highly validated tests, each patient being his/her own control. It is nevertheless important to be aware of the test–retest effects that could be avoided by using parallel versions.
- **Forensic evaluation.** The aim of this evaluation is to infer the effective disturbances in real life situations (personal and professional) resulting from neuropsychological disorders. Therefore a trend to assess the patient with more 'ecological tests' has emerged (Alderman *et al.* 2003). However this approach remains complementary to more classical and well-established tests.

2.2.1.2 Evaluation of a rehabilitation procedure

This sort of evaluation has two aims. First, as during clinical evaluation, an appreciation of the patient's cognitive status across time is needed (improvement or deterioration). Second, the specifics of the effects of rehabilitation should be evaluated. Furthermore, it is important to establish whether rehabilitation effects have generalized to non-trained items within the rehabilitated domain or to non-rehabilitated cognitive domains. The results of this evaluation may ultimately lead to modifications of the rehabilitation programme. During this type of assessment the examiner will face three pitfalls.

- **Test–retest effect.** This may lead to a false-positive result for the rehabilitation programme. However, some tests are sophisticated enough to avoid this effect, e.g. by using parallel lists of items tested.
- **Spontaneous variability and the natural history of the cognitive performance.** For example, it will sometimes be difficult to evaluate the beneficial effect of speech therapy administered to an aphasic patient after a stroke as recovery is part of the natural history. To avoid this confounding factor in the rehabilitation programme assessment it is therefore necessary to evaluate the patient several times at baseline before any treatment. These baseline evaluations will then be averaged and compared to the subsequent evaluations.
- **Test specificity to the rehabilitated cognitive processes programme**. Here it is important to choose, on the one hand, tests specific to the cognitive functions that are at stake in the rehabilitation programme and, on the other hand, tests independent of the former (e.g. constructive apraxia tests in an aphasic patient being rehabilitated with a phonological paradigm).

2.2.1.3 In research

In this case, tests will be chosen or even elaborated in order to match the aim of the study, i.e. describing a cognitive process, evaluating the natural history of the cognitive deficit, establishing a specific rehabilitation procedure, or assessing the influence of a specific pharmacological compound. Neuropsychological but also behavioural or quality of life tests will be chosen or elaborated to investigate specific dissociations within or between processes. A qualitative approach to the results obtained will be of particular importance, and focusing on the type of errors will enable the researcher to decipher the cognitive disturbance underlying the performance deficit. These research approaches will sometimes require the formation of groups of patients rigorously selected on specific inclusion criteria. Patients fulfilling the criteria will subsequently be systematically assessed with a set of tests predefined on the basis of the study hypothesis.

2.3 **Test classification**

Since clinicians need to measure the cognitive performance of patients, a very large body of tests has accumulated over the past century ranging from tests administered by the examiner to the patient (California Verbal Learning Test; Delis *et al.* 1983, 1987, 2000) to self-questionnaires for the carer (Neuropsychiatric Inventory; Cummings *et al.* 1994).

The ideal test would be reproducible, valid in practice, and readily comprehensible and the 'best battery' would encompass a set of modules of tests assessing specifically different cognitive domains that one can use or combine to meet the patient/research protocol's specific needs.

Tests can be classified in different ways as the following example shows.

- Cognitive (Stroop test; Stroop 1935), behavioural (Lebert *et al.* 1998), and quality of life (Naglie *et al.* 2006) tests and questionnaires.
- Global (Mini Mental State Examination; Folstein *et al.* 1975), multidomain tests sensitive to different cognitive processes (categorical fluency involving both executive functions, working memory, and semantic memory) or domain-specific tests (Grober and Buschke memory test; Grober *et al.* 1988).
- A psychometric approach in which the performance of a subject is compared to a validated norm (IQ measurement with WAIS; Wechsler 1997*a*) versus concept-driven cognitive evaluation (dissociated performance for producing proper names compared to common names).

In the following tables we provide the reader with some example with batteries, tests, and questionnaires frequently used in the neuropsychological assessment. Tables 2.1and 2.2 list some ability and neuropsychological assessment batteries, respectively. Table 2.3 and 2.4 list some dementia batteries. Tables 2.5–2.11 give examples of frequently used single-domain tests (memory, attention, perception, language, construction, reasoning, executive function).

Table 2.1 Batteries testing ability

Battery (reference)	**Description**	**Comments**
WAIS-R, Wechsler Adult Intelligence Scale—Revised (Wechsler 1981)	Global cognitive functioning: verbal tests (information, comprehension, arithmetic, similarities, digit span, vocabulary) & non-verbal tests of performance (digit symbol, picture completion, block design, picture arrangement, object assembly)	Complete and representative standardization; verbal intelligence and performance intelligence scores
WAIS-III, Wechsler Adult Intelligence Scale III (Wechsler 1997*a*)	Global cognitive functioning: same as WAIS-R, plus letter/number sequencing, symbol search, matrix reasoning	Same as for WAIS-R

Table 2.2 Neuropsychological assessment batteries

Battery (reference)	Description	Comments
NAB, Neuropsychological Assessment Batteries (Stern and White 2003)	Attention, spatial, language, memory, executive 'modules' in 36 tests	Norms for ages from 18 to 97 (tested on 1400 subjects); norms given for each of the 36 tests; evaluation time up to 4 hours

Table 2.3 Dementia assessment batteries: general

Battery (reference)	Description	Comments
MMSE, Mini Mental State Examination (Folstein *et al.* 1975)	Brief screening instrument for dementia evaluating 5 domains: concentration or working memory; language; praxis; orientation memory; attention span	Strongly influenced by age & education; rapid to administer (10 minutes); total score, 30
ACE, Addenbrooke's Cognitive Examination (Mathuranath *et al.* 2000)	Global cognitive functioning: orientation; attention/mental tacking, episodic & semantic memory; verbal fluency; visuospatial ability	15–20 minutes, score from 0 to 100; MMSE score can be calculated from the global score. Cut-off score, 88/100
DRS or MDRS, Dementia Rating Scale or Mattis Dementia Rating Scale (Mattis 1988)	Designed for Alzheimer patients: attention; initiation and perseveration; construction; conceptual, memory	Healthy volunteers, 20 minutes, Alzheimer patient, up to 45 minutes. Maximum score, 144; cut-off, 125 for Alzheimer's disease
CERAD, Consortium to Establish a Registery for Alzheimer Disease (Morris *et al.* 1989)	Designed for Alzheimer patients: verbal fluency: animals; 15 pictures of the Boston Naming Tests; Mini Mental State; word list memory test; constructional praxis; word list recall; word list recognition	Rigorous standardization procedure; brief evaluation. Used as a diagnosis and to follow patient's course
SIB, Severe Impairment Battery (Saxton and Swihart 1989)	Designed to provide documentation of residual cognitive function at the lowest levels (one step question, use of gestural cues): social interaction; orientation; visuospatial ability; constructional ability; language; memory; attention; orienting to name; praxis	20 minute evaluation; standardization on Alzheimer patients with MMSE lower than 14. Sensitive to disease progression
ADAS-Cog, Alzheimer Disease Assessment Scale, Cognitive subscale (Rosen *et al.* 1984)	Scale used in research for Alzheimer disease drug approval. Language abilities, memory, praxis, orientation	30–35 minutes to administer. Maximum–minimum scores, 0–70 (higher scores indicating higher impairment)

Table 2.4 Dementia assessment batteries: neuropsychiatric and behavioural assessments

Battery (reference)	Description	Comments
NPI, Neuropsychiatric Inventory (Cummings *et al.* 1994)	Designed to assess behavioural disturbance in dementia patients by asking the caregiver about: delusion; hallucination; dysphoria; agitation/aggression; apathy; irritability/lability; disinhibition; aberrant motor behaviour	Frequency and severity are assessed on 4- and 3-point scales, respectively
Clinical Dementia Rating (http://www.adrc.wustl.edu/cdrScale.html)	Rates dementia on a 5-point scale where 0 = no dementia. This rating is based on memory, orientation, judgement, & problem solving; community and home activities; and hobbies and determined via a semi-structured questionnaire of the patient & his/her carer separately	CDR 0.5 is qualified 'questionable impairment', CDR1 'mild impairment', CDR2 'impairment dementia', & CDR3 'severe impairment'

Table 2.5 Tests of attention

Test (reference)	Description	Comments
Reaction time	A set of various tests ranging from simple reaction time (target detection) to more complex tasks (including complex visual target detection)	Test processing speed; speed is recorded
Digit span	The subject is asked to repeat a list of digits forward and backward	Tests short-term memory storage . capacity Individual scores (number of digits repeated in each task) give more information than the combined one as done in the WAIS-R
Sentence repetition	Repeating from easy and short to complicated and long sentences	Ecological test more related than the previous one to everyday functioning
Alpha span (Craik 1990)	Repeating a list of words in alphabetical order	Performance in this test is correlated with digit forward, backward and category fluency
N-back task	This task asks the subject to report when a stimulus item presented serially is the same as an item 'n' steps back from the items at hand	Mainly used in research
Stroop test (Jensen and Rohwer 1966)	3 phases: (1) read words of colours printed in black; (2) name the colour of coloured patches; (3) name the colour of the ink of words designating colours (where the meaning of the words & colour of ink are different)	Based upon the fact that it takes longer to find the name of the colour of an ink than to read the word written with this ink. Errors made and time to read/name the list of words/colours are recorded

Table 2.5 (continued) Tests of attention

Test (reference)	Description	Comments
Trail making test A and B	The subject is asked in part A to connect consecutively circled numbers. In part B, the subject has to perform the same task but alternating numbers and letters in an increasing and alphabetical order	Tests visuomotor tracking, divided attention, & mental flexibility. Subject is required to perform the task as fast as he/she can as time is recorded as well as errors

Table 2.6 Tests of visual inattention

Test (reference)	Description	Comments
Line bisection test (Schenkenberg *et al.* 1980)	The subject is shown a set of 20 horizontal lines of different size on an A4 format page & is asked to 'cut each line in half by placing a pencil mark through each line as close to its centre as possible'. Test is performed alternately with both hands & with the page at 0° & at 180°	Test for unilateral inattention. A percent deviation score is then calculated & is positive for marks placed right & negative for marks placed left of the centre
Cancellation tasks (Gauthier *et al.* 1989)	The patient is asked to cross out all the designated targets (bells, letters, balloons, etc.)	Test for visual inattention. Performance (omissions & errors) & speed are recorded
Drawing and copying test for inattention (Strub and Black 2000)	Patient is asked to draw (e.g. a clock, a daisy in a pot, a house in perspective) & to copy (e.g. a diamond, a cross, a cube, a pipe, a triangle within a triangle)	Test for visual unilateral inattention

Table 2.7 Tests of visual perception

Test (reference)	Description	Comments
Counting dots	The subject is asked to count dots widely scattered over a piece of paper	Visual scanning
Farnswoth's dichotomous test for colour blindness (D15)	Coloured caps of different brightness but slight differences of hue have to be rearranged in a consistent colour continuum starting with a cap fixed on a horizontal tray	Color perception. This test does not require colour naming & helps to distinguish colour agnosia from colour anomia
Judgement of line orientation (Benton *et al.* 1994)	Patient is asked to match a line segment shown to one of 11 radii forming a semi-circle. The task is repeated 30 times	Visual recognition. Estimates angular relationship of line segments to models

Table 2.7 (continued) Tests of visual perception

Test (reference)	Description	Comments
Test of facial recognition (Benton *et al.* 1994)	Patient is shown a face and asked to match it to the same face, either with identical or different light conditions or rotation	Face recognition. Ability to recognize faces with no memory involvement
Visual form discrimination (Benton *et al.* 1994)	Patient is asked in this multiple choice test to recognize a target among stimuli with very little variation from the target	Visual form recognition. Because of its multiple choice format, this test can be converted to a memory test
Gestalt completion tests (McCarty & Warrington 1990)	Incomplete pictures are presented & patient has to recognize and name the picture	Perceptual closure capacity. Test can be done on faces or object with varying difficulties
Visual object and space (Warrington & James 1991)	Shape detection screening, incomplete letters, silhouettes, object decision, progressive silhouettes, dot counting, number location, cube analysis	9-test battery exploring object & space perception; each test can be administered on its own. Normative data & cutting scores are provided for each subtest's perception battery
Overlapping figures tests (Gainotti *et al.* 1989)	Overlapping figures are presented to the patient & he/she is asked to name as many as possible	

Table 2.8 Tests of memory

Test (reference)	Description	Comments
Auditory verbal learning test (Rey 1964; Schmidt 1996)	The examiner reads list A (15 words) & patient is asked to recall them. Same procedure is done 5 times. Then 15 words of a second (interference) list (B) are read & the patient is asked to recall them. Finally, the patient is asked to recall as many words as possible from previously learned list A. A recognition trial of list A words can also be given	Tests verbal memory and does not control for encoding; The score for each trial is the number of words correctly recalled; it is also of interest to note words repeated during the recall, words from the other list, or errors (intrusions)
California verbal learning test & California verbal learning test—2nd edition (Delis *et al.* 1983, 1987; 2000)	Lists of 16 words (list A) belonging to 4 different categories (spices, vegetables, etc.) are read in a random order as in the auditory verbal learning test. Then list B is read after 5 trials. Patient after a 'short delay' has to recall as many words as possible and is then semantically cued ('free' and 'cued' recalls). The same procedure is done after a 'long delay' (20 minutes). Then a recognition task is administered mixing words from lists A & B and words not presented	Designed to assess the use of spontaneous semantic association as strategy for learning words. This is not a specific memory test but evaluates the interaction between memory & conceptual ability

Table 2.8 (continued) Tests of memory

Test (reference)	Description	Comments
Grober et Buschke test (Grober *et al.* 1988)	Patient is shown 4 × 4 written words belonging to 16 different semantic categories. He/she is asked to read aloud the word related to the category given by the examiner and immediately recall the words. 3 free recalls each followed by a semantically cued recall	This test is designed to assess the influence of semantic cuing in word retrieval. It is more specific to memory than the previous test & does not require patient to organize semantically the items to be remembered
Story recall (Wechsler 1997*b*)	A story is read aloud to the patient. After a delay, the patient is asked to recall as many details from the story as possible	Resembles everyday demand on memory
Complex figure test (Rey 1941; Corwin & Bylsma 1993)	A complex figure (Rey–Osterrieth) is copied by patient. After a delay, patient is asked to recall the complex figure	Test is designed to assess visual memory
Benton visual retention test (Sivan 1992)	3 figures are presented to the patient & he/she has to draw them, once hidden	This test is sensitive to unilateral spatial neglect & reflects of span of recall

Table 2.9 Tests of language

Test (reference)	Description	Comments
Western aphasia battery (Kertesz 1988) Kaplan	4 oral subtests: spontaneous speech; auditory comprehension; repetition; naming	Battery adapted from the Boston diagnostic aphasia examination (Goodglass & 1983, 2000)
Token test (Boller and Vignolo 1966)	Shapes (circle and squares) of different sizes (big or little) & colours (5 different) are placed in front of patient. He/she is asked to perform 62 different tasks from simple ('touch the green circle') to complex ('when I touch the green circle, you take the white square')	Test simple to administer and score that is sensitive to aphasia. Good performance relies mainly on auditory comprehension. It has been adapted in a short version (De Renzi & Faglioni 1978)
Boston naming test (Goodglass & Kaplan 2001)	Patient is shown 60 black & white ink pictures from common to less common & is asked to name them. When patient not able to name drawing, examiner gives him/her semantic then phonetic cues	Naming test simple to administer both in aphasic patients with left brain damage & in patients with a neurodegenerative disorder such as Alzheimer's disease
Control oral word association test (Benton & Hamsher 1994)	Patient is asked to give in 1 minute as many words as possible starting with a designated letter (e.g. F, then A and S) excluding proper nouns, numbers, & same words with different suffix	For each of the letters norms are provided except for the letters X and Z. Scores at this test are usually compared to the scores obtained in a similar test in which a patient is asked to give words belonging to a designated category

Table 2.10 Tests of construction

Test (reference)	Description	Comments
Complex figure test (Rey 1941; Corwin & Bylsma 1993)	A complex figure (Rey–Osterrieth) is copied by patient. After a delay, patient is asked to recall the complex figure	Test is designed to assess perceptual organization & visual memory. Each time a portion of the drawing is completed, the examiner gives patient a different-coloured pen in order to keep a record of the sequence used
Clock drawing (Battersby *et al.* 1956)	Examiner asks patient to draw a clock showing the number and 2 hands, set to 11:10	This test is very sensitive but not specific as it requires from the patient visuospatial abilities, numerical knowledge, working memory, executive function
Block design (Wechsler 1955, 1981, 1997*a*)	Subject is given red & white blocks & is asked to use them to replicate printed designs	This test is included in WAIS-III

Table 2.11 Tests of reasoning and executive functions

Test (reference)	Description	Comments
Similarities (Wechsler 1955, 1981, 1997*a*)	The subject is asked to explain what a pair of words have in common	This test has 2 levels of difficulty
Proverbs	Patient is asked to translate meaning of proverbs into concrete statements	Material used in this test must be familiar to patient
Raven's progressive matrices (Raven 1996)	Patient is asked to match visual patterns & analogy problems pictured in non-representational designs	This test does not require language & has been adapted to both young subjects & older patients (Raven's Coloured Progressive Matrices; Raven 1995)
Wisconsin card sorting test (Berg 1948; Milner 1964)	Subject is given cards on which are printed 1–4 identical symbols (triangle, circle, star, or cross) of different colours (red, blue, green, yellow). One color and type of symbol is printed on each given card. The task is to place the card according to a principle that the patient must deduce from the examiner's response. The rule changes during the test; therefore, patient must change the way he/she places the cards (the rule can be 'colour', 'number', 'form')	For example, patient has card with 4 blue circles. He/she can choose 3 different strategies to classify the card: circle; blue; or number (4.) According to the examiner's answer ('right' or 'wrong'), patient will have to keep the good strategy or continue to deduce the appropriate one
Tower of London (Shallice 1982)	The patient must look ahead to determine the order of moves necessary to arrange 3 coloured rings from their initial position on 2 of 3 sticks to a new set of predetermined positions on 1 or more of the sticks	

Table 2.11 (continued) Tests of reasoning and executive functions

Test (reference)	Description	Comments
Frontal assessment battery (Dubois *et al.* 2000)	Conceptualization (similarities), letter fluency, Luria motor sequence (fist-edge, palm), sensitivity to interference, inhibitory control, & environmental autonomy	Test takes no more than 10 minutes to administer

References

Alderman, N., Burgess, P.W., *et al.* (2003). Ecological validity of a simplified version of the multiple errands shopping test. *J. Int. Neuropsychol. Soc.* **9** (1), 31–44.

Battersby, W.S., Bender, M.B., *et al.* (1956). Unilateral spatial agnosia (inattention) in patients with cerebral lesions. *Brain* **79** (1), 68–93.

Benton, A.L. and Hamsher, K. (1994). *Multilingual aphasia examination.* AJA, Iowa City.

Benton, A.L., Sivan, A.B., *et al.* (1994). *Contribution to neuropsychological assessment. A clinical manual.* Oxford University Press, New York.

Berg, E.A. (1948). A simple objective technique for measuring flexibility in thinking. *J. Gen. Psychol.* **39**, 15–22.

Boller, F. and Vignolo, L.A. (1966). Latent sensory aphasia in hemisphere-damaged patients: an experimental study with the token test. *Brain* **89** (4), 815–30.

Boller, F. and Grafman, J. (2000). *Handbook of neuropsychology.* Elsevier, Amsterdam.

Coltheart, V., Avons, S.E., *et al.* (1991). The role of assembled phonology in reading comprehension. *Mem. Cognit.* **19** (4), 387–400.

Corwin, J. and Bylsma, F.W. (1993). Translations of the excerpts from André Rey's 'Psychological examination of traumatic encephalopathy' and P.A. Osterrieth's 'The complex figure copy test'. *Clin. Neuropsychologist* **7**, 3–15.

Craik, F.I. (1990). Changes in memory with normal aging: a functional view. *Adv. Neurol.* **51**, 201–5.

Cummings, J.L., Mega, M., *et al.* (1994). The neuropsychiatric inventory: comprehensive assessment of psychopathology in dementia. *Neurology* **44** (12), 2308–14.

De Renzi, E. and Faglioni, P. (1978). Normative data and screening power of a shortened version of the token test. *Cortex* **14** (1), 41–9.

Delis, D.C., Kramer, J.H., *et al.* (1983, 1987). *California verbal learning test (CVLT). Adult version.* Psychological Corporation, San Antonio, Texas.

Delis, D. C., Kramer, J.H., *et al.* (2000). *California verbal learning test*, 2nd edn (CVLT-II). Psychological Corporation, San Antonio, Texas.

Dubois, B., Slachevsky, M.D., Litvan, I., and Pillon, B. (2000). The FAB: a frontal assessment battery at bedside. *Neurology* **55**, 1621–6.

Folstein, M.F., Folstein, S.E., *et al.* (1975). 'Mini-mental state'. A practical method for grading the cognitive state of patients for the clinician. *J. Psychiatr. Res.* **12** (3), 189–98.

Gainotti, G., D'Erme, P., *et al.* (1989). Composant of visual attention disrupted in unilateral neglect. In *Neuropsychology of visual perception* (ed. J.W. Brown). IRBN Press, New York.

Gauthier, L., Dehaut, F., *et al.* (1989). The bells test: a quantitative and qualitative test for visual neglect. Int. *J. Clin. Neuropsychol.* **11**, 49–54.

Goodglass, H. and Kaplan, E. (1983). *Boston diagnostic aphasia examination (BDAE).* Lea and Febiger, Philadelphia.

Goodglass, H. and Kaplan, E. (2000). *Boston diagnostic aphasia examination (BDAE-3).* Lea and Febiger, Philadelphia.

Goodglass, H. and Kaplan, E. (2001). *Boston naming test.* Lea and Febiger, Philadelphia.

Grober, E., Buschke, H., *et al.* (1988). Screening for dementia by memory testing. *Neurology* **38** (6), 900–3.

Jensen, A.R. and Rohwer, W.D., Jr (1966). The Stroop color–word test: a review. *Acta Psychol. (Amst.)* **25** (1), 36–93.

Kertesz, A. (1988). *Western aphasia battery.* Psychological Corporation, San Antonio, Texas.

Lebert, F., Pasquier, F., *et al.* (1998). Frontotemporal behavioral scale. *Alzheimer Dis. Assoc. Disord.* **12** (4), 335–9.

Lezak, M.D., Howieson, D.B., *et al.* (2004). *Neuropsychological assessment.* Oxford University Press, Oxford.

Mathuranath, P.S., Nestor, P.J., *et al.* (2000). A brief cognitive test battery to differentiate Alzheimer's disease and frontotemporal dementia. *Neurology* **55** (11), 1613–20.

Mattis, S. (1988). *Dementia rating scale.*Psychological Assessment Resources, Odessa, Florida.

McCarty, S.M. and Warrington, E.K. (1990). *Cognitive neuropsychology: a clinical introduction.* Academic Press, San Diego.

Morris, J.C., Heyman, A., *et al.* (1989). The Consortium to Establish a Registry for Alzheimer's Disease (CERAD). Part I. Clinical and neuropsychological assessment of Alzheimer's disease. *Neurology* **39** (9), 1159–65.

Naglie, G., Tomlinson, G., *et al.* (2006). Utility-based quality of life measures in Alzheimer's disease. *Qual. Life Res.* **15** (4), 631–43.

Rey, A. (1941). L'examen psychologique dans les cas d'encephalopathie traumatique. *Arch. Psychol. (Paris)* **28**, 286–340.

Rey, A. (1964). *L'examen clinique en neuropsychologie.* Presses Universitaires de France, Paris.

Rosen, W.G., Mohs, R.C., *et al.* (1984). A new rating scale for Alzheimer's disease. *Am. J. Psychiatry* **141** (11), 1356–64.

Saxton, J. and Swihart, A.A. (1989). Neuropsychological assessment of the severely impaired elderly patients. In *Clinics in geriatric medicine* (ed. F.J. Pirozzolo). Saunders, Philadelphia.

Schenkenberg, T., Bradford, D.C., *et al.* (1980). Line bisection and unilateral visual neglect in patients with neurologic impairment. *Neurology* **30** (5), 509–17.

Schmidt, M. (1996). *Rey auditory and verbal learning test. A handbook.* Western Psychological Services, Los Angeles.

Shallice, T. (1982). Specific impairments of planning. *Phil. Trans. R. Soc. (Lond.) B* **298**, 199–209.

Shallice, T. (1988). *From neuropsychology to mental structure.* Cambridge University Press, Cambridge.

Sivan, A.B. (1992). *Benton visual retention test.* The Psychological Corporation, San Antonio, Texas.

Stern, R.A. and White, T. (2003). *Neuropsychological assessment battery.* Psychological Assessment Resources, Lutz, Florida.

Stroop, J.R. (1935). Studies of interference in serial verbal reaction. *J. Exp. Psychol.* **18**, 643–62.

Strub, R.L. and Black, F.W. (2000). *The mental status examinationin neurology.* Davis, Philadelphia.

Warrington, E.K. and James, M. (1991). A new test of object decision: 2D silhouettes featuring a minimal view. *Cortex* **27** (3), 370–83.

Wechsler, D. (1955). *Manual for the Wechsler adult intelligence scale.* The Psychological Corporation, New York.

Wechsler, D. (1981). *WAIS-R manual.* The Psychological Corporation, New York.

Wechsler, D. (1997*a*). *Wechsler adult intelligence scale-III.* The Psychological Corporation, San Antonio, Texas.

Wechsler, D. (1997*b*). *Wechsler memory scale. Third edition manual.* The Psychological Corporation, San Antonio, Texas.

Chapter 3

Neurophysiological examination methods: electrophysiology and neuroimaging

Guillaume Thierry

This chapter introduces some of the neuroimaging and electrophysiological methods that have proved useful for neuropsychological diagnosis. Rather than being exhaustive, examples will be given of applications using electrophysiology and structural/functional neuroimaging. The focus will be on selected domains, such as language pathology, epilepsy, and dementia, where these techniques have already provided valuable insight.

3.1 Introduction to neuroimaging and electrophysiological methods

There is no clear consensus on whether the brain exploration tools available today can all be considered 'neuroimaging techniques'. For practical reasons, the following working definitions will be used here.

- *Neuroimaging* is taken to refer to methods for which the output is fundamentally an image, whether structural (e.g. computerized tomographic scanner (CT scan), magnetic resonance imaging (MRI)) or functional (e.g. positron emission tomography (PET), functional MRI (fMRI)).
  - *Functional* here relates to metabolic signals on variations in the cerebral blood flow, which is considered a reliable indirect index of neural activity.
- Techniques that measure the electromagnetic activity of the brain, e.g. electroencephalography (EEG) and magnetoencephalography (MEG), will be referred to as *electrophysiological techniques.*

3.1.1 Structural imaging: principles of the CT scan and MRI

CT scan imaging is based on the differential absorption of X-rays by biological tissues. Modern CT scans produce fairly high resolution images in which dense structures like bone appear white (maximum absorption) and liquids such as the cerebrospinal fluid look black (minimum absorption). Although it is invasive, the CT scan is relatively cheap to implement and allows fast screening of major brain trauma, lesions, sizeable tumours, and haemorrhages. The injection of a contrasting agent makes it possible to visualize brain vessels and highlight the extent of haemorrhages.

A priori much less invasive, MRI requires a homogeneous magnetic field of large magnitude that forces hydrogen protons to 'line up'. Electromagnetic impulsions of defined radiofrequency then have the power to temporarily disturb this line-up and, during the relaxation that follows an impulsion, protons return to their default orientation in the ambient field whilst emitting signals that are characteristic of the surrounding macromolecular composition. The recording of these signals coupled with their localization makes it possible to construct images of high resolution (in the range of millimetres) and high contrast.

Amongst recent developments in MRI structural analysis, two important ones need to be highlighted.

- *Voxel-based morphometry* (VBM; Ashburner and Friston 2000, 2001) is a method used for comparing the local concentration of grey matter in two groups of subjects such as patients with the same aetiology and matched controls (e.g. see Honea *et al.* 2005 for a review of VBM in schizophrenia research).
- *Diffusion tensor imaging* (DTI) is a technique that permits the visualization of the structure, orientation, and anisotropy of axon bundles (i.e. white matter) in the brain (Le Bihan *et al.* 2001). Since water molecules tend to diffuse along the main direction of these bundles rather than across, it is possible to describe the diffusion pattern of water molecules using dedicated diffusion gradients. A colour-coded output then allows visualization of white matter anisotropy in three dimensions. DTI is beginning to be extensively used to evaluate connectivity deterioration in mild cognitive impairment (MCI) and neurodegenerative diseases such as dementia of the Alzheimer type (DAT) or dementia with Lewy bodies (DLB).

3.1.2 Functional imaging: the principles of PET and fMRI

Positron emission tomography (PET) and SPECT (single-photon emission computerized tomography) measure the incidence of photons of high energy received by gamma emission-sensitive crystals or detectors arranged around a living biological tissue. SPECT is a relatively widely available technique and the use of appropriate radiotracers (often using ^{99}technetium as emitting isotope) might be helpful in the diagnosis and management of several neurological diseases especially dementias and epilepsy (for reviews see Dougall *et al.* 2004; Knowlton 2006). Though less expensive, SPECT has poorer spatial resolution than PET. In the latter technique, gamma emissions are produced by the collision of an electron and a positron derived from the disintegration of positron-emitting isotopes (e.g. ^{18}F or ^{15}O) labelling biological molecules (e.g. deoxyglucose or water) injected into the systemic blood supply. By measuring the number of photons received in coincidence (i.e. at the same time) by detectors over time, it is possible to evaluate the concentration of the isotope in the volume of the organ and further calculate indices of interest such local consumption or variations in blood flow.

fMRI measures variations in the local magnetic susceptibility in biological tissues, i.e. the capacity of molecules to distort the ambient magnetic field. Haemoglobin is an endogenous marker since its magnetic susceptibility varies depending on whether it carries oxygen or carbon dioxide (Ogawa *et al.* 1990). The local variation of magnetic susceptibility over time can therefore be used as an index of oxygenated blood concentration (blood oxygen-level dependent or BOLD signal), which, in turn, indexes blood flow variations.

In the case of the brain, measuring the concentration of an exogenous tracer such as ^{15}O (PET) or an endogenous tracer such as haemoglobin (fMRI) provides an estimate of the regional cerebral blood flow (rCBF), which is an indirect index of neural activity in tissues surrounding microvessels (Logothetis *et al.* 2001; Magistretti and Pellerin 1996; Ts'o *et al.* 1990; Yacoub *et al.* 2001). PET and fMRI have a spatial resolution on the order of a cubic millimetre, which corresponds to roughly 105 neurons in the human cortex and remains rather coarse considering the fine and intricate structure of neural networks in the brain.

However, given that higher cognitive functions involve widely distributed networks across the entire brain, images with a resolution of 1 mm are already very informative. The temporal resolution of PET and fMRI, on the other hand, is quite poor relative to the typical speed of neural communication (on the order of a millisecond): PET images require continuous acquisition for 30–90 s and fMRI acquisition typically requires 50–100 ms. Even though acquiring one functional slice with fMRI can be pushed down to a few tenths of milliseconds, the slow coupling between neural activity and BOLD signal variations makes fMRI's temporal resolution inherently coarse. To overcome the slowness of vessel-dependent functional imaging, advances in diffusion imaging makes it possible to record functionally relevant variations in diffusion signals that indicate much earlier cellular changes following neural activity shift in the living brain such as stimulus perception (Le Bihan *et al.* 2006).

3.1.3 **Electrophysiological techniques**

Brain neural activity constantly generates local electrical and magnetic variations that can be measured on or in the proximity of the scalp. Whereas the electromagnetic fields generated by transient action potentials (temporary depolarizations of the axon's membrane) have a rapid decay rate (Wikswo 1983), post-synaptic potentials (whether excitatory or inhibitory) result in ion gradients of greater magnitude at the macrocellular level that are resilient for several tenths of milliseconds. As a consequence, post-synaptic potentials can 'polarize' whole cells and groups of cells similarly oriented in space, which is sufficient to influence the electromagnetic state of the scalp (Lopes de Silva and Van Rotterdam 1987; Rockel *et al.* 1980).

- Electroencephalography (EEG) measures the variations of the electrical potential at different locations on the scalp. Highly conductive electrodes are bridged with the scalp using an electrolytic gel and signals are amplified on the order of 105 times before the signal is printed or digitized and stored on a computer.
- Magnetoencephalography (MEG) records the magnetic variations that are a mandatory correlate of electrical currents. A set of highly sensitive superconducting sensors arranged around the head measures the minute magnetic variations induced by neural activity, which can be visualized or stored similarly to EEG signals.

The temporal resolution of EEG and MEG can go below a millisecond and is therefore very satisfactory *vis-à-vis* neuronal firing rate. The spatial resolution of these methods, however, is considerably limited by the complex diffusion/transmission of currents through the various layers that separate the brain from the surfaces of the scalp. Predicting the pattern of electromagnetic activity based on known generators in the brain (forward modelling) is a tough mathematical challenge but inferring the location, orientation, and strength of brain sources based on surface activity (backward modelling) is theoretically impossible because there is an infinite number of solutions for a given surface topography. Nevertheless, when source analysis is guided by *a priori* neuroanatomical hypotheses or when the properties of brain sources are constrained based on biological models, source localization can provide rough spatial information (Grave de Peralta Menendez *et al.* 2001, 2004; Scherg and Berg 1991; Scherg and Ebersole 1994).

Electromagnetic signals can be decomposed into their constituent frequencies using a Fourier transform. The quantitative study of the various frequencies in the signal, known as quantitative EEG (or qEEG), can provide insight into the neurophysiological state of the brain and has particular applications in epilepsy (cf. Section 3.2.1). More recently, the study of high frequencies (40–80 Hz, gamma band) has proved promising for the study of human cognition and this may become a promising neuropsychological investigation tool in the future (Crone *et al.* 2001; Krause *et al.* 1998; Rodriguez *et al.* 1999; Singer 1999; Tallon-Baudry and Bertrand 1999).

Event-related potentials (ERPs) and evoked magnetic fields (EMFs) are also derived from EEG and MEG. ERPs and EMFs are derived from continuous recordings by averaging a large number of recording sections time-locked to an external event (stimulus or participant's response). Averaging over a number of trials (1000 for the most subtle components of ERPs to 30 for the largest) progressively cancels out electrical or magnetic activity that bears no relation to the processing of the event. This simple procedure reveals the mean activity produced by the brain in response to/resulting in the event in the form of a series of positive and negative deflections (see Rugg *et al.* 1995). Some ERP components have been consistently shown to index specific aspects of human cognition. The P300, for instance, is a positive variation that reflects aspects of executive function that are impaired in Alzheimer's disease (AD), such as shifts of attention and working memory updating mechanisms (Donchin *et al.* 1984; Johnson 1986; Polich and Kok 1995).

3.2 Diagnosis and electrophysiology: EEG; qEEG; MEG; and ERPs

The longstanding tradition of clinical EEG examination based on the visual assessment of EEG print-outs needs no introduction. Clinical EEG has been in use for over 50 years and provides good complementary clinical insight in fields as varied as epilepsy, dementia, traumatic brain injury, acute ischaemic stroke, sleep disorders, and depression. More recently and despite the greater costs involved, some advantages of MEG have become apparent that make MEG an excellent complementary or alternative diagnostic tool. Here two domains are considered in which electrophysiology provides key elements to the clinical diagnostic: (1) epilepsy and (2) dementia.

3.2.1 Electrophysiology and epilepsy

An epileptic seizure is a transient manifestation of signs or symptoms induced by excessive and/or synchronous activity of neural networks in the brain (Fisher *et al.* 2005). Interictal spikes are the result of synchronous bursts of activity that last for less than 70 ms in a group of neurons and do not constitute a seizure by themselves (de Curtis and Avanzini 2001). The diagnosis of epilepsy is based on the observation of interictal epileptic activity that features interictal spikes, sharp waves, and spike–wave discharges (for a review see Duncan *et al.* 2006). EEG is one of the best suited tools for the diagnosis and study of epilepsy since it directly records electrical activity produced by the brain over the scalp. The fact that EEG is totally non-invasive, relatively low cost, and potentially mobile (ambulatory EEG) allows recording over long periods. As pointed out by Duncan *et al.* (2006), in patients presenting with frequent seizures, it is possible to make direct recordings during seizure, which provides invaluable insight complementary to routine clinical examination (e.g. 30 minute rest EEG).

Bressler and Kelso (2001) have conceptualized the brain as a metastable dynamic system, the different parts of which have a tendency to function autonomously but, at the same time, are maintained in a state of global coordinated activity (for a review see Fingelkurts 2004). Perez Velazquez *et al.* (2003) have proposed that chronic epilepsy can be seen as a new, metastable level of activity that can be adapted to. One consequence of this hypothesis is that brain activity in chronic epileptic patients in the interictal period should be somewhat different from normal brain activity. A number of EEG studies investigating interictal EEG characteristics tend to lend support to this hypothesis. Gelety *et al.* (1985), for instance, have shown that alpha-range signals (7.5±; 12.5 Hz) tend to be slowed down. This observation has been made for other frequency bands (Drake *et al.* 1998), and interictal EEG signals in chronic epilepsy have been shown to display regional slow-waves (Gastaut *et al.* 1985; Koutroumanidis *et al.* 1998; Massa *et al.* 2001). Moreover, decreases in synchronization have been found well before a seizure occurs (Mormann *et al.* 2000) and the complexity of the EEG spectrum is overall reduced at most recording sites (Bhattacharya 2000; Jing and Takigawa 2000; Ravelli and Antolini 1992; Weber *et al.* 1998). A view commonly held, however, is that, in the majority of cases, the interictal EEG without epileptiform patterns is normal (Desai *et al.* 1988). Fingelkurts and Kaplan (2006) propose that the use of averaged EEG measures over extended time windows might explain why differences between the interictal EEG of chronic epileptics and that of controls may be masked. More specifically, Finglekurts and Kaplan (2003) showed that the total power spectrum of a recording does not characterize the power spectra measured for each of the EEG subsegments separately. Finglekurts and Kaplan (2006) therefore proposed to study the exact composition of the EEG spectrum based on a probability-classification analysis of short-term EEG spectral patterns (Fingelkurts *et al.* 2006). Amongst their observations, they found evidence for a shift toward higher frequency throughout the EEG spectrum, an increase in polyrhythmic activity, and a decrease in spectral pattern diversity.

The main advantages of MEG over EEG for the study of epilepsy are: (1) the minimum distortion of magnetic relative to electrical fields by tissues between the cortex and the external surface of the scalp (scalp, skull, cerebrospinal fluid, meninges, parenchyma); (2) the absence of a reference; (3) superior sensitivity (particularly in neocortical epilepsy); and (4) the greater reliability of source localization procedures (Barkley 2004; but see Baumgartner 2004), particularly in the case of patients with non-lesional neocortical epilepsies, in whom invasive recordings are systematically required (Stefan 2000; Barkley and Baumgartner 2003; Cascino 2001; Knowlton *et al.* 1997; Smith *et al.* 2000; Wheless *et al.* 1999). EEG remains far cheaper to operate, is far more available, is portable, and can be implemented during most everyday patient activities. EEG also remains superior to MEG in localizing deep sources. MEG, however, has shown great potential in finding the optimal placement of intracranial electrodes when they are required (Stefan *et al.* 2000). In the case of patients who have had brain surgery or head trauma involving cortical lesions, MEG might be very helpful because scalp EEG recordings are particularly difficult to interpret (Kirchberger *et al.* 1998).

3.2.2 **EEG and dementia (both frontal and Alzheimer types)**

Visual inspection of EEG in patients presenting with DAT classically shows general slowing of resting activity and a decrease in EEG coherence between recording sites (for a review see Jeong 2004). More specifically, the power of signals of higher frequency such as alpha (7.5 ±; 12.5 Hz) and beta (12.5 ±; 20 Hz) is reduced, whereas lower frequency bands, i.e. delta (1.5 ±; 3.5 Hz) and theta (3.5 ±; 7.5 Hz), increase in power (Brenner *et al.* 1986; Coben *et al.* 1983; Giaquinto and Nolfe 1986). This shift in the relative power of EEG frequencies is accompanied by a decline of EEG coherence, particularly in the alpha and beta bands (Dunkin *et al.* 1994; Leuchter *et al.* 1987; Locatelli *et al.* 1998), and has been shown to correlate with the level of cognitive impairment (Elmstahl and Rosen 1997; Filipovic *et al.* 1989; Leuchter *et al.* 1987, but see Hughes *et al.* 1989; Kowalski *et al.* 2001; Prinz and Vitiello 1989; Strijers *et al.* 1997). As is the case for functional neuroimaging investigation of dementia (see Section 3.3.2), however, it is important to distinguish between the effects of normal ageing and the early impact of the disease. Although the existence of age-related changes in EEG profile is debated (Duffy *et al.* 1984; Giaquinto and Nolfe 1986; Pollock *et al.* 1990), ageing has been associated with a slowing of alpha activity over the temporal regions (Torres *et al.* 1983) and a more even distribution of EEG activity across the scalp (Dustman *et al.* 1985).

Despite the resistance of various professional organizations to the use of quantitative EEG (qEEG) as a clinical assessment tool (Hoffman *et al.* 1999; Nuwer 1997), this quantitative approach to clinical EEG is now widely used to compare psychiatric patients with matched control groups (Hughes and John 1999). In qEEG, a 1–2 minute long EEG recording at rest is acquired from a set of 15 to 20 electrodes placed at standard recording sites and analysed using the fast Fourier transform (FFT) to determine the power of EEG signals in each of the four frequency bands defined above (i.e. alpha, beta, delta, and theta). In addition to the absolute and relative power spectra in each frequency band, qEEG often includes a measure of EEG coherence (level of signal synchronization between two recording sites). Leuchter *et al.* (1994) have derived another qEEG measure, cordance, which is based on the relationship between the absolute and relative spectral power at each recording site (Cook and Leuchter 1996). Congruent with visual inspection of the electroencephalogram, qEEG shows a slowing down of background EEG rhythm positively correlated with the degree of cognitive impairment in demented patients. In the case of delirium tremens, though, the EEG has normal characteristics with fast rhythms (Reilly *et al.* 1979; Small 1993), and slowing down of activity generally indicates associated pathology such as Wernicke encephalopathy (Kelley and Reilly 1983). Delirium is fairly well discriminated from dementia based on increased theta activity and delta relative power (Jacobson *et al.* 1993). The general consensus in the literature regarding DAT diagnosis using EEG is that slow background activity is increased and the decrease in mean EEG frequency correlates with cognitive deficits measured using neuropsychological testing (Brenner *et al.* 1986; Duffy *et al.* 1984; Fisch and Pedley 1989; Hughes 1995; Hughes *et al.* 1989; Leuchter *et al.* 1987; Prinz and Vitiello 1989). Some authors have proposed that the earliest EEG indicator of DAT might be increased slow activity before any significant reduction in the relative power of alpha activity can be detected (Brenner *et al.* 1989; Coben *et al.* 1985; Duffy *et al.* 1995; Hughes 1995; Prichep *et al.* 2006; Soininen *et al.* 1991; Veldhuizen *et al.* 1993; Williamson *et al.* 1990). On the other hand, theta band power seem to be the measurement that best correlates with cognitive impairment (Dierks *et al.* 1991; Duffy *et al.* 1993; Prichep *et al.* 1994; Rae-Grant *et al.* 1987; Richards *et al.* 1993; Valdes *et al.* 1992). Significant increases in the delta band are an indication of advanced stages of dementia (Hier *et al.* 1991; Hughes *et al.* 1989; Prichep *et al.* 1994; Rae-Grant *et al.* 1987). Several qEEG studies have shown that DAT can be differentiated from other pathologies such as multi-infarct dementia (Besthorn *et al.* 1994; Hier *et al.* 1991; John *et al.* 1988; Martin-Loeches *et al.* 1991; Matsuura *et al.* 1993), depression (Brenner *et al.* 1986; Duffy *et al.* 1984; Leuchter *et al.* 1992; O'Connor *et al.* 1979; Robinson *et al.* 1994), and fronto-temporal dementia (FTD, Yener *et al.* 1996).

Event-related potentials (ERPs) have also been used in an attempt to discriminate DAT patients from matched controls. One of the prominent ERP paradigms used is the P300 oddball paradigm, in which a series of stimuli with high local probability (standard) is interrupted by stimuli of low local probability (deviants; for reviews see Polich and Herbst 2000). Numerous variants of the P300 paradigm have been employed but most authors report differences between DAT patients and controls. The P300 is generally of lesser amplitude and its peaking latency delayed in DAT (for a review see Polich and Corey-Bloom 2005). According to Polich and Corey-Bloom (2005) the most discriminative P300 tasks are easy discrimination tasks, particularly in the visual modality.

3.3 Diagnosis and brain imaging: PET and fMRI

In this section two fields are considered where neuroimaging already plays a key role and has promising applications: (1) the presurgical assessment of language cortical representation; and (2) the subtyping and predictive diagnosis of dementias.

3.3.1 Presurgical assessment of language lateralization: Wada versus fMRI

The intracarotid amobarbital test also known as Wada test was first introduced by John Wada at the end of the 1940s (Wada 1949). This test classically consists of an injection of amobarbital (intermediate acting barbiturate) in the internal carotid artery via a catheter routed through the femoral artery so as to anaesthetize selectively one hemisphere (Wada 1997). Although it is widely used, the Wada test is fundamentally invasive and is generally preceded by a cerebral angiography which carries with it the risk of neurological complications (incidence 1.3%, with 0.5% permanent; Willinsky *et al.* 2003). In most patients, the test offers radical insight into global language lateralization in the brain since the injection in the language-dominant hemisphere totally disrupts simple language tasks such as semantic decision on words, word generation, verbal fluency, or sentence repetition. However, beyond the fact that it is invasive, the test has inherent limitations such as the total lack of spatial resolution within the hemisphere and a very short time window for testing (3–5 minutes is the recommended test duration). In addition, it is worth noting that cross-flow to the contralateral hemisphere has been reported with a relatively high incidence rate (e.g. 30% of the cases in Simkins-Bullock 2000), which casts a shadow over the hemispheric specificity of the diagnosis. Finally, different centres use a variety of barbiturate dosage, type of task used, latency between injection and testing, resting period between left- and right-side injections, etc. (Meador and Loring 1999). Because of these limitations, the search is on for a less invasive method that would make a good alternative to the Wada test.

In the last decade, there have been attempts to find an alternative using functional transcranial Doppler sonography (Knake *et al.* 2003), near infrared spectroscopy (Watson *et al.* 2004), and synthetic aperture magnetometry (Hirata *et al.* 2004). Since it is now widely available in hospital settings, fMRI has already been substantially tested as an alternative (Kloppel and Büchel 2005). Most studies have used a range of cognitive tasks tapping into language processing and memory function with the aim of comparing the outcome since fMRI is far less invasive, is much less constrained in terms of time, allows measurement of test–retest reliability (Fernandez *et al.* 2003), and is substantially less expensive than the Wada test (Medina *et al.* 2004). The agreement between Wada and fMRI testing in the same individuals is in the range of 90% (Binder *et al.* 1996; Brockway 2000; Gaillard *et al.* 2004; Lehericy *et al.* 2000; Sabsevitz *et al.* 2003; Woermann *et al.* 2003). There remains approximately 10% of at least partial inconsistency between Wada and fMRI assessments of language lateralization, e.g. in patients who have had a cluster of focal cortical seizures (e.g., Jayakar *et al.* 2002). The assessment of language distribution in atypical patients, in particular, is a difficult task both when using the Wada or the fMRI procedure. The advantage of fMRI in the latter case is that many different tests tapping different aspects of language comprehension and production can be conducted.

The ultimate goal here is to obtain reliable presurgical assessment of core cognitive function. As noted by Kloppel and Büchel (2005), it must be kept in mind that the Wada test and fMRI differ fundamentally in the information they provide. The Wada test is an inactivation procedure that sheds light on the territories that are necessary for the tested cognitive functions. FMRI, on the other hand, is an activation procedure that offers insight into the involvement of brain structures. Some regions activated during test might not be critical for language or memory, and patients may compensate well after surgical removal of such regions. The predictive value of fMRI for postsurgical outcome is also inherently limited by the problem of finding adequate statistical thresholds, especially in the case of single-case data (see Kloppel and Büchel 2005). Nevertheless, the correlation between fMRI measures and postsurgical outcome remains good overall for both language and memory function. In fact, fMRI testing using visual memory encoding tasks has proved more reliable in establishing lateralization of memory function than the Wada test in several studies (Janszky *et al.* 2005; Rabin *et al.* 2004). In sum, fMRI is a promising tool for assessing the preoperative functional status of brain regions involved in high-level cognitive operations but further investigations using standardized tests and exploring more systematically the correlations between activation indices and postsurgical outcomes are needed before the Wada test becomes obsolete.

3.3.2 Neuroimaging of dementia

It is well established that ageing affects both the functional status and the structure of the human brain as it does other organs (Kemper 1994; Raz *et al.* 1998). Comparing old adults without signs of dementia and young control adults has revealed differences in executive functioning and a global slowing down of processing (Craik and Byrd 1982; Greenwood 2000; Moscovitch and Winocur 1995; Nyberg *et al.* 1996; Salthouse 1996). It is therefore not an easy task to distinguish normal ageing from the onset of dementia. Neuroimaging, whether structural or functional, is on the front line of new investigation methods to find sensitive markers of dementia and particularly dementia of the Alzheimer type (DAT).

3.3.2.1 Structural imaging of dementia

For two decades at least, a good consensus has emerged in the literature that key structures affected in DAT but also in mild cognitive impairment (MCI) are located within the medial temporal lobe (MTL) including the hippocampus and the entorhinal, perirhinal, and parahippocampal cortices (Amaral *et al.* 1987; Insausti *et al.* 1995). It is well-established that one of the first reliable clinical symptoms of DAT is a declarative memory loss (Reisberg *et al.* 1982) and it is as well-established that the hippocampus is one of the core structures mediating declarative memory encoding, consolidation, and retrieval (Squire and Zola 1996). It is therefore in the MTL in general and in the hippocampus in particular that signs of degeneration are sought (Braak and Braak 1991). DAT is associated with general MTL atrophy (Mosconi *et al.* 2004*a*), and the severity of cognitive impairment has been shown to correlate with cerebral atrophy (de Leon *et al.* 1989; Fox and Freeborough 1997; Fox *et al.* 1996). Hippocampal volume reduction, in particular, allows good discrimination of patients with DAT from controls matched in age (Convit *et al.* 1995; Jack *et al.* 2002; Kesslak *et al.* 1991; Killiany *et al.* 1993) but also from individuals with MCI (Convit *et al.* 1997; de Leon *et al.* 2001; Jack *et al.* 2005). Even more interestingly, longitudinal studies have shown that hippocampal volume reduction predicts conversion from MCI to DAT with very good accuracy (> 80%; Convit *et al.* 2000; Jack *et al.* 1999, 2000; Kaye et *al.* 1997). Similar observations have been made for the entorhinal cortex, although the diagnostic value of this measure is less widely accepted (Bobinski *et al.* 1999; Erkinjuntti *et al.* 1993; Killiany *et al.* 2002). In sum, structural imaging of individuals presenting with MCI and/or at risk of DAT has proved a useful element of the clinical diagnosis.

By providing microstructural maps of tissue orientation *in vivo*, diffusion tensor imaging (DTI) offers new insight into neural degeneration mechanisms in dementia (Moseley *et al.* 2002). In particular, the degree of anisotropy measured in white matter by DTI (Basser 1995; Pierpaoli and Basser 1996) has been shown to correlate with memory performance (Charlton *et al.* 2006; Muller *et al.* 2005; Salat *et al.* 2005). In patients presenting with cognitive decline (probable DAT), Naggara *et al.* (2006) have shown deterioration of frontal and temporal white matter anisotropy significantly superior to that in age-matched controls, whilst no such differences were found in subcortical white matter tracts. Furthermore, Kalus *et al.* (2006) have recently shown that DTI of the perforant pathway can successfully discriminate MCI patients from normal controls where more traditional high-resolution MRI volumetry and measurement of intervoxel coherence of the hippocampus and the entorhinal cortex fail. In sum, DTI is a very promising diagnostic tool since it allows the detection of structural anomalies that cannot be detected based on conventional MRI scans.

3.3.2.2 Functional imaging of dementia

A number of studies have found significant correlation between cerebral atrophy in dementia and hypofunction of glucose transporters (Kalaria *et al.* 1988; Simpson *et al.* 1994), defective glutamate signalling of glucose metabolism (Magistretti *et al.* 1999), dysfunctional glycolytic cycles (Marcus *et al.* 1989), and impaired peripheral glucoregulation (Hoyer *et al.* 1994; Vanhanen and Soininen 1998). Fluorodeoxyglucose (FDG)-PET provides an index of brain glucose metabolism that correlates with synaptic activity and density (Herholz 2003) and seems therefore suitable for studying the functional correlates of DAT as well as other types of dementia (for a review see Mosconi 2005). At first sight, however, results from FDG-PET studies in patients presenting with DAT are not straightforwardly consistent with results from structural MRI investigations. Dysfunctional glucose metabolism has been found predominantly in the parieto-temporal cortex and the posterior cingulate cortex as well as frontal regions in advanced degenerative stages, whereas primary cortices, cerebellum, and subcortical nuclei appear to be less affected (Hoyer *et al.* 1994; Kalaria *et al.* 1988; Killiany *et al.* 2002; Marcus *et al.* 1989; Minoshima *et al.* 1997; Simpson *et al.* 1994; Vanhanen and Soininen 1998). Although hypometabolism of the parieto-temporal and posterior cingulate cortex is considered a good indicator of DAT, hypometabolism in the hippocampus and parahippocampal region, which is expected from structural MRI studies, has seldom been reported. This is not true of all FDG-PET studies, however, with the most significant exceptions being studies that have used MRI co-registration targeting the hippocampus (de Leon *et al.* 2001; for a review see Mosconi 2005; Nestor *et al.* 2003). A number of studies have drawn direct comparisons between FDG-PET profiles of patients and the gold standard of AD diagnosis, which remains post-mortem histopathology (McKhann *et al.* 1984). Results obtained by Hoffman *et al.* (2000) for instance were encouraging with 79% of correct positive diagnosis and 88% of correct negative diagnosis. In a large cohort study by Silverman *et al.* (2001), the correct identification of DAT reached 88%. Moreover, several studies have demonstrated that FDG-PET examination successfully discriminated between DAT patients and patients presenting with dementia with Lewy bodies (DLB), based on marked primary visual cortex hypometabolism in DLB that is not found in DAT (Albin *et al.* 1996; Minoshima *et al.* 2001). One other interesting observation is that the transition to DAT can be predicted with an accuracy of 75–100% by glucose metabolism reduction in the parieto-temporal cortex/MTL of patients diagnosed with MCI (Chetelat *et al.* 2003; Herholz *et al.* 1999; Mosconi *et al.* 2004*b*). To sum up, FDG-PET is already established as an excellent complementary diagnostic tool for MCI, DAT, and DLB. Its sensitivity is good but its specificity remains unsatisfactory (Mosconi 2005).

Dementia is fundamentally a process of cognitive degradation. Therefore, a method susceptible of providing a quantitative physiological index of cognitive processing has great diagnostic potential. Activation studies of dementia have used various cognitive tasks and manipulated task difficulty to investigate cognitive function in demented or at-risk patients and age-matched controls (for reviews see Almkvist 2000; Prvulovic *et al.* 2005). There is a fairly good agreement between functional activation studies of memory encoding/retrieval. Relative to age-matched controls, DAT patients consistently show reduced activation in the hippocampus as well as temporal and frontal cortices (Kato *et al.* 2001; Machulda *et al.* 2003; Sperling *et al.* 2003). Results from studies tapping working memory (e.g. Becker *et al.* 1996; Grady *et al.* 2001) and visual object matching/discrimination (e.g. Grady *et al.* 1993; Prvulovic *et al.* 2002) have provided more confused difference patterns. Becker *et al.* (1996), for instance, found significant differences between DAT patients and controls in an eight-word repetition task but not in the same task requiring repetition of three words. In a passive visual task, Mentis *et al.* (1996) found hypoactivation of the middle temporal and occipital cortices in patients presenting with DAT relative to controls, but Grady *et al.* (1993) found hyperactivation in the frontal eye fields and occipital cortex in a face-matching task and Prvulovic *et al.* (2002) found decreased activation in the parietal cortex and simultaneous increased activation in the occipito-temporal cortex in an angle discrimination task. The use of different tasks with varying levels of difficulty between laboratories makes comparisons difficult. The same overall confusion arises from investigations in subjects at genetic risk of developing DAT. Some authors have reported overactivation in the hippocampal, parietal, and frontal cortices in high-risk compared to low-risk participants performing a verbal learning task (Bookheimer *et al.* 2000). Consistent increased activation in the parietal cortex of at-risk subjects has been found by Smith *et al.* (2002) using a verbal fluency task. However, Burggren *et al.* (2002), using an auditory attention task, failed to find such differences. Although systematic longitudinal investigations using large subject cohorts and parametric designs are still missing, the few functional activation studies reported so far are promising because they approach dementia from a different perspective. Indeed, investigations solely based on structural damage are blind to pathological overactivations and palliative mechanisms, particularly in the early stages of the disease, when patients can still compensate for subclinical deficits.

3.4 **Conclusion**

Although new technical breakthroughs are announced regularly, always bringing new insight helping the clinical diagnosis, old and well-established methods have the powerful advantage of a long history of use, which comes with considerable amounts of data allowing statistical testing and validation. This makes the transition to new approaches relatively slow, which should be seen as positive because it is the only safe way, but can sometimes be seen as frustrating because one would like to see diagnostic tools with better sensitivity and selectivity constantly appear. Some alternative neuroimaging techniques such as near infrared spectroscopy and some neurointervention techniques such as transcranial magnetic stimulation are beginning to be used to study neuropsychological patients. The lack of perspective regarding these methods is due to the need for a scientifically established rationale for their clinical use, which will probably arise from fundamental research. In any case, one core idea that, it is hoped, comes from this chapter is that converging evidence from different methods offers the best opportunity for accurate clinical diagnosis. This, however, entails interdisciplinary exchanges in which specialists in different fields recognize the complementary power of techniques other than their own. Such exchange is definitely good, in principle, for clinical practice but also for fundamental research.

References

Albin, R.L., Minoshima, S., D'Amato, C.J., Frey, K.A., Kuhl, D.A., and Sima, A.A. (1996). Fluoro-deoxyglucose positron emission tomography in diffuse Lewy body disease. *Neurology* **47**, 462–6.

Almkvist, O. (2000). Functional brain imaging as a looking-glass into the degraded brain: reviewing evidence from Alzheimer disease in relation to normal aging. *Acta Psychol. (Amst.)* **105**, 255–277.

Amaral, D.G., Insausti, R., and Cowan, W.M. (1987). The entorhinal cortex of the monkey: I. Cytoarchitectonic organization. *J. Comp. Neurol.* **264**, 326–55.

Ashburner, J. and Friston, K.J. (2000). Voxel-based morphometry—the methods. *Neuroimage* **11**, 805–21.

Ashburner, J., and Friston, K.J. (2001). Why voxel-based morphometry should be used. *Neuroimage* **14**, 1238–43.

Barkley, G.L. (2004). Controversies in neurophysiology. MEG is superior to EEG in localization of interictal epileptiform activity: pro. *Clin. Neurophysiol.* **115**, 1001–9.

Barkley, G.L. and Baumgartner, C. (2003). MEG and EEG in epilepsy. *J. Clin. Neurophysiol.* **20**, 163–78.

Basser, P.J. (1995). Inferring microstructural features and the physiological state of tissues from diffusion-weighted images. *NMR Biomed.* **8**, 333–44.

Baumgartner, C. (2004). Controversies in clinical neurophysiology. MEG is superior to EEG in the localization of interictal epileptiform activity: con. *Clin. Neurophysiol.* **115**, 1010–20.

Becker, J.T., Mintun, M.A., Aleva, K., Wiseman, M.B., Nichols, T., and DeKosky, S.T. (1996). Compensatory reallocation of brain resources supporting verbal episodic memory in Alzheimer's disease. *Neurology* **46**, 692–700.

Besthorn, C., Forstl, H., Geiger-Kabisch, C., Sattel, H., Gasser, T., and Schreiter-Gasser, U. (1994). EEG coherence in Alzheimer disease. *Electroencephalogr. Clin. Neurophysiol.* **90**, 242–5.

Bhattacharya, J. (2000). Complexity analysis of spontaneous EEG. *Acta Neurobiol. Exp. (Wars.)* **60**, 495–501.

Binder, J.R., Swanson, S.J., Hammeke, T.A., Morris, G.L., Mueller, W.M., Fischer, M., Benbadis, S., Frost, J.A., Rao, S.M., and Haughton, V.M. (1996). Determination of language dominance using functional MRI: a comparison with the Wada test. *Neurology* **46**, 978–84.

Bobinski, M., de Leon, M.J., Convit, A., De Santi, S., Wegiel, J., Tarshish, C.Y., Saint Louis, L.A., and Wisniewski, H.M. (1999). MRI of entorhinal cortex in mild Alzheimer's disease. *Lancet* **353**, 38–40.

Bookheimer, S.Y., Strojwas, M.H., Cohen, M.S., Saunders, A.M., Pericak-Vance, M.A., Mazziotta, J.C., and Small, G.W. (2000). Patterns of brain activation in people at risk for Alzheimer's disease. *N. Engl. J. Med.* **343**, 450–6.

Braak, H. and Braak, E. (1991). Neuropathological stageing of Alzheimer-related changes. *Acta Neuropathol. (Berl.)* **82**, 239–59.

Brenner, R.P., Ulrich, R.F., Spiker, D.G., Sclabassi, R.J., Reynolds, C.F., 3rd, Marin, R.S., and Boller, F. (1986). Computerized EEG spectral analysis in elderly normal, demented and depressed subjects. *Electroencephalogr. Clin. Neurophysiol.* **64**, 483–92.

Brenner, R.P., Reynolds, C.F., 3rd, and Ulrich, R.F. (1989). EEG findings in depressive pseudodementia and dementia with secondary depression. *Electroencephalogr. Clin. Neurophysiol.* **72**, 298–304.

Bressler, S.L. and Kelso, J.A. (2001). Cortical coordination dynamics and cognition. *Trends Cogn. Sci.* **5**, 26–36.

Brockway, J.P. (2000). Two functional magnetic resonance imaging f(MRI) tasks that may replace the gold standard, Wada testing, for language lateralization while giving additional localization information. *Brain Cogn.* **43**, 57–9.

Burggren, A.C., Small, G.W., Sabb, F.W., and Bookheimer, S.Y. (2002). Specificity of brain activation patterns in people at genetic risk for Alzheimer disease. *Am. J. Geriatr. Psychiatry* **10**, 44–51.

Cascino, G.D. (2001). Epilepsy surgery in non-substrate-directed partial epilepsy. In *Epilepsy surgery* (ed. H. Luders and Y.G. Comair), pp. 1020–5. Lippincott, Williams and Wilkins, Philadelphia.

Charlton, R.A., Barrick, T.R., McIntyre, D.J., Shen, Y., O'Sullivan, M., Howe, F.A., Clark, C.A., Morris, R.G., and Markus, H.S. (2006). White matter damage on diffusion tensor imaging correlates with age-related cognitive decline. *Neurology* **66**, 217–22.

Chetelat, G., Desgranges, B., de la Sayette, V., Viader, F., Eustache, F., and Baron, J.C. (2003). Mild cognitive impairment: can FDG-PET predict who is to rapidly convert to Alzheimer's disease? *Neurology* **60**, 1374–7.

Coben, L.A., Danziger, W.L., and Berg, L. (1983). Frequency analysis of the resting awake EEG in mild senile dementia of Alzheimer type. *Electroencephalogr. Clin. Neurophysiol.* **55**, 372–80.

Coben, L.A., Danziger, W., and Storandt, M. (1985). A longitudinal EEG study of mild senile dementia of Alzheimer type: changes at 1 year and at 2.5 years. *Electroencephalogr. Clin. Neurophysiol.* **61**, 101–12.

Convit, A., de Leon, M.J., Tarshish, C., De Santi, S., Kluger, A., Rusinek, H., and George, A.E. (1995). Hippocampal volume losses in minimally impaired elderly. *Lancet* **345**, 266.

Convit, A., De Leon, M.J., Tarshish, C., De Santi, S., Tsui, W., Rusinek, H., and George, A. (1997). Specific hippocampal volume reductions in individuals at risk for Alzheimer's disease. *Neurobiol. Aging* **18**, 131–8.

Convit, A., de Asis, J., de Leon, M.J., Tarshish, C.Y., De Santi, S., and Rusinek, H. (2000). Atrophy of the medial occipitotemporal, inferior, and middle temporal gyri in non-demented elderly predicts decline to Alzheimer's disease. *Neurobiol. Aging* **21**, 19–26.

Cook, I.A. and Leuchter, A.F. (1996). Synaptic dysfunction in Alzheimer's disease: clinical assessment using quantitative EEG. *Behav. Brain Res.* **78**, 15–23.

Craik, F.I.M. and Byrd, M. (1982). Aging and cognitive deficits: the role of attentional resources. In *Aging and cognitive processes* (ed. F.I.M. Craik, and S. Trehub), pp. 191–221. Plenum, New York.

Crone, N.E., Boatman, D., Gordon, B., and Hao, L. (2001). Induced electrocorticographic gamma activity during auditory perception. *Clin. Neurophysiol.* **112**, 565–82.

de Curtis, M. and Avanzini, G. (2001). Interictal spikes in focal epileptogenesis. *Prog. Neurobiol.* **63**, 541–67.

de Leon, M.J., George, A.E., Stylopoulos, L.A., Smith, G., and Miller, D.C. (1989). Early marker for Alzheimer's disease: the atrophic hippocampus. *Lancet* **2**, 672–3.

de Leon, M.J., Convit, A., Wolf, O.T., Tarshish, C.Y., DeSanti, S., Rusinek, H., Tsui, W., Kandil, E., Scherer, A.J., Roche, A., *et al.* (2001). Prediction of cognitive decline in normal elderly subjects with 2-[(18)F]fluoro-2-deoxy-D-glucose/poitron-emission tomography (FDG/PET). *Proc. Natl. Acad. Sci. USA* **98**, 10966–71.

Desai, B., Whitman, S., and Bouffard, D.A. (1988). The role of the EEG in epilepsy of long duration. *Epilepsia* **29**, 601–6.

Dierks, T., Perisic, I., Frolich, L., Ihl, R., and Maurer, K. (1991). Topography of the quantitative electroencephalogram in dementia of the Alzheimer type: relation to severity of dementia. *Psychiatry Res.* **40**, 181–94.

Donchin, E., Heffley, E., Hillyard, S.A., Loveless, N., Maltzman, I., Ohman, A., Rosler, F., Ruchkin, D., and Siddle, D. (1984). Cognition and event-related potentials. II. The orienting reflex and P300. *Ann. NY Acad. Sci.* **425**, 39–57.

Dougall, N., Bruggink, S., and Ebmeier, K.P. Systematic review of the diagnostic accuracy of 99mTc-HMPAO-SPECT in dementia. *Am. J. Geriatr. Psychiatry* **12** (6), 554–70.

Drake, M.E., Padamadan, H., and Newell, S.A. (1998). Interictal quantitative EEG in epilepsy. *Seizure* **7**, 39–42.

Duffy, F.H., Albert, M.S., McAnulty, G., and Garvey, A.J. (1984). Age-related differences in brain electrical activity of healthy subjects. *Ann. Neurol.* **16**, 430–8.

Duffy, F.H., McAnulty, G.B., and Albert, M.S. (1993). The pattern of age-related differences in electrophysiological activity of healthy males and females. *Neurobiol. Aging* **14**, 73–84.

Duffy, F.H., Jones, K.J., McAnulty, G.B., and Albert, M.S. (1995). Spectral coherence in normal adults: unrestricted principal components analysis; relation of factors to age, gender, and neuropsychologic data. *Clin. Electroencephalogr.* **26**, 30–46.

Duncan, J.S., Sander, J.W., Sisodiya, S.M., and Walker, M.C. (2006). Adult epilepsy. *Lancet* **367**, 1087–100.

Dunkin, J.J., Leuchter, A.F., Newton, T.F., and Cook, I.A. (1994). Reduced EEG coherence in dementia: state or trait marker? *Biol. Psychiatry* **35**, 870–9.

Dustman, R.E., LaMarche, J.A., Cohn, N.B., Shearer, D.E., and Talone, J.M. (1985). Power spectral analysis and cortical coupling of EEG for young and old normal adults. *Neurobiol. Aging* **6**, 193–8.

Elmstahl, S. and Rosen, I. (1997). Postural hypotension and EEG variables predict cognitive decline: results from a 5-year follow-up of healthy elderly women. *Dement. Geriatr. Cogn. Disord.* **8**, 180–7.

Erkinjuntti, T., Lee, D.H., Gao, F., Steenhuis, R., Eliasziw, M., Fry, R., Merskey, H., and Hachinski, V.C. (1993). Temporal lobe atrophy on magnetic resonance imaging in the diagnosis of early Alzheimer's disease. *Arch. Neurol.* **50**, 305–10.

Fernandez, G., Specht, K., Weis, S., Tendolkar, I., Reuber, M., Fell, J., Klaver, P., Ruhlmann, J., Reul, J., and Elger, C.E. (2003). Intrasubject reproducibility of presurgical language lateralization and mapping using fMRI. *Neurology* **60**, 969–75.

Filipovic, S., Gueguen, B., Derouesne, C., Ancri, D., Bourdel, M.C., and Plancon, D. (1989). Dementia of the Alzheimer type: some features of the posterior cerebral electrical activity. *Psychiatry Res.* **29**, 409–10.

Fingelkurts, A.A. (2004). Making complexity simpler: multivariability and metastability in the brain. *Int. J. Neurosci.* **114**, 843–62.

Fingelkurts, A.A. and Kaplan, A.Y. (2003). The regularities of the discrete nature of multi-variability of EEG spectral patterns. *Int. J. Psychophysiol.* **47**, 23–41.

Fingelkurts, A.A. and Kaplan, A.Y. (2006). Interictal EEG as a physiological adaptation. Part I. Composition of brain oscillations in interictal EEG. *Clin. Neurophysiol.* **117**, 208–22.

Fingelkurts, A.A., Ermolaev, V.A., and Kaplan, A.Y. (2006). Stability, reliability and consistency of the compositions of brain oscillations. *Int. J. Psychophysiol.* **59**, 116–26.

Fisch, B.J. and Pedley, T.A. (1989). The role of quantitative topographic mapping or 'neurometrics' in the diagnosis of psychiatric and neurological disorders: the cons. *Electroencephalogr. Clin. Neurophysiol.* **73**, 5–9.

Fisher, R.S., van Emde Boas, W., Blume, W., Elger, C., Genton, P., Lee, P., and Engel, J., Jr. (2005). Epileptic seizures and epilepsy: definitions proposed by the International League Against Epilepsy (ILAE) and the International Bureau for Epilepsy (IBE). *Epilepsia* **46**, 470–2.

Fox, N.C. and Freeborough, P.A. (1997). Brain atrophy progression measured from registered serial MRI: validation and application to Alzheimer's disease. *J. Magn. Reson. Imaging* **7**, 1069–75.

Fox, N.C., Warrington, E.K., Freeborough, P.A., Hartikainen, P., Kennedy, A.M., Stevens, J.M., and Rossor, M.N. (1996). Presymptomatic hippocampal atrophy in Alzheimer's disease. A longitudinal MRI study. *Brain* **119**, 2001–7.

Gaillard, W.D., Balsamo, L., Xu, B., McKinney, C., Papero, P.H., Weinstein, S., Conry, J., Pearl, P.L., Sachs, B., Sato, S., *et al.* (2004). fMRI language task panel improves determination of language dominance. *Neurology* **63**, 1403–8.

Gastaut, H., Santanelli, P., and Salinas Jara, M. (1985). [Interictal EEG activity specific for a particular variety of temporal epilepsy. Epileptic temporal theta rhythm]. *Rev. Electroencephalogr. Neurophysiol. Clin.* **15**, 113–20.

Gelety, T.J., Burgess, R.J., Drake, M.E., Jr., Ford, C.E., and Brown, M.E. (1985). Computerized spectral analysis of the interictal EEG in epilepsy. *Clin. Electroencephalogr.* **16**, 94–7.

Giaquinto, S. and Nolfe, G. (1986). The EEG in the normal elderly: a contribution to the interpretation of aging and dementia. *Electroencephalogr. Clin. Neurophysiol.* **63**, 540–6.

Grady, C.L., Haxby, J.V., Horwitz, B., Gillette, J., Salerno, J.A., Gonzalez-Aviles, A., Carson, R.E., Herscovitch, P., Schapiro, M.B., and Rapoport, S.I. (1993). Activation of cerebral blood flow during a visuoperceptual task in patients with Alzheimer-type dementia. *Neurobiol. Aging* **14**, 35–44.

Grady, C.L., Furey, M.L., Pietrini, P., Horwitz, B., and Rapoport, S.I. (2001). Altered brain functional connectivity and impaired short-term memory in Alzheimer's disease. *Brain* **124**, 739–56.

Grave de Peralta Menendez, R., Gonzalez Andino, S., Lantz, G., Michel, C.M., and Landis, T. (2001). Noninvasive localization of electromagnetic epileptic activity. I. Method descriptions and simulations. *Brain Topogr.* **14**, 131–7.

Grave de Peralta Menendez, R., Murray, M.M., Michel, C.M., Martuzzi, R., and Gonzalez Andino, S.L. (2004). Electrical neuroimaging based on biophysical constraints. *Neuroimage* **21**, 527–39.

Greenwood, P.M. (2000). The frontal aging hypothesis evaluated. *J. Int. Neuropsychol. Soc.* **6**, 705–26.

Herholz, K. (2003). PET studies in dementia. *Ann. Nucl. Med.* **17**, 79–89.

Herholz, K., Nordberg, A., Salmon, E., Perani, D., Kessler, J., Mielke, R., Halber, M., Jelic, V., Almkvist, O., Collette, F., *et al.* (1999). Impairment of neocortical metabolism predicts progression in Alzheimer's disease. *Dement. Geriatr. Cogn. Disord.* **10**, 494–504.

Hier, D.B., Mangone, C.A., Ganellen, R., Warach, J.D., Van Egeren, R., Perlik, S.J., and Gorelick, P.B. (1991). Quantitative measurement of delta activity in Alzheimer's disease. *Clin. Electroencephalogr.* **22**, 178–82.

Hirata, M., Kato, A., Taniguchi, M., Saitoh, Y., Ninomiya, H., Ihara, A., Kishima, H., Oshino, S., Baba, T., Yorifuji, S., and Yoshimine, T. (2004). Determination of language dominance with synthetic aperture magnetometry: comparison with the Wada test. *Neuroimage* **23**, 46–53.

Hoffman, D.A., Lubar, J.F., Thatcher, R.W., Sterman, M.B., Rosenfeld, P.J., Striefel, S., Trudeau, D., and Stockdale, S. (1999). Limitations of the American Academy of Neurology and American Clinical Neurophysiology Society paper on QEEG. *J. Neuropsychiatry Clin. Neurosci.* **11**, 401–7.

Hoffman, J.M., Welsh-Bohmer, K.A., Hanson, M., Crain, B., Hulette, C., Earl, N., and Coleman, R.E. (2000). FDG PET imaging in patients with pathologically verified dementia. *J. Nucl. Med.* **41**, 1920–8.

Honea, R., Crow, T.J., Passingham, D., and Mackay, C.E. (2005). Regional deficits in brain volume in schizophrenia: a meta-analysis of voxel-based morphometry studies. *Am. J. Psychiatry* **162**, 2233–45.

Hoyer, S., Muller, D., and Plaschke, K. (1994). Desensitization of brain insulin receptor. Effect on glucose/energy and related metabolism. *J. Neural Transm. Suppl.* **44**, 259–68.

Hughes, J.R. (1995). The EEG in psychiatry: an outline with summarized points and references. *Clin. Electroencephalogr.* **26**, 92–101.

Hughes, J.R. and John, E.R. (1999). Conventional and quantitative electroencephalography in psychiatry. *J. Neuropsychiatry Clin. Neurosci.* **11**, 190–208.

Hughes, J.R., Shanmugham, S., Wetzel, L.C., Bellur, S., and Hughes, C.A. (1989). The relationship between EEG changes and cognitive functions in dementia: a study in a VA population. *Clin. Electroencephalogr.* **20**, 77–85.

Insausti, R., Tunon, T., Sobreviela, T., Insausti, A.M., and Gonzalo, L.M. (1995). The human entorhinal cortex: a cytoarchitectonic analysis. *J. Comp. Neurol.* **355**, 171–98.

Jack, C.R., Jr., Dickson, D.W., Parisi, J.E., Xu, Y.C., Cha, R.H., O'Brien, P.C., Edland, S.D., Smith, G.E., Boeve, B.F., Tangalos, E.G., *et al.* (2002). Antemortem MRI findings correlate with hippocampal neuropathology in typical aging and dementia. *Neurology* **58**, 750–7.

Jack, C.R., Jr., Petersen, R.C., Xu, Y.C., O'Brien, P.C., Smith, G.E., Ivnik, R.J., Boeve, B.F., Waring, S.C., Tangalos, E.G., and Kokmen, E. (1999). Prediction of AD with MRI-based hippocampal volume in mild cognitive impairment. *Neurology* **52**, 1397–403.

Jack, C.R., Jr., Petersen, R.C., Xu, Y., O'Brien, P.C., Smith, G.E., Ivnik, R.J., Boeve, B.F., Tangalos, E.G., and Kokmen, E. (2000). Rates of hippocampal atrophy correlate with change in clinical status in aging and AD. *Neurology* **55**, 484–9.

Jack, C.R., Jr., Shiung, M.M., Weigand, S.D., O'Brien, P.C., Gunter, J.L., Boeve, B.F., Knopman, D.S., Smith, G.E., Ivnik, R.J., Tangalos, E.G., and Petersen, R.C. (2005). Brain atrophy rates predict subsequent clinical conversion in normal elderly and amnestic MCI. *Neurology* **65**, 1227–31.

Jacobson, S.A., Leuchter, A.F., and Walter, D.O. (1993). Conventional and quantitative EEG in the diagnosis of delirium among the elderly. *J. Neurol. Neurosurg. Psychiatry* **56**, 153–8.

Janszky, J., Jokeit, H., Kontopoulou, K., Mertens, M., Ebner, A., Pohlmann-Eden, B., and Woermann, F.G. (2005). Functional MRI predicts memory performance after right mesiotemporal epilepsy surgery. *Epilepsia* **46**, 244–50.

Jayakar, P., Bernal, B., Santiago Medina, L., and Altman, N. (2002). False lateralization of language cortex on functional MRI after a cluster of focal seizures. *Neurology* **58**, 490–2.

Jeong, J. (2004). EEG dynamics in patients with Alzheimer's disease. *Clin. Neurophysiol.* **115**, 1490–505.

Jing, H. and Takigawa, M. (2000). Comparison of human ictal, interictal and normal non-linear component analyses. *Clin. Neurophysiol.* **111**, 1282–92.

John, E.R., Prichep, L.S., Fridman, J., and Easton, P. (1988). Neurometrics: computer-assisted differential diagnosis of brain dysfunctions. *Science* **239**, 162–9.

Johnson, R., Jr. (1986). A triarchic model of P300 amplitude. *Psychophysiology* **23**, 367–84.

Kalaria, R.N., Gravina, S.A., Schmidley, J.W., Perry, G., and Harik, S.I. (1988). The glucose transporter of the human brain and blood–brain barrier. *Ann. Neurol.* **24**, 757–64.

Kalus, P., Slotboom, J., Gallinat, J., Mahlberg, R., Cattapan-Ludewig, K., Wiest, R., Nyffeler, T., Buri, C., Federspiel, A., Kunz, D., *et al.* (2006). Examining the gateway to the limbic system with diffusion tensor imaging: the perforant pathway in dementia. *Neuroimage* **30**, 713–20.

Kato, T., Knopman, D., and Liu, H. (2001). Dissociation of regional activation in mild AD during visual encoding: a functional MRI study. *Neurology* **57**, 812–16.

Kaye, J.A., Swihart, T., Howieson, D., Dame, A., Moore, M.M., Karnos, T., Camicioli, R., Ball, M., Oken, B., and Sexton, G. (1997). Volume loss of the hippocampus and temporal lobe in healthy elderly persons destined to develop dementia. *Neurology* **48**, 1297–304.

Kelley, J.T. and Reilly, E.L. (1983). EEG, alcohol, and alcoholism. In *EEG and evoked potentials in psychiatry and behavioral neurology* (ed. J.R. Hughes and W.P. Wilson), pp. 55–77. Butterworth, London.

Kemper, T.L. (1994). Neuroanatomical and neuropathological changes during aging and dementia. In *Clinical neurology of aging* (ed. M.L. Albert and J. Kusefel), pp. 3–67. Oxford University Press, New York.

Kesslak, J.P., Nalcioglu, O., and Cotman, C.W. (1991). Quantification of magnetic resonance scans for hippocampal and parahippocampal atrophy in Alzheimer's disease. *Neurology* **41**, 51–4.

Killiany, R.J., Moss, M.B., Albert, M.S., Sandor, T., Tieman, J., and Jolesz, F. (1993). Temporal lobe regions on magnetic resonance imaging identify patients with early Alzheimer's disease. *Arch. Neurol.* **50**, 949–54.

Killiany, R.J., Hyman, B.T., Gomez-Isla, T., Moss, M.B., Kikinis, R., Jolesz, F., Tanzi, R., Jones, K., and Albert, M.S. (2002). MRI measures of entorhinal cortex vs hippocampus in preclinical AD. *Neurology* **58**, 1188–96.

Kirchberger, K., Hummel, C., and Stefan, H. (1998). Postoperative multichannel magnetoencephalography in patients with recurrent seizures after epilepsy surgery. *Acta Neurol. Scand.* **98**, 1–7.

Kloppel, S. and Büchel, C. (2005). Alternatives to the Wada test: a critical view of functional magnetic resonance imaging in preoperative use. *Curr. Opin. Neurol.* **18**, 418–23.

Knake, S., Haag, A., Hamer, H.M., Dittmer, C., Bien, S., Oertel, W.H., and Rosenow, F. (2003). Language lateralization in patients with temporal lobe epilepsy: a comparison of functional transcranial Doppler sonography and the Wada test. *Neuroimage* **19**, 1228–32.

Knowlton, R.C. (2006). The role of FDG-PET, ictal SPECT, and MEG in the epilepsy surgery evaluation. *Epilepsy Behav.* **8**, 91–101.

Knowlton, R.C., Laxer, K.D., Aminoff, M.J., Roberts, T.P., Wong, S.T., and Rowley, H.A. (1997). Magnetoencephalography in partial epilepsy: clinical yield and localization accuracy. *Ann. Neurol.* **42**, 622–631.

Koutroumanidis, M., Binnie, C.D., Elwes, R.D., Polkey, C.E., Seed, P., Alarcon, G., Cox, T., Barrington, S., Marsden, P., Maisey, M.N., and Panayiotopoulos, C.P. (1998). Interictal regional slow activity in temporal lobe epilepsy correlates with lateral temporal hypometabolism as imaged with 18FDG PET: neurophysiological and metabolic implications. *J. Neurol. Neurosurg. Psychiatry* **65**, 170–6.

Kowalski, J.W., Gawel, M., Pfeffer, A., and Barcikowska, M. (2001). The diagnostic value of EEG in Alzheimer disease: correlation with the severity of mental impairment. *J. Clin. Neurophysiol.* **18**, 570–5.

Krause, C.M., Korpilahti, P., Porn, B., Jantti, J., and Lang, H.A. (1998). Automatic auditory word perception as measured by 40 Hz EEG responses. *Electroencephalogr. Clin. Neurophysiol.* **107**, 84–7.

Le Bihan, D., Mangin, J.F., Poupon, C., Clark, C.A., Pappata, S., Molko, N., and Chabriat, H. (2001). Diffusion tensor imaging: concepts and applications. *J. Magn. Reson. Imaging* **13**, 534–46.

Le Bihan, D., Urayama, S., Aso, T., Hanakawa, T., and Fukuyama, H. (2006). Direct and fast detection of neuronal activation in the human brain with diffusion MRI. *Proc. Natl. Acad. Sci. USA* **103** (21), 8263–8.

Lehericy, S., Cohen, L., Bazin, B., Samson, S., Giacomini, E., Rougetet, R., Hertz-Pannier, L., Le Bihan, D., Marsault, C., and Baulac, M. (2000). Functional MR evaluation of temporal and frontal language dominance compared with the Wada test. *Neurology* **54**, 1625–33.

Leuchter, A.F., Spar, J.E., Walter, D.O., and Weiner, H. (1987). Electroencephalographic spectra and coherence in the diagnosis of Alzheimer's-type and multi-infarct dementia. A pilot study. *Arch. Gen. Psychiatry* **44**, 993–8.

Leuchter, A.F., Newton, T.F., Cook, I.A., Walter, D.O., Rosenberg-Thompson, S., and Lachenbruch, P.A. (1992). Changes in brain functional connectivity in Alzheimer-type and multi-infarct dementia. *Brain* **115**, 1543–61.

Leuchter, A.F., Cook, I.A., Lufkin, R.B., Dunkin, J., Newton, T.F., Cummings, J.L., Mackey, J.K., and Walter, D.O. (1994). Cordance: a new method for assessment of cerebral perfusion and metabolism using quantitative electroencephalography. *Neuroimage* **1**, 208–19.

Locatelli, T., Cursi, M., Liberati, D., Franceschi, M., and Comi, G. (1998). EEG coherence in Alzheimer's disease. *Electroencephalogr. Clin. Neurophysiol.* **106**, 229–37.

Logothetis, N.K., Pauls, J., Augath, M., Trinath, T., and Oeltermann, A. (2001). Neurophysiological investigation of the basis of the fMRI signal. *Nature* **412**, 150–7.

Lopes de Silva, F.H. and Van Rotterdam, A. (1987). Biophysical aspects of EEG and MEG generation. In *Electroencephalography: basic principles, clinical applications and related fields* (ed. E. Niedermeyer, and F.H. Lopes da Silva), pp. 15–28. Urban and Schwarzenberg, Baltimore.

Machulda, M.M., Ward, H.A., Borowski, B., Gunter, J.L., Cha, R.H., O'Brien, P.C., Petersen, R.C., Boeve, B.F., Knopman, D., Tang-Wai, D.F., *et al.* (2003). Comparison of memory fMRI response among normal, MCI, and Alzheimer's patients. *Neurology* **61**, 500–6.

Magistretti, P.J. and Pellerin, L. (1996). Cellular bases of brain energy metabolism and their relevance to functional brain imaging: evidence for a prominent role of astrocytes. *Cereb. Cortex* **6**, 50–61.

Magistretti, P.J., Pellerin, L., Rothman, D.L., and Shulman, R.G. (1999). Energy on demand. *Science* **283**, 496–7.

Marcus, D.L., de Leon, M.J., Goldman, J., Logan, J., Christman, D.R., Wolf, A.P., Fowler, J.S., Hunter, K., Tsai, J., Pearson, J., *et al.* (1989). Altered glucose metabolism in microvessels from patients with Alzheimer's disease. *Ann. Neurol.* **26**, 91–4.

Martin-Loeches, M., Gil, P., Jimenez, F., Exposito, F.J., Miguel, F., Cacabelos, R., and Rubia, F.J. (1991). Topographic maps of brain electrical activity in primary degenerative dementia of the Alzheimer type and multiinfarct dementia. *Biol. Psychiatry* **29**, 211–23.

Massa, R., de Saint-Martin, A., Carcangiu, R., Rudolf, G., Seegmuller, C., Kleitz, C., Metz-Lutz, M.N., Hirsch, E., and Marescaux, C. (2001). EEG criteria predictive of complicated evolution in idiopathic rolandic epilepsy. *Neurology* **57**, 1071–9.

Matsuura, M., Okubo, Y., Toru, M., Kojima, T., He, Y., Hou, Y., Shen, Y., and Lee, C.K. (1993). A cross-national EEG study of children with emotional and behavioral problems: a WHO collaborative study in the Western Pacific Region. *Biol. Psychiatry* **34**, 59–65.

McKhann, G., Drachman, D., Folstein, M., Katzman, R., Price, D., and Stadlan, E.M. (1984). Clinical diagnosis of Alzheimer's disease: report of the NINCDS-ADRDA Work Group under the auspices of Department of Health and Human Services Task Force on Alzheimer's Disease. *Neurology* **34**, 939–44.

Meador, K.J. and Loring, D.W. (1999). The Wada test: controversies, concerns, and insights. *Neurology* **52**, 1535–6.

Medina, L.S., Aguirre, E., Bernal, B., and Altman, N.R. (2004). Functional MR imaging versus Wada test for evaluation of language lateralization: cost analysis. *Radiology* **230**, 49–54.

Mentis, M.J., Horwitz, B., Grady, C.L., Alexander, G.E., VanMeter, J.W., Maisog, J.M., Pietrini, P., Schapiro, M.B., and Rapoport, S.I. (1996). Visual cortical dysfunction in Alzheimer's disease evaluated with a temporally graded 'stress test' during PET. *Am. J. Psychiatry* **153**, 32–40.

Minoshima, S., Giordani, B., Berent, S., Frey, K.A., Foster, N.L., and Kuhl, D.E. (1997). Metabolic reduction in the posterior cingulate cortex in very early Alzheimer's disease. *Ann. Neurol.* **42**, 85–94.

Minoshima, S., Foster, N.L., Sima, A.A., Frey, K.A., Albin, R.L., and Kuhl, D.E. (2001). Alzheimer's disease versus dementia with Lewy bodies: cerebral metabolic distinction with autopsy confirmation. *Ann. Neurol.* **50**, 358–65.

Mormann, F., Lehnertz, K., David, P., and Elger, C.E. (2000). Mean phase coherence as a measure for phase synchronization and its application to the EEG of epilepsy patients. *Physica D* **144**, 358–69.

Mosconi, L. (2005). Brain glucose metabolism in the early and specific diagnosis of Alzheimer's disease. FDG-PET studies in MCI and AD. *Eur. J. Nucl. Med. Mol. Imaging* **32**, 486–510.

Mosconi, L., De Santi, S., Rusinek, H., Convit, A., and de Leon, M.J. (2004*a*). Magnetic resonance and PET studies in the early diagnosis of Alzheimer's disease. *Expert Rev. Neurother.* **4**, 831–49.

Mosconi, L., Perani, D., Sorbi, S., Herholz, K., Nacmias, B., Holthoff, V., Salmon, E., Baron, J.C., De Cristofaro, M.T., Padovani, A., *et al.* (2004*b*). MCI conversion to dementia and the APOE genotype: a prediction study with FDG-PET. *Neurology* **63**, 2332–40.

Moscovitch, M. and Winocur, G. (1995). Frontal lobes, memory, and aging. *Ann. NY Acad. Sci.* **769**, 119–50.

Moseley, M., Bammer, R., and Illes, J. (2002). Diffusion-tensor imaging of cognitive performance. *Brain Cogn.* **50**, 396–413.

Muller, M.J., Greverus, D., Dellani, P.R., Weibrich, C., Wille, P.R., Scheurich, A., Stoeter, P., and Fellgiebel, A. (2005). Functional implications of hippocampal volume and diffusivity in mild cognitive impairment. *Neuroimage* **28**, 1033–42.

Naggara, O., Oppenheim, C., Rieu, D., Raoux, N., Rodrigo, S., Dalla Barba, G., and Meder, J.F. (2006). Diffusion tensor imaging in early Alzheimer's disease. *Psychiatry Res.* **146** (3), 243–9.

Nestor, P.J., Fryer, T.D., Smielewski, P., and Hodges, J.R. (2003). Limbic hypometabolism in Alzheimer's disease and mild cognitive impairment. *Ann. Neurol.* **54**, 343–51.

Nuwer, M. (1997). Assessment of digital EEG, quantitative EEG, and EEG brain mapping: report of the American Academy of Neurology and the American Clinical Neurophysiology Society. *Neurology* **49**, 277–92.

Nyberg, L., Backman, L., Erngrund, K., Olofsson, U., and Nilsson, L.G. (1996). Age differences in episodic memory, semantic memory, and priming: relationships to demographic, intellectual, and biological factors. *J. Gerontol. B Psychol. Sci. Soc. Sci.* **51**, P234–40.

O'Connor, K.P., Shaw, J.C., and Ongley, C.O. (1979). The EEG and differential diagnosis in psychogeriatrics. *Br. J. Psychiatry* **135**, 156–62.

Ogawa, S., Lee, T.M., Kay, A.R., and Tank, D.W. (1990). Brain magnetic resonance imaging with contrast dependent on blood oxygenation. *Proc. Natl. Acad. Sci. USA* **87**, 9868–72.

Perez Velzaquez, J.L., Cortez, M.A., Snead, C.O., and Wennberg, R. (2003). Dynamical regimes underlying epileptiform events: role of instabilities and bifurcations in brain activity. *Physica D* **186**, 205–20.

Pierpaoli, C. and Basser, P.J. (1996). Toward a quantitative assessment of diffusion anisotropy. *Magn. Reson. Med.* **36**, 893–906.

Polich, J. and Corey-Bloom, J. (2005). Alzheimer's disease and P300: review and evaluation of task and modality. *Curr. Alzheimer Res.* **2**, 515–25.

Polich, J. and Herbst, K.L. (2000). P300 as a clinical assay: rationale, evaluation, and findings. *Int. J. Psychophysiol.* **38**, 3–19.

Polich, J. and Kok, A. (1995). Cognitive and biological determinants of P300: an integrative review. *Biol. Psychol.* **41**, 103–46.

Pollock, V.E., Schneider, L.S., and Lyness, S.A. (1990). EEG amplitudes in healthy, late-middle-aged and elderly adults: normality of the distributions and correlations with age. *Electroencephalogr. Clin. Neurophysiol.* **75**, 276–88.

Prichep, L.S., John, E.R., Ferris, S.H., Reisberg, B., Almas, M., Alper, K., and Cancro, R. (1994). Quantitative EEG correlates of cognitive deterioration in the elderly. *Neurobiol. Aging* **15**, 85–90.

Prichep, L.S., John, E.R., Ferris, S.H., Rausch, L., Fang, Z., Cancro, R., Torossian, C., and Reisberg, B. (2006). Prediction of longitudinal cognitive decline in normal elderly with subjective complaints using electrophysiological imaging. *Neurobiol. Aging* **27**, 471–81.

Prinz, P.N. and Vitiello, M.V. (1989). Dominant occipital (alpha) rhythm frequency in early stage Alzheimer's disease and depression. *Electroencephalogr. Clin. Neurophysiol.* **73**, 427–32.

Prvulovic, D., Hubl, D., Sack, A.T., Melillo, L., Maurer, K., Frolich, L., Lanfermann, H., Zanella, F.E., Goebel, R., Linden, D.E., and Dierks, T. (2002). Functional imaging of visuospatial processing in Alzheimer's disease. *Neuroimage* **17**, 1403–14.

Prvulovic, D., Van de Ven, V., Sack, A.T., Maurer, K., and Linden, D.E. (2005). Functional activation imaging in aging and dementia. *Psychiatry Res.* **140**, 97–113.

Rabin, M.L., Narayan, V.M., Kimberg, D.Y., Casasanto, D.J., Glosser, G., Tracy, J.I., French, J.A., Sperling, M.R., and Detre, J.A. (2004). Functional MRI predicts post-surgical memory following temporal lobectomy. *Brain* **127**, 2286–98.

Rae-Grant, A., Blume, W., Lau, C., Hachinski, V.C., Fisman, M., and Merskey, H. (1987). The electroencephalogram in Alzheimer-type dementia. A sequential study correlating the electroencephalogram with psychometric and quantitative pathologic data. *Arch. Neurol.* **44**, 50–4.

Ravelli, F. and Antolini, R. (1992). Complex dynamics underlying the human electrocardiogram. *Biol. Cybern.* **67**, 57–65.

Raz, N., Gunning-Dixon, F.M., Head, D., Dupuis, J.H., and Acker, J.D. (1998). Neuroanatomical correlates of cognitive aging: evidence from structural magnetic resonance imaging. *Neuropsychology* **12**, 95–114.

Reilly, E.L., Glass, G., and Faillace, L.A. (1979). EEGs in an alcohol detoxification and treatment center. *Clin. Electroencephalogr.* **10**, 69–71.

Reisberg, B., Ferris, S.H., de Leon, M.J., and Crook, T. (1982). The Global Deterioration Scale for assessment of primary degenerative dementia. *Am. J. Psychiatry* **139**, 1136–9.

Richards, M., Folstein, M., Albert, M., Miller, L., Bylsma, F., Lafleche, G., Marder, K., Bell, K., Sano, M., Devanand, D., *et al.* (1993). Multicenter study of predictors of disease course in Alzheimer disease (the 'predictors study'). II. Neurological, psychiatric, and demographic influences on baseline measures of disease severity. *Alzheimer Dis. Assoc. Disord.* **7**, 22–32.

Robinson, D.J., Merskey, H., Blume, W.T., Fry, R., Williamson, P.C., and Hachinski, V.C. (1994). Electroencephalography as an aid in the exclusion of Alzheimer's disease. *Arch. Neurol.* **51**, 280–4.

Rockel, A.J., Hiorns, R.W., and Powell, T.P. (1980). The basic uniformity in structure of the neocortex. *Brain* **103**, 221–44.

Rodriguez, E., George, N., Lachaux, J.P., Martinerie, J., Renault, B., and Varela, F.J. (1999). Perception's shadow: long-distance synchronization of human brain activity. *Nature* **397**, 430–3.

Rugg, M.D., Doyle, M.C., and Wells, T. (1995). Word and nonword repetition within- and across-modality: an event-related potential study. *J. Cogn. Neurosci.* **7**, 209–27.

Sabsevitz, D.S., Swanson, S.J., Hammeke, T.A., Spanaki, M.V., Possing, E.T., Morris, G.L., 3rd, Mueller, W.M., and Binder, J.R. (2003). Use of preoperative functional neuroimaging to predict language deficits from epilepsy surgery. *Neurology* **60**, 1788–92.

Salat, D.H., Tuch, D.S., Greve, D.N., van der Kouwe, A.J., Hevelone, N.D., Zaleta, A.K., Rosen, B.R., Fischl, B., Corkin, S., Rosas, H.D., and Dale, A.M. (2005). Age-related alterations in white matter microstructure measured by diffusion tensor imaging. *Neurobiol. Aging* **26**, 1215–27.

Salthouse, T.A. (1996). The processing-speed theory of adult age differences in cognition. *Psychol. Rev.* **103**, 403–428.

Scherg, M. and Berg, P. (1991). Use of prior knowledge in brain electromagnetic source analysis. *Brain Topogr.* **4**, 143–50.

Scherg, M. and Ebersole, J.S. (1994). Brain source imaging of focal and multifocal epileptiform EEG activity. *Neurophysiol. Clin.* **24**, 51–60.

Silverman, D.H., Small, G.W., Chang, C.Y., Lu, C.S., Kung De Aburto, M.A., Chen, W., Czernin, J., Rapoport, S.I., Pietrini, P., Alexander, G.E., *et al.* (2001). Positron emission tomography in evaluation of dementia: Regional brain metabolism and long-term outcome. *J. Am. Med. Assoc.* **286**, 2120–7.

Simkins-Bullock, J. (2000). Beyond speech lateralization: a review of the variability, reliability, and validity of the intracarotid amobarbital procedure and its nonlanguage uses in epilepsy surgery candidates. *Neuropsychol. Rev.* **10**, 41–74.

Simpson, I.A., Chundu, K.R., Davies-Hill, T., Honer, W.G., and Davies, P. (1994). Decreased concentrations of GLUT1 and GLUT3 glucose transporters in the brains of patients with Alzheimer's disease. *Ann. Neurol.* **35**, 546–51.

Singer, W. (1999). Neurobiology. Striving for coherence. *Nature* **397**, 391–3.

Small, J.G. (1993). Psychiatric disorders and EEG. In *Electroencephalography: basic principles, clinical applications, and related fields* (ed. E. Niedermeyer, and F. Lopes da Silva), pp. 581–96. Williams and Wilkins, Baltimore.

Smith, C.D., Andersen, A.H., Kryscio, R.J., Schmitt, F.A., Kindy, M.S., Blonder, L.X., and Avison, M.J. (2002). Women at risk for AD show increased parietal activation during a fluency task. *Neurology* **58**, 1197–202.

Smith, J.R., King, D.W., Park, Y.D., Lee, M.R., Lee, G.P., and Jenkins, P.D. (2000). Magnetic source imaging guidance of gamma knife radiosurgery for the treatment of epilepsy. *J. Neurosurg.* **93** (suppl. 3), 136–40.

Soininen, H., Partanen, J., Laulumaa, V., Paakkonen, A., Helkala, E.L., and Riekkinen, P.J. (1991). Serial EEG in Alzheimer's disease: 3 year follow-up and clinical outcome. *Electroencephalogr. Clin. Neurophysiol.* **79**, 342–8.

Sperling, R.A., Bates, J.F., Chua, E.F., Cocchiarella, A.J., Rentz, D.M., Rosen, B.R., Schacter, D.L., and Albert, M.S. (2003). fMRI studies of associative encoding in young and elderly controls and mild Alzheimer's disease. *J. Neurol. Neurosurg. Psychiatry* **74**, 44–50.

Squire, L.R. and Zola, S.M. (1996). Memory, memory impairment, and the medial temporal lobe. *Cold Spring Harb. Symp. Quant. Biol.* **61**, 185–95.

Stefan, H., Hummel, C., Hopfengartner, R., Pauli, E., Tilz, C., Ganslandt, O., Kober, H., Moler, A., and Buchfelder, M. (2000). Magnetoencephalography in extratemporal epilepsy. *J. Clin. Neurophysiol.* **17**, 190–200.

Strijers, R.L., Scheltens, P., Jonkman, E.J., de Rijke, W., Hooijer, C., and Jonker, C. (1997). Diagnosing Alzheimer's disease in community-dwelling elderly: a comparison of EEG and MRI. *Dement. Geriatr. Cogn. Disord.* **8**, 198–202.

Tallon-Baudry, C. and Bertrand, O. (1999). Oscillatory gamma activity in humans and its role in object representation. *Trends Cogn. Sci.* **3**, 151–62.

Torres, F., Faoro, A., Loewenson, R., and Johnson, E. (1983). The electroencephalogram of elderly subjects revisited. *Electroencephalogr. Clin. Neurophysiol.* **56**, 391–8.

Ts'o, D.Y., Frostig, R.D., Lieke, E.E., and Grinvald, A. (1990). Functional organization of primate visual cortex revealed by high resolution optical imaging. *Science* **249**, 417–20.

Valdes, P., Bosch, J., Grave, R., Hernandez, J., Riera, J., Pascual, R., and Biscay, R. (1992). Frequency domain models of the EEG. *Brain Topogr.* **4**, 309–19.

Vanhanen, M., and Soininen, H. (1998). Glucose intolerance, cognitive impairment and Alzheimer's disease. *Curr. Opin. Neurol.* **11**, 673–7.

Veldhuizen, R.J., Jonkman, E.J., and Poortvliet, D.C. (1993). Sex differences in age regression parameters of healthy adults—normative data and practical implications. *Electroencephalogr. Clin. Neurophysiol.* **86**, 377–84.

Wada, J. (1949). A new method for determination of the side of cerebral speech dominance: a preliminary report on the intracarotid injection of sodium amytal in man. *Iqakaa te Seibutzuqaki* **14**, 221–2.

Wada, J.A. (1997). Clinical experimental observations of carotid artery injections of sodium amytal. *Brain Cogn.* **33**, 11–13.

Watson, N.F., Dodrill, C., Farrell, D., Holmes, M.D., and Miller, J.W. (2004). Determination of language dominance with near-infrared spectroscopy: comparison with the intracarotid amobarbital procedure. *Seizure* **13**, 399–402.

Weber, B., Lehnertz, K., Elger, C.E., and Wieser, H.G. (1998). Neuronal complexity loss in interictal EEG recorded with foramen ovale electrodes predicts side of primary epileptogenic area in temporal lobe epilepsy: a replication study. *Epilepsia* **39**, 922–7.

Wheless, J.W., Willmore, L.J., Breier, J.I., Kataki, M., Smith, J.R., King, D.W., Meador, K.J., Park, Y.D., Loring, D.W., Clifton, G.L., *et al.* (1999). A comparison of magnetoencephalography, MRI, and V-EEG in patients evaluated for epilepsy surgery. *Epilepsia* **40**, 931–41.

Wikswo, J.P. (1983). Cellular action currents. In *Biomagnetism, an interdisciplinary approach* (ed. S.J. Williamson, G.L. Romani, L. Kaufman, and L. Modena), pp. 173–207. Plenum Press, New York.

Williamson, P.C., Merskey, H., Morrison, S., Rabheru, K., Fox, H., Wands, K., Wong, C., and Hachinski, V. (1990). Quantitative electroencephalographic correlates of cognitive decline in normal elderly subjects. *Arch. Neurol.* **47**, 1185–8.

Willinsky, R.A., Taylor, S.M., TerBrugge, K., Farb, R.I., Tomlinson, G., and Montanera, W. (2003). Neurologic complications of cerebral angiography: prospective analysis of 2,899 procedures and review of the literature. *Radiology* **227**, 522–8.

Woermann, F.G., Jokeit, H., Luerding, R., Freitag, H., Schulz, R., Guertler, S., Okujava, M., Wolf, P., Tuxhorn, I., and Ebner, A. (2003). Language lateralization by Wada test and fMRI in 100 patients with epilepsy. *Neurology* **61**, 699–701.

Yacoub, E., Shmuel, A., Pfeuffer, J., Van De Moortele, P.F., Adriany, G., Ugurbil, K., and Hu, X. (2001). Investigation of the initial dip in fMRI at 7 Tesla. *NMR Biomed.* **14**, 408–12.

Yener, G.G., Leuchter, A.F., Jenden, D., Read, S.L., Cummings, J.L., and Miller, B.L. (1996). Quantitative EEG in frontotemporal dementia. *Clin. Electroencephalogr.* **27**, 61–8.

Part 2

Neuropsychological syndromes associated with focal brain damage

Introduction to Part 2

Julien Bogousslavsky

Stroke yearly affects nearly one million Europeans and one million North Americans (Mackay and Mensah 2005). It is the second cause of death in most countries and the first cause of acquired disability in active adults. At least 80% of strokes affect the brain hemispheres, which translates into a high frequency of acute or persisting cognitive and behavioural manifestations. Moreover, even in strokes limited to the brainstem or cerebellum, recent work has emphasized the significant prevalence of attentional and other disorders (Carota *et al.* 2002) that may greatly impact on cognitive performances, for example, post-stroke fatigue in patients who are otherwise recovering well (Staub and Bogousslavsky 2001). Indeed, systematic assessment of cognitive function shows that significant disturbances may be found in patients with strokes that are small in size involving 'non-cognitive' areas of the brain hemispheres (Annoni *et al.* 2003). Examples include pure sensory stroke from lateral thalamic damage and other lacunar syndromes.

My personal experience of over 25 years of seeing patients immediately upon referral to an acute stroke unit has also made it obvious to me that cognitive dysfunction in acute stroke is a very dynamic and evolving process that has little to do with the much better studied chronic disorders found in stabilized patients 1 or 2 weeks later (Croquelois *et al.* 2003). In fact, large chapters of acute stroke cognitive neurology remain to be written. This would be very timely, since at present a large number of patients are admitted to acute units with sophisticated facilities for functional and anatomical neuroimaging, which allows a previously unrivalled understanding of brain–symptom correlations as well as providing useful bases for predicting recovery.

In more chronic phases after stroke, the development of post-insult depression or dementia in patients who are otherwise recovering well is a previously overlooked major problem that is now better recognized. While vascular dementia remains a controversial topic, post-stroke dementia is a critical issue, including unmasking previously unrecognized Alzheimer's disease (Bogousslavsky 2003). Post-stroke depression, which may affect one-third of patients, bears a strong relationship to cognitive dysfunction (Carota *et al.* 2005).

These facts underline the importance of routine cognitive testing and mood evaluation in stroke patients, both in the acute and chronic stages. Besides providing help in diagnosis and in delineating prognosis, systematic assessment may also allow us to adapt specific treatments, such as selecting patients for starting early antidepressant drug therapy.

Finally, since stroke is both a frequent and a focal process that affects the brain, it provides a unique material for research studies on brain function and adaptation to injury. It is striking how little stroke specialists still know about cognition and behaviour, while neuropsychologists commonly have only a vague understanding of the pathophysiology and mechanisms of stroke. Stroke units, teams, and clinics provide a unique opportunity to unify expertise in these fields, with the emergence of a useful, new, domain—cognitive and behavioural stroke neurology.

References

Annoni, J.M., Khateb, A., Gramigna, S., Staub, F., Carota, A., Maeder, P., and Bogousslavsky, J. (2003). Chronic cognitive impairment following laterothalamic infarcts. A study of 9 cases. *Arch. Neurol.* **60**, 1439–43.

Bogousslavsky, J. (2003). J. William Feinberg lecture 2002: emotions, mood, and behavior after stroke. *Stroke* **34**, 1046–50.

Carota, A., Staub, F., and Bogousslavsky, J. (2002). Emotions, behaviors and mood changes in stroke. *Curr. Opin. Neurol.* **15**, 57–69.

Carota, A., Berney, A., Aybek, S., Iaria, G., Staub, F., Ghika-Schmid, F., Annable, L., Guex, P., and Bogousslavsky, J. (2005). A prospective study of predictors of poststroke depression. *Neurology* **64**, 428–33.

Croquelois, A., Wintermark, M., Reichhart, M., Meuli, R., and Bogousslavsky, J. (2003). Aphasia in hyperacute stroke: language follows brain penumbra dynamics. *Ann. Neurol.* **54**, 321–9.

Mackay, J. and Mensah, G.A. (2005). *The atlas of heart disease and stroke*. WHO, Geneva.

Staub, F. and Bogousslavsky, J. (2001). Fatigue after stroke. A major but neglected issue. *Cerebrovasc. Dis.* **12**, 75–81.

Chapter 4

Language disorders

Jubin Abutalebi and Stefano F. Cappa

4.1 Introduction

This chapter focuses on the acquired language disorders (aphasias) that are due to focal damage, typically a stroke, involving the left hemisphere. The chapter is organized as follows. After a brief definition of language in Section 4.2, Section 4.3 describes the main clinical aspects of aphasia and of aphasic syndromes. Section 4.4 then reconsiders the clinical manifestations of aphasia from the vantage point of cognitive neuropsychology. Finally, Section 4.5 provides an overview of the neuroanatomy of language, based not only on the evidence provided by the traditional anatomo-clinical correlation approach, but also on recent evidence from functional neuroimaging studies.

4.2 Language

Language is the main tool that humans use to represent and communicate mental states. It must be clearly distinguished from 'speech', which refers to the distinct, audible manner of communicating language. Even if most of us think of words as the basic building blocks of language, linguists more properly consider 'morphemes' as the smallest meaningful units. Morphemes are built by the combination of 'phonemes', which are the abstract representation of language sounds. The combination of phonemes, in particular concatenation, produces 'morphemes'. Some morphemes may be by themselves words (such as 'go'), while others may be an affix (such as 're' in 'review'), an inflection (such as 'ing' in 'reviewing'), or a base form (such as 'view' in 'review'). The words in a given language form the 'lexicon' of that language. More properly, the lexicon is the storage of word forms, and hence includes all the word-specific information, including the morphological and syntactic specifications of a given word. The lexicon interfaces with the conceptual knowledge expressed by words, which is represented in the semantic system. Words are combined in strings conforming to the specific rules of grammar, resulting in phrases and sentences; this is known as 'syntax'. Finally, the combination of sentences into narratives is referred to as the 'discourse' level, while the system of vocal intonations that can modify the meaning of words and sentences is referred to as 'prosody'.

The subdivision of language components just described bears important practical implications, since aphasia can selectively affect some of them while leaving others spared. For instance, it is not infrequent to observe patients with anomic aphasia due to impaired access to the lexicon, while their semantic system is spared. Likewise, aphasics may have selective deficits at the syntactical level, while the lexical–semantic level is spared. At the theoretical level, the observation of aphasic deficits selectively affecting a language component is the main source of evidence supporting the idea that the levels of language organization proposed by linguistic theory have a psychological reality, and that they are subserved by specific brain circuitries.

4.3 The clinical syndromes of aphasia

The aphasias are disorders of language due to acquired cerebral lesions occurring in subjects who have enjoyed a normal linguistic development.

The aphasias must then be distinguished from developmental disorders of language acquisition, which are due to congenital neurological dysfunction.

The main features of aphasias are impairments in the ability to generate linguistic messages from mental contents, and vice versa. Aphasias must be distinguished from other disorders that can affect the communication system, of which language is only one, albeit the most important, aspect. In particular, aphasia must be distinguished from impairments in the motor realization of language, i.e. from disorders of articulation (dysarthria) or phonation (dysphonia). While these speech disorders may be associated with aphasia, they can be observed in isolation, and aphasia can be present without any speech disorder. Actually, aphasia is totally independent from the motor and sensory channels used for linguistic production and comprehension by individual subjects. For example, aphasia can be observed after left hemispheric brain lesions in deaf people, who use manual signing instead of vocal articulation to produce language (Hickok *et al.* 1996).

Cerebrovascular lesions are the leading cause of adult aphasia, and aphasia due to stroke has been most intensively investigated since the nineteenth century.

This fact has had important consequences for research. Infarctions and haemorrhages do not occur randomly in the brain, but tend to affect a set of brain regions. In the case of ischaemia these are the vascular territories, such as the branches of the middle cerebral artery. In the case of haemorrhages, these are the 'typical' locations, such as the basal ganglia or the thalamus. The traditional aphasic syndromes, recognized in clinical neurology from the end of the nineteenth century, are thus constellations of linguistic symptoms associated with a set of specific lesion sites. From this it follows that the aphasic syndromes are clusters of symptoms that tend to co-occur more frequently than by chance, because they result from damage in regions typically affected by strokes (Poeck 1983). The traditional syndromic labels do not denote theoretically meaningful entities, but continue to be used by clinicians as a shorthand to convey the main feature of the language disorder observed in a patient.

The most widely used classification system is based on the Lichtheim–Wernicke anatomo-clinical model (see the Section 4.3.1 for a description) as revised by prominent aphasia researchers such as Geschwind, Goodglass, and Benson (Benson 1979; Goodglass and Kaplan 1983). In many patients, the syndromic classification may represent only the first diagnostic step, and can be supplemented by a cognitive diagnosis, based on models of normal language processing, that attempts to pinpoint the 'locus' of the impairment within the normal processing system. This approach, which will be briefly described in Section 4.4, has been very fruitful at the research level as a tool to investigate language function and its neural substrates. At the clinical level, a 'cognitive diagnosis' may be useful for the development of theoretically grounded rehabilitation programmes (Hillis 1993; Gainotti *et al.* 2000).

4.3.1 The classical aphasic syndromes

The classification of aphasic syndromes (Table 4.1) is based on the clinical assessment of three main aspects of language performance. They are the characteristics of language production (in particular the fluency), the ability to understand, and the ability to repeat.

Table 4.1 Classification of the aphasias

	Production	Comprehension	Repetition
Perisylvian aphasias			
Broca	Non-fluent	+	—
Global	Non-fluent	—	—
Wernicke	Fluent	—	—
Conduction	Fluent	+	—
Extrasylvian aphasias			
Transcortical motor	Non-fluent	+	+
Transcortical sensory	Fluent	—	+
Mixed transcortical	Non-fluent	—	+
Anomic	Fluent	+	+

These three aspects may be easily examined at the bedside, without the need to use specialized test materials. The initial diagnosis must then be confirmed by a standard aphasia test.

- *Language production.* Simply listening to the patient speaking provides a lot of crucial information. An adequate evaluation requires extended production samples, which can be elicited by an open conversation or by specific requests to narrate an event or a complex picture. The analysis of production is easier to perform on-line, using video or audio taping. The transcription of the sample can be used for an in-depth analysis of error types. A basic feature of production is its 'fluency', a concept introduced by Goodglass *et al.* (1964) to define a 'global' dimension of production based on the assessment of a number of linguistic and extralinguistic features. The assessment of fluency is based on a quantitative measure (phrase length, i.e. the longest uninterrupted sequence of words produced by the patients), combined with several parameters that are assessed only qualitatively. These include speech articulation, the presence of phonological and lexical errors (paraphasias), the grammatical abilities, and the melodic line (intonational contour). On the basis of these parameters, aphasic patients can be subdivided into two large groups, i.e. fluent and non-fluent.
    - Non-fluent patients produce short sentences or even only single words, usually have articulation disorders, may produce paraphasias and grammatical errors, and have an altered melodic line.
    - Conversely, fluent patients produce grammatically well-structured, longer sentences, with phonological and lexical errors; their articulation is unimpaired, and the melodic line sounds normal.

  The examination of production is completed by an assessment of the naming abilities. In a clinical setting, this can be accomplished using common objects or parts of objects, by asking the patient to provide their name.

- *Language comprehension.* The ability to understand language produced by others is the second crucial aspect of language performance to be assessed. At the single word level, the clinical test can be based on the same set of objects or parts of objects used for naming. The examiner puts three of four items in front of the subject, pronounces a word, and asks the patient to point to the corresponding item. Sentence comprehension is usually assessed with verbal commands; another possibility is to ask yes–no questions.

- *Repetition*. This aspect of language performance does not play a crucial role in communicative language use, but has a central importance for aphasia classification. To be able to repeat indicates preserved phonological abilities, and suggests an integrity of the immediately perisylvian language areas (Broca, Wernicke, supramarginal gyrus) and their connections. Conversely, a disproportionate impairment of repetition in an aphasic patient points to a disruption of the same circuit.

4.3.1.1 Non-fluent aphasias with impaired repetition

Broca's aphasia

Broca's aphasia is characterized by non-fluent language production. Morphology is affected with omissions and, less frequently, substitutions of 'function words' including free-standing flectional and derivational morphemes.

The speech is effortful and hesitant, the articulation is defective, and prosody is affected, resulting in a monotonous melodic line. Word-finding difficulties and phonological errors can be typically observed. The morphological disorder and the simplification of sentence structure are the main features of 'agrammatism' in production. The ability to name is also affected, often more for naming actions rather than objects. The comprehension of single words and declarative sentences is preserved, but the ability to understand more complex syntactic structures, such as semantically reversible passive sentences (such as 'the boy is followed by the girl') is often affected. Repetition is impaired, and shows the same features of spontaneous production, i.e. defective articulation and phonological errors. The ability to read aloud and write spontaneously or to dictation is also often affected.

The complete syndrome of Broca's aphasia is associated with large lesions, which are not limited to Broca's area but extend to neighbouring regions such as the precentral gyrus, the anterior insula, the underlying white matter tracts, and sometimes the basal ganglia and the anterior temporal lobe (Mohr *et al.* 1978). This is the vascular territory of the superior branches of the left middle cerebral artery. The observation of the consequences of smaller lesions, involving only parts of the broad region described above, has led to attempts to 'fractionate' the neural correlates of the different component of the syndrome. The articulation impairment has been attributed to damage affecting the rolandic region, with the underlying white matter (Lecours and Lhermitte 1976), or to involvement of the anterior insula (Dronkers 1996). Damage limited to Broca's area proper has been associated with word-finding disturbances (Mohr *et al.* 1978) or has been considered as the crucial determinant of defective syntactic processing (Grodzinsky 2000). The complexities of Broca's area and Broca's aphasia have been addressed from multiple perspectives in a recent book (Grodzinsky and Amunts 2006).

Global aphasia

Global aphasia is the most severe aphasic syndrome, and is characterized by reduced, severely non-fluent speech and by a profound impairment of language comprehension.

In the early stages after the stroke, the patient may be mute, or produce only isolated syllables. Sometimes, the only vocalization is a predilection word a profanity that is used repetitively in all verbal exchanges (stereotypies). The impairment of comprehension is by definition severe, and may extend to the ability to understand single words. Repetition, as well as the abilities to read and write, is often impossible. Global aphasia is typically observed as a consequence of massive strokes, destroying the entire vascular territory of the left middle cerebral artery. After the acute stage, an improvement in comprehension can usually be observed, while production remains severely affected, leading to a clinical picture of Broca's aphasia. On the other hand, there is evidence that persistent global aphasia can follow from lesions that do not involve the whole middle cerebral artery territory, but only the region typically involved in Broca's aphasia, or even subcortical structures (Vignolo *et al.* 1986). These observations are compatible with the idea of interindividual variability in the localization of language areas. In atypical global aphasia associated with partial lesions of the MCA territory hemiparesis may be absent (Hanlon *et al.* 1999).

4.3.1.2 Fluent aphasias with impaired repetition

Wernicke's aphasia

The clinical picture of Wernicke's aphasia is characterized by a language production that is fluent but marred by phonological and lexical errors. Auditory comprehension is severely affected in the acute stage and may remain impaired at follow-up, in particular for sentences.

The patient produces sentences of normal length, with preserved morphology, but he/she makes many mistakes in the selection and production of lexical items. Typical of acute Wernicke's aphasia are the neologisms, which can be either recognizable phonological distortions of words (target-related neologisms) or completely novel words. When they are abundant, the production has been defined as 'phonemic jargon'. Less frequently, the dominant errors are real words, which can be semantically or phonologically related to a target, or apparently unrelated. In this case, the patient is said to produce a verbal jargon, or a "word salad". Similar errors are produced in naming tasks. Repetition is impaired, sometimes even at the single word level. A striking phenomenon that has recently been reported is that repetition may be improved if the task is disguised, i.e. if the patient is asked to repeat the word while engaged in an auditory word–picture matching task (Otsuki *et al.* 2005). Written language is also affected. Reading aloud is usually impossible, and the comprehension of written text is severely defective. Written production can display the same features as spoken language, with abundant, unintelligible output (jargonagraphia). The typical lesion involves the superior temporal lobe, including Wernicke's area (Ba 22), and usually extends to the neighbouring temporal and parietal regions. In acute stroke, the severity of hypoperfusion in Wernicke's area, as assessed by perfusion-weighted MR, correlates with the degree of word comprehension impairment (Hillis *et al.* 2001).

Conduction aphasia

The syndrome of conduction aphasia is characterized by the disproportionate impairment of repetition contrasting with a relatively preserved auditory comprehension and with a fluent production with mostly phonological errors.

The theoretical possibility of observing an isolated impairment of repetition had been predicted by Lichtheim (1885) as the consequence of interruption of the connections between an intact 'centre of motor images of words' (Broca's area) and a 'centre of auditory images of words'

(Wernicke's area). The actual observation of this clinical picture provided considerable support for the anatomo-clinical model of Wernicke–Lichtheim.

The errors in production were explained by the classical theory as the consequence of defective 'control' of speech production by the posterior regions.

While relatively infrequent in clinical practice, conduction aphasia enjoys a special status among aphasic syndromes. While, as said above, Broca's or Wernicke's aphasia are considered as symptom aggregates due to lesions affecting multiple areas involved in different aspects of language processing, conduction aphasia may represent a relatively 'pure' consequence of a selective dysfunctional mechanism. Cognitive neuropsychological studies have suggested that there may be more than one mechanism resulting in impaired repetition. Some patients are defective in repetition because of impaired functioning of phonological planning mechanisms; others are impaired as the consequence of defective short-term memory (Kohn 1992; Bartha and Benke 2003).

The typical lesion in conduction aphasia damages the posterior sylvian region, usually involving the parietal operculum (supramarginal gyrus) and the underlying white matter. The latter includes the arcuate fasciculus, classically considered as the transmission pathway between Broca's and Wernicke's areas. However, classical conduction aphasia has also been observed after lesions involving Wernicke's area, the insular region, and underlying white matter, or the angular gyrus and underlying white matter (Damasio and Damasio 1980). It has been proposed that 'suprasylvian' and infrasylvian conduction aphasias may be associated with different profiles of linguistic performance (Axer *et al.* 2001).

4.3.1.3 Aphasias with preserved repetition

Transcortical aphasias

> The main feature of the transcortical aphasias is the preservation of repetition, which stands in contrast with the severe impairment of the other aspects of language performance.

The preserved repetition indicates that the phonological abilities are intact, and suggests that the lesion spares the perisylvian cortex. It is thus surprising that 'transcortical-type' language disturbances have been reported following electrical interference in Wernicke's area during presurgical cortical mapping (Boatman *et al.* 2000). An alternative interpretation is that spared repetition abilities are subserved by the right hemisphere (Berthier 2000).

There are three varieties of transcortical aphasia.

- *Transcortical motor (or dynamic) aphasia* is characterized by reduced language production. The naming ability is often preserved, and auditory comprehension is unaffected. The responsible lesion involves the prefrontal cortex, anterior to Broca's area, which is typically spared. The disorder may not be specific for language, but rather reflect a general reduction of spontaneous activity (Freedman *et al.* 1984; Robinson *et al.* 2006).
- *Transcortical sensory aphasia* is characterized by fluent production replete with verbal and semantic paraphasias and by the severe impairment of auditory comprehension. The responsible lesion typically involves the watershed area between the vascular territories of the middle and posterior cerebral artery. A severe hypotension may result in damage to this region (Howard *et al.* 1987).
- *Mixed transcortical aphasia*, or isolation of the language area, is characterized by non-fluent speech, severely impaired comprehension, and echolalia. This unusual clinical picture has been reported as a consequence of extensive anoxic cortical lesions, sparing the immediately

perisylvian cortex (Geschwind and Kaplan 1962), or following acute internal carotid artery occlusion (Bogousslavsky *et al.* 1988).

Anomic aphasia

> Anomic aphasia is defined by the presence of a severe disorder of word finding in the context of fluent speech, good repetition, and preserved comprehension.

This clinical picture is infrequent in acute stroke patients, as it often represents the evolution of other aphasic syndromes. All aphasics are impaired in lexical retrieval, and this core feature may represent the residual deficit when other aspect of language performance have recovered. On the other hand a selective word-finding disorder is frequently observed in patients with degenerative dementia, head injury, or intracranial hypertension There is ample evidence that the left temporal lobe is crucial for naming, and that a selective anomia may reflect damage to this brain region (Coughlan and Warrington 1978).

Selective disorders of oral and written language

> In most aphasic patients the language impairment affects both oral and written production and comprehension. Typically, the disorder is more severe in the written than in the oral modality.

There are, however, some unusual situations in which the two main modalities of language use show a conspicuous dissociation. These disorders are due to selective impairments of the input and output channels that allow language utilization, rather than to a language disorder.

- *Alexia without agraphia.* Alexia without agraphia, or 'pure' alexia, is the only selective disorder that can be observed relatively frequently in clinical practice. Pure alexia has classically been interpreted as a 'disconnection syndrome', due to the interruption of the connections between visual and linguistic areas (Catani and Ffytche 2005). In the patient originally described by Dejerine (1914), the responsible lesion was an ischaemic stroke in the territory of the left posterior cerebral artery that damaged the left occipital cortex and the splenium of the corpus callosum, thus separating the right occipital cortex from the left hemisphere. The pure alexic patient's reading performance is quite characteristic. They read using a 'letter by letter' strategy, and their reading times are much longer than those observed in normal readers, increasing linearly with word length (Patterson and Kay 1982). Recent studies have underlined the important role of damage to a specific region in the occipito-temporal cortex, i.e. the midportion of the left fusiform gyrus (Gaillard *et al.* 2006; Leff *et al.* 2006), which is considered to play a crucial role in parallel letter recognition.
- *Alexia with agraphia.* The syndrome of selective impairment of written language, without any disorder of oral production and auditory comprehension, is very seldom observed in the acute stage after a stroke. Most patients with reading and writing impairment in the absence of other features of aphasia are recovering from other aphasic syndromes. A possible exception is the syndrome of alexia with agraphia for Kanji, which can be attributed to a selective disorder for ideographic reading due to a posterior-inferior temporal lesion in Japanese patients (Sakurai 2004).

- *Pure agraphia.* A selective disorder of writing in the absence of language impairment is very rare. It has been reported as a selective form of apraxia for writing movements, following a lesion affecting the superior parietal lobule (Alexander *et al.* 1992). In acute stroke, lesions affecting the posterior frontal cortex have been associated with isolated agraphia (Hillis *et al.* 2004).
- *Anarthria (aphemia).* A selective disorder of speech production, in the absence of any other linguistic impairment, can follow not only from peripheral causes, but also from a brain lesion. The traditional European label for this condition is 'anarthria' or 'aphemia', which are clearly confusing terms, as the condition is not associated with a total lack of articulation, but only with a speech disorder due to a brain lesion. The same condition is called 'speech apraxia' in the USA. The differential diagnosis with Broca's aphasia is easy, as the patient has a totally preserved ability to communicate by writing.

The location of the lesion is debated. Possible candidates as cortical centre for articulation are the opercular portion of Broca's area with the neighbouring left precentral gyrus (Lecours and Lhermitte 1976; Schiff *et al.* 1983) and the anterior insular cortex (Dronkers 1996).

- *Pure word deafness.* This very unusual condition is characterized by the selective impairment of the ability to understand spoken language, with normal oral production and written language. The disorder has been traditionally attributed to a 'disconnection' between auditory processing and language areas, and the few patients for whom pathological information is available have had bilateral temporal strokes (Szirmai *et al.* 2003).

Subcortical aphasia

Language disorders can also be observed in patients whose strokes apparently spare the cortex of the left hemisphere. These 'subcortical aphasias' have been reported after lesions involving the thalamus, the basal ganglia, and the neighbouring white matter tracts. They are extremely heterogeneous in term of clinical features and recovery pattern. These anatomo-clinical observations have been taken to indicate the participation of the subcortical nuclei of the left hemisphere in language processing. An alternative interpretation is that these disorders are simply the consequence of the functional involvement of the structurally unaffected cortex overlying the subcortical lesions (Perani *et al.* 1987; Hillis *et al.* 2002).

4.3.2 Acute aphasia

The classical modality for the study of vascular aphasia was to deal with 'stable' patients, typically examined several weeks after stroke. Only in the latter case was the clinical picture considered to be the faithful reflection of the site and extent of the brain damage. This approach has drastically changed in recent years. The advancements in the management of acute stroke and the advent of the stroke units has kindled interest in the assessment of aphasia, as well as of other aspects of cognition, in the first hours after stroke onset. It is now possible to assess the site of reduced blood flow immediately after stroke, by means of perfusion weighted magnetic resonance imaging (for a review see Hillis, 2007), and correlate the imaging results with the clinical findings. If the hypoperfusion recovers, spontaneously or as a consequence of treatment, the regression of the correlated clinical findings provides additional evidence for the essential role of a specific brain area in the task under consideration.

The clinical picture in the acute stage after a massive stroke involving the middle cerebral artery territory is often characterized by mutism associated with impaired single word comprehension. Less extensive damage leads to clinical pictures that show the features of Broca's or Wernicke's aphasia. It has been repeatedly observed that fluent, jargonaphasic production is more frequently observed in elderly patients (Ferro 2001; Pedersen *et al.* 2004). In a large series of patients studied in a stroke unit, about 50% of patients had a global aphasia, or could not be classified as having a specific syndrome (Godefroy *et al.* 2002).

4.4 The cognitive approach to aphasia

The cognitive neuropsychological approach was born in the second half of the last century, and reflects the important developments in the fields of cognitive psychology and cognitive science (Gardner 1985).

> In its application to the study of language disorders cognitive neuropsychology is based on a careful analysis of the quantitative and qualitative aspects of language impairment in the individual patient.

The results of this analysis are interpreted on the basis of models of normal processing, derived from psycholinguistic investigations in normal subjects. The main goal of this approach is theoretical, rather than clinical, i.e. the understanding of the normal functional architecture of language. However, an increased knowledge of 'language physiology' can be expected to benefit clinical studies, as well as to provide a rational foundation to treatment methods (Gainotti *et al.* 2000). The large body of knowledge derived from this approach is summarized in excellent textbooks (Caplan 1992; Hillis 2002); here we present selected examples of the application to clinical studies.

4.4.1 Disorders of single word processing

As in the case of the Wernicke-Lichtheim model, much of the effort of the cognitive neuropsychology enterprise has been devoted to single-word processing and, in particular, to spoken word production (Goldrick and Rapp 2007). However, from an historical point of view, the first application of a cognitive model of language processing to a neuropsychological case study dealt with written language. The observations of patients producing semantic errors in reading aloud (Marshall and Newcombe 1966), who could not read non-words (Dérouesné and Beauvois 1979), or were impaired in reading irregular words (Marshall and Newcombe 1973) were puzzling for classical models of reading, which generally assumed a phonological mediation (silent reading) as a necessary processing step. The 'multiple pathways' model of reading, proposed by cognitive psychologists provided an elegant way to interpret the clinical observations. According to the model, a word could be read by a conversion process of graphemic unitis into phonemes, or by a global process of lexical recognition. In the case of new or non-existent words, which do not have a lexical representation, only the conversion process allows reading. Conversely, words that include irregular mapping of graphemes to phonemes can be correctly pronounced only by means of the lexical route. It is easy to derive the observed pattern of dysfunctions from theoretical lesions to the model (Fig. 4.1). The interpretation of semantic errors in reading requires the assumption of a complete abolition of the conversion pathways associated to dysfunction of the lexical reading mechanisms.

In the following decades the same approach, based on the information-processing concept, was extended to other aspects of single word processing. The most successful attempt to formulate a comprehensive model of lexical processing has been pursued by Caramazza and his co-workers (Caramazza 1988; Miceli 2001)

As an introduction to this approach, let us consider the case of spoken word production (Fig. 4.1). The model assumes that the normal performance of speaking a word is the result of a number of

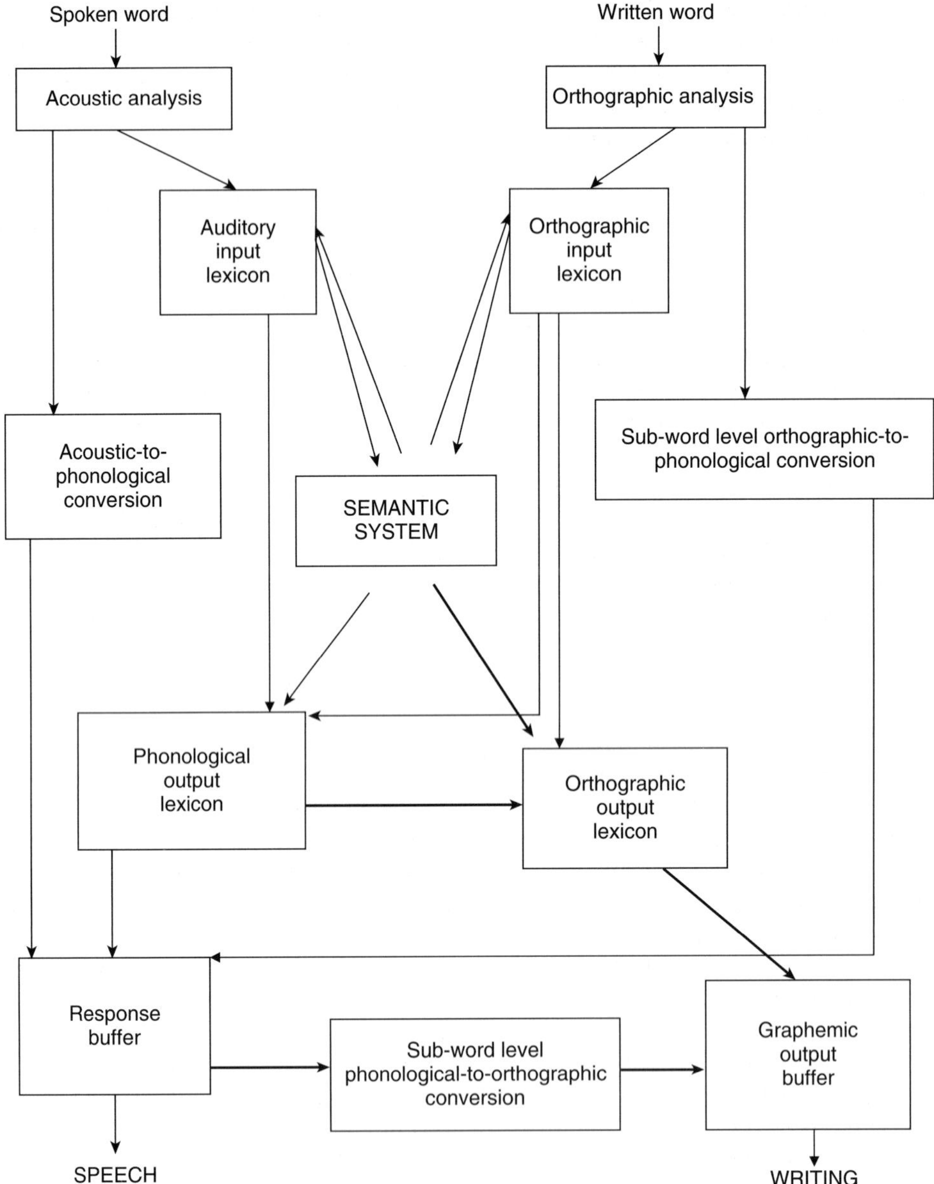

Fig. 4.1 A model of single-word processing.

sequential stages. Each of them can be affected by pathology, resulting in distinctive patterns of dysfunction.

The first, input stage depends upon the nature of the task: the spoken word can be elicited in response to a written input (reading), to a spoken input (repetition), or to a non-verbal input, such as a picture. Both reading and repeating can be performed without understanding the meaning of the word: they are thus called transcoding modalities. On the other hand, naming a picture requires its identification, i.e. the activation of the semantic system.

The hallmark of semantic disorders is the presence of impairment in all auditory or visual tasks that require semantic mediation: in other words, the patient fails not only in oral naming, but also in written naming, in auditory word comprehension, and written word comprehension.

Of course, this does not mean his/her performance is abolished in all these tasks: as any clinician knows, the disorder is almost never complete. What is truly interesting about semantic disorders is that they can be selective, affecting some entities but not others. This kind of observation offers an unique window on the organization of the semantic system. The most extensively studied distinction is between living and non-living entities. After the original observations of patients affected by semantic disorders that involved biological entities but not artefacts and vice-versa, many other reports have confirmed the existence of selective semantic disorders, and enormously complicated the phenomenology and the interpretation of these clinical observations (Capitani *et al.* 2003; Tyler *et al.* 2000; Vinson *et al.* 2003). The main issues under discussion are related to the unitary or multiple nature of the semantic system, and to its organization along knowledge domains, or according to the properties of the entities that are represented in the semantic system (perceptual, motor, functional, etc.).

The subsequent stage is lexical selection. In the model this is accomplished by access to the phonological output lexicon: the correctly assigned word meaning is associated to the corresponding word form. The specific content of this store is a matter of intense debate. In particular, not only meaning and form are involved in lexical selection, but also grammatical information (for example, word class), as well as morphological structure which is typically represented at the phonological level (for example, the -s ending of the third person in English present tense; Levelt 1989). A selective disorder of lexical retrieval is exemplified by patients who perform normally in auditory comprehension tasks but are anomic, or produce semantic errors in oral production. Lexical disorders are often characterized by grammatical category effects. Some patients are impaired in naming actions and not objects, while others present with the reverse pattern of impairment (Cappa and Perani 2003; Shapiro and Caramazza 2003). It has been suggested that a difference in the cerebral localization of lesions underlies this behavioural dissociation: patients with a selective disorder for object naming have usually had lesions centred on the left temporal lobe; conversely, a selective impairment in action naming has been associated with large lesions, usually extending to the left frontal cortex.

The stages following lexical retrieval are relatively less controversial. In order to produce the item selected in the phonologic output lexicon pre-articulatory planning is needed. The latter process is supposed to take place in the phonological buffer, a short-term memory component that stores the output of both the lexical system (addressed phonology, i.e. the representations coming from the phonological output lexicon) as well as the product of non-lexical conversion procedures (assembled phonology, as in the case of non-words; Levelt 1989).

Phonological disorders can be easily diagnosed in production tasks: if the patient produces phonological approximations to the target word that can be recognized, the disorder can be attributed to processes that follow the selection of the semantically appropriate lexical item. On the other hand, if the patient produces abstruse neologisms, it is not possible to decide if the disorder is purely phonological on the basis of the speech errors.

A disorder of the phonological buffer can explain the clinical observations of patients who are impaired in all production tasks, involving both word and non-word processing. These patients are usually among those labelled clinically as conduction aphasics. The study of patients with phonological disorders has provided important information on the nature of the phonological representations. For example, it has been shown that 'segmental' phonemic errors, for example, phonemic substitutions, do not affect other levels of phonological representation, such as the syllable or the stress (Beland *et al.* 1990). Disorders of another suprasegmental phonological aspect, that is sentence prosody, are usually observed in the context of impaired articulatory production.

The serial model of lexical retrieval delineated here is not without alternatives. Other models allow for interaction of phonological and lexical–semantic levels in single-word processing and have been applied to the interpretation of qualitative aspects of error production (for example, to interpret errors that are related both phonologically and semantically to the target, e.g. 'rat' for 'cat'; Dell *et al.* 1997). Interactive models still postulate the existence of 'local' representations of phonemes and lexical units. Connectionist modelling disposes of these symbolic representations, and attempts to simulate lexical retrieval as the result of a statistical process mapping input to output by means of neural networks. Well-described examples are the model applied by Plaut and Shallice (1993) to the simulation of error pattern in deep dyslexia and the simulation of relearning after damage to a network (Plaut 1996).

4.4.2 **Sentence-level disorders**

The presence of morphological and syntactic disorders in speech production is the hallmark of the clinical syndrome of agrammatism, which is characterized in particular by the omission of function words and bound morphemes in the context of a non-fluent production. The label of paragrammatism, on the other hand, is used to characterize the presence of substitutions of morphological elements and function words in the context of fluent speech.

Recent developments in the linguistic investigation of aphasia indicate that different mechanisms of impairment can result in agrammatic production. These include selective disorders in the retrieval of 'grammatical' elements, disorders in the generation of syntactic form, and defective mapping of thematic roles.

The latter mechanism is particularly interesting, because it is based on one of the basic concepts of modern syntactic theory. A verb is considered to assign thematic role, such as agent, theme, and goal, at the semantic level, for example, 'to kill' implies an actor (the killer) and a theme (the killed); 'to send' implies an actor, a theme, and a goal. Each verb is also associated with an argument structure that specifies the syntactic roles, i.e. the external argument (subject), and the internal arguments (direct object, dative object, etc.). For example, the verb 'to love' assigns the role of agent to the external argument (John loves Mary); but if it is used in the passive form, the external argument is the theme of the action (John is loved by Mary). In other words, the same semantic content can map on to two different sentences by means of the application of different movement rules. A disorder in the interpretation of the mapping can produce errors both in sentence production and sentence comprehension (Linebarger 1995).

Another interesting linguistic hypothesis is the 'pruning of the syntactic tree'(Friedmann 2006), which is based on the observation that agrammatism does not involve all syntactic structures and all functional elements, with some interesting cross-linguistic differences. The impaired and preserved aspects do not seem to be random, but rather to follow from the inaccessibility of higher nodes in the abstract representation of sentence structure provided by the syntactic tree.

Along similar lines, syntactic comprehension failures have been attributed to 'trace deletion' (Grodzinsky 1990). For example, compare the sentence 'The girl is followed by the boy' with the sentence 'The boy follows the girl'. The non-canonical sentence is the result of movement of the object of the verb 'follow' from its original position after the verb to an initial position. This syntactic phenomenon is supposed to leave a trace (a phonologically empty position marker): 'The girl$_i$ is followed$_{ti}$ by the boy'. A 'deletion' of the trace would result in a defective interpretation of the sentence, and the attribution of the role of agent to the noun in the initial position.

There is, however, evidence that a disorder in the comprehension of syntactically complex sentences can be due to several other mechanisms, such as the reduction of general cognitive resources required for syntactic processing and sentence 'parsing', or a disorder of phonological memory (Friederici and Kotz 2003).

4.5 The neurology of language

4.5.1 The beginnings

The traditional doctrine of language organization in the brain was born in the XIXth century on the basis of the anatomo-clinical observations of Broca and Wernicke. The neural model of language based on the concept of multiple localized 'centres' connected by fibre pathways has remained influential to the present day.

Since the mid-eighteenth century, clinicians have proposed that several different parts of the brain are specifically involved with language. In the nineteenth century there was a rapid expansion of knowledge, due to the systematic investigation of the effects of localized brain damage on language processing (the anatomo-clinical method). This marked the beginning of the era of localization of mental functions in the brain. Although earlier authors had proposed that the substance of the brain, as opposed to the ventricles, had specific functions, the main localization theories began with the phrenologists. Gall (1815) speculated that the human brain was composed of many organs, in which various human faculties resided. The speculations of phrenologists were soon superseded by empirically-grounded localization theories, based on clinical observations. The French surgeon Paul Broca (1861) made the claim that there was an area in the brain specially devoted to speech production, based on his observation of a patient with loss of speech. The story of Broca's achievements has been well-recorded, and the subsequent designation of the foot of the third frontal convolution of the dominant hemisphere as 'Broca's area' is widely known. However, it was Karl Wernicke (1874) who wrote what may be considered the most influential paper on aphasia, *Der aphasische Symptomencomplex*. In this article Wernicke contrasted Broca's ('motor') aphasia with the form of 'sensory' aphasia that is currently called Wernicke's aphasia. Unlike patients with Broca's aphasia, whose speech was impaired, patients with 'sensory' aphasia had normal articulation. Moreover, unlike patients with Broca's aphasia, patients with this form of aphasia had impaired comprehension. Like the patients with Broca's aphasia, their naming and repetition was impaired. Whereas patients with Broca's aphasia had anterior perisylvian lesions, patients with Wernicke's aphasia had posterior perisylvian lesions. Wernicke suggested that the critical area might be the posterior portion of the superior temporal lobe, a portion of auditory association cortex (now known as Wernicke's area). He proposed that this area contains the memories of how words sound (i.e. what nowadays is considered to be the phonological lexicon). According to this formulation, Wernicke not only suggested a second speech/language-specific region, but also was the first to posit an information-processing network when he suggested that the area that contains the memories of how words sound (Wernicke's area) provides information to the area where the sounds of these words are programmed (Broca's area). Therefore, he suggested that the posterior portion of the superior temporal gyrus must be anatomically connected to Broca's area. Based on this simple information-processing system, Wernicke further postulated that, in the case of a lesion disconnecting Broca's area from the posterior portion of the superior temporal gyrus, the patient's production would also be impaired. Because the phonological lexicon cannot entirely inform Broca's area about the sounds (phonemes) by which words are constructed, the production of words would be impaired, with patients making phonological errors. However, unlike the patients with sensory (Wernicke's) aphasia, whose phonological lexicon is destroyed and who therefore cannot monitor their errors, patients with this disconnection disorder would be able to monitor their errors and might attempt to correct them. In the years after Wernicke's postulation of this aphasic picture based on his model, patients demonstrating the constellation of behaviours he predicted were actually reported. The term used for this aphasic syndrome is 'conduction aphasia'.

In the following years, many different cerebral centres dedicated to various functions were defined by neurologists, comprising centres for writing, reading, calculating, etc. In general, these implicated the left side of the brain. These observations gave scientists the first glimpses of the distributed nature of language function in the brain. The brain seemed to have no single location where language is created or stored. Instead, multiple regions of the brain are involved in the control of different aspects of speech and language. In the next section, we will provide a brief overview of language organization as formulated by the classical anatomo-clinical approach.

4.5.2 **Language areas before the advent of modern imaging techniques**

On the basis of the patient findings, we know that the language areas include large zones of the associative cortex and of the subcortical white matter of the frontal, parietal and temporal lobes around the sylvian fissure of the left hemisphere (only one-third of left-handed individuals have language sites located in the right hemisphere). Language areas can be subdivided into perisylvian and extraperisylvian. The former include Broca's area (Ba 44), Wernicke's area (Ba 22), and the arch-shaped fasciculus arcuatus that connects Wernicke's area to Broca's area. This set of areas has been traditionally thought to be important for the phonological and phonetic–articulatory level of language processing (Vignolo 1986). Wernicke's area is crucial for the identification and correct selection of phonemes; Broca's area for the combination of phonemes into verbal–motor speech sequences. It is noteworthy that the perisylvian areas are also the first to mature during development. Indeed, infants below the age of 1 year are generally only capable to generate isolated syllables, such as 'ta-ta' or 'ba-ba'.

The 'marginal' language areas are located around the perisylvian areas. In the frontal lobe they include Ba 45, which was thought to be important for the combination of words into appropriate morpho-syntactical sequences in order to construct coherent sentences. In posterior brain areas of the left hemisphere the 'marginal' language areas comprise the posterior parts of the middle and inferior temporal lobe (Ba 37), the supramarginal gyrus (Ba 40), and the angular gyrus (Ba 39) located at the temporal–parietal–occipital transition area. The angular gyrus is a multimodal associative region of the brain and connects Wernicke's area with other associative cortices, playing a central role in the functioning of the semantic code, making it possible to understand and evoke meaningful words. A role of subcortical structures of the dominant hemisphere, such as the caudate and the thalamus, in language function has not yet been clearly defined. It has been hypothesized that they play a role in semantic decision processes (Cappa and Abutalebi 1999).

> An important functional distinction based on lesion studies is between the perisylvian language areas of the left hemisphere, which are engaged in articulatory–phonetic, phonological, and morphosyntactic processing, and the surrounding associative areas, which are responsible for lexical–semantic processing.

4.5.3 The limits of the anatomo-clinical approach

The present concept of the neural architecture of language is much more extended and complex than the system described above. Our current knowledge derives largely from the new insights gained by the application of functional neuroimaging techniques in healthy normal subjects. The observation that specific lesions may give rise to specific linguistic deficits provided the foundation of classical aphasiology. However, it should be underlined that the classical aphasia model based on the anatomo-clinical method is far from being adequate when it comes to deriving representations of brain functions. Although some of the first lesion-related findings have never been totally invalidated (e.g. the involvement of Broca's area in speech production), there are several reasons that make the interpretation of lesion studies complex and, in some cases, quite impossible (for review see Demonet *et al.* 2005). In the first place, language is a most complex cognitive function and as such it is embedded in complex and highly interconnected networks. Anatomo-clinical studies may demonstrate whether a certain brain region is necessary for a given language component, but not the broader network of which that region may form a part. These networks may be specialized for distinct language functions such as syntactical or lexical processing (Neville and Bavelier 1998). It is unlikely that an accidental lesion in a certain brain region knocking out a given linguistic function such as syntactical processing may permit us to localize that function at the lesion site.

> The possibility of studying the neural correlates of language processing in normal subjects by means of functional neuroimaging has considerably expanded our knowledge of the 'language areas'. While lesion evidence remains crucial to delineate the structures that are necessary for any given aspect of language performance, imaging studies delineate the complex networks involved in each aspect of language processing.

Consider, for instance, that syntactical processing may be carried out by the interplay of a neural network containing at least three brain areas, i.e. Broca's area, the left basal ganglia, and to a certain degree Wernicke's area. A single lesion in each of these structures or even in the connections among these structures could give rise to the same linguistic deficit and, hence, a sufficient correspondence between a specific lesion site and a symptom may not be established. As mentioned above, language like other higher cognitive functions, is thought to rely on the interplay of many different brain areas (Mesulam 1990), and hence the classical lesion–symptom relationships are likely to be influenced by a set of distributed regions rather than a single, circumscribed area (Alexander *et al.* 1989).

A further weak point of the anatomo-clinical approach to language–brain relationships in aphasic patients is its static nature. Consider that dynamic changes in both language behaviour and brain functions may take place after brain injury such as a stroke. This brain reorganization may depend on the nature and extent of the lesion and may also be influenced by various therapeutic interventions. These rearrangements give birth to a 'brain architecture' that may not be just the 'normal' network minus the damaged component. In fact, the observed clinical picture may often be the result of neural reorganization following the brain injury that caused the disruption. In other words, this means that, when the patient comes to our observation, his/her linguistic performance may not be due to the lesion itself but rather to the reorganization. Moreover, even in the case of acute aphasia post-stroke, when no therapeutic intervention has yet taken place, the relationship between a lesion location and linguistic deficit is quite complex, because variables such as the 'penumbra effect' may overestimate the real cognitive defict (Cappa 1998).

Likewise, numerous subject-dependent factors, such as gender, age, handedness, and literacy, whose precise effects are still poorly understood, can substantially influence aphasic symptoms (Cappa 1998). For instance, stroke more frequently affects elderly patients; therefore, the influence of age on aphasic symptoms cannot easily be dissociated from the aetiology of the lesion.

4.5.4 The anatomy of language: new vistas

Given the complexity and the limitations of the classical anatomo-clinical approach to the study of the neural basis of language, functional neuroimaging techniques constitute an independent source of evidence. The value that functional neuroimaging brings to language research is to improve the perspective on the distributed anatomy of language. Thus, it can be used in normal subjects to identify where the different domains of language processing are localized with considerable precision. In general, functional neuroimaging studies have not only confirmed the anatomical knowledge gained from lesion studies, but have indeed opened a number of new discoveries, leading to to substantial revisions of traditional concepts. Consider, for instance, Broca's area: recent imaging evidence reports that the traditional Broca's area in the left inferior frontal gyrus can be functionally subdivided into three regions: one that is posterior and superior and is involved in the sound structure (phonology) of language; a second, anterior and ventral that is concerned with the meaning of words (semantics); and a third, lying in-between the first two regions, that is involved in meaning conveyed by sentence structure (syntax; Bookheimer S. 2002). Broca's area has been proposed as the main neural correlate of morphosyntactical aspects of language processing (Moro *et al.* 2001; Tettamanti *et al.* 2002).

As in the case of Broca's area, also for Wernicke's area and the superior temporal gyrus, new discoveries are challenging the classical view of language areas. Indeed, new observations on auditory processing with functional activation studies in normal subjects during speech perception are producing a fundamental shift away from the standard neurological model of language: Wernicke's area connected to Broca's area by the arcuate fasciculus. An important review of functional activation studies (Wise 2003) proposed that there are two connections between posterior and anterior language areas. Similar to the ventral and dorsal streams of visual processing, one involves a 'rostral route' from the anterior temporal cortex via the uncinate fasciculus to ventral and rostral prefrontal cortex, while the other involves a 'caudal route' via the well-known arcuate fasciculus to dorsolateral prefrontal cortex (Fig. 4.2). Although these two routes are unlikely to be independent, the former may process word meaning and the latter, carried out by the arcuate fasciculus, word sound structure (phonetics and phonology). New developments in magnetic resonance (MR) scanning are even challenging the exact anatomical structure of the *arcuate fasciculus*. Diffusion tensor imaging (DTI) through tractography provides *in vivo* information about the trajectories of white matter tracts. In one such study (Catani *et al.* 2005), it was shown that the arcuate fasciculus itself may be subdived into two main pathways: a direct pathway linking Wernicke's area to Broca's area and an indirect pathway consisting of a posterior segment linking Wernicke's area to the inferior parietal lobule (angular and supramarginal gyrus) and an anterior segment linking the inferior parietal lobule to Broca's area (Fig. 4.2). It is noteworthy that Catani and Ffytche (2005) ascribed distinct functions to these two pathways. While the direct pathway would be responsible for phonological processing, the indirect pathway is hypothesized to be responsible with its posterior segment for auditory comprehension and with its anterior segment for vocalization of semantic contents. The subdivision of the arcuate fasciculus may have also clinical implications. A lesion of both pathways may lead to global aphasia; a lesion of the direct pathway may lead to a classical conduction aphasia leaving auditory comprehension intact. A lesion to the anterior segment of the indirect pathway may result in a non-fluent aphasia

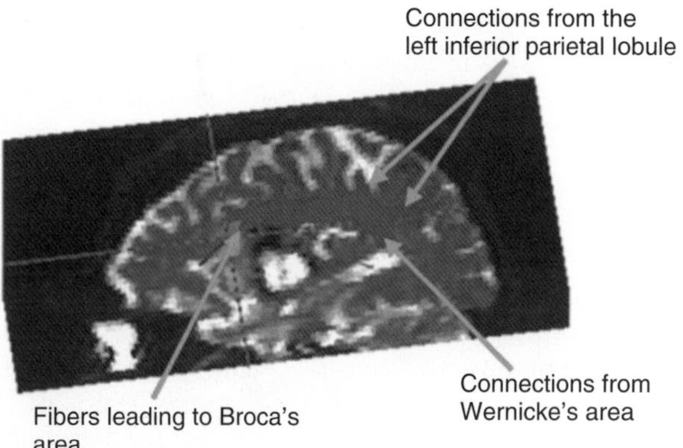

Fig. 4.2 Diffusion tensor imaging (DTI) and the reconstruction of the left arcuate fasciculus in a patient with a left basal ganglia haemorrhage causing transcortical sensory aphasia. Apart from showing the two components of the arcuate fasciculus (see text), the image shows that in this patient the subcortical haemorrhage itself did not lesion the connection between Wernicke's area and Broca's area. This is a black and white version of Plate 1.

with spared repetition and comprehension, while a lesion to the posterior segment may result in a fluent aphasia with impaired comprehension and repetition. A lesion to the entire indirect pathway may thus result in an aphasia of the mixed transcortical type, with normal repetition but with reduced fluency and comprehension.

It is also worth citing that language-related activations have also been reported outside the classical language areas, such as in the left prefrontal cortex, the temporal pole, or in the lingual and fusiform gyri (see reviews in Price 1998; Indefrey and Levelt 2000).

> Brain imaging has not only allowed a deeper insight into the functional role of Broca's and Wernicke's areas in language processing but has also indicated the participation of other structures such as Ba47, the fusiform gyrus, and the temporal pole.

An example in the left prefrontal cortex is *Brodmann's area 47* (Ba 47). This prefrontal area is located more rostral and ventral to Broca's area and, in the classical aphasiological literature, was not considered to have a specific role in language. Functional MRI (fMRI) studies have consistently reported that this area is activated in tasks such as semantic retrieval (Wagner *et al.* 2001; Poldrack *et al.* 1999). This result was in apparent contrast with the findings from the classical anatomo-clinical approach that ascribed semantic functions to posterior brain areas.

The temporal pole activity was frequently reported in studies aimed at characterizing the neural architecture involved in connected speech. These studies are important because a major drawback of imaging studies is that they are mostly focused on the single-word processing level, which is obviously not the natural context of language processing. Early studies involving story listening (Perani *et al.* 1998) attempted to identify subparts of the language network that are specific to coherent, connected language samples. The authors reported the involvement of the anterior polar aspects of the superior temporal gyrus. Since then, various studies (Humphries *et al.* 2001; Scott *et al.* 2000) have confirmed the crucial involvement of this portion of the brain for processing discourse. Interestingly, in addition to anterior temporal activation, Maguire *et al.* (1999)

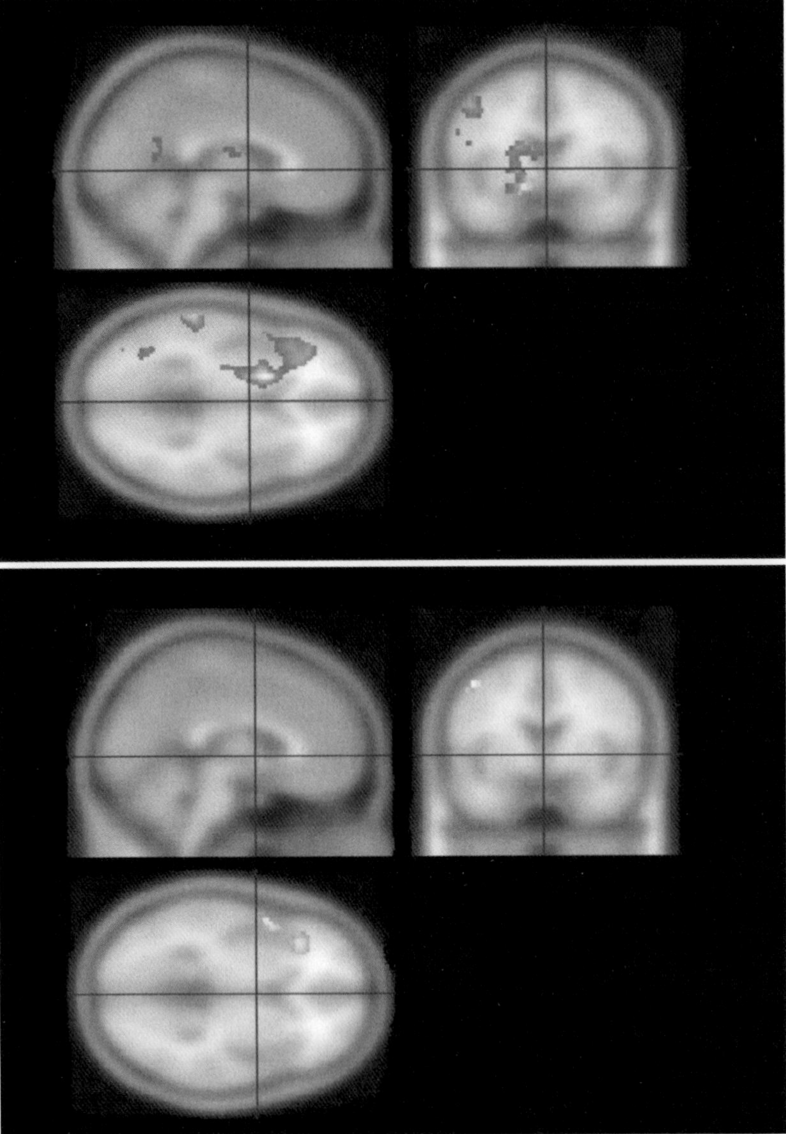

Fig. 4.3 Brain plasticity as observed during learning to read a native language in late learners. These subjects, whose native language is a dialect that is not formally learned at school, were scanned while learning to read words belonging to their dialect. During the initial learning phase, brain activity was observed in learning-related brain areas, such as the left anterior hippocampal formation and the left caudate nucleus, and in the left prefrontal cortex (top image). After having reached a sufficient proficiency in reading, this network disappeared, highlighting learning-related brain plasticity. This is a black and white version of Plate 2.

found activation in the medial parietal posterior cingulate cortex and proposed that the latter was involved in linking the current understanding of a story with prior knowledge.

Another example of how functional neuroimaging was successful in revealing the neural underpinnings of specific aspects of language processing comes from the field of reading. Consider that, until the approach of functional neuroimaging, not much was known of the neural pathways of reading. Following, the classical anatomo-clinical approach we only knew that lesion to the left occipital lobe or to the temporo–parieto–occipital junction could give rise to acquired disorders of reading (see, for instance, Dejerine 1914). The simple assumption that these areas were responsible for reading proved to be too vague. fMRI has been successful in subdividing the reading process into basic aspects and allocating these aspects to specific neural pathways. For instance, word reading is carried out through a left-hemispheric network comprising frontal, temporal, occipito-temporal, and parietal areas (Price *et al.* 1996; Abutalebi *et al.* 2007; Price and Mechelli 2005). Reading-related visual information is transferred via a ventral pathway linking striate and extrastriate cortices to the left fusiform gyrus, where the interplay between orthographic and phonological codes may take place (Price and Devlin 2003). In addition, a dorsal pathway including the left inferior parietal lobule, superior temporal gyrus, and the inferior frontal gyrus is engaged in retrieving and assembling phonological codes and in associating these to semantic representations.

Another field in which the contribution of functional neuroimaging has been fruitful is the study of bilinguals, who were supposed to have particular and language specific representations in the brain (Albert and Obler 1978). Before the advent of functional neuroimaging, many researchers postulated that bilinguals may have languages represented in different brain areas or even in different hemispheres. This picture was essentially based on the fact that it is not rare to observe a bilingual aphasic who recovers only with one language, while the other is lost. The latter observation gave rise to the hypothesis that the brain area for one language was damaged and that for the other was not. However, fMRI studies have contradicted this assumption (see for review Abutalebi *et al.* 2001; Perani and Abutalebi 2005). Functional neuroimaging studies have shown that bilinguals use identical brain areas for their languages; differences are only observed in areas linked to cognitive control such as the anterior cingulate cortex, basal ganglia, and prefrontal cortex. This control circuitry may be important when processing a weaker language. In the case of brain damage, recovery may be more problematic for a weaker language because of decreased input (i.e. such as appropriate activation) from this control circuitry. The study on bilinguals is an elegant example of how the approach to the study of language changed with the advent of functional neuroimaging: the brain and language relationship is no longer considered to be a mere question of representation but rather that of neural processing and functioning.

Finally, fMRI is a suitable tool to investigate neural plasticity of language areas, an issue that was totally impossible to address until 20 years ago (Fig. 4.3). Plastic changes may be observed, for instance, following learning of an artificial language (Opitz and Friederici 2004) or following the acquisition of literacy (Abutalebi *et al.* 2007). In both cases, there is evidence that, at the initial stages, the role of the left hippocampus is predominant, underlining its role for language learning. In the later stages, activity shifts more to left hemispheric language areas, while, once the consolidation of learning is achieved, these left hemispheric language areas decrease their level of activity.

Plasticity may also be studied directly in recovering aphasics, which is another fruitful field of functional neuroimaging applications. This can be done in two distinct ways. One possible approach is to scan recovered aphasics during the performance of a task whose functional anatomy is well known, in order to assess the modifications of brain activation associated to recovery. A more informative approach is based on follow-up studies that compare brain activity at two different times after stroke (Saur *et al.* 2006) or before and after speech therapy. The available evidence indicates that, in the initial stages of recovery, right homologous areas may be more important, while, in later stages, the role of left perilesional areas becomes prevailing and is correlated with superior recovery.

4.6 **Conclusions**

Language impairment remains one of the most severe consequences of stroke, with a large negative impact on the prognosis for functional recuperation after acute brain damage (Paolucci *et al.* 2005). An adequate neuropsychological diagnosis, which goes beyond the attribution of a syndromic label, is thus an important component of the neurological assessment in clinical practice. In particular, serial assessments in the acute stage provides crucial information about the evolution of tissue damage in the language areas of the left hemisphere (Hillis, 2007). When the patient is stabilized, the evaluation of strength and weaknesses in the different aspects of language processing is useful for the definition of functional prognosis and of optimal patient management. Besides these clinical considerations, the study of aphasia remains one of the cornerstones of the cognitive neuroscience of language. In combination with functional imaging, the observation of selective deficits of language processing after localized damage offers a unique tool for the investigation of the brain mechanisms subserving this central and uniquely human component of cognition.

References

Abutalebi, J., Cappa, S.F., and Perani, D. (2001). The bilingual brain as revealed by functional neuroimaging. Bilingualism: *Lang. Cogn.* **4**, 179–90.

Abutalebi, J., Keim, R., Brambati, S.M., Tettamanti, M., Cappa, S.F., De Bleser, R., and Perani, D. (2007). Late acquisition of literacy in a native language. *Hum. Brain Map.* **28**, 19–33.

Albert, M.L. and Obler, L.K. (1978). *The bilingual brain.* Academic Press, New York.

Alexander, M.P., Hildbrunner, B., and Fisher, R.S. (1989). Distributed anatomy of transcortical sensory aphasia. *Arch. Neurol.* **46**, 885–92.

Alexander, M.P., Fisher, R.S., and Friedman, R.B. (1992). Lesion localization in apractic agraphia. *Arch. Neurol.* **49**, 246–51.

Axer, H., von Keyserlingk, A., Berks, G., and von Keyserlingk, D. (2001). Supra- and infrasylvian conduction aphasia. *Brain Lang.* **76**, 317–31.

Bartha, L. and Benke, T. (2003). Acute conduction aphasia: an analysis of 20 cases. *Brain Lang.* **85**, 93–108.

Beland, R., Caplan, D., and Nespoulous, J.L. (1990). The role of abstract phonological representations in word production: evidence from phonemic paraphasias. *J. Neurolinguistics* **5**, 125–64.

Benson, D.F. (1979). *Aphasia, alexia and agraphia.* Churchill Livingstone, New York.

Berthier, M. (2000). *Transcortical aphasias.* Psychology Press, Hove.

Boatman, D., Gordon, B., Hart, J., Selnes, O., Miglioretti, D., and Lenz, F. (2000). Transcortical sensory aphasia: revisited and revised. *Brain* **123** (8), 1634–42.

Bogousslavsky, J., Regli, F., and Assal, G. (1988). Acute transcortical mixed aphasia. A carotid occlusion syndrome with pial and watershed infects. *Brain* **111**, 631–41.

Bookheimer, S. (2002). Functional MRI of language: new approaches to understanding the cortical organization of semantic processing. *Annu. Rev. Neurosci.* **25**, 151–88.

Broca, P. (1861). Remarques sur la siège de la faculté du langage articulé, suivies d'une observation d'aphémie. *Bulletin Société d'Anthropologie, Paris* 2e série,**VI,** 330–57.

Capitani, E., Laiacona, M., Mahon, B., and Caramazza, A. (2003). What are the facts of semantic category specific deficits? A critical review of clinical evidence. *Cogn. Neuropsychol.* 20, 213–61.

Caplan, D. (1992). *Language.* MIT Press, Cambridge, Massachusetts.

Cappa, S.F. (1998). Spontaneous recovery from aphasia. In *Handbook of neurolinguistics* (ed. B. Stemmer and H. Withaker), pp. 535–45. Academic Press, San Diego.

Cappa, S.F. and Abutalebi, J. (1999). Subcortical aphasia. In *Concise Encyclopedia of Language Pathology* (ed. F. Fabbro), pp. 319–27. Pergamon Press, Oxford.

Cappa, S.F. and Perani, D. (2003). The neural correlates of noun and verb processing. *J. Neurolinguisitcs* **16**, 183–9.

Caramazza, A. (1988). Some aspects of language processing revealed through the analysis of acquired aphasia: the lexical system. *Annu. Rev. Neurosci.* **11**, 395–421.

Catani, M. and Ffytche, D.H. (2005). The rises and falls of disconnection syndromes. *Brain* **128**, 2224–39.

Catani, M., Jones, D.K., and Ffytche, D.H. (2005). Perisylvian language networks of the human brain. *Ann. Neurol.* **57**, 8–16

Coughlan, A.K. and Warrington, E.K. (1978). Word comprehension and word retrieval in patients with localized cerebral lesions. *Brain* **101**, 163–85.

Damasio, H. and Damasio, A.R. (1980). The anatomical basis of conduction aphasia. *Brain* **103**, 337.

Dejerine, J. (1914). *Sémiologie des affections du systéme nerveux.* Masson, Paris.

Dell, G.S., Schwartz, M.F., Martin, N., Saffran, E.M., and Gagnon, D.A. (1997). Lexical access in aphasic and nonaphasic speakers. *Psychol. Rev.* **104**, 801–38.

Demonet, J.F., Thierry, G., and Cardebat, D. (2005). Renewal of the neurophysiology of language: functional neuroimaging. *Physiol. Rev.* **85**, 49–95.

Dérouesné, J. and Beauvois, M.F. (1979). Phonological processing in reading: data from alexia. *J. Neurol. Neurosurg. Psychiatry* **42**, 1125–32.

Dronkers, N.F. (1996). A new brain region for coordinating speech articulation. *Nature* **384**, 159–61.

Ferro, J. (2001). Hyperacute cognitive stroke syndromes. *J. Neurol.* **248**, 841–9.

Freedman, M., Alexander, M.P., and Naeser, M.A. (1984). Anatomical basis of transcortical motor aphasia. *Neurology* **34**, 409–17.

Friederici, A.D. and Kotz, S. (2003). The brain basis of syntactic processes: functional imaging and lesion studies. *Neuroimage* **20**, S8–S17.

Friedmann, N. (2006). Generalizations on variations in comprehension and production: a further source of variation and a possible account. *Brain Lang.* **96**, 151–3; discussion 157–70.

Gaillard, R., Naccache, L., Pinel, P., Clemenceau, S., Volle, E., Hasboun, D., Dupont, S., Baulac, M., Dehaene, S., Adam, C., and Cohen, L. (2006). Direct intracranial, FMRI, and lesion evidence for the causal role of left inferotemporal cortex in reading. *Neuron* **50**, 191–204.

Gainotti, G., Basso, A., and Cappa, S.F. (2000). *Cognitive neuropsychology and language rehabilitation.* Psychology Press, Hove.

Gall, F.J. (1815). In Leischner, A. (1987). *Aphasien und Sprachentwicklungsstoerungen.*Thieme Verlag, Stuttgart.

Gardner, H. (1985). *The mind's new science: a history of the cognitive revolution.* Basic Books, New York.

Geschwind, N. and Kaplan, E. (1962). A human cerebral disconnection syndrome. A preliminary report. *Neurology* **12**, 65–75.

Godefroy, O., Dubois, C., Debachy, B., Leclerc, M., and Kreisler, A. (2002). Vascular aphasias: main characteristics of patients hospitalized in acute stroke units. *Stroke* **33**, 702–5.

Goldrick, M. and Rapp, B. (2007). Lexical and post-lexical phonological representations in spoken production. *Cognition* **102**, 219–60.

Goodglass, H. and Kaplan, E. (1983). *Assessment of aphasia and related disorders.* Lea and Febiger, Philadelphia.

Goodglass, H., Quadfasel, F.A., and Timberlake, W.H. (1964). Phrase length and the type and severity of aphasia. *Cortex* **1**, 133–53.

Grodzinsky, Y. (1990). *Theoretical perspectives on language deficits.* MIT Press, Cambridge, Massachusetts.

Grodzinsky, Y. (2000). The neurology of syntax: language use without Broca's area. *Behav. Brain Sci.* **23** (1), 1–71.

Grodzinsky, Y. and Amunts, K. (2006). *The Broca's region.* Oxford University Press, New York.

Hanlon, R.E., Lux, E.W., and Dromerick, A.W. (1999). Global aphasia without hemiparesis: language profiles and lesion distribution. *J. Neurol. Neurosurg. Psychiatry* **66**, 365–9.

Hickok, G., Bellugi, U., and Klima, E.S. (1996). The neurobiology of sign language and its implications for the neural basis of language. *Nature* **381**, 699–702.

Hillis, A.E. (1993). The role of models of language processing in rehabilitation of language impairments. *Aphasiology* **7**, 5–26.

Hillis, A.E. (2002). *The handbook of adult language disorders.* Psychology Press, New York.

Hillis, A.E. (in press). Magnetic resonance perfusion imaging in the study of language. *Brain Lang.*

Hillis, A.E, Wityk, R.J, Tuffiash, E., Beauchamp, N.J., Jacobs, M.A., Barker, P.B., and Selnes, O.A. (2001). Hypoperfusion of Wernicke's area predicts severity of semantic deficit in acute stroke. *Ann. Neurol.* **50**, 561–6.

Hillis, A.E., Wityk, R.J., Barker, P.B., Beauchamp, N.J., Gailloud, P., Murphy, K., Cooper, O., and Metter, E.J. (2002). Subcortical aphasia and neglect in acute stroke: the role of cortical hypoperfusion. *Brain* **125**, 1094–104.

Hillis, A.E., Chang, S., Breese, E., and Heidler, J. (2004). The crucial role of posterior frontal regions in modality specific components of the spelling process. *Neurocase* **10**, 175–87.

Howard, R., Trend, P., and Ross-Russel, R.W. (1987). Clinical features of ischemia in cerebral arterial border zones after periods of reduced cerebral blood flow. *Arch. Neurol.* **44**, 934–40.

Humphries, C., Willard, K., Buchsbaum, B., and Hickok, G. (2001). Role of anterior temporal cortex in auditory sentence comprehension: an fMRI study. *Neuroreport* **12**, 1749–52.

Indefrey, P. and Levelt, P. (2000). The neural correlates of language production. In *The new cognitive neurosciences* (ed. M.S. Gazzaniga), pp. 845–65. MIT Press, Cambridge, Massachusetts.

Kohn, S.E. (1992). *Conduction aphasia.* Lawrance Erlbaum Associates, Hillsdale, New Jersey.

Lecours, A.R. and Lhermitte, F. (1976). The pure form of the phonetic disintegration syndrome (pure anarthria): anatomo-clinical report of an historical case. *Brain Lang.* **3**, 88–113.

Leff, A.P., Spitsyna, G., Plant, G.T., and Wise, R.J. (2006). Structural anatomy of pure and hemianopic alexia. *J. Neurol. Neurosurg. Psychiatry* **77**, 1004–7.

Levelt, W.J.M. (1989). *Speaking: from intention to articulation.* MIT Press, Cambridge, Massachusetts.

Lichtheim, L. (1885). On aphasia. *Brain* **7**, 433–84.

Linebarger, M.C. (1995). Agrammatism as evidence about grammar. *Brain Lang.* **50**, 52–91.

Maguire, E.A., Frith, C.D., and Morris, R.G. (1999). The functional neuroanatomy of comprehension and memory: the importance of prior knowledge. *Brain* **122**, 1839–50.

Marshall, J.C. and Newcombe, F. (1966). Syntactic and semantic errors in paralexia. *Neuropsychologia* **4**, 169–76.

Marshall, J.C. and Newcombe, F. (1973). Patterns of paralexia: a psycholinguistic approach. *J. Psycholinguistic Res.* **2**, 175–99.

Mesulam, M.-M. (1990). Large-scale neurocognitive networks and distributed processing for attention, language, and memory. *Ann. Neurol.* **28**, 597–613.

Miceli, G. (2001). Disorders of single word processing. *J. Neurol.* **248**, 658–64.

Mohr, J.P., Pessin, M.S., Finkelstein, S., Funkestein, H.H., Duncan, G.W., and Davis, K.R. (1978). Broca aphasia. Pathologic and clinical. *Neurology* **28**, 311–24.

Moro, A., Tettamanti, M., Perani, D., Donati, C., Cappa, S.F., and Fazio, F. (2001). Syntax and the brain: disentangling grammar by selective anomalies. *Neuroimage* **13**, 110–18.

Neville, H.J. and Bavelier, D. (1998). Neural organization and plasticity of language. *Curr. Opin. Neurobiol.* **8**, 254–8.

Opitz, B. and Friederici, A.D. (2004). Brain correlates of language learning: the neuronal dissociation of rule-based versus similarity-based learning. *J. Neurosci.* **24**, 8436–40.

Otsuki, M., Soma, Y., Yoshimura, N., Miyashita, K., Nagatsuka, K., and Naritomi, H. (2005). How to improve repetition ability in patients with Wernicke's aphasia: the effect of a disguised task. *J. Neurol. Neurosurg. Psychiatry* **76**, 733–5.

Paolucci, S., Matano, A., Bragoni, M., Coiro, P., De Angelis, D., Fusco, F.R., Morelli, D., Pratesi, L., Venturiero, V., and Bureca, I. (2005). Rehabilitation of left brain-damaged ischemic stroke patients: the role of comprehension language deficits. A matched comparison. *Cerebrovasc. Dis.* **20**, 400–6.

Patterson, K.E. and Kay, J. (1982). Letter by letter reading: psychological description of a neurological syndrome. *Quart. J. Exp. Psychol.* **34A**, 411–41.

Pedersen, P.M., Vinter, K., and Olsen, T.S. (2004). Aphasia after stroke: type, severity and prognosis. The Copenhagen aphasia study. *Cerebrovasc. Dis.* **17**, 35–43.

Perani, D. and Abutalebi, J. (2005). Neural basis of first and second language processing. *Curr. Opin. Neurobiol.* **15**, 202–6.

Perani, D., Vallar, G., Cappa, S.F., Messa, C., and Fazio, F. (1987). Aphasia and neglect after subcortical stroke. *Brain* **110**, 1211–29.

Perani, D., Paulesu, E., Sebastian Galles, N., Dupoux, E., Dehaene, S., Bettinardi, V., Cappa, S.F., Fazio, F., and Mehler, J. (1998). The bilingual brain. Proficiency and age of acquisition of the second language. *Brain* **121**, 1841–52.

Plaut, D. (1996). Relearning after damage to a connectionist network: toward a theory of rehabilitation. *Brain Lang.* **52**, 25–82.

Plaut, D.C. and Shallice, T. (1993). Deep dyslexia: a case study of connectionist neuropsychology. *Cogn. Neuropsychol.* **10**, 377–500.

Poeck, K. (1983). What do we mean by aphasia syndromes? A neurologist's view. *Brain Lang.* **20**, 79–89.

Poldrack, R.A., Wagner, A.D., Prull, M.W., Desmond, J.E., Glover, G.H., and Gabrieli J.D. (1999). Functional specialization for semantic and phonological processing in the left inferior prefrontal cortex. *Neuroimage* **10,** 15–35.

Price, C.J. (1998). The functional anatomy of word comprehension and production. *Trends Cogn. Sci.* **2**, 281–8.

Price, C.J. and Devlin, J.T. (2003). The myth of the visual word form area. *Neuroimage* **19**, 473–81.

Price, C.J. and Mechelli, A. (2005). Reading and reading disturbance. *Curr. Opin. Neurobiol.* **15**, 231–8.

Price, C.J., Wise, R.S.J., and Frackowiak, R.S.J. (1996). Demonstrating the implicit processing of visually presented words and pseudowords. *Cereb. Cortex* **6**, 62–70.

Robinson, G., Shallice, T., and Cipolotti, L. (2006). Dynamic aphasia in progressive supranuclear palsy: a deficit in generating a fluent sequence of novel thought. *Neuropsychologia* **44**, 1344–60.

Sakurai, Y. (2004). Varieties of alexia from fusiform, posterior inferior temporal and posterior occipital gyrus lesions. *Behav. Neurol.* **15**, 35–50.

Saur, D., Lange, R., Baumgaertner, A., Schraknepper, V., Willmes, K., Rijntjes, M., and Weiller, C. (2006). Dynamics of language reorganization after stroke. *Brain* **129**, 1371–84.

Schiff, H.B., Alexander, M.P., Naeser, M.A., and Galaburda, A.M. (1983). Aphemia: clinical-anatomic correlations. *Arch. Neurol.* **40**, 720–7.

Scott, S.K., Blank, C.C., Rosen, S., and Wise, R.J. (2000). Identification of a pathway for intelligible speech in the left temporal lobe. *Brain* **123**, 2400–6.

Shapiro, K. and Caramazza, A. (2003). The representation of grammatical categories in the brain. *Trends Cogn. Sci.* **7**, 201–6.

Szirmai, I., Farsang, M., and Csuri, M. (2003). Cortical auditory disorder caused by bilateral strategic cerebral bleedings. Analysis of two cases. *Brain Lang.* **85**, 159–65.

Tettamanti, M., Alkadhi, H., Moro, A., Perani, D., Kollias, S., and Weniger, D. (2002). Neural correlates for the acquisition of natural language syntax. *Neuroimage* **17**, 700–9.

Tyler, L.K., Moss, H.E., Durrant-Peatfield, M.R., and Levy, J.P. (2000). Conceptual structure and the structure of concepts: a distributed account of category-specific deficits. *Brain Lang.* **75**, 195–231.

Vignolo, L.A. (1986). Le basi anatomiche del linguaggio: ipotesi tratte dallo studio dell'afasia. *Boll. Med. Chir. Bresciana* **37**, 7–19.

Vignolo, L.A., Boccardi, E., Caverni, L., and Frediani, F. (1986). Unexpected CT-scan findings in global aphasia. *Cortex* **22**, 55–70.

Vinson, D.P., Vigliocco, G., Cappa, S., and Siri, S. (2003). The breakdown of semantic knowledge: insights from a statistical model of meaning representation. *Brain Lang.* **86**, 347–65.

Wagner, A.D., Paré-Blagoev, E.J., Clark, J., Poldrack, R.A. (2001). Recovering Meaning: Left Prefrontal Cortex Guides Controlled Semantic Retrieval. *Neuron* **31,** 329–38.

Wernicke, C. (1874). *Der aphasische Symptomencomplex.* Cohn und Weigert, Breslau.

Wise, R.J.S. (2003). Language systems in normal and aphasic human subjects: functional imaging studies and inferences from animal studies. *Br. Med. Bull.* **65**, 95–119.

Chapter 5

Apraxia

Ferdinand Binkofski and Kathrin Reetz

5.1 Introduction

In 1891 the term apraxia (Greek: inactivity) was first used by Heyman Steinthal to describe failures in the performance of purposeful actions and the incorrect use of objects by patients with aphasia (Steinthal 1871, 1881). Apraxias are higher motor dysfunctions that affect performance and imitation of actions or action sequences as well as the appropriate use of objects. The observed deficits do not result from paresis, ataxia, dyskinesia, paraesthesia, or impairment of language understanding or recognition of objects.

The most complex forms of apraxia are the ideational and ideomotor apraxia syndromes defined by Liepmann (1920). They are derived from lesions of the language dominant hemisphere, though the manifestation is bilateral (i.e. contra- as well as ipsilateral).

In rare cases, with a lesion of the callosal fibres, a unilateral ideomotor apraxia in the extremities ipsilateral to the language dominant hemisphere can be observed. In those forms of apraxia defined by Liepmann, the disturbance of execution of complex movements results either from incorrect action planning (ideational apraxia) or from the incorrect conversion of correct planning into correct performance of actions or action sequences (ideomotor apraxia). Thus (simplifying) two main components of action planning and execution are distinguished: (1) an action concept system, containing knowledge of the tool use and of the basic mechanical constraints (impaired by ideational apraxia); and (2) an action production system, with information about the motor programmes and their conversion into learned movement patterns (damage leads to ideomotor apraxia; Roy and Hall 1992). Liepmann (1920) also differentiated a third component, the 'kinetic memory' of the 'sensomotorium', in which overlearned movement patterns are stored and whose damage leads to an isolated limb-kinetic apraxia of the opposite hand. Traditionally, investigations of patients with such complex forms of apraxia concentrate on disturbances in the three most important domains of action performance: imitation of meaningless gestures; performance of meaningful gestures on verbal command; and the use of tools and objects.

The simpler forms of apraxia include purely executive or production apraxias (limb-kinetic, speech), which are predominantly caused by frontal lesions, and unimodal apraxias (tactile, visuomotor), which are predominantly associated with lesions of the superior parietal lobule and the adjacent structures. Apraxic deficits manifest themselves not only in the arms and legs, but can also affect the face musculature (buccofacial or face apraxia).

Aphasia and apraxia often occur simultaneously, but their grades of severity do not correlate. Some studies appear to demonstrate a (double) dissociation of language functions and practice, which suggests that the neural organization of these two functions is organized, at least in part, in structurally different networks.

With careful clinical examination apraxia can quite often be found in patients with stroke. According to De Renzi (1989) apraxic disorders can be found as a result of applied testing in

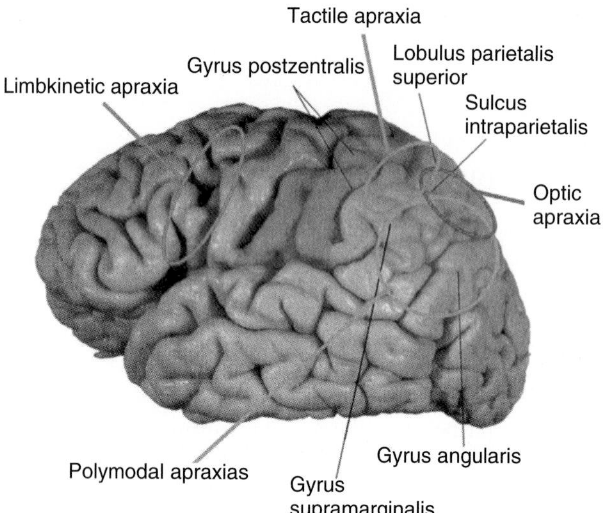

Fig. 5.1 Schematic drawing demonstrating the predominant localizations of lesions in the individual forms of apraxia. This is a black and white version of Plate 3.

30–50% of left brain damaged patients and in 2–9 % of right brain damaged patients. The natural history of apraxia is quite heterogeneous—of those patients, who were apraxic in the first week post-onset of infarction, approximately half were still apraxic after 3 months and approximately 20% remained apraxic (Basso *et al.* 1987; Kertesz and Ferro 1984).

5.2 **Classification of apraxias**

With reference to the work of De Renzi and colleagues (De Renzi and Luchelli 1988), Freund (1992) proposed the following classification of apraxias (Fig. 5.1).

- The executive (production) apraxias concern mainly effector-specific execution of movements and are derived predominantly from frontal lesions (limb-kinetic apraxia from contralateral premotor lesions, speech apraxia from frontal insular lesions).
- Posterior apraxias, stemming predominantly from lesions of the parietal lobe, include unimodal and polymodal apraxias.
    - Unimodal apraxias are caused by deficits in the elementary somatosensory or visual functions and affect predominantly the contralesional extremity (examples: optic apraxia (ataxia), tactile apraxia).
    - The disturbed motor behaviour in polymodal apraxias is not anchored in one modality only, but instead the ideation and conception of motor actions on a more global level are affected (ideational and ideomotor apraxia).

Polymodal apraxias are observed predominantly after lesions of the parietal lobes but disturbances of pantomime and real object use may occur after frontal lesions as well.

5.3 **Executive apraxias**

The frontal or executive apraxias are characterized by deficits in the execution (production) of complex movement components. Representative forms are limb-kinetic apraxia and speech apraxia.

They are the consequence of disturbed 'premotor' functions of the caudal frontal lobe, which acts as a store and a processor of complex actions. Lesion-induced interruptions of the parieto-premotor information flow often play an important causal role.

5.3.1 **Limb-kinetic apraxia**

5.3.1.1 Diagnosis

Limb-kinetic (also 'innervation' or 'melokinetic') apraxia manifests itself as the inability to accomplish finely coordinated and precise hand movements (Kleist 1911; Liepmann 1920). The higher the demand on finely tuned motor control, the more awkward is the movement execution. Luria (1966) described the characteristic feature of limb-kinetic apraxia as the loss of 'kinetic melody'. This syndrome is rarely diagnosed, mainly because the distinction from paresis resulting from a lesion of the pyramidal tract is difficult. There is also as yet no standardized test for limb-kinetic apraxia.

The characteristic clinical diagnostic features are awkwardness of arm and hand movements and disturbance of fine motor skills, dexterity, coordination of exploratory finger movements, writing, and joint coordination, all that is associated with preserved force production and individual finger movements. One useful diagnostic procedure is the alternating fist closure test after Osseretzki (Luria 1966). Patients are asked to open and close the fists alternating at a comfortable pace (open right, close left, and vice versa). Usually the patients cannot keep pace and lose track. Bimanual coordination can be tested also by means of a rhythm production task. When patients are asked to knock simple rhythms with both hands they fail to do so after a short while (Halsband *et al.* 1993).

The diagnosis can be made when the integrity of the primary motor cortex and the pyramidal tract is demonstrated by means of structural and functional neuroimaging and/or electrophysiological procedures. If the lesion is located clearly before the gyrus precentralis, the task is rather easy. For example, transcranial magnetic stimulation can demonstrate the intact central motor latencies to, and normal amplitudes of, the motor action potentials (MAP) in the muscles of the affected extremity, indicating that the pyramidal tract is intact.

The advantage of the combined use of clinical investigation and auxiliary diagnostics is demonstrated by an example of a patient with limb-kinetic apraxia associated with a lesion within the right frontal operculum (Fig. 5.2).

5.3.1.2 Pathophysiology

During the translation of sensory information into suitable movement patterns the inferior parietal cortex and the ventral premotor cortex interact closely with each other. In the parietal cortex (for example, in the anterior intraparietal area (AIP); Binkofski *et al.* 1998; Grefkes *et al.* 2002) multisensory information is integrated and several alternative motor programmes for the hand are prepared. The programme that is needed for the execution of a specific movement is selected in the ventral premotor cortex (Jeannerod *et al.* 1995; Rumiati *et al.* 2004) and executed via the primary motor cortex (M1; Fig. 5.3). Since there are no direct anatomical connections between the area AIP and the primary motor cortex, a 'deafferentation' of M1 can occur after a lesion of the premotor cortex (whereby the sensory afferents from SI, etc. are still well preserved). The consequence is insufficient movement control, because the access to motor programmes is no longer possible (Binkofski and Buccino 2004).

Limb-kinetic apraxias may also develop with basal ganglia diseases such as corticobasal degeneration or Parkinson's disease (Leiguarda and Marsden 2000). This indicates that the fine tuning of movements on the cortical level is subject to constant control by the basal ganglia.

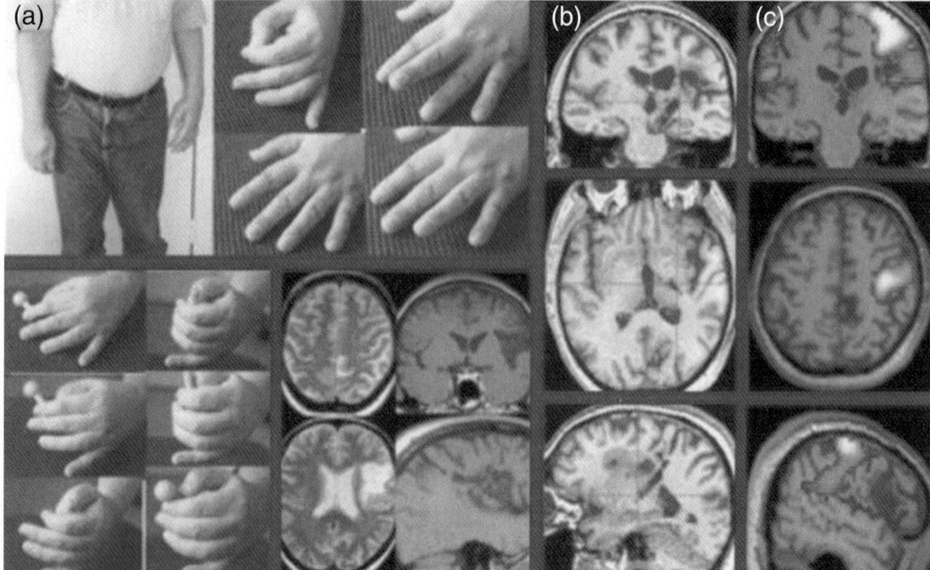

Fig. 5.2 Limb-kinetic apraxia. (a) A patient with a pronounced disturbance of dexterity and the skilled movements of the left hand (a, bottom left), with well preserved individual finger movements (a, above right), and normal force production due to a chronic ischaemic lesion of the premotor cortex in the right-sided frontal operculum (a, lower right). (b) The continuity of the pyramid tract on the lesion side could be demonstrated by means of the diffusion tensor tractography (in blue). (c) fMRI: During the execution of an exploratory sensorimotor task with the affected hand not only the bilateral secondary somatosensory cortex, but also the primary sensorimotor as well as the intra-parietal cortex on the lesion side are activated. This is a black and white version of Plate 4.

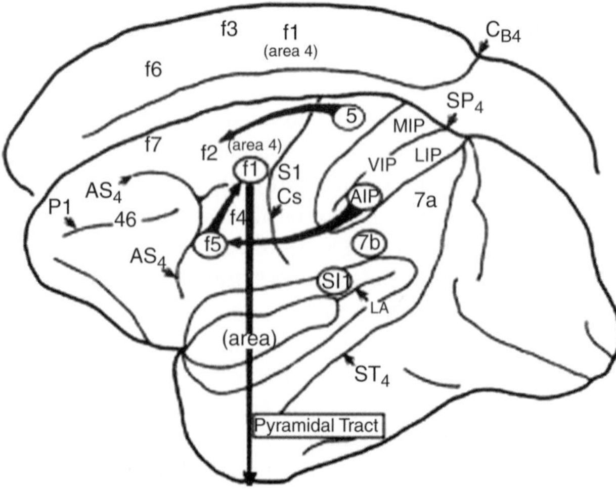

Fig. 5.3 The parieto-premotor circuit for the control of hand actions (after Jeannerod *et al.* 1995; explanations in the text).

5.3.1.3 Localization

Limb-kinetic apraxias result in most cases from lesions of the premotor cortex and manifest themselves contralaterally.

5.3.1.4 Therapy and relevance

Limb-kinetic apraxia is frequently misdiagnosed as paresis and therefore often not recognized. However, this form of apraxia is quite responsive to physiotherapeutic measures, much more so than many forms of paresis. The patients profit considerably from intensive exercise patterns such as constraint-induced therapy (CIT; Taub *et al.* 2002). Also new 'top-down' oriented approaches (e.g. by motor imagery or movement observation), such as mirror therapy and video training (Binkofski *et al.* 2004), promise to provide good results.

5.3.2 Speech apraxia

5.3.2.1 Diagnosis

In speech apraxia the composition of articulatory movements to produce language sounds and words is disturbed. The patient's speech seems weary; it is slow and disfigured by phonetic deviations. When speaking, the patients give the impression that they must consciously control their mouth movements, the coordination of the speech apparatus, and respiration.

The diagnosis of speech apraxia is based on analysis of the linguistic utterances of the patient, particularly in the absence of symptoms of aphasia or dysarthria. In German-speaking countries there exists a standardized test battery for the diagnosis of speech apraxias (Liepold *et al.* 2002). Advanced planning of speech movements is disturbed and sounds are badly coordinated. With speech apraxia individual movements of the mouth can be accomplished with normal strength and speed, but they cannot be coordinated for fluent execution of speech. The disturbed articulation of speech, in combination with an absence of structural lesions of the speech apparatus, indicates that a defect of higher motor language control is present in speech apraxia. Thus, speech apraxia can be classified as an executive (productive) deficit.

5.3.2.2 Localization

Speech apraxia results most frequently from left frontal lesions, in or around the gyrus precentralis (parts of Broca's area); subcortical structures may also be affected (Schiff *et al.* 1983; Alexander *et al.* 1989). Other data suggest a predominant participation of the intrasylvian structures, above all of the anterior insula (Dronkers 1996).

5.3.2.3 Therapy and relevance

Patients who are moderately to heavily affected should begin the therapy with the pronunciation and intonation of simple syllables. Performance of correct movements of the lips and the tongue might be helpful. Some patients may improve their articulation by rhythmic knocking or clapping. The exercise of pronunciation should be aligned to the natural speech rhythm in order to improve comprehension.

5.4 Posterior apraxias

The parietal cortex, as the key structure of the so-called 'dorsal' (or 'how') way of the data processing, functions as a sensorimotor 'interface'. Lesions of the parietal lobes are often associated with posterior apraxias. The superior parts of the parietal lobes are engaged in direct and modality-bound movement control; lesions in this region lead to unimodal apraxias.

The inferior parts of the parietal lobes and the parieto-temporal junction process complex polymodal sensorimotor information (Rizzolatti *et al.* 1997; Bremmer *et al.* 2001) and integrate spatial and temporal information for the execution of complex movements (Assmus *et al.* 2003; Binkofski *et al.* 1998; Liepmann 1920). Lesions in this area are associated with polymodal apraxias.

5.4.1 Unimodal apraxias: introduction

Unimodal apraxias are localized within one sensory system and manifest themselves predominantly on the contralateral side to the lesion. Typical representatives are tactile apraxia and optical (visuomotor) apraxia (also optic ataxia).

5.4.2 Unimodal apraxias: tactile apraxia

5.4.2.1 Diagnosis

In tactile apraxia (Klein 1931), exploratory finger movements are mainly affected (with simultaneous absence of paresis or sensory deficits). The finger movements seem uncoordinated and inadequate in relation to size and shape of objects to be explored (Binkofski *et al.* 2001; see Fig. 5.4). Typically, the intransitive (not object-related) and expressive movements (e.g. gestures) are well preserved. Delay (1935) referred to the association between apraxic and agnostic deficits.

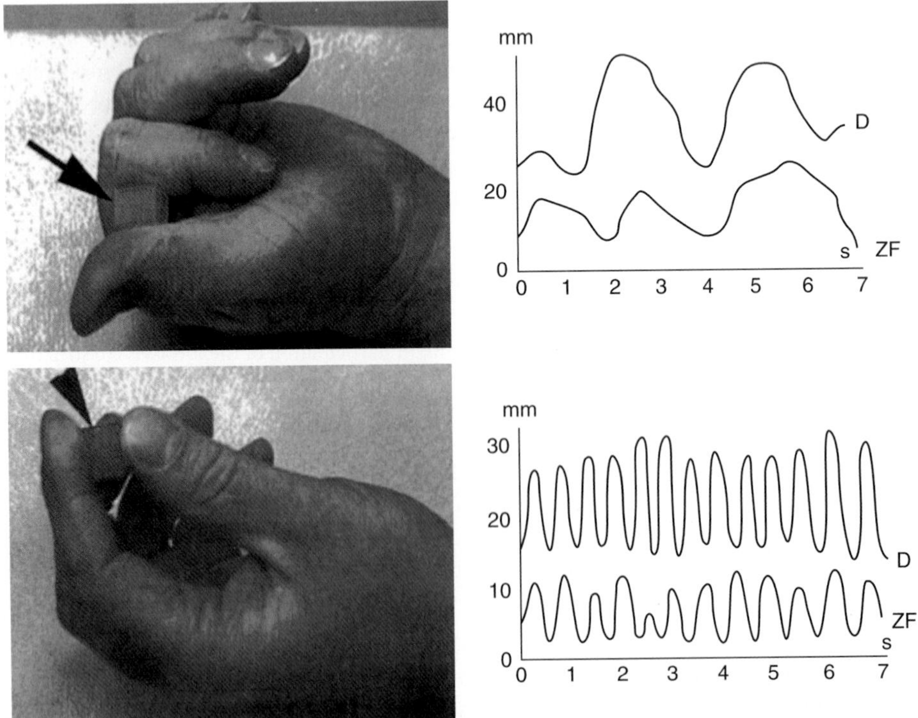

Fig. 5.4 Tactile apraxia. Exploratory finger movements are poorly coordinated and (in relation to the object size) inadequate (left above) with clearly increased range and delayed speed of the finger movements (right above). An example of well coordinated finger movements of a normal person is presented in the lower part of the picture. D, Thumb; ZF, index finger.

Accordingly, tactile apraxia is often accompanied by astereognosia (inability to recognize objects by tactile exploration, despite the well preserved basic sensory and motor functions; Binkofski *et al.* 2001; Wernicke 1876).

5.4.2.2 Pathophysiology

Similarly to limb-kinetic apraxia, a disturbance of the interaction between specialized parietal and premotor areas might be inferred as one cause of tactile apraxia. The parietal cortex serves as sensorimotor 'interface' for coordination of exploratory movements. Object characteristics trigger appropriate finger movement patterns that serve the perception of object's features ('action for perception', 'feedback'). At the same time the object properties determine the movement extent—perception in the service of action ('perception for action', 'feedforward'; Lederman and Klatzky 1997). Although many steps in the processing of tactile object recognition occur in the anterior and posterior parietal lobes (Bodegård *et al.* 2000; Caselli 1993; Head and Holmes 1911; Servos *et al.* 2001), it is still unclear whether tactile recognition of objects is processed by the parietal lobes alone. It appears that, during the process of tactile object recognition, an exchange of information with the inferior temporal lobe, a region that is known to be important for visual recognition of objects, takes place (Rossetti and Pisella 2002).

5.4.2.3 Localization

Tactile apraxia typically results from lesions of the contralateral superior parietal lobulus and/or the more anterior part of the intraparietal sulcus. If the caudal parts of the gyrus postcentralis are affected, accompanying disturbances of somatosensory qualities can occur. The important roles of the superior parietal lobulus and the anterior part of the sulcus intraparietalis (area AIP) for controlling the manipulation of objects were proven in several functional imaging studies (Binkofski *et al.* 1998; Grefkes *et al.* 2002; Rumiati *et al.* 2004).

5.4.2.4 Therapy and relevance

Since the disturbed handling of objects is the central failure in tactile apraxia and there is frequently a concomitant disturbance of tactile object recognition (in particular if the area AIP is also damaged; Rizzolatti and Luppino 2001), the patients are often significantly impaired in daily life (Delay 1935; Binkofski *et al.* 1999*b*). In particularly severe cases, the hand can be useless despite intact motor and sensory function. Dedicated intensive physiotherapeutic measures and learning alternative strategies can provide good results.

5.4.3 **Unimodal apraxias: optic (visuomotor) apraxia (ataxia)**

5.4.3.1 Diagnosis

In 1909 optic ataxia was first described by Balint (1909) as part of a broader visuoperceptive deficit. Optic ataxia is characterized by inaccuracy when reaching for visually located objects (Garcin *et al.* 1967; Perenin and Vighetto 1988; Ratcliff and Davies-Jones 1972). The terms visuomotor ataxia or optic apraxia are used synonymously.

The typical behaviour of a patient with optic apraxia includes misreaching for objects, in particular when the objects are not centrally fixated by the patient. The finger aperture is clearly increased and inadequately scaled in relation to the object's size, although visual object recognition is intact (Jeannerod 1986; Milner and Goodale 1995; Perenin and Vighetto 1988). In some patients misreaching is present in only one arm but in both hemifields (hand effect; rare); in others it is present in both arms in the contralesional visual field (field effect). The most frequent deficit is present in the contralesional arm and in the contralesional hemifield. This disturbance arises rarely in both arms and both hemifields (and then mostly after extensive bilateral parietal lesions).

Typically, the patients are capable of reaching towards their own body parts or towards objects that are localized on the body surface. For the diagnosis of optic apraxia goal-directed reaching should be examined with each arm and in both peripheral hemifields under simultaneous central fixation (Fig. 5.5).

A related disorder is mirror-apraxia, a result of lesions of the right or left posterior parietal lobe (Binkofski *et al.* 1999*a*, 2003). If patients with mirror-apraxia are presented with an object that they can see only through a mirror and are asked to reach for the real object, these patients reach constantly for the virtual object in the mirror. Even if the arm of the patient is guided under constant visual control in the mirror to the real object position, these patients continue to reach for the virtual object in the mirror directly afterwards. On the other hand, despite the presence of the mirror, reaching for objects in the direct proximity of the body or reaching for their own body parts is intact. These patients also have no problems in reaching for objects they view directly.

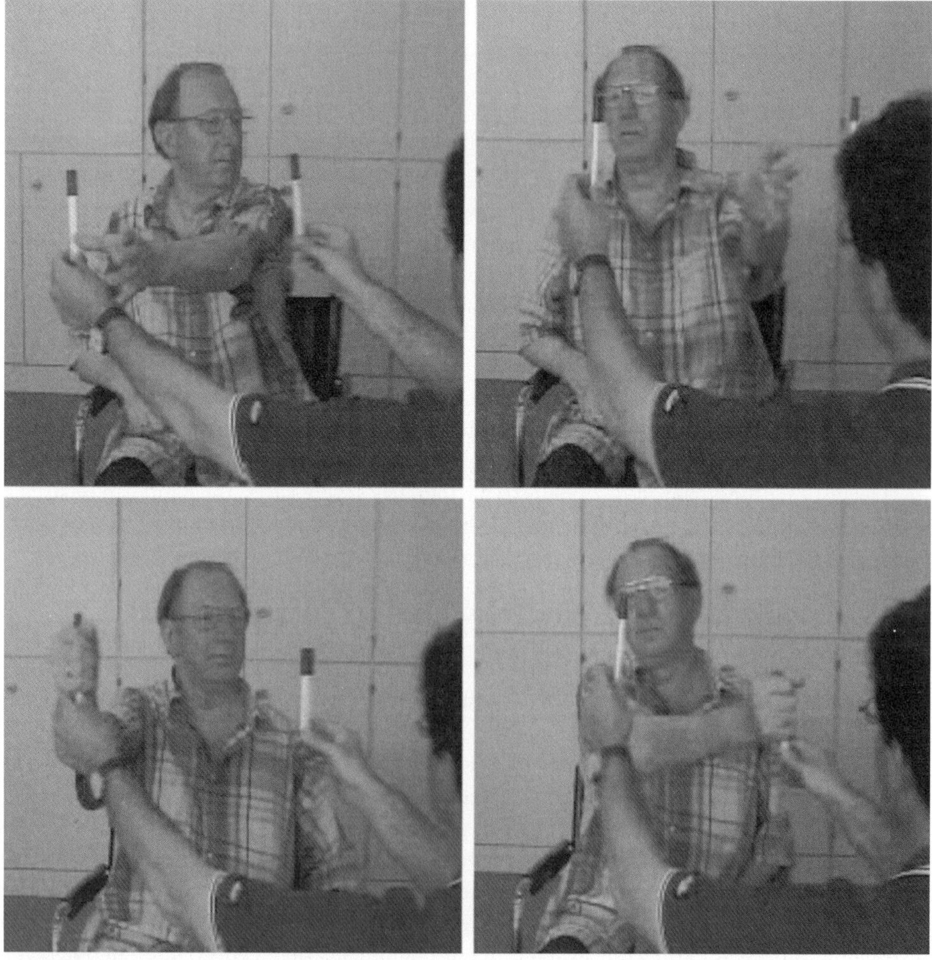

Fig. 5.5 Optic apraxia. The patient misreaches the target object with the contralesional left arm in both peripheral visual fields (hand effect, upper picture). There is no misreaching with the right arm in both visual hemifields (lower picture).

5.4.3.2 Pathophysiology

Haaxma and Kuypers (1975) assumed a visuomotor disconnection as a cause of optic apraxia. New studies involving visuomotor behaviour imply an extended interpretation of the function of the dorsal stream in the pathophysiology of optic apraxia (Pisella *et al.* 2000; Gréa *et al.* 2002). While in normal subjects reaching for objects after a delay becomes worse, a delay between the presentation of the object and the initiation of the reaching movement can improve the accuracy of reaching in patients with optic apraxia (Pisella *et al.* 2000). This finding can be explained with the help of new ideas about the structure of the dorsal (or 'where') stream of visual data processing. Hereafter, the dorsal stream is divided into two substreams: the dorso-dorsal stream for direct ('on-line') movement control and the ventro-dorsal stream for slower movement processing. The latter also contains more time-consuming components of movement programming (Rizzolatti and Matelli 2003; Rossetti *et al.* 2003; Ferro 1984; Fig. 5.6). Therefore, optic apraxia is defined as a deficit of direct, on-line visuomotor control. The improvement after a delay is interpreted as compensation via the ventro-dorsal stream, due to interactions with the ventral stream.

5.4.3.3 Localization

Many studies of optic apraxia have reported lesions of the superior parietal lobulus that tend to centre around the sulcus intraparietalis (Buxbaum and Coslett 1998; Ferro 1984; Ratcliff and Davies-Jones 1972; Perenin and Vighetto 1988; see Fig. 5.7). It is, however, possible that the MIP (medial intraparietal) area (Grefkes *et al.* 2004) plays an important role.

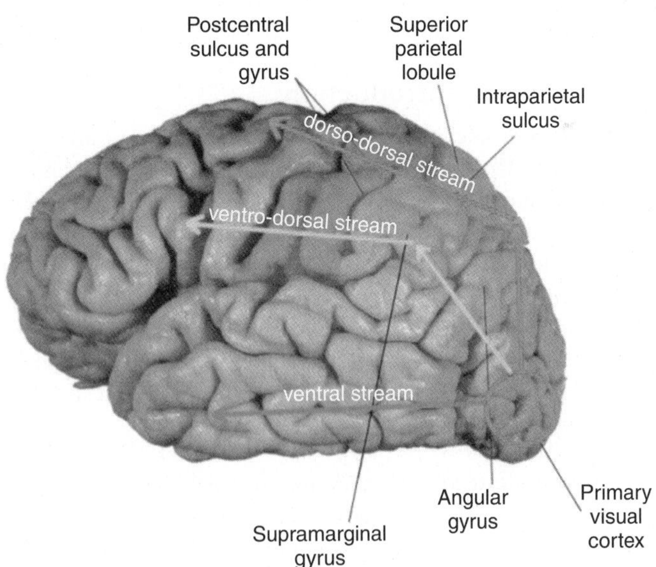

Fig. 5.6 Schematic representation of the dorsal ('where') way and the ventral ('what') streams. The dorsal way can be subdivided into the dorso-dorsal stream (red) and the ventro-dorsal (green) stream. The dorso-dorsal stream leads over the superior parietal lobulus to the dorsal premotor cortex and is responsible for the fast 'online' control of visually guided movements. The ventro-dorsal stream goes through the inferior parietal lobulus towards the ventral premotor cortex and is responsible for the complex spatio-temporal planning of movements. The ventral stream (blue) is responsible for the visual object recognition (Rizzolatti and Matelli 2003). This is a black and white version of Plate 5.

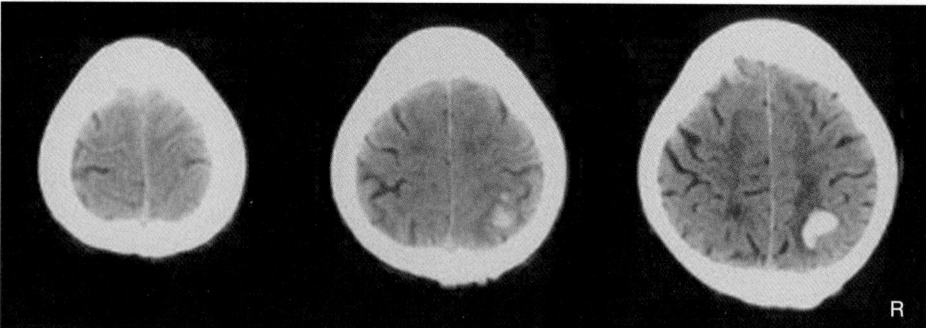

Fig. 5.7 An example of a small bleeding in the region of the right middle intraparietal sulcus, which is associated with optic apraxia (see Fig. 5.5).

5.4.3.4 Therapy and relevance

The most severely affected patients also show misreaching for centrally fixated objects. These rather rare cases are usually associated with larger or bilateral lesions. Patients with optic apraxia in the context of a Balint syndrome have difficulties getting along in unusual environments. Simultanagnosia and optical apraxia lead to a severe deficit of the visual exploration—the patients cannot detect objects or have difficulties in judging their own position in relation to objects. Patients with smaller and one-sided lesions are often mildly affected. If the optic apraxia is limited to the periphery of the visual field, patients can practise compensatory strategies in which they first learn to turn their gaze to objects and then to reach for them under central fixation.

5.4.4 Polymodal apraxias: introduction

The execution of simple movement components is not affected in polymodal apraxias. The deficits of action execution depend rather on the context in which the motor action is implemented. An important feature of polymodal apraxias is that the disturbance of action execution manifests itself on both sides of the body (ipsi- and contralateral to the lesion). The disorder affects mechanisms of action conception that operate on a hierarchically higher level than the purely contralateral action execution and sensorimotor control. The most important representatives of these forms of apraxia are ideomotor and ideational apraxia. Such apraxias can manifest themselves both in the extremities and in the face. In the latter case it is called apraxia of face or buccofacial apraxia. Up to 80% of all aphasic patients have a buccofacial apraxia.

5.4.4.1 Pathophysiology of ideomotor and ideational apraxia

Apraxic patients cannot imitate because they are not able to convert the characteristics of the perceived (observed) actions into adequate, own action patterns (Barbieri and De Renzi 1988). A deficit in the so-called 'mirror neuron' system may possibly play a substantial role here (Rizzolatti *et al.* 2001). The mirror neurons, which are localized in parts of the ventral premotor and the inferior parietal cortex, code both movement perception and movement execution and serve the creation of internal movement representations and understanding of movement contents (Rizzolatti *et al.* 2001; Umilta *et al.* 2001).

In order to perform a pantomime of object use, the parameters of the object (its physical characteristics, its position in space) and the related movement programme must be evoked together and combined. Besides the explicit knowledge about the correct use of an object, the pantomime also requires the ability to emphasize distinct and explicit aspects of its use and express them by hand movements (Goldenberg 2003). The impairment of pantomime of object use can originate either from deficient access to information about the object or from faulty initiation of the appropriate movement sequence or the combination of both.

There is evidence that many different respective 'movement schemas' are stored *a priori*. It is less a matter of a 'movement formula' (Liepmann 1920), but rather of specific movement 'replicas' that are focused on the acting extremity, on the interaction with objects, and/or on certain situations (Buccino *et al.* 2001; Rizzolatti *et al.* 2001). Results from several neuroimaging studies on action observation and motor imagery support the existence of such effector-specific representations of movements (Buccino *et al.* 2001; Ehrsson *et al.* 2003).

The use of common objects or tools or the sequential use of different tools in order to perform a complex action requires the ability to recall the concepts of use of these objects or of sequential actions. In the case of individual objects it can require the recall of explicit 'instructions of use' from the semantic memory or the ability to solve mechanical problems by inferring possible functions from the structure (Goldenberg and Hagmann 1998; Norman 1989). 'Instructions for use' of single familiar tools can be conceptualized as associations between the tool, its purpose, its recipient, and a motor action (Buxbaum *et al.* 1997; Hartmann *et al.* 2005; Hodges *et al.* 2000). New findings show that objects themselves are also stored at a conceptual level in the human brain (Johnson-Frey *et al.* 2003).

Complex multistep actions that include the use of several objects also require more complex instructions of use that integrate several simpler action object units (Cooper and Shallice 2000; Mayer *et al.* 1990). Complex actions with several objects challenge the working memory and the ability for serial planning. 'Trial and error' strategies are used to find out causal contexts that are not directly derivable from the structure or if the necessary technical knowledge is lacking.

5.4.5 **Polymodal apraxias: ideomotor apraxia**

5.4.5.1 Diagnosis

Limb-kinetic apraxia manifests itself in three domains of motor behaviour: imitation of meaningless gestures; execution of meaningful gestures on verbal command; and use of tools and objects. Since each of them can vary depending on the localization and lateralization of the lesion, Goldenberg (2006) proposes that they be examined separately. While deficiencies in imitation of meaningless gestures and execution of meaningful gestures are characteristic of ideomotor apraxia, disturbance of the individual and serial usage of objects appears to be characteristic of ideational apraxia. In everyday life patients with ideomotor apraxia are rather inconspicuous; their deficit is revealed predominantly in the experimental situation, mostly if they are requested to perform a pantomime of object use after verbal or visual presentation of the object. Whereas most errors occur during the pantomime of the object use, the patients clearly show less remarkable findings during the real use of objects (see Fig. 5.8).

Types of errors The cardinal symptom of ideomotor apraxia is parapraxia (Liepmann 1908). It contains a combination of deficient action selection with errors of sequencing of actions and spatial orientation errors. The most frequently observed parapraxic errors are the following (after Poeck 2002).

- Perseveration. The patient repeats either complete movements or elements of movements that she/he was performing previously during the investigation.
- Substitution. A requested movement is replaced by another movement.

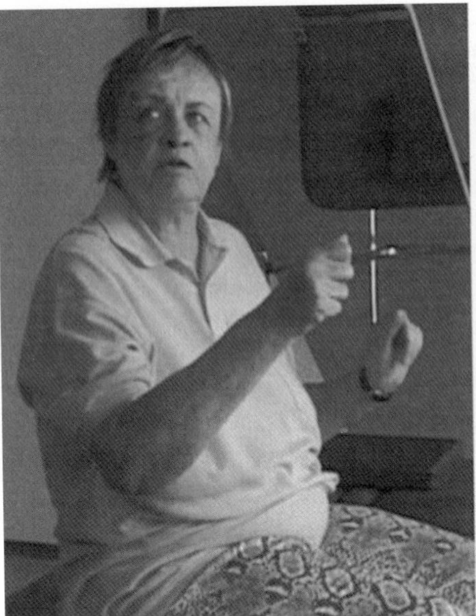
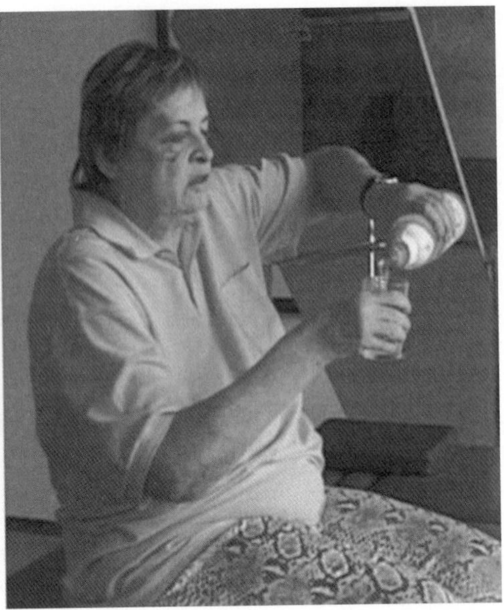

Fig. 5.8 Example of a female patient with ideomotor apraxia, after lesion of the left inferior parietal lobe. The attempt to perform a pantomime, in which she is requested to represent pouring of water from a bottle into a glass, leads to confusion and perseveration of an incomplete movement. When using real objects the complex action is executed without errors.

- Surplus movements. Movements that exceed the range of the requested movement are executed. Example: instead of only wrinkling the nose, the patient also purses the lips, or the patient firmly closes his/her eyes while whistling.
- 'Verbal overflow'. Aphasic patients try to explain how to handle the object instead of demonstrating its use or they accompany the use with comments and noises.
- Omission. Movements are performed only incompletely. Example: instead of making a combing movement, the patient runs his/her hand through the hair.
- *Conduite d'approche*. The patient approaches the requested goal movement in several different attempts, until he/she succeeds in performing the correct movement. If this attempt remains futile, it may come to a '*conduite d'ecart*' error where the patient drifts away from the requested goal movement.
- 'Body-part-as-object' (BPO) error. During the demonstration of the pantomimed object use, body parts are used as tools. BPO can be considered as pathological errors if they are produced despite repeated corrections and if they are referred to objects, which are for BPO uncommon and have little communicative load (e.g. to hammer with the fist, where the fist strikes like the head of a hammer on the table or to suck a finger for the pantomime of smoking).

Testing the imitation of gestures A native imitation of gestures can only take place when novel gestures that have no connection to stored movement representations are examined (Goldenberg 2001). It has been proven to be useful to test finger and hand gestures separately. The two functions are differently distributed over the hemispheres (Goldenberg 1996); therefore apraxic

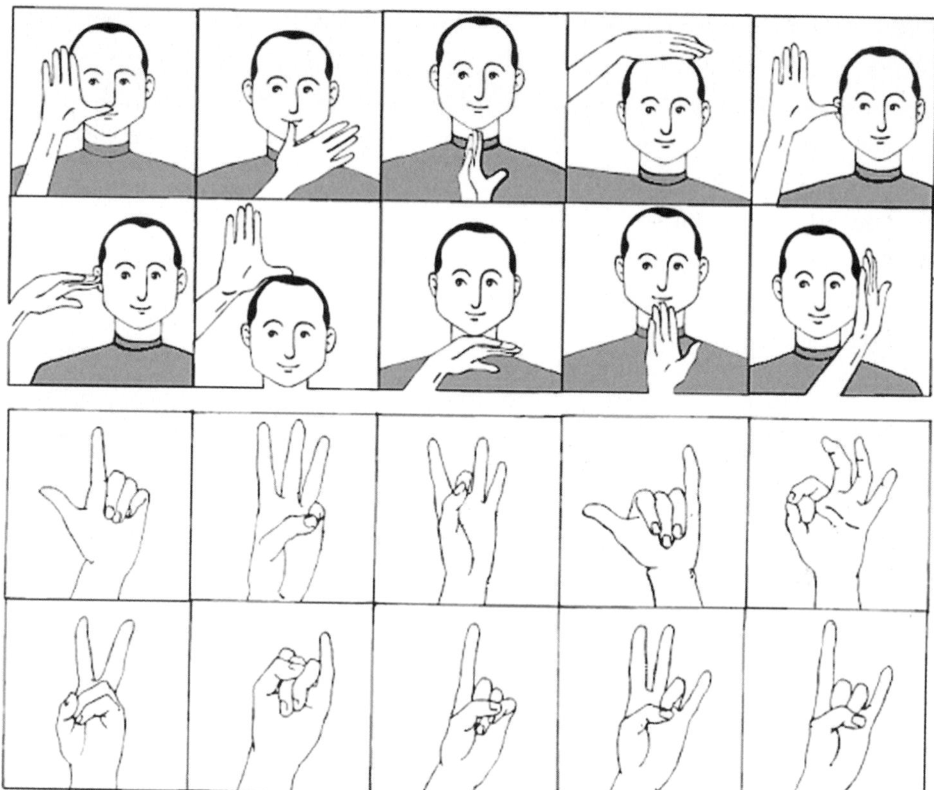

Fig. 5.9 A set of meaningless hand and finger postures for the examination of imitation. As a rule, the patients should use the hand ipsilateral to the lesion. The gestures are presented to the patient in a mirror-like fashion, i.e. if the patient imitates with the left hand, the examiner is presenting with the right and vice versa. The imitation follows the presentation after a short delay, but is not performed simultaneously. Only the final position of the hand and the fingers is subject to evaluation; hesitant movements and self-corrections are not taken into account. When testing the imitation of finger postures, only the final position of the fingers (but not of the hand) is evaluated. If the required end position is not reached in the first attempt, a second attempt is undertaken. For correct imitation in the first run two points are granted and in the 2nd only one point. The cut-off score for the hand-positions is 18 and for the finger-positions is 17; lower values are regarded as pathological (Goldenberg 1996, 2003).

errors can also be observed in patients with right-hemispherical lesions. For testing of visual imitation of hand and finger gestures, a set of 10 (more or less) meaningless hand and finger gestures (Fig. 5.9) can be used (Goldenberg 1996).

The investigation of imitation in 'mirror-like' fashion has proven to be most effective (see Fig. 5.9). The right hand of the examiner is imitated with the left hand of the patient (and vice versa). According to Poeck (2002) the commands to perform meaningless gestures shown in the box can also be used to test the ability to pantomime.

A set of commands for meaningless gestures to test the ability to pantomime (Poeck 2002)

- After performing a wide bow in the air place open hand on the contralateral shoulder
- Place back of hand on forehead
- Place palm close to left ear
- Place fist on chest
- Make a cross in the air with hand
- Make a circle in the air with fist
- Place closed hand on top of head
- Place the open hand on the neck
- Bend elbow and place hand on hip
- Touch chin with fingertips

Performance of meaningful gestures on command Pantomime of object use belongs to the category of meaningful gestures that can be tested on command. The form of these gestures is determined by the pragmatic characteristics of the object and the situational context. Furthermore, gestures with a communicative character or with a predefined meaning in a certain cultural context can be tested (e.g. 'to drive by hitchhikers' or 'to tap one's head at somebody').

While testing the pantomime of object use, the examiner verbally asks the patients to demonstrate the use of certain objects spontaneously and without seeing them. If the patients, in particular aphasic patients, are not able to understand the command, an object can be presented to them. Despite the considerable variance in the individual strategies of pantomime of object use and the occasionally difficult distinction between a normal and a pathological performance, the typical errors in the movement execution listed here are still suitable for diagnosis of apraxia. A section from the 'pantomime and drawing' test designed by Goldenberg (2003) is validated for the quantitative assessment of pantomime of object use (see box). Standard values have been worked out for this test and it contains exact guidelines for the evaluation of pantomimes.

Screening test for pantomine of object use

Criteria are given for the evaluation of four different pantomimes of object use that are part of the 'pantomine and drawing' test (Goldenberg 2003; Goldenberg *et al.* 2003). When naming an object, the real object or a picture thereof should also be demonstrated. If the pantomine fails at the first attempt, the examiner should demonstrate the correct performance, in order to facilitate the understanding for the task. Coarse deviations and the absence of several characteristic components of several pantomines are pathological.

The four pantomimes of object use and their characteristic components are as follows.

- Drinking from glass:
  - wide cylinder grasp;
  - movement until just before mouth;
  - tilting motion.

Screening test for pantomine of object use *(continued)*

- Brushing teeth:
  - lateral grasp or narrow cylinder grasp;
  - repetitive movement;
  - distance from mouth.
- Ironing:
  - narrow cylinder grasp, pronation;
  - large amplitude movement parallel to the table;
  - distance from the table.
- Cutting paper with scissors:
  - finger bent, opposition of the thumb;
  - opening and closing;
  - finger movement perpendicular to the table;
  - movement of the whole hand parallel to the table.

Poeck (2003) suggested another set of 10 gestures involving object use or with a conventional meaning that can be used in examining the ability to execute meaningful gestures (see box).

Examination of the ability to execute meaningful gestures on verbal command (suggested by Poeck 2003)

- Imitate a movement as when smoking a cigarette!
- Imitate, as if you were drinking alcohol!
- Tap your head!
- Cock a snook!
- Make a movement as when combing!
- Wave!
- Perform a rejecting hand movement!
- Make a threatening gesture with the hand!
- Perform a movement as when brushing teeth!
- Salute like soldiers!

Finally, the following box lists some instructions that can be used in testing for buccofacial apraxia.

Testing for buccofacial apraxia (Poeck 2002)

- Please wrinkle your nose!
- Bare your teeth!
- Stick out your tongue!
- Lick your lips!
- Blow out your cheeks!
- Smack!
- Click your tongue making a sound like a horse galloping!
- Purse your lips!
- Make a hissing sound!
- Clear your throat!

5.4.5.2 Localization

Ideomotor apraxia is generally associated with lesions of the language dominant hemisphere. The imitation of simple and complex movements can be affected after lesions of the left frontal and parietal cortex; this deficit can be seen more frequently after lesions of the parietal cortex (De Renzi *et al.* 1983). Many patients with lesions of the left parietal lobe seem to have difficulties in executing and analysing movements that refer to their own body schema (Halsband *et al.* 2001). The lateralization of the deficiency in imitation of meaningless movements is specific for the body part. Left brain lesions affect imitation of hand and foot postures more than that of finger postures. Right brain lesions do not have an influence on hand postures and only a slight one on foot postures, but may cause marked deficits in imitation of finger postures (Goldenberg 1996). Within the left hemisphere, lesions of the lower parietal lobe (supramarginal gyrus) are particularly important.

Deficits of pantomime of transitive (object-related) movements are seen predominantly after left hemispheric lesions. Conversely, deficits in the pantomime of intransitive (not object-related) movements seem to be distributed over both hemispheres (Haaland and Flaherty 1984). Patients with right hemisphere lesions do not have problems with pantomiming meaningful gestures.

5.4.5.3 Therapy and relevance

Many patients with ideomotor apraxia are impaired in their everyday life (Ochipa and Gonzales-Rothi 2000) and therefore need significantly more assistance than non-apraxic patients (Sundet *et al.* 1988). The deficit in the ability to imitate can also have a negative influence on motor learning in physical and occupational therapy. The inability to express the meaning of objects or actions by gestures reduces the ability of patients with severe aphasia to compensate for their language deficits by non-verbal communication (Borod *et al.* 1989). Therefore 'gesture training' can provide positive results.

5.4.6 Polymodal apraxias: ideational apraxia

5.4.6.1 Diagnosis

The impairment of object and tool use is a cardinal symptom of ideational apraxia (De Renzi and Luchelli 1988; Morlaas 1928; Poeck 1982). There is still uncertainty as to whether the impairment of the use of single objects belongs to the symptom complex of ideational apraxia so that ideational apraxia can be defined as a specific disturbance of the object use or whether the ideational apraxia is rather characterized by the inability to perform purposeful serial movements or movement sequences (Liepmann 1908; Pick 1905). Patients with ideational apraxia are severely impaired in their daily life.

In the clinical routine it is important to examine the use of objects intensively. The use of tools and objects embraces a broad spectrum from the routine use of everyday simple tools (e.g. a comb or a toothbrush) up to solving complex mechanical problems or organizing complex actions with several objects or handling technical and electronic equipment.

In order to accomplish an object-oriented action, we need to know about the semantic context (in which the object is used) or to derive the object's function from its mechanical characteristics. In the neurological investigation, it is best to stick to the routine use of familiar tools and objects. The patient is given the necessary objects, e.g. scissors and paper, a lock with a key, a hammer and a nail, and is asked to demonstrate their use. In the case of patients with hemiplegia, the objects must be prepared for one-handed use (e.g. the nail is already positioned in the block). Apraxic errors can be recognized easily. For example, patients press the hammer on the nail instead of pounding or try to cut with closed scissors. As an example of a complex movement sequence patients can try punching holes into a sheet of paper and putting it into a file. It is important that the patients show the ability to perform sequential actions with several objects in a logical order so that the aim of the action can be recognized.

Typical examples of complex 'naturalistic' actions that can be used for detailed testing of ideational apraxia (Poeck and Lehmkuhl 1980) are the following.

- Making coffee. A pot with water, a cup on a saucer, a spoon, a jar of instant coffee, and an immersion heater are to be used in the correct order in order to make coffee.
- Put a letter into an envelope and address and frank the letter. Fold a letter, put it into an envelope, seal the envelope, address, and frank the letter.

Actions that require some technical knowledge, such as insertion of batteries and of a cassette into a tape recorder in order to hear music, can also be employed (Hartmann *et al.* 2005).

The typical errors of patients with ideational apraxia during the execution of complex movements are the following.

- The logical sequence of individual movements is not kept, e.g. objects are used in the wrong order.
- Individual movements that belong to the complex action are omitted or repeated in a perserverative manner.

5.4.6.2 Localization

Most patients with ideational apraxia have large lesions that include the temporo-parietal region in the language dominant hemisphere. Comparative studies on patients with right- and left-hemispheric lesions that examined the use of individual objects or tool–object pairs revealed deficits in these activities only in left-hemispheric patients (De Renzi *et al.* 1968; Goldenberg and Hagmann 1998). Patients with left-hemispheric lesions have difficulties in selecting objects appropriate to movements that are shown to them as pantomimes of the object's use (Gainotti and Lemmo 1976; Vaina *et al.* 1995; Varney 1978). They also have difficulties in pantomiming object-associated movements (Barbieri and De Renzi 1988; Goldenberg and Hagmann 1998; Goodglass and Kaplan 1963) or with the selection of objects that are to serve the same purpose (De Renzi *et al.* 1969; Rumiati *et al.* 2001; Vignolo 1990). The integrity of the left hemisphere is crucial for establishing the association of tools with purpose, recipient, and action, and the inference of function from structure.

While deficits in the use of simple and familiar objects occur exclusively after lesions of the left hemisphere, patients with right-hemispheric lesions have problems in performing complex actions with several objects, in particular, if the objects are unfamiliar and the correct use has to be found (Hartmann *et al.* 2005; Schwartz *et al.* 1999). 'Naturalistic' multistep actions, like making coffee, can be even more impaired in right-hemispheric patients.

5.4.6.3 Therapy and relevance

Of those patients, who were apraxic in the first week post-onset of infarction, approximately half were still apraxic after 3 months and approximately 20% remained apraxic (Basso *et al.* 1987; Kertesz and Ferro 1984). In a study regarding the efficacy of training in activities of daily living (ADL), Goldenberg and Hagmann (1998) found that patients with a right hemiparesis, aphasia, and apraxia did not show any tendency to improve in everyday activities, such as putting on a sweater or brushing teeth, within a period of 3 months. So-called 'strategy training', in which the patients were asked, for example, to verbalize or to write notes about their own actions or to point at pictures of an already existing action sequence in the correct order, showed positive effects in comparison to a conventional physiotherapeutical treatment (Donkervoort *et al.* 2001; van Heugten *et al.* 2000).

In a 'cross- over' study Goldenberg *et al.* (2001) compared the direct exercise of daily activities with 'exploratory training', in which patients learned to derive possible functions of objects from their structural characteristics. A clear reduction in faulty actions and the patient's need for assistance could be found only after the direct training, in which concrete ADL activities were learned. On the other hand, the patients could not concretely use the new insights about object use they gained from the exploration training. Also, the abilities gained in direct training could not be generally transferred to situations outside of the therapeutic framework (Goldenberg *et al.* 2001). Apparently, only those patients who practise on a regular basis can keep the level of improvement high (Goldenberg and Hagmann 1998); patients who stop practising deteriorate. The therapeutic aims for patients with ideational apraxia should be strongly oriented towards the domestic environment and based on the desires of the patients and their family members.

5.5 **Summary**

Apraxias are deficits of higher motor behaviour that are not primarily caused by elementary deficits of the sensorimotor system, communication problems, or dementia. The patients present with deficits in imitating meaningful or meaningless gestures, purposeful use of objects, or dexterity. The different forms of apraxia originate from lesions of different levels/structures of the motor system, reflecting its complexity. Apraxias are caused by deficits in motor programmes generated in the frontal motor areas (executive apraxias, e.g. limb-kinetic apraxia), in the modality-specific higher sensorimotor control (unimodal apraxias, e.g. tactile apraxia, optic apraxia), or at the highest level of motor planning and motor conception (polymodal apraxias, i.e. ideomotor and ideational apraxias). Polymodal apraxias typically result from left hemisphere lesions and are therefore often, but not necessarily, observed in combination with aphasia. The different types of apraxia differentially affect the activities of daily living and hence show marked differences in the prognosis of recovery and the need of physiotherapeutic treatment. Therefore, diagnosis and appropriate treatment of the different forms of apraxia is of foremost clinical importance.

Acknowledgements

The authors thank Professor Georg Goldenberg, Professor Gereon R. Fink, Dr Peter Weiss-Blankenhorn, and Adam McNamara for valuable suggestions concerning this chapter.

References

Alexander, M.P., Benson, D.F., and Stuss, D.T. (1989). Frontal lobes and language. *Brain Lang.* **37**, 656–91.

Assmus, A., Marshall, J.C., Ritzl, A., Noth, J., Zilles, K., Fink, G.R. (2003). Left inferior parietal cortex integrates time and space during collision judgments. *Neuroimage* **20**, S82–8.

Balint, R. (1909). Seelenhamung des 'Schauens', optische Ataxie, räumlische Störung des Aufmerksamkeit. *Monatsschr. Psychiatrie Neurol.* **25**, 51–81.

Barbieri, C. and De Renzi, E. (1988). The executive and ideational components of apraxia. *Cortex* **24**, 535–44.

Basso, A., Capitani, E., Della Sala, S., *et al.* (1987). Recovery from ideomotor apraxia—a study on acute stroke patients. *Brain* **110**, 747–60.

Binkofski, F. and Buccino, G. (2004). Motor functions of the Broca's region. *Brain Lang.* **89**, 362–9.

Binkofski, F., Dohle, C., Posse, S., Hefter, H., Seitz, R.J., and Freund, H-J. (1998). Human anterior intraparietal area subserves prehension. A combined lesion and fMRI study. *Neurology* **50**, 1253–9.

Binkofski, F., Buccino, G., Dohle, C., Seitz, R.J., and Freund, H-J. (1999*a*). Mirror agnosia and mirror ataxia constitute different parietal lobe disorders. *Ann. Neurol.* **46**, 51–61.

Binkofski, F., Buccino, G., Posse, S., Seitz, R.J., Rizzolatti, G., and Freund, H-J. (1999*b*). A fronto-parietal circuit for object manipulation in man. Evidence from a fMRI-study. *Eur. J. Neurosci.* **11**, 3276–86.

Binkofski, F., Kunesch, E., Classen, J., Seitz, R.J., and Freund, H-J. (2001). Tactile apraxia: an unimodal disorder of tactile object exploration associated with parietal lesions. *Brain* **124**, 132–44.

Binkofski, F., Butler, A.J., Buccino, G., Heide, W., Freund, H-J., Fink, G.R., and Seitz, R.J. (2003). Mirror apraxia is affecting the peripersonal mirror space. A combined lesion and cerebral activation study. *Exp. Brain Res.* **153**, 210–19.

Binkofski, F., Ertelt, D., Dettmers, C., and Buccino, G. (2004). The role of the mirror neuron system in neurorehabilitation. *Neurol. Rehabil.* **10**, 1–10.

Bodegård, A., Ledberg, A., Geyer, S., Naito, E., Zilles, K., and Roland PE (2000). Object shape differences reflected by somatosensory cortical activation. *J. Neurosci.* **20**, RC51.

Borod, J.C., Fitzpatrick, P.M., Helm-Estabrooks, M., and Goodglass, H. (1989). The relationship between limb apraxia and the spontaneous use of communicative gesture in aphasia. *Brain Cogn.* **10**, 121–31.

Bremmer, F., Schlack, A., Shah, N.J., *et al.* (2001). Polymodal motion processing in posterior parietal and premotor cortex: a human fMRI study strongly implies equivalencies between humans and monkeys. *Neuron* **29**, 287–96.

Buccino, G., Binkofski, F., Fink, G.R., *et al.* (2001). Action observation activates premotor and parietal areas in a somatotopic manner: an fMRI study. *Eur. J. Neurosci.* **13**, 400–4.

Buxbaum, L.J. and Coslett, H.B. (1998). Spatio-motor representations in reaching: evidence for subtypes of optic ataxia. *Cogn. Neuropsychol.* **15**, 279–312.

Buxbaum, L.J., Schwartz, M.F., and Carew, T.G. (1997). The role of semantic memory in object use. *Cogn. Neuropsychol.* **14**, 219–54.

Caselli, R.J. (1993). Ventrolateral and dorsomedial somatosensory association cortex damage produces distinct somesthetic syndromes in humans. *Neurology* **43**, 762–71.

Cooper, R. and Shallice, T. (2000). Contention scheduling and the control of routine activities. *Cogn. Neuropsychol.* **17**, 297–338.

Delay, J-P.L. (1935). *Les astéréognosies: pathologie du toucher.* Masson, Paris.

De Renzi, E. (1989). Apraxia. In *Handbook of neuropsychology* (ed. F. Boller and J. Grafman), pp. 245–63. Elsevier, Amsterdam.

De Renzi, E. and Luchelli, F. (1988). Ideational apraxia. *Brain* **111**, 1173–85.

De Renzi, E., Pieczuro, A., and Vignolo, L.A. (1968). Ideational apraxia: a quantitative study. *Neuropsychologia* **6**, 41–55.

De Renzi, E., Scotti, G., and Spinnler, H. (1969). Perceptual and associative disorders of visual recognition. *Neurology* **19**, 634–42.

De Renzi, E., Faglioni, P., Lodesani, M., *et al.* (1983). Performance of left brain damaged patients on imitation of single movements and motor sequences. Frontal and parietal injured patients compared. *Cortex* **19**, 333–43.

Donkervoort, M., Dekker, J., Stehmann-Saris, J.C., and Deelman, G.B. (2001). Efficacy of strategy training in left hemisphere stroke with apraxia: a rendomized clinical trial. *Rehabil. Psychol.* **11**, 549–66.

Dronkers, N.F. (1996). A new brain region for coordinating speech articulation. *Nature* **384**, 159–61.

Ehrsson, H.H., Geyer, S., and Naito, E. (2003). Imagery of voluntary movement of fingers, toes, and tongue activates corresponding body-part-specific motor representations. *J. Neurophysiol.* **90**, 3304–16.

Ferro, J. (1984). Transient inaccuracy in reaching caused by a posterior parietal lobe lesion. *J. Neurol. Neurosurg. Psychiatry* **47**, 1016–19.

Freund, H-J. (1992). The apraxias. In *Diseases of the nervous system: clinical neurobiology* (ed. A.K. Asbury, G.M. McKhan, and W.I. McDonald), pp. 751–67. W.B. Saunders, Philadelphia.

Gainotti, G. and Lemmo, M.A. (1976) Comprehension of symbolic gestures in aphasia. *Brain Lang.* **3**, 451–60.

Garcin, R., Rondot, P., and de Recondo, J. (1967). Optic ataxia localized in 2 left homonymous visual hemifields (clinical study with film presentation). *Rev. Neurol. (Paris)*, **116**, 707–14.

Goldenberg, G. (1996). Defective imitation of gestures in patients with damage in the left or right hemisphere. *J. Neurol. Neurosurg. Psychiatry* **61**, 176–80.

Goldenberg, G. (2001). Imitation and matching of hand and finger postures. *Neuroimage* **14**, S132–36.

Goldenberg, G. (2003). The neuropsychological assessment and treatment of disorders of voluntary movement. In *Handbook of clinical neuropsychology* (ed. P. Halligan, U. Kischka, and J.C. Marshall), pp. 340–52. Oxford University Press, Oxford.

Goldenberg, G. (2006). Apraxie. In *Klinische neuropsychologie* (ed. H.O. Karnath and P. Thier), pp. 337–50. Springer, Berlin.

Goldenberg, G. and Hagmann, S. (1998). Tool use and mechanical problem solving in apraxia *Neuropsychologia* **36**, 581–9.

Goldenberg, G., Daumüller, M., and Hagmann, S. (2001). Assessment and therapy of complex ADL in apraxia. *Rehabil. Psychol.* **11**, 147–68.

Goldenberg, G., Hartmann, K., and Schlott, I. (2003). Defective pantomime of object use in left brain damage: apraxia or asymbolia? *Neuropsychologia* **41**, 1565–73.

Goodglass, H. and Kaplan, E. (1963). Disturbance of gesture and pantomime in aphasia. *Brain* **86**, 703–20.

Gréa, H., Pisella, L., Rossetti, Y., Desmurget, M., Tilikete, C., Prablanc, C., and Vighetto, A. (2002). A Lesion of the posterior parietal cortex disrupts on-line adjustments during aiming movements. *Neuropsychologia* **40**, 2471–80.

Grefkes, C., Weiss, P.H., Zilles, K., and Fink, G.R. (2002). Crossmodal processing of object features in human anterior intraparietal cortex: an fMRI study implies equivalencies between humans and monkeys. *Neuron* **35**, 173–84.

Grefkes, C., Ritzl, A., Zilles, K., and Fink, G.R. (2004). Human medial intraparietal cortex subserves visuomotor coordinate transformation. *Neuroimage* **23**, 1494–506.

Haaland, K.Y. and Flaherty, D. (1984). The different types of limb apraxia errors made by patients with left vs. right hemisphere damage. *Brain Cogn.* **3**, 370–84.

Haaxma, R. and Kuypers, H.G. (1975). Intrahemispheric cortical connexions and visual guidance of hand and finger movements in the rhesus monkey. *Brain* **98**, 239–60.

Halsband, U., Ito, N., Tanji, J., and Freund, H-J. (1993). The role of premotor cortex and the supplementary motor area in the temporal control of movements in man. *Brain* **116**, 243–66.

Halsband, U., Schmitt, J., Weyers, M., Binkofski, F., *et al.* (2001). Recognition and imitation of pantomimed motor acts after unilateral parietal and premotor lesions: a perspective on apraxia. *Neuropsychologia* **39**, 200–16.

Hartmann, K., Goldenberg, G., Daumüller, M., and Hermsdörfer, J. (2005). It takes the whole brain to make a cup of coffee: the neuropsychology of naturalistic actions involving technical devices. *Neuropsychologia* **43**, 625–37.

Head, H. and Holmes, G. (1911). Sensory disturbances from cerebral lesions. *Brain* **34**, 102–254.

Hodges, J.R., Bozeat, S., Lambon Ralph, M.A., *et al.* (2000). The role of conceptual knowledge in object use—evidence from semantic dementia. *Brain* **123**, 1913–25.

Jeannerod, M. (1986). Mechanisms of visuo-motor coordination: a study of normal and brain-damaged subjects. *Neuropsychologia* **24**, 41–78.

Jeannerod, M., Arbib, M.A., Rizzolatti, G., and Sakata, H. (1995). Grasping objects: the cortical mechanism of visuomotor transformation. *Trends Neurosci.* **18**, 314–20.

Johnson-Frey, S.H., Maloof, F.R., Newman-Norlund, R., *et al.* (2003). Actions or hand–object interactions? Human inferior frontal cortex and action observation. *Neuron* **39**, 1053–8.

Kertesz, A. and Ferro, J.M. (1984). Lesion size and location in ideomotor apraxia. *Brain* **107**, 921–33.

Klein, R. (1931). Zur Symptomatologie des Parietallappens. *Z. Gesamte Neurol. Psychiatrie* **135**, 589–608.

Kleist, K. (1911). Der Gang und der gegenwärtige Stand der Apraxieforschung. *Ergeb. Neurol. Psychiatrie* **1**, 342–452.

Lederman, J.L. and Klatzky, R.L. (1997). Haptic aspects of motor control. In *Handbook of neuropsychology* (ed. F. Boller and J. Grafman), Vol. 11, pp. 131–47. Elsevier, Amsterdam.

Leiguarda, R.C. and Marsden, C.D. (2000). Limb apraxias. Higher order disorders of sensorimotor integration. *Brain* **123**, 860–79.

Liepmann, H. (1908). *Drei Aufsätze aus dem Apraxiegebiet.* Karger, Berlin.

Liepmann, H. (1920). Apraxie. In *Ergebnisse der gesamten Medizin* (ed. H. Brugsch), pp. 516–43. Urban and Schwarzenberg, Vienna.

Liepold, M., Ziegler, W., and Brendel, B. (2002). *Hierarchische Wortlisten: Ein Nachsprechtest für die Sprechapraxiediagnostik.* Verlag Modernes Lernen Borgmann KG, Dortmund.

Luria, A.R. (1966). *Higher cortical functions in man.* Basic Books, New York.

Mayer, N.H., Reed, E., Schwartz, M.F., *et al.* (1990). Buttering a hot cup of coffee: an approach to the study of errors of action in patients with brain damage. In *The neuropsychology of everyday life: assessment and basic competencies* (ed. D.E. Tupper and K.D. Cicerone), pp. 259–84. Kluwer Academic Publishers, Boston.

Milner, A.D. and Goodale, M.A. (1995). *The visual brain in action.* Oxford University Press, Oxford.

Morlaas, J. (1928). *Contribution à l'etude de l'apraxie.* Amèdèe Legrand, Paris.

Norman, D.A. (1989). *The design of everyday things.* Doubleday, New York.

Ochipa, C. and Gonzales-Rothi, L.J. (2000). Limb apraxia. *Semin. Neurol.* **20**, 471–8.

Perenin, M-T. and Vighetto, A. (1988). Optic ataxia: a specific disruption in visuomotor mechanisms. I. Different aspects of the deficit in reaching for objects. *Brain* **111**, 643–74.

Pick, A. (1905). *Studien zur motorischen Apraxia und ihr nahestende Erscheinungen; ihre Bedeutung in der Symptomatologie Psychopathischer Symptomenkomplexe.* Franz Deuticke, Leipzig.

Pisella, L., Gréa, H., Tiliket, C., Vighetto, A., Desmurget, M., Rode, G., Boisson, D., and Rossetti, Y. (2000). An automatic pilot for the hand in the human posterior parietal cortex toward a reinterpretation of optic ataxia. *Nature Neurosci.* **3**, 729–36.

Poeck, K. (1982). The two types of motor apraxia. *Arch. Ital. Biol.* **120**, 361–9.

Poeck, K. (2002) Apraxie. In *Klinische Neuropsychologie* (ed. W. Hartje and K. Poeck), pp. 227–38. Thieme, Stuttgart.

Poeck, K. and Lehmkuhl, G. (1980). Das Syndrom der ideatorischen Apraxie und seine Lokalisation. *Nervenarzt* **51**, 217–25.

Ratcliff, G. and Davies-Jones, G.A. (1972). Defective visual localization in focal brain wounds. *Brain* **95**, 49–60.

Rizzolatti, G. and Luppino, G. (2001). The cortical motor system. *Neuron* **31**, 889–901.

Rizzolatti, G. and Matelli, G. (2003). Two different streams form the dorsal visual system: anatomy and functions. *Exp. Brain Res.* **153**, 146–57.

Rizzolatti, G., Fogassi, L., and Gallese, V. (1997). Parietal cortex: from sight to action. *Curr. Opin. Neurobiol.* **7**, 562–7.

Rizzolatti, G., Fogassi, L., and Gallese, V. (2001). Neurophysiological mechanisms underlying the understanding and imitation of action. *Nature Rev. Neurosci.* **2**, 661–70.

Rossetti, Y. and Pisella, L. (2002) Several 'vision for action' systems: A guide to dissociating and integrating dorsal and ventral functions. In *Attention and performance XIX: common mechnisms in perception and action* (ed. W. Prinz and B. Hommel), pp. 62–119. Oxford University Press, Oxford.

Rossetti, Y., Pisella, L., and Vigheto, A. (2003). Optic ataxia revisited: visually guided action versus immediate visuomotor control. *Exp. Brain Res.* **153**, 171–9.

Roy, E.A. and Hall, C. (1992). Limb apraxia: a process approach. In *Vision and Motor Control* (ed. L. Proteau and D. Elliott), pp. 261–82. Elsevier, Amsterdam,

Rumiati, R.I., Zanini, S., Vorano, L., and Shallice, T. (2001). A form of ideational apraxia as a selective deficit of contention scheduling. *Cogn. Neuropsychol.* **18**, 617–42.

Rumiati, R.I., Weiss, P.H., Shallice, T., Ottoboni, G., Noth, J., Zilles, K., and Fink, G.R. (2004). Neural basis of pantomiming the use of visually presented objects. *Neuroimage* **21**, 1224–31.

Schiff, H.B., Alexander, M.P., Naeser, M.A., and Galaburda, A.M. (1983). Aphemia: clinical-anatomic correlations. *Arch. Neurol.* **40**, 720–7.

Schwartz, M.F., Buxbaum, L.J., Montgomery, M.W., *et al.* (1999). Naturalistic action production following right hemisphere stroke. *Neuropsychologia* **37**, 51–66.

Servos, P., Lederman, S., Wilson, D., and Gati, J. (2001). fMRI-derived cortical maps for haptic shape, texture, and handedness. *Brain Res. Cogn. Brain Res.* **12**, 307–13.

Steinthal, H. (1871, 1881). *Einleitung in die Psychologie und Sprachwissenschaft (Band I): Abriss der Sprachwissenschaft.* Duemmler, Berlin.

Sundet, K., Finset, A., and Reinvang, I. (1988). Neuropsychological predictors in stroke rehabilitation. *J. Clin. Exp. Psychol.* **10**, 363–79.

Taub, E., Useatte, G., and Elbert, T. (2002). New treatments in neurorehabilitation founded on basic research. *Nature Rev. Neurosci.* **3**, 226–36.

Umilta, M.A., Kohler, E., Gallese, V., Fogassi, L., Fadiga, L., Keysers, C., and Rizzolatti, G. (2001). I know what you are doing, a neurophysiological study. *Neuron* **31**, 155–65.

Vaina, L.M., Goodglass, H., and Daltroy, L. (1995). Inference of object use from pantomimed actions by aphasics and patients with right hemisphere lesions. *Synthese* **104**, 43–57.

van Heugten, C.M., Dekker, J., Deelman, B.G., *et al.* (2000). Rehabilitation of stroke patients with apraxia: the role of additional cognitive and motor impairments. *Disabil. Rehabil.* **22**, 547–54.

Varney, N.R. (1978). Linguistic correlates of pantomime recognition in aphasic patients. *J. Neurol. Neurosurg. Psychiatry* **41**, 564–8.

Vignolo, L.A. (1990) Non-verbal conceptual impairment in aphasia. In *Handbook of clinical neuropsychology* (ed. F. Boller and J. Grafman), pp. 185–206. Elsevier, Amsterdam.

Wernicke, C. (1876). Das Urwindungssystem den menschlichen Gehirns. *Arch. Psychiatrischen Nervenkrankh.* **6**, 298–326.

Chapter 6

Spatial disorders

Angelo Maravita

6.1 Introduction

Our daily life is characterized by continuous interactions with the space around us. For example, when we see an object of interest or hear the voice of a friend, we may wish to orient our eyes or head towards that sensory stimulation. We may even want to stand up from our chair, walk around the desk, and reach a person on the other side of the room to shake his/her hand or go out from our office and orient through city streets in order to reach a given place. Also, many times in the day, we grasp and manipulate objects of interest or tasty foods.

In order to accomplish all these tasks we must keep a constantly updated representation of our own body and the external, or extrapersonal, space. Such critical functions can be severely affected by brain damage. In this chapter some of the deficits of spatial cognition that can be observed in clinical practice will be described and related to current knowledge about the neural substrates of space representation in the human and animal brain.

6.1.1 Space representation through multiple frames of reference

Space representation is a very complex neurological function. Spatial locations are coded relative to different 'perspectives' that are usually referred to as **frames of reference**. In particular, any object in external space is represented relative to the observer's body midline, or better still to the observer's midsagittal plane. This is the so-called *egocentric* reference frame. Usually, when we say that something is on the left or on the right, we imply this kind of reference frame where space is coded relatively to the whole body of the observer. In other cases egocentric space representation may be referred to a single body part. Typically, for example, although the left hand can be moved from the left to the right side across the body midline, its little finger always remains the leftmost finger of the hand. By contrast, the little finger of the left hand may assume the rightmost position within the hand, when the hand is placed palm-up.

Furthermore, any object placed on the left or the right of a hypothetical observer's midsagittal plane has its own left and right. For instance, a mug may have its handle oriented towards the left or right, regardless of its position relative to an observer. This is called *allocentric* or *object-centred* reference frame.

Thanks to anatomical and electrophysiological studies in animals, it is now known that different neural structures code space in different perspectives and work in parallel to give us a unitary representation of the external space. In anatomical terms, the first cortical representation of visual space is that occurring in V1. This is the so-called *retinotopic* representation, whereby any stimulus in the visual field is projected to a given location in V1. In this case, the anatomical correspondence of the left and right visual fields is relative to the different hemispheres, with a contralateral representation of each visual field. This kind of representation is, of course, completely linked to eye position since the first map that is formed, and then transferred to V1, is that on the retina. However, other neurons represent space relative to the head while totally (or partially) ignoring the absolute spatial projection of the stimulus on the retina. For example, neurons in parietal cortex may represent left and right space relative to the animal's head, while eye position may be largely irrelevant (e.g. Duhamel *et al.* 1997; Rizzolatti *et al.* 1997) or only partially modulate the neuronal response (see, for example, Andersen *et al.* 1997). In this case, a more *egocentric, non-retinotopic* space representation occurs.

Recent neuroimaging data in humans have helped to clarify the neural networks subserving space representation according to egocentric versus allocentric frames of reference. Galati and colleagues (2000) asked normal observers to judge the position (left or right) of a vertical segment drawn over an horizontal line. The lines could be overall shifted to the left or to the right relative to the observer's midsagittal plane and the segments could be placed to the left or right of the line's objective midpoint. Two different tasks were required. In the first task subjects had to evaluate the spatial position of the vertical segment relatively to the observer's body midline ('egocentric' frame of reference). In the second task, the position of the vertical segment had to be performed relative to the objective midpoint of the horizontal line ('allocentric' frame of reference). The patterns of brain activation showed the existence of rather overlapping, but different cortical circuits for the two tasks. In the first (egocentric) task activations included the parietal cortex (superior and inferior parietal lobules) from the medial surface down to the temporo-parietal junction, and the lateral premotor cortex (superior and inferior frontal gyri; see also Vallar *et al.* 1999). Activations were observed bilaterally, although those in the right hemisphere were found to be much wider. In the second task, again a fronto-parietal network was activated, this time centred on the superior parietal and intraparietal region and superior frontal sulcus of the right hemisphere.

However, space coding may require different neural mechanisms depending on the space sector considered. In particular, in the last 20 years, thanks to the neurosciences and neuropsychology, the notion of space representation has been progressively integrated with that of action planning and execution. In this view space representation has been considered less and less as the mere construction of a 'map' of external space, where we can represent objects of interest, and more and more as the locus of integration between perception, action, and awareness. In this view, the neural coding of an object in external space is closely linked to the neural processing necessary to grasp or manipulate that particular object (e.g. see Rizzolatti *et al.* 1997, 1998). To this aim a critical distinction has to be made between a near or *peripersonal* space, where objects can be reached and manipulated, and a far or *extrapersonal* space that is beyond hand's grasp. Since the 1980s, the difference between these representations of space has been made clear by cortical ablation studies in the monkey. For example, while the ablation of the frontal prearcuate area 8 of the macaque monkey would produce a lack of awareness and reaction to contralateral stimuli in far space, ablation of the postarcuate area 6 would produce similar deficits but limited to the space near the animal's body (Rizzolatti *et al.* 1983). Now it is known that these frontal areas represent space according to the kind of action that can be performed in different space sectors (reaching, grasping, eye movements), thanks to their rich interconnections with selective portions of the parietal cortex (e.g. Rizzolatti *et al.* 1998).

6.1.2 Space representation through multisensory integration

In recent years there is a key aspect of space representation that has received much interest from the point of view of the cognitive neurosciences. In natural conditions, the majority of stimuli in external space, both far from and near to the body, present to our senses as a combination of multisensory information (e.g. Calvert *et al.* 2004). Often, when we see a dog or a car the visual stimulation is accompanied by a barking or roaring sound. Furthermore, when we catch a ball the vision of the approaching ball is accompanied by a tactile sensation when the ball contacts our hand. Our brain is equipped to integrate multisensory input in order to give us a seamless, unitary perception of the outside world. The importance of such an effective multisensory integration is that of increasing our efficiency in orienting towards, detecting, and manipulating external objects. For example, it is faster and easier to visually detect and orient towards a bird hidden among tree branches if we can also hear it twittering. Here integration of vision and audition is critical. On the other hand, when we want to reach and manipulate an object, tactile and proprioceptive inputs are critically integrated with visual ones.

The fundamental work by Berry Stein and co-workers has shown extensively that neurons in the deep layers of the cat's superior colliculus (SC) typically respond to multiple sensory modalities (vision, touch, audition; Stein and Meredith 1993). For example, both acoustic and visual stimuli can make the same SC neuron discharge (multisensory neuron). One critical feature of such multisensory responses is that they occur at their best when visual and auditory stimulation are in spatial register (the so-called *spatial rule*) or temporally synchronous (*temporal rule*). In these conditions some multisensory neurons discharge at a higher frequency than the sum of the discharge rates produced by the same neuron to each single unimodal stimulus (*supra-additive multisensory enhancement*). In behavioural studies, it has been shown that this enhanced neural discharge observed with spatially coincident multisensory stimuli corresponds to a faster and more accurate orienting of the animal towards the spatial location of a given stimulus. The SC is then a key structure for multisensory integration, but the role of a number of cortical structures is also critical in this respect. For example, in the cat, the ectosylvian cortex and the lateral suprasylvian sulcus include neurons discharging in response to both unimodal and multisensory stimuli, and critically exert a descending modulation of the activity of multisensory SC neurons (Stein 2005; Wallace and Stein 1994).

Much work has also been conducted on the nature of cortical multisensory integration in the monkey brain. In particular, a very intriguing set of studies has addressed the issue of multisensory space coding in near peripersonal space. Peripersonal acoustic (Graziano *et al.* 1999), visual, and tactile (for a recent review see Maravita *et al.* 2003*b*) stimuli are all specifically coded and integrated in the brain. In particular, in order to control object reaching and manipulation, vision and touch are highly interdependent. In the macaque monkey, around 50% of neurons in ventral premotor cortex (area F4; Fogassi *et al.* 1996), 70% of neurons in the ventral intraparietal area (VIP; Duhamel *et al.* 1998), 20–30% of neurons in the posterior parietal cortex area 7b, and 24% of cells in the putamen (Graziano and Gross 1994) show receptive fields both in the visual (vRF) and the somatosensory (sRF) modalities, meaning that they discharge in response to both visual and tactile stimuli. Typically, also, visual and somatosensory responses are in the spatial register. For instance, if a neuron responds to a touch or a joint displacement on the hand region, a visual response will also occur for stimuli near that hand. A similar pattern of discharge is found for most neurons in areas F4, 7b, and the putamen and for around one-half of VIP neurons (Graziano and Gross 1994; Rizzolatti *et al.* 1981). Critically, each one of these cells codes for a region of peripersonal visual space that is spatially aligned to the preferred sRF of that cell. For example, VIP neurons with somatosensory receptive fields on the right upper face will respond to stimuli presented to the right upper quadrant of the visual field or a premotor neuron with a tactile receptive field on the arm or hand will discharge in response to visual stimuli approaching that body part. These cells constitute a functional network of bimodal neurons subserving a common representation of the body surface and the visual space nearby the body.

Another critical finding is that the spatial selectivity of visual responses for some such multisensory neurons in areas F4, VIP, and putamen is not merely retinotopic. For instance, for many premotor neurons and some neurons in the putamen with a sRF on the arm, the corresponding vRF may shift along with the arm if this is moved in space (e.g. Graziano *et al.* 2002). Also, shifting gaze position while the spatial location of the visual stimulus is kept constant, does not affect (or minimally affects) the firing rate of most neurons in ventral premotor cortex (e.g. Rizzolatti *et al.* 1997) and of a subset of neurons in area VIP that respond to visual stimuli very close (ultra-near stimuli: Colby *et al.* 1993) to the body (Duhamel *et al.* 1998).

This system may be critical for coding space in egocentric coordinates centred on single body parts, thus putting each body part in strict spatial relationship to any visual event that may occur nearby. In this view, it is important that the brain keeps a constantly updated representation of the body surface and position together with that of the space immediately around the body (Graziano and Botvinick 2002; Maravita 2006; Maravita *et al.* 2003*b*).

Much work has also been devoted to multisensory space representation in humans (Calvert *et al.* 2004; Spence and Driver 2004). For example, Frassinetti and co-workers (2002) showed that spatially congruent unattended sounds can improve the perception of below-threshold visual targets in a fashion that is reminiscent, though without any neurophysiological support, of the response enhancement shown by SC audiovisual neurons in response to spatially coincident multisensory stimuli. With functional neuroimaging it has been shown that crossmodal binding of audiovisual stimuli may be critical for cognitive functions of higher order than the simple spatial localization. For example, recent fMRI data in humans have shown that delivering semantically congruent versus incongruent audiovisual speech stimuli significantly modulates the activity in the superior temporal sulcus (Calvert *et al.* 2000, 2004). Within peripersonal space, the neuroimaging work of Macaluso and co-workers (Macaluso and Driver 2003) has highlighted the functional link between vision and touch for spatial attention. In a seminal work, tactile unattended stimuli have been shown to significantly enhance responses in extrastriate visual cortex to attended, spatially coincident visual targets (Macaluso *et al.* 2000). This result suggests that multimodal stimuli may have the effect of increasing the response of unimodal cortical areas via back-projections from multisensory areas thus enhancing spatial perceptual processing.

The knowledge about the integrated neural coding of space and body in the animal and human brain outlined above may be used as a fundamental theoretical framework for interpreting the neural substrates of some spatial disorders that can follow a damage to the human brain. In the following paragraphs, a clinical–functional view of some such neuropsychological conditions, i.e. unilateral spatial neglect (USN), extinction to double stimulation, optic ataxia, Balint's syndrome, and disorders of spatial orientation, will be discussed in order to try and illustrate the nature of spatial representation and body–space interactions. The description of each neuropsychological disorder will be given while trying to merge data from neuropsychology and the neurosciences into a unitary framework.

6.2 **Unilateral spatial neglect**

Unilateral spatial neglect (USN) or neglect is one of the most studied neuropsychological syndromes. This syndrome typically occurs after stroke, neoplastic lesions, and head injury. It has also been reported in cases of Alzheimer's dementia (e.g. Bartolomeo *et al.* 1998). The importance of this syndrome is not only theoretical but also clinical. Indeed, neglect is very frequent after stroke, and its presence can strongly affect the patient's outcome. The incidence of neglect has been recently studied in a large group study involving more than a thousand stroke patients (Ringman *et al.* 2004). Neglect in the acute stage was present in 43% of patients suffering a right brain stroke and in 20% of patients with a left hemispheric stroke. This seems to support the typical bias for neglect after right hemispheric stroke reported in the literature (e.g. Bisiach and Vallar 2000). A similar, although reduced bias was present 3 months after the stroke, when neglect was present in 17% of the right brain-damaged group as compared to the 5% in the left hemispheric group.

Furthermore, neglect has a strongly negative impact on stroke patients' outcome (Jehkonen *et al.* 2006). In particular, the presence of anosognosia has been shown to greatly limit the effect of rehabilitation of hemiplegia (Gialanella *et al.* 2005). Although there is recent evidence for non-spatial deficits in neglect (e.g. Husain and Rorden 2003; Husain *et al.* 1997), this syndrome offers a unique opportunity to explore the effect of brain damage on spatial cognition and awareness (Karnath *et al.* 2002). USN is a complex syndrome where many different symptoms can be present at the same time or double dissociated in different patients. In this presentation the syndrome will be described in its main clinical features, each one of them casting light on a different aspect of space representation. USN can be characterized by a variable degree of *perceptual* impairment. Patients ignore sensory stimulation delivered to the side of space or body that is contralateral to the damaged hemisphere (the so-called *contralesional* space). Perceptual deficits can involve different sensory modalities, as shown below. Furthermore, neglect patients can be affected on the *motor* side, failing to move the contralesional limbs (*motor neglect*) or showing a reluctance to execute movements towards the contralesional space (*directional hypokinesia*).

In all cases, these symptoms cannot simply be explained by a primary sensory (e.g. haemianopia) or motor (e.g. hemiplegia) deficit, although excluding the influence of coexisting primary sensory deficits on neglect may be a challenge for the clinician (see the box).

Primary sensory impairment or neglect?

Although simple sensory deficits cannot explain neglect *per se*, these can often coexist with neglect and, in some patients, their contribution to the overall clinical picture of contralesional imperception may be hard to assess. In particular, sensory deficits have been found to be more frequent after right than left brain damage. This difference suggests a role of neglect, more frequent after right brain damage, in the occurrence of left-sided sensory deficits (Sterzi *et al.* 1993). In recent years it has been shown that, through different kinds of external stimulation, such as caloric vestibular stimulation, optokinetic stimulation, prismatic adaptation, and neck vibration, some sensory deficits occurring after brain damage may show a temporary relief. It is likely that sensory deficits in such cases are due to neglect and not to the lesion of primary sensory pathways that would show no benefit from such external stimulations (Bottini *et al.* 2005; Maravita *et al.* 2003*a*; Vallar *et al.* 1990, 1993*a*,*b*, 1995*b*).

Of course, event-related brain potentials, or even functional imaging, can be used to unequivocally bear witness to the integrity of sensory pathways, since electrical or metabolic brain responses can be observed even if the patient denies any conscious perception (see, for example, Eimer *et al.* 2002; Vuilleumier *et al.* 2001). However, these techniques are not usually suitable for clinical assessment, and simpler clinical procedures can be used at bedside.

In general terms, giving a warning to the patient prior to each stimulation is a helpful strategy to increase stimulus detection in neglect patients (Robertson *et al.* 1998) and show that not all the impairment is due to peripheral, sensory problems.

More specifically, different techniques can be used to asses the relative contribution of hemianopia or hemianaesthesia to contralesional sensory deficits. In order to differentiate between hemianopia and neglect one can change the spatial position of visual stimuli relatively to the patient. This procedure is illustrated in Fig. 6.1. One can first test perception of left-sided visual stimuli while the patient keeps his/her gaze in primary position (straight gaze, i.e. aligned with the midsagittal plane of the patient's body). In case of manual stimulation, the patient is asked to keep his/her gaze fixed straight at the examiner's nose, while the examiner

Primary sensory impairment or neglect? *(continued)*

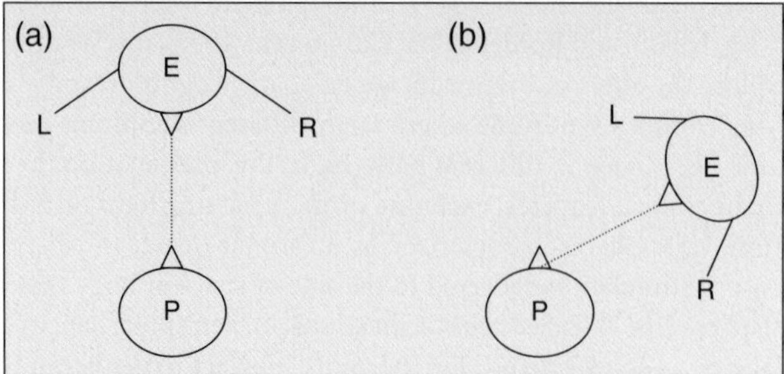

Fig. 6.1 (a) The examiner (E) is positioned in front of the patient (P) who looks straight ahead towards the examiner (dotted line). Left and right visual stimuli are manually delivered and, in this arrangement, fall in the left and right hemifield, but are also to the left and right spatial positions relative to the body's midsagittal plane. (b) The patient looks straight towards the examiner who has now moved towards the patient's right side. In this arrangement, stimuli that fall in the left and right hemifields are both included in the patient's right ipsilesional field. With this arrangement perception of left-sided stimuli may improve if misperception is due to neglect, but does not improve if it is due to hemianopia.

sits in front of him/her. Then the patient can be asked to gaze towards the right side, where the examiner has now moved. Now visual stimuli delivered to the left visual field will be positioned within the right hemifield relatively to the patient's body midline. Since perception in neglect typically improves along a horizontal gradient that goes from the left towards the right extreme, with this manipulation visual perception of contralesional stimuli could now improve, pointing to a contribution of neglect to the visual deficit (Kooistra and Heilman 1989; Vuilleumier *et al.* 1999).

A recent study suggests that using the Müller–Lyer illusion in the version proposed by Brentano can be of help in differentiating between neglect and hemianopia (Daini *et al.* 2002). In particular, in patients with neglect and hemianopia (assessed with visual field examination and visual evoked potentials), no effect of the illusion on bisection error was found, while in those patients without hemianopia the error was influenced (i.e. increased or reduced) depending on the direction of the illusion. Therefore, this test may be usefully used to help assessing the presence of any visual field defect coexisting with neglect.

Within the somatosensory modality again, the relative contributions of neglect and primary somatosensory impairment to contralesional imperception can be hard to assess in some patients. Apart from vestibular stimulation, which is helpful in this instance but rather invasive and often unpleasant for the patient, some clinical manipulations can be of help. First, one can use strong tactile stimuli to start with, while the patient's attention is oriented towards the stimulated body part. The use of von Frey hairs with progressively weaker stimuli is a good way of obtaining a perceptual threshold. Furthermore, in some patients with tactile extinction it has been observed that moving the contralesional hand towards the ipsilesional side can improve tactile detection on that hand (e.g. Aglioti *et al.* 1999); however this may not work in all patients (Bartolomeo *et al.* 2004), as discussed in the section on extinction. The opposite but logically related finding, i.e. that perception of ipsilesional

Primary sensory impairment or neglect? *(continued)*

right touches may be impaired by moving the hand to the left side, has recently been studied by Valenza and colleagues with an fMRI experiment. These authors have found that a decrease of metabolic activation of right primary somatosensory and posterior parietal cortex and middle frontal gyrus bilaterally follows the reduced awareness of stimuli delivered to the distal part of the right arm when this is a shift across the midline. This finding suggests the presence of a high-level attentional circuit responsible for the integration of proprioceptive and somatosensory information into a body-centred reference frame (Valenza *et al.* 2004*b*).

The independence of neglect and extinction from pure sensory deficit is intriguingly demonstrated by work on *implicit processing* of neglected or extinguished stimuli (Berti 2002). In these studies it is shown that stimuli that are not consciously perceived, can nonetheless modulate the patient behavior in several perceptual tasks (e.g. Berti *et al.* 1992, 1994, 1999; Berti and Rizzolatti 1992; Maravita 1997; Marshall and Halligan 1988; Marzi *et al.* 1996) or leave neural traces as shown by electrophysiology (e.g. Deouell *et al.* 2000*b*; Eimer *et al.* 2002; Marzi *et al.* 2000) or neuroimaging (e.g. Driver *et al.* 2001; Rees *et al.* 2000; Vuilleumier 2002; Vuilleumier *et al.* 2001).

A typical aspect of this complex neuropsychological syndrome is the unawareness of the deficit, a deficit named *anosognosia* by Babinski (1914). A typical dialogue between a caregiver (C) and a neglect patient (P) could be the following.

C: 'Why do you keep on ignoring items on the left side?'

P: 'Do I miss anything on the left? I can see perfectly on my left side!'

C: 'Are you not aware that something on your left side is missing when you look around?'

P: 'According to me, what I see is a *complete* space, with its left and right. Nothing is missing ...'

Patients may become aware of the deficit with time and rehabilitation. Very often, however, they may acquire knowledge of their deficit through the reports of their relatives or caregivers, without becoming really aware of such problems. Anosognosia may be present for one sensory modality (e.g. visual) but not for another, or selectively for motor or sensory deficits or vice versa and may be variously related with primary sensory or motor deficits (Detailed accounts on anosognosia can be found in Berti *et al.* 1996; Bisiach and Vallar 2000; Vallar *et al.* 2003*b*; Vallar and Ronchi 2006.)

As anticipated before, lesions responsible for this complex syndrome are multiple in nature. Vascular and neoplastic are more typical, but also traumatic brain injuries and even degenerative diseases (e.g. Bartolomeo *et al.* 1998) can result in neglect. Also the locus of the lesion responsible for neglect may vary across patients. Although neglect is more often found after right hemispheric damage, left-sided lesions can also produce contralesional neglect for right space (for a discussion about this point see Bisiach and Vallar 2000). Brain structures more often damaged in the case of neglect are the inferior parietal lobule, the subcortical parietal white matter, the superior temporal and frontal cortex plus the basal ganglia (see discussion in Bisiach and Vallar 2000; Vallar and Perani 1986). Although the more typical focus of cortical damage responsible for neglect seems to be the temporo-parietal cortex (e.g. Mort *et al.* 2003; Vallar *et al.* 2003*a*), recent evidence suggests the importance of the superior temporal gyrus (Karnath *et al.* 2001).

6.2.1 Perceptual aspects of USN

Perceptual aspects of neglect are usually more evident and call for the attention of the patient's caregivers as soon as they occur. Given the multisensory nature of perceptual experience, USN can be shown by testing different sensory modalities. Different patients may show a variable degree of impairment of each sensory modality, and complete dissociations (e.g. neglect in vision but not in the somatosensory modality) can be shown. Since the visual modality is by far the more studied, a more detailed account of deficits in this modality will be given.

6.2.1.1 Visuospatial neglect

The patient tends to ignore any stimulation presented in the side of space contralateral to the brain damage. Typically the space side affected is the left one, following right brain damage. While eating, patients may leave food on the contralesional side of the dish or fail to find items placed on the contralesional side of the table. Typically, the patient cannot be convinced in any way that there is food left, and the only strategy to make them eat all the food is to turn the dish by 180°. If their clinical condition allows them to read, patients may find this task impossible since they fail to read the left page of a newspaper, or the left side of each single page or word, including titles written in bold characters, thus losing the meaning of the text completely (*neglect dyslexia*).

Many different tests can be used to assess visuospatial neglect. At bedside, the examiner may ask the patient to describe the room or collect objects scattered on a tray, noticing any omission of items in the contralesional space. Also patients may be asked to read a newspaper headline, looking for neglect dyslexia.

Many 'pencil and paper' tests are available to formally test for neglect. The simplest one is line bisection (Bisiach *et al.* 1990; Milner *et al.* 1993). The patient is asked to mark the midpoint of lines of various length. Typically the subjective midline is placed at various degrees more towards the ipsilesional extreme of the line as compared to the objective midline. This test is usually influenced by the line length. A stronger neglect is observed for longer lines (length effect), while a paradoxical deviation towards the contralesional side can be observed with short lines (around 1–2 cm), a sign called *cross-over* (Chatterjee, 1995; Halligan and Marshall 1988). A useful test of line bisection, included in the battery called the Behavioural Inattention Test (BIT), can help in distinguishing whether neglect is due to a disruption of 'object-centred' versus 'egocentric' space representation (see discussion above). In a single sheet of paper, three lines of the same length are drawn one above the other. Each line is shifted from the one above by a few centimetres to the left (see Fig. 6.2). The patient is asked to mark the midpoint of each line. Basically, two behaviours can be observed. In one case all the marks are placed one below the other at the same distance from the sheet's right margin. In this case the error takes into account the absolute position of the sheet of paper relative to the patient's body midline, regardless of the relative position of each line on the paper (so-called 'egocentric' neglect; see Fig. 6.2(a)). In the second case the marks are drawn at the same distance from the right extreme of each line (so-called position effect: Halligan and Marshall 1995), independent of the relative position of each line on the paper ('object-centred neglect'; see Fig. 6.2(b)).

Copying line drawings is another typical test for neglect. At bedside any simple line drawing can easily be created for the patient to copy. Again, the main frame of reference on to which visuospatial neglect is centred, i.e. 'object-centred' or 'egocentric' neglect, can be well distinguished by choosing line drawings consisting of more items. In the case of 'egocentric' neglect, only right-sided items will be copied, while in the case of 'object-centred' neglect the left part of each single line drawing will be omitted. Figure 6.3 shows cases of 'egocentric' or 'object-centred' neglect obtained by using the line-drawings proposed by Marshall and Halligan (1993). In this test, copying a complex figure (a pot with two flowers) gives a similar result for 'egocentric' and 'object-centred'

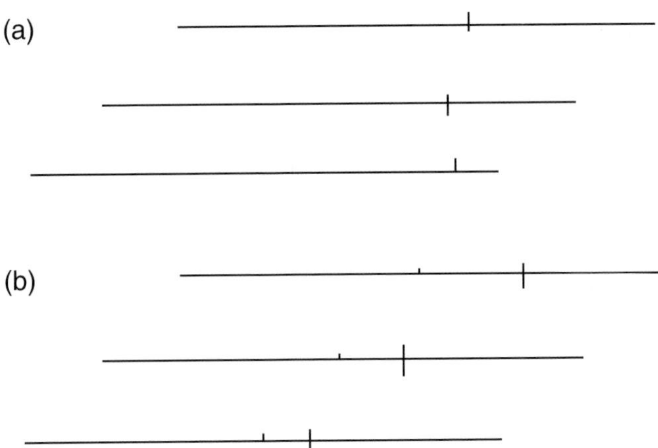

Fig. 6.2 (a) Line bisection: 'egocentric' neglect: Each mark is roughly at the same distance from the right side of the sheet of paper. (b) Line bisection: 'object-centred' neglect: Each mark is placed at roughly the same distance from the right extreme of the line, but at a different distance from the right side of the sheet, according to absolute spatial position of each line.

neglect (Fig. 6.3(a)). However, when the central part of the drawing is omitted, while patients with 'object-centred' neglect will omit left-sided details of each pot and flower (Fig. 6.3(b)), patients with 'egocentric' neglect will omit the left side of the whole figure (Fig. 6.3(c)).

Further assessment can be performed by means of cancellation tasks (see Fig. 6.4). Circle (Bisiach *et al.* 1986a) or line cancellation, the Albert test (Albert 1973; Fig. 6.4(a)), are easy tests suitable for all patients, including those in the acute stage who may not be fully cooperative. A number of circles or lines is drawn on a sheet of paper and the patient is asked to mark each one of them. Typically, the patient omits items on the left side to a variable extent. Patients may also show perseverative behaviours (Manly *et al.* 2002; Rusconi *et al.* 2002). They may recurrently mark the same lines on the right side, or even add elements to the testing sheet (e.g. more items to cancel, line drawings from memory, or their own signature), a behaviour that has been associated with frontal or subcortical lesions (Rusconi *et al.* 2002). More sensitive cancellation tasks are those consisting of more difficult visual search displays including both targets and distractors. For example, the Mesulam random shape cancellation task (Mesulam 1985; Fig. 6.4(b)) and the star cancellation test (Wilson *et al.* 1987) include non-verbal and a mixture of verbal and non-verbal distractors, respectively. As shown in Fig. 6.4(b), these tests are sometimes more sensitive than those without distractors, thus resulting in worse performance (as in the example shown in the figure) or even disclosing neglect that would have gone undiagnosed by simpler tests.

Reading tests can also be used to disclose neglect. Reading of newspaper titles or columns may be useful at bedside. Sometimes reading of simple sentences or words may be enough to show neglect. Again, 'object-centred' or 'egocentric' neglect may be suspected if the patient omits to read the left (initial) part of each word in a sentence or the left part of the sentence, respectively. In a famous study Caramazza and co-workers (Caramazza and Hillis 1990) gave a strong demonstration of object-centred neglect in reading. Their patient was shown to neglect the final part of a word (right-sided neglect), not only when the word was written horizontally from left to right, but also when it was written vertically or mirror-reversed. The authors hypothesized that word orthography is coded in a prototypical left–right horizontal orientation. Their neglect patient was likely to show a specific object-centred, or better word-centred, neglect relative to such

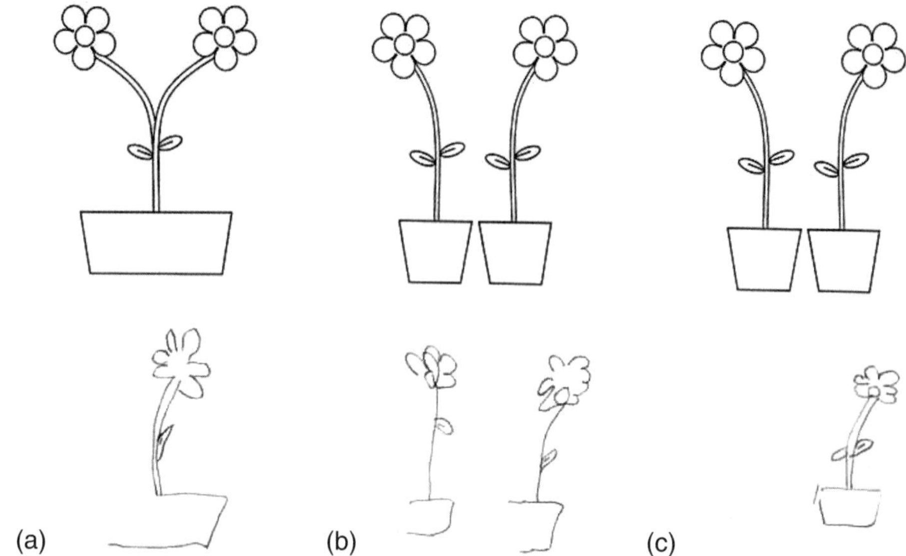

Fig. 6.3 Copy of line drawings (Marshall and Halligan 1993) may disclose 'egocentric' or 'object-centred' omissions in neglect patients. While copying the complex figure in (a) will give similar results for all patients, a different figure (b, c) may show some differences across patients. (b) While patients with 'object-centred' neglect will omit left-sided details of each pot and flower, (c) patients with 'egocentric' neglect will omit the left side of the whole figure.

a specific spatial representation of words. In particular, words would be first automatically coded in the prototypical left–right orientation, and then the contralesional part would be neglected. By contrast, if a purely egocentric left–right code was the critical reference, no neglect with vertically oriented words would have occurred.

In some patients it is possible to find a distinction between the performances in near versus far extrapersonal space. Cases are reported of patients showing a relatively more severe neglect in the far extrapersonal space (Cowey *et al.* 1994; Vuilleumier *et al.* 1998) or in the near extrapersonal space (Berti and Frassinetti 2000; Halligan and Marshall 1991), although this may not always be the case and might be task-dependent (Berti and Frassinetti 2000; Pizzamiglio *et al.* 1989). The existence of a similar dissociation suggests that neural structures coding for the two sectors of space are different (see Section 6.1 plus discussion in Berti and Frassinetti 2000), although the transition between near and far space performance may not be always clear-cut (Cowey *et al.* 1999).

One striking feature of USN is its occurrence when non-external sensory stimulation is involved, such as in visual imagery situations. Bisiach and co-workers famously demonstrated that neglect patients requested to mentally describe the main square of Milan (*Piazza del Duomo*) neglected items located in the contralesional side of the mentally reconstructed image (Bisiach and Luzzatti 1978). Intriguingly, if patients were asked to rotate their subjective viewpoint by 180°, the items that were previously described in the ipsilesional side of the image fell on the contralesional side of the image and were thus neglected. Following this discovery, an explanation of visual neglect in terms of a deficit of space representation was proposed (which was then further characterized with neuroanatomical considerations taken from the neurophysiological literature, e.g. Rizzolatti and Berti 1990) in contrast with purely sensory (e.g. Denny-Brown *et al.* 1952)

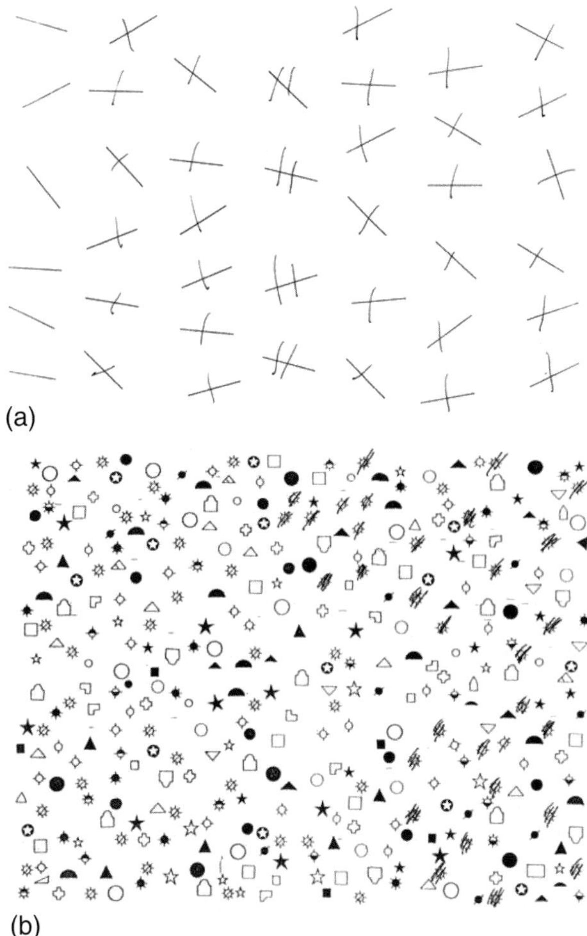

Fig. 6.4 Cancellation tasks. In the same patient, neglect is often less evident when using simple cancellation tasks like the Albert line cancellation (Albert 1973), as shown in (a), than with more difficult visual search tasks including targets and distractors, like the Mesulam random shape cancellation task (Mesulam 1985), as shown in (b).

or attentional (such as the failure to orient towards the contralesional space proposed by Heilman (Heilman and Valenstein 1979) or the imbalance between hemispheric vectors directing attention contralaterally as proposed by Kinsbourne 1977) accounts. (For discussion about different theoretical accounts of neglect see Bisiach and Vallar 2000.)

Apart from description of mental images, representational neglect can be disclosed by asking patients to produce drawings from memory, for example, a clock face with numbers and hands, or any other object familiar to the patient. In this test, the left part of the drawing is typically omitted (Fig. 6.5). Representational neglect can be double dissociated by personal and extrapersonal neglect, and cases of selective representational neglect have been reported (e.g. Guariglia *et al.* 1993).

6.2.1.2 Auditory neglect

Auditory space is also abnormally represented in patients with USN. Clinically, the patient spontaneously ignores people addressing him/her from the contralesional side, failing to respond to

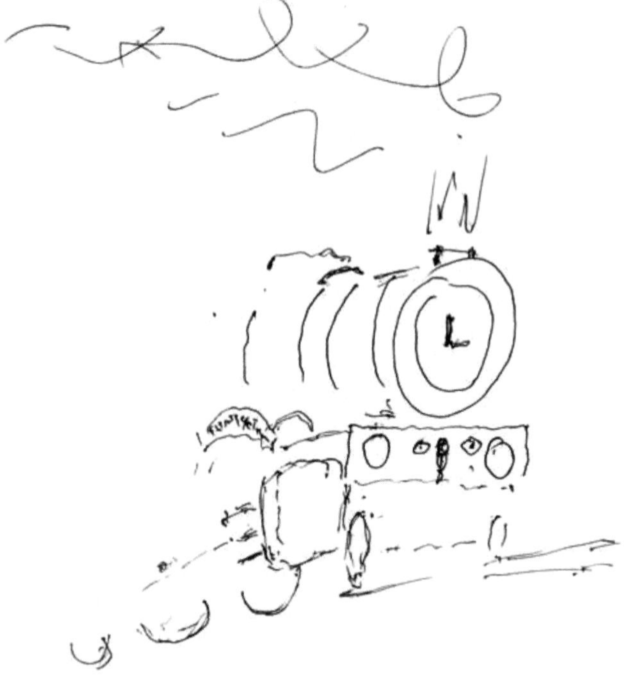

Fig. 6.5 Spontaneous drawing from memory. The left part of the drawing is omitted.

questions or answering as if the speaker were placed on the ipsilesional side (a disturbance also called *alloacousia*; Heilman and Valenstein 1972). Asking the patient to report left and right finger snaps is a simple clinical test for auditory neglect. Again, the patient may either ignore stimuli completely, or perceive such stimuli, but localize them on the ipsilesional side.

In the early 1980s Bisiach and co-workers showed that auditory localization of dichotic stimuli is typically defective in right brain damaged patients who mislocalize sounds towards the right side (Bisiach *et al.* 1984). An ipsilesional shift in sound localization is also observed in free-field pointing tasks, or in the positioning of a continuous phantom sound generated through loudspeakers (for a recent review see Pavani *et al.* 2003). Intriguingly, the finding that auditory stimuli are mislocalized towards the ipsilesional side both in front and back space in several patients has suggested that a lateral shift of the perceived body midsagittal plane, rather than a rotation of the body midline along a vertical axis, may occur in neglect patients (Vallar *et al.* 1995*a*).

The above deficits are likely to follow a high-level deficit of spatial localization of sounds rather than the simple suppression of input coming from the left ear. A neat demonstration of this hypothesis was provided by Soroker and colleagues (1995) who showed that identification of a syllable presented in free-field on the left side was improved by showing a visible, though inactive, sound source on the right side. This setting produced a ventriloquist-like effect that made left sounds, which were in fact perceived, appear as if they were delivered from the right side, thus improving the patient's auditory performance.

Given that auditory neglect can be tested in several ways and that different auditory deficits may be found in different patients, the interpretation of the underlying mechanism of auditory neglect is challenging. In a recent paper Bellmann and colleagues (2001) showed different levels of impairment of auditory attention in four patients showing left extinction of auditory targets in dichotic listening. While two patients showed an ipsilesional bias in a dichotic task based on the interaural time difference but no deficit in sound localization, the other two patients showed the opposite pattern. In analogy to the dichotomic 'what' and 'where' system analysing the meaning versus the spatial position of visual stimuli (Ungerleider and Mishkin 1982), it has been proposed that a deficit in a putative 'what' auditory system was present in the first two patients, whose brain damage was centred on the basal ganglia, and a disrupted 'where' system was present in the latter two with cortical, fronto-temporo-parietal lesions (Clarke and Thiran 2004).

Furthermore, the ipsilateral displacement of perceived sound location found in several patients may be due to an increased uncertainty of sound localization on the contralesional side rather than to a simple horizontal shift in sound localization. In this respect, a recent study has shown a worse performance of speeded localization of contralesional free-field sounds in the vertical axis, suggesting a general impairment of sound localization in the contralesional space (Pavani *et al.* 2002). A similar finding has been found for same/different elevation judgements relative to contralesional sounds (Pavani *et al.* 2001; Tanaka *et al.* 1999). Congruently with the above idea, it has been shown that neglect patients show a reduced 'mismatch negativity', an electrophysiological marker of a sudden change in sound position, specifically for contralesional auditory stimuli (Deouell *et al.* 2000*a*).

Furthermore, auditory neglect is likely to be part of a wider deficit of space representation, as confirmed by a recent meta-analysis showing a significant positive correlation between different measures of auditory neglect and visuospatial neglect. This finding suggests that a disruption of multisensory space representation may often occur in these patients as a consequence of brain lesions that typically involve areas devoted to multisensory processing (Pavani *et al.* 2004).

6.2.1.3 Body-related neglect

Neglect patients may show defective awareness, not only relative to contralesional extrapersonal space, but also to contralesional body parts or somatosensory stimuli. This aspect may not seem strictly related to spatial cognition but more to body awareness. However, since these deficits have the same spatial lateralization as the typical NSU visual deficits (thus, interestingly, the contralesional side of 'personal space'), they can be considered as one of the core features of the neglect syndrome. Bodily manifestations of neglect are not always associated with extrapersonal neglect, and double dissociations can be found (Bisiach *et al.* 1986*a*).

First, patients may be unaware of somatosensory stimuli delivered to contralesional body parts. This deficit is not determined by primary sensory deficit, although this may be present and add on to the neuropsychological disorder (e.g. Eimer *et al.* 2002), and the relative importance of primary sensory deficits and neglect could be difficult to assess (see the box in Section 6.2). For example, somatosensory evoked potentials and skin conductance responses from somatosensory stimuli delivered to the contralesional side have been shown to be present even without conscious awareness (Vallar *et al.* 1991*a*,*b*), while external sensory stimulations, such as vestibular stimulation, may influence contralesional somatosensory unawareness especially in right brain damaged patients, suggesting that neglect may play an important role in such deficits (see the box in Section 6.2, page 93).

In analogy to what is found for auditory stimuli (see above), patients may sometimes perceive contralesional somatosensory stimuli, but mislocalize them towards the ipsilesional side (*alloaesthesia*: see discussion in Meador *et al.* 1991). Further details on contralateral somatosensory imperception will be given in the section about extinction.

Patients may show defective awareness about their body parts (*personal neglect*). A typical test to disclose this deficit is to ask the patient to touch his/her contralesional hand with the ipsilesional one. A variety of behaviours can be observed: from misreaching of the body part (e.g. touching the forearm instead of the hand) to a confused groping with the ipsilesional hand, which may not even cross the body midline (Bisiach *et al.* 1986*a*). In another test, the 'fluff test', several little markers are attached to the blindfolded patient's body. Afterwards, the patient, still blindfolded, is asked to collect all the items using his/her ipsilesional hand. The number of omitted items on the contralesional half of the body is taken as a measure of personal neglect (Cocchini *et al.* 2001).

In some instances, patients may show striking delusional, pseudopsychiatric confabulations about their contralesional limbs (*somatoparaphrenia*) and deny the ownership of those limbs, attributing their ownership to a caregiver, a relative, or even the patient who was lying in the same bed before them (e.g. Bisiach *et al.* 1991; Bisiach and Vallar 2000; Halligan *et al.* 1995). The delusion may even include extrapersonal objects usually linked to the body part that the patient feels as alien (Aglioti *et al.* 1996). Described cases of somatoparaphrenia are not numerous (around 30 reported in the literature) since a clear somatoparaphrenia is usually present only in the acute stage, and tends to remit within a few hours or days (see the box for a report of chronic somatoparaphrenia).

The arm in the cupboard: a case of chronic somatoparaphrenia

What follows is a report of a patient (Mr S.) whom I had the occasion of interviewing, together with my colleague, Dr Patrick Vuilleumier, in a London hospital. The patient had a stroke a few weeks prior to the interview, and showed a florid visuospatial neglect together with a profound left hemiplegia.

Doctors: 'How are you?'

Mr S.: 'Not so bad, in general, but I still have that acute pain where the prosthesis is.'

Doctors: 'Which prosthesis?'

Mr S.: 'Don't you see? This thing here [indicating his left arm]! The doctors have attached this tool to my body in order to help me to move … but it's completely useless and very painful. I asked the nurses several times to take it away and put it in the cupboard!'

Doctors [pointing to the patient's left arm]: 'If this is a prosthesis, where is your left arm?'

Mr S. [smiling]: 'Well … what do you think? It should be there!' [pointing towards his left side].

Doctors: 'Can you move it?'

Mr S.: 'I am very tired. Furthermore, this prosthesis is so painful that I cannot do anything at all …'

After several weeks of rehabilitation, Mr. S. became apparently aware of his hemiplegia. We interviewed him one last time prior to his discharge from the ward.

Doctors: 'Mr S., how are you?'

Mr S.: 'Very well thanks. Now I feel much better than before. I have some problems with my left side [pointing to the leg and arm] and some pain here [pointing to the shoulder] but no more such silly feelings about my left arm and the prosthesis …'

Doctors: 'Very well! So you are ready to go home.'

Mr S.: 'Yes … but before leaving … could I ask you something? Once home, could I ask my wife, from time to time, to remove this left arm and put it in the cupboard for a few hours, in order to have some relief from pain?'

In a recent intriguing single-case study, a neglect patient attributed her left arm to her niece. Surprisingly, tactile perception over that arm, which was very poor, was substantially improved by asking the patient to imagine that her niece's arm, and not her own arm, was actually touched (Bottini *et al.* 2002). This evidence suggest that awareness of somatosensory stimulation in right brain damaged patients may be highly modulated by the patients' personal beliefs about their own body. Furthermore, rare cases of chronic somatoparaphrenia (see report in the box) may show that bodily awareness can be hard to regain for neglect patients and that it is likely to be conditioned by several factors, including information coming from external sources, as well as the internal representation and awareness of one's own body.

6.2.2 **Motor aspects**

Neglect may not only be confined within the sensory or mental imagery domain. Patients without motor deficit can show a reluctance in using the contralesional limbs, a phenomenon called *motor neglect*. Such patients may show underutilization of contralesional limbs not only during spontaneous activities, but also in response to painful stimulations (e.g. Castaigne *et al.* 1972). In a group study including 20 patients, motor neglect was found without sensory neglect as a consequence of brain damage to different brain structures, such as frontal and parietal lobes plus the thalamus (Laplane and Degos 1983), suggesting the importance of a cortical network for intentional control of contralesional limbs in neglect, either due to the lesion itself or to diaschisis (Fiorelli *et al.* 1991; von Giesen *et al.* 1994).

A more subtle disorder is the reluctance of neglect patients to move towards the contralesional space, a condition also called *directional hypokinesia* (Heilman *et al.* 1985). In this case the deficit is visible not only for contralesional limbs, as in the case of motor neglect, but also for leftward-directed movements with the unaffected ipsilesional limb. Controlled experiments have shown that this deficit is not due to perceptual but rather to directional/intentional motor programming towards targets that are put to the left relative to the acting limb, regardless of their position relative to the patient's body midline. A key role of the inferior parietal lobe has been suggested for this deficit, underlying the role of that brain region in motor programming (Husain *et al.* 2000; Mattingley *et al.* 1998).

Different strategies have been adopted in order to distinguish motor-intentional from perceptual aspects of neglect. The general strategy of such studies was to put perceptual and motor aspects of a given task into conflict (Bisiach *et al.* 1990; Husain *et al.* 2000; Tegner and Levander 1991). A simple pencil and paper task to distinguish between the two components of neglect is the so-called landmark task (Milner *et al.* 1993). In this test, pre-bisected lines are shown to the patient who is asked to judge which half is shorter/longer by means of a forced-choice response. In this condition, which is purely perceptual, neglect patients tend to indicate the right segment as longer than the left one even when this is not the case, suggesting that they are actually underestimating the length of the left segment. In a motor version of the task, a different performance can be observed in some patients if they are asked to make their judgement by manually pointing (Bisiach *et al.* 1999). In particular, patients may keep on indicating the right segment regardless of whether they are asked to show the longer or the shorter segment of the pre-bisected line. This behaviour suggests that a motor bias towards the right side, or a reluctance to move towards the left side, is present.

6.3 **Extinction to double stimulation**

There is a particular neuropsychological condition called *extinction*, in which patients ignore contralesional stimuli. This condition differs from neglect because contralesional stimuli are normally, or nearly normally, detected when presented in isolation, but omitted when presented together with ipsilesional ones. Although extinction seems to be more frequent after right than left hemispheric damage, its lateralization seems to be weaker than that observed in neglect (for discussion see Bisiach and Vallar 2000). Subcortical lesions (thalamus, basal ganglia, or white matter) are present in around 50% of extinction patients, while in the remaining patients, frontal or temporo-parietal cortical regions are typically involved, with some specificities for visual versus tactile extinction (see details in Vallar *et al.* 1994). The specific importance of temporo-parietal junction for visual extinction has recently been underlined (Karnath *et al.* 2003).

Extinction is often present together with neglect, but can be double dissociated from it and is considered by different authors to be a different disorder (Bisiach 1991; Bisiach *et al.* 1986*a*; Bisiach and Vallar 2000; Liu *et al.* 1992; Ogden 1985). While extinction is often observed without neglect, and in some instances this occurs after an initial neglect syndrome has recovered (hence the idea that extinction may be a sort of residual feature of neglect), neglect without extinction has also been reported (Cocchini *et al.* 2001).

Extinction can be easily tested by using the clinical procedure called confrontation (see Fig. 6.6). In vision, the examiner delivers to the patient single unilateral and bilateral brief finger movements in each hemifield, while the patient keeps his/her eyes fixed on the examiner's nose. In the tactile modality, light touches on the hands, face, or feet can be delivered to blindfolded patients. In audition, brief unilateral or bilateral finger snaps can be used to assess auditory extinction. An easy and useful standardized protocol is that proposed by Bisiach and co-workers (1986*b*) where a list of unilateral and bilateral stimuli to assess visual and tactile sensation and extinction are provided. The score range is between 0 (no deficit) and 3 (maximum deficit). Extinction is defined as the condition where at least 3 out of 10 bilateral stimuli are omitted, while at least 8 out of 10 single contralesional stimuli are correctly reported. In some instances a computerized examination may give more reliable results and, by making it possible to

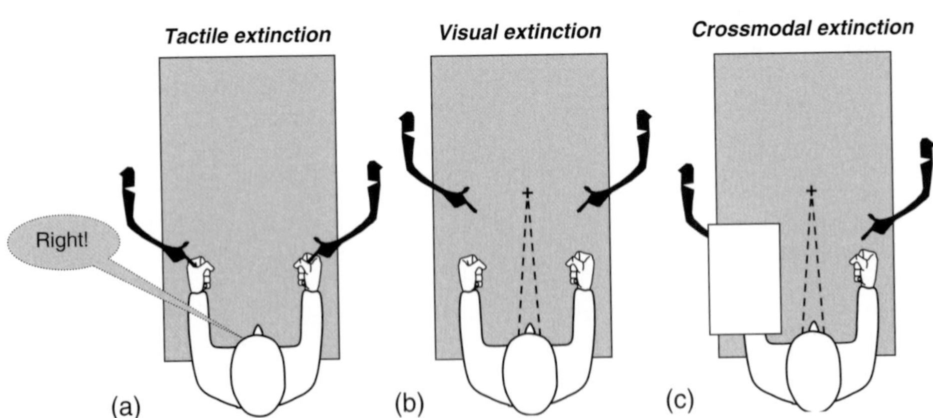

Fig. 6.6 Clinical testing for extinction. (a) Tactile extinction. With the patient blindfolded light, brief touches are delivered to symmetrical positions of the patient's body. (b) Visual extinction. Brief finger movements are presented to the patient who keeps eyes fixed straight ahead (typically towards the examiner's nose). (c) Crossmodal visual–tactile extinction. Light touches are delivered to the contralesional hand (hidden from the patient's direct view as schematized by the white rectangle) while visual stimuli (brief finger movements) are delivered close to the ipsilesional hand. Extinction may be stronger for ipsilesional visual stimuli close to the hand than for those far away from the hand (see text for further details).

precisely modulate stimulus intensity and duration, it may be more sensitive in disclosing extinction (see examples in Maravita *et al.* 2001; Marzi *et al.* 2000).

Extinction may be observed in different sensory modalities and may co-occur with primary sensory deficits. Although an interpretation of extinction as a simple effect of primary sensory deficit seems nowadays implausible, nonetheless the role of sensory deficits may be relevant as witnessed by cases of tactile extinction following spinal cord damage (Bender 1945) and by the typical observation of slower reaction times (e.g. Marzi *et al.* 1996, 2000) and altered contralateral hemispheric electrophysiological responses (e.g. Eimer *et al.* 2002; Marzi *et al.* 2000) to single contralesional stimuli. At present, an influential account of extinction is that derived from theories of competitive spatial attention (Bundesen 1990; Desimone and Duncan 1995). A common suggestion is that the lesion confers an advantage in terms of 'weighting' to ipsilesional stimuli whenever multiple concurrent stimuli compete for spatial attention (e.g. Driver *et al.* 1997). Interestingly, in different laboratories, neuroimaging results have put the accent on the reduced event-related potential (ERP) or fMRI activations of brain regions that are typically modulated by attention in trials with extinctions as compared to trials where contralesional stimuli are detected. Such effects may occur at an earlier (Marzi *et al.* 2000) versus later (Eimer *et al.* 2002; Vuilleumier *et al.* 2001) stage, possibly depending on the nature of the lesion and the task. In particular, the importance of damage to cortical networks controlling stimulus-driven attention for extinction has been recently postulated (Corbetta *et al.* 2000; Corbetta and Shulman 2002).

Extinction can be modulated by a variety of manipulations. Although extinction is typically observed for simultaneous bilateral stimuli, it may also occur following asynchronous stimulation (di Pellegrino *et al.* 1997*a*; Rorden *et al.* 1997). However, in some instances, when the contralesional stimulus precedes the right one by a few hundred milliseconds (thus avoiding competition with the ipsilesional stimulation during that interval), an improvement of performance may be observed (Rorden *et al.* 1997).

Furthermore, a number of perceptual, pre-attentive mechanisms can effectively reduce extinction. For example, in a figure–ground segregation task where symmetric figures are typically chosen as foreground by normal observers, the patient correctly named as the foreground colour that filling the symmetrical shapes even if, due to his neglect, he was unable to consciously identify the symmetrical foreground figures (Driver *et al.* 1993). Also, bilateral stimuli that can be perceptually grouped in a single unit have been shown to effectively reduce visual extinction, suggesting that some early attentional ('pre-attentive') processing of the stimulus can still process the whole visual display in extinction patients (Mattingley *et al.* 1997*a*; Ward *et al.* 1994).

As far as the coordinate system within which extinction can occur is concerned, there is evidence that this phenomenon may occur relative to multiple frames of reference. Extinction is typically present for stimuli that are at the opposite side of the patient's midsagittal plane, but this is not always the case. For instance, visual stimuli have been shown to be extinguished following this prototypical left–right orientation even when they are vertically aligned, one above and one below the patient's head. In this case, the stimulus in the examiner's right hand (left side for the patient) was lost, even if its real spatial position was physically above the patient's head (Rafal 1994). This suggests that a coordinate transformation of the vertical arrangement into an horizontal representation had occurred before the pathological extinction of one item. Furthermore, there are cases of within-field extinction, where the leftmost stimulus is missed even when both stimuli are presented in the right visual field (Bisiach and Geminiani 1991; di Pellegrino and De Renzi 1995; Rapcsak *et al.* 1987).

Within the tactile domain, extinction can be reduced if hands are crossed, even if these are both placed within the right or left hemispace, suggesting a critical role for the relative position of the limbs in external space in somatosensory spatial representation, and not only of the position of the limbs relatively to the body midline (Aglioti *et al.* 1999; but see Bartolomeo *et al.* 2004). Spatial coding of touch can even be centred on single sections of a limb, as witnessed by cases of extinction for bilateral stimuli delivered across the wrist or a single finger. In these cases the extinguished stimuli were those delivered to the contralesional side of the stimulated wrist (regardless of the position being palm-up or palm-down; Moschowitch and Behrmann 1994) or finger (Tinazzi *et al.* 2000).

As mentioned before, extinction can involve single sensory modalities in different patients (De Renzi *et al.* 1984; Marzi *et al.* 2000; Vallar *et al.* 1994). However, a single patient may present with extinction in more than one sensory modality (Heilman and Valenstein 1972; Inhoff *et al.* 1992) or even for multiple stimuli belonging to different sensory modalities, as already shown by the pioneering work of Bender (1970). For example, a right visual stimulus can extinguish awareness of a touch on the left hand that would otherwise have been felt (Mattingley *et al.* 1997*b*). This kind of extinction, also named *crossmodal extinction*, can occur between vision, touch, and audition (di Pellegrino *et al.* 1997*b*; Farnè and Ladàvas 2002; Làdavas 2002; Sarri *et al.* 2006). The most studied combination is that between vision and touch. For visual–tactile crossmodal extinction, di Pellegrino and co-workers (1997*b*) have also shown that crossmodal visual–tactile extinction of left-hand touch by a right visual stimulus is more pronounced when the right visual stimulus falls close in three-dimensional space to the right hand. This has led to the suggestion that a visual stimulus near one hand may activate a multimodal (visual–tactile) representation of the space near that hand (analogous to the representations of peripersonal space provided by multimodal neurons in the primate brain discussed in the introduction), in addition to a purely visual response. Activating a multimodal representation of the right hand in this way might then, in turn, compete with the activation of the contralesional left hand by touch, hence producing extinction of that contralesional touch. By contrast, when the right visual stimulus is located further away from the right hand, it may no longer activate a multimodal representation of the space near that hand, hence producing less extinction of touch on the other hand (di Pellegrino *et al.* 1997*b*; Làdavas 2002).

Interesting modulations of crossmodal extinction have recently been obtained with tool use. In these experiments crossmodal extinction was used as a paradigm to test the effect of prolonged activity with tools in modulating crossmodal body representation (for review see Maravita 2006; Maravita and Iriki 2004). The general outcome of these studies is that wielding or using a tool in extrapersonal far space can increase the impact of far ipsilesional visual stimuli on contralesional tactile extinction (as if far space were rendered akin to near space by becoming reachable with the tool; Farnè and Làdavas 2000; Maravita *et al.* 2001). By contrast, using a tool with the contralesional hand to operate in the ipsilesional space may reduce tactile extinction by right visual flashes, possibly by constructing a common visual–tactile representation of the two sides of space, hence reducing the competition between multiple stimuli (Maravita *et al.* 2002).

6.3.1 Extinction and neglect for special senses

A few reports are available of neglect and extinction in olfaction and taste, although these sensory modalities are technically difficult to study, and their testing for any sign of extinction or neglect in the clinical environment is often omitted. Neglect and extinction of contralesional olfactory stimuli have been reported (Bellas *et al.* 1988*a*,*b*, 1989), although their nature as true neglect manifestations has recently been criticized (Berlucchi *et al.* 2004). Extinction of contralesional gustative stimuli has also been reported together with other signs of neglect and extinction (Andre *et al.* 2000; Bender and Feldman 1952; Berlucchi *et al.* 2004), and sometimes within a more complex picture of oropharyngeal deficits (Andre *et al.* 2000). Berlucchi and colleagues have recently suggested that the independence between gustative perception and tactile extinction on the tongue may rely on the different mapping of tactile (contralateral) and gustative (mainly ipsilateral) cortical input (Berlucchi *et al.* 2004).

The main features of the neglect syndrome

- **Perceptual–spatial disorders:** unawareness of stimuli in different sensory modalities (visual, tactile, auditory, gustative, olfactory)
- **Motor disorders:** failure to move the contralesional limbs (*motor neglect*) or reluctance to move towards the contralesional space (*directional hypokinesia*)
- **Specific body-related symptoms**:
  - *personal neglect*: ignoring contralesional body parts
  - *somatoparaphrenia*: denial of the ownership of contralesional limbs with delusional, pseudo-psychiatric confabulations about the person's contralesional limbs
- **Anosognosia**: unawareness of sensory and motor deficits

6.4 Non-lateralized spatial disorders

A number of spatial disorders do not show the typical lateralization, both for the occurrence of the clinical deficits and for the hemispheric prevalence of the critical brain damage, that occurs for unilateral neglect and extinction. Furthermore, these disorders do not imply the unawareness of the deficit and the productive manifestations typically observed in neglect, although associations between these different disorders are possible due to the anatomical proximity of the critical brain regions.

An account of spatial disorders affecting visuomotor performance and spatial orientation will now be given (for comprehensive reviews of other spatial deficits see e.g. Heilman and Valenstein 2003; Walsh and Darby 1999).

6.4.1 Visuomotor–spatial perceptual disorders and Balint's syndrome

While patients with unilateral lesions (mainly centred in the inferior parietal lesion of the right hemisphere) may show the neuropsychological conditions of contralesional neglect and extinction, other patients with unilateral or bilateral parietal or occipito-parietal damage may show different kinds of spatial disorders. First, these disorders may include misreaching for extrapersonal objects, characterized by a deficit in both reaching to the object location and grasping it (so-called *optic ataxia*). This deficit can follow unilateral parietal lesions and can be present independently of neglect. Both left and right parietal lesions can give rise to this deficit. According to Perenin and colleagues (e.g. Perenin and Vighetto 1988) different kinds of behaviour may result from right versus left parietal lesions. In particular, after right parietal damage patients show misreaching with both hands in the contralesional visual field, while after a left parietal lesion the misreaching is limited to the right hand but occurs in both hemifields. At odds with neglect, the locus of the lesion typical of optic ataxia is the superior parietal cortex. This underlines a critical functional–anatomical distinction within the parietal cortex in humans (for a useful discussion about homologies and differences between human and monkey parietal areas see Milner 1997). While the superior aspect of the parietal cortex would be important for unconscious and automatic integration of spatial information necessary for visuomotor programming, the inferior aspect may be more critical for the construction of conscious, stable spatial awareness (for further discussion see Perenin 1997).

Recently, an intriguing form of misreaching towards objects observed in mirrors (named by the authors 'mirror ataxia') has been described following parietal lesions (Binkofski *et al.* 1999). There would be different grades of impairment due to more posterior and larger or more anterior and smaller parietal lesions underlying deeper or lighter impairment, respectively. Interestingly, similarly to the anatomical differences found between neglect and optic ataxia, mirror ataxia can be distinguished from a tendency to reach towards an object's reflection in a mirror instead of the real object, a deficit named 'mirror agnosia', which would be more specifically linked to inferior parietal lesions (Binkofski *et al.* 1999).

Otpic ataxia and mirror ataxia have been recently put together into an organic framework interpreting visuomotor impairments as dependent on the disruption of specific fronto-parietal networks for action. While optic ataxia would reflect a disruption of a more dorso-dorsal parieto-frontal network, mirror apraxia as well as limb apraxia would follow the disruption of a more ventro-dorsal pathway (with possible commonalities with spatial neglect; Pisella *et al.* 2006; Rossetti *et al.* 2003). In association with optic ataxia, patients may also show an inability to voluntarily direct their gaze towards spatial objects, the so-called *gaze apraxia*, originally named as 'psychic paralysis of gaze' (Balint 1909). Furthermore, some patients may present with a pathological narrowing of the field of spatial attention, and seem to be able to detect only one stimulus at a time while analysing complex scenes, a condition also known as *simultaneous agnosia*. The above three signs can be found in association in the same patient, giving rise to the so-called *Balint* (or Balint–Holmes) syndrome (for a review see Rafal 1997). The typical lesion underlying this complex disorder involves the occipito-parietal cortex bilaterally. At odds with neglect and extinction, errors in Balint's syndrome are not spatially lateralized, and misguided actions can occur on both sides of space, although different patterns of lateralized bias can be shown across patients. Furthermore, although the inability to perceive multiple stimuli at the same time observed in simultaneously agnosic patients may be reminiscent of extinction on double stimulation, the two deficits are clearly different since, again, the deficit here involves both sides of the whole visual scene (see discussion in Driver *et al.* 1997; Rafal 1997).

Another notable difference with the neglect syndrome is that optic ataxia or Balint's syndrome do not include body-related disorders. Patients showing a notable deficit in reaching for objects in external space do not show similar problems when they are asked to point to parts of their own bodies (Robertson *et al.* 1997).

Similarly to what is shown by extinction or neglect patients, patients with Balint's syndrome can show some sort of unconscious processing for stimuli that they poorly process because of their simultagnosia or misreaching. For example, a patient studied by Robertson and colleagues (1997) showed an interference effect on reaction times for the word 'up' written in the lower visual field and vice versa ('down' written in the upper visual field), although he was unable to explicitly locate the words in the upper or lower visual field. Following this experimental evidence, one can argue that some forms of spatial coding are still functioning in these patients, although they are not sufficient to guide perception and action correctly (for further discussion on the importance of Balint's syndrome for the understanding of visual attention mechanisms see Robertson and Rafal 2000).

Finally, recent evidence shows that Balint's syndrome can affect not only the coding of stimuli in unimodal conditions, but also multisensory integration. Valenza and co-workers (2004*a*) have recently shown that a patient with Balint's syndrome showing a stronger deficit in the left side of space also showed reduced crossmodal visual–tactile interference for the left hand held in the left visual field, while crossmodal interference was shown for the right hand in the right visual field, congruently with what is typically found in normal subjects (Spence *et al.* 2004). Interestingly, crossmodal interference increased for the left hand when this was moved in the right visual space, suggesting that such a crossmodal interference requires a functional interaction between a hand-centred and an egocentric space representation (Valenza *et al.* 2004*a*).

6.4.2 Disorders of spatial localization and orientation

If we want to walk through city streets in order to reach a place of interest, we have to perform a number of operations that can be critically damaged by brain lesions. First, some patients may show a general deficit in *spatial localization* and find it difficult to describe the spatial location of an object or even point to that object. These patients may be impaired in orienting inside the hospital environment or their own house, since they cannot judge the absolute spatial position of visual objects in the environment. In these patients abnormal performances in tests of absolute or relative spatial localization of visual or tactile stimuli are described and lesions of the parietal-occipital areas are typically reported (e.g. Bender and Teuber 1947), with a prevalence for right hemisphere in some studies (De Renzi *et al.* 1971; Faglioni *et al.* 1971).

A more complex deficit is that specifically involving spatial orientation, or *topographical disorientation*. This deficit, for example, impairs the patient's ability to reproduce a given path (e.g. walking on the floor following a visual map; Semmes *et al.* 1955). This deficit may be found for both visual and tactile modalities, thus suggesting that brain damage may impair a supramodal mechanism of spatial orientation, not limited to the visual modality and independent from a pure deficit of visuospatial localization. Furthermore, in these patients an impaired ability to reproduce a 'route' on their own bodies by indicating different body parts in succession has also been found. While 'personal' spatial disorientation would be more frequent after anterior, mainly left-sided lesions, 'extrapersonal' impairments would more often follow posterior right-sided lesions (Semmes *et al.* 1963). Importantly, in cases of pure topographical disorientation patients can correctly report the absolute position of objects in space and can also correctly indicate the location of landmark buildings and sites along a route. In other words, their abilities for absolute spatial localization and their memory function are intact. However, they are specifically unable to follow or reconstruct the route necessary to go from one spatial location to another, i.e. holding what Takahashi and colleagues (1997) refer to as the 'sense of direction'. Although cases of topographical disorientation may follow lesions of different brain areas (for a more detailed account see Walsh and Darby 1999), these more often involve the right hemisphere in the retrosplenial cingulate cortex and medial parietal cortex (Takahashi *et al.* 1997).[1]

Spatial disorders can also involve memory components. Visuospatial short- and long-term memory may both be affected by specific lesions. Although the detailed description of such disorders goes beyond the limits of this chapter, it is worth noting here that memory for topographical information can be selectively impaired. A patient described by Bottini and co-workers (1990) showed a selective loss of retrograde topographic memory for well-known routes, while he retained a good performance in other tests of topographic orientation. The authors concluded that this patient suggests a dissociation between 'agnosic' and 'amnesic' components of topographical orientation (Bottini *et al.* 1990).

By contrast with deficits of retrograde topographic memory, a selective deficit in learning new routes, i.e. a deficit of anterograde topographic memory, has been described. These patients show a pure deficit in learning a novel route, while still being able to remember routes learned before

[1] A deficit in describing routes or even orienting in spatial environments can be shown by neglect patients. In this case, however, the deficit is typically lateralized, so that patients miss any landmark placed on their contralesional side (thus, for example, missing their room door in the ward and getting lost) plus which they show a reluctance in making left turns in route descriptions (Bisiach *et al.* 1993).

the brain injury and performing to a normal level in other tests of spatial knowledge. Patients with this clinical picture are affected by lesions of the parahippocampal cortex in the right cerebral hemisphere (Habib and Sirigu 1987). These neuropsychological data seem to converge with recent imaging data in showing the critical role of parahippocampal gyrus in topographical learning. Such anatomical data are reminiscent of those found in animals. The medial, deep aspect of the temporal lobe seems important for topographical orientation in rats, where specific neurons, called 'place cells', have been found. The function of such cells seems to be to code for the absolute position of the animal in space during navigation (e.g. see essays in Burgess *et al.* 1999). However, at partial odds with what is found in animals, in humans the parahippocampal gyrus on the medial temporal cortex, more than the hippocampus, seems important for learning to navigate in spatial environments (Aguirre *et al.* 1996).

6.5 **Conclusion**

The complexity of space representation for perception and action in the human brain is being fruitfully explored by a complex multidisciplinary approach. On the one hand, neurophysiological and neuroimaging data can show how the intact brain normally processes spatial information about extrapersonal objects and our own body. On the other hand, further critical clues come from the study of neuropsychological syndromes specifically affecting patients' spatial skills.

In this chapter the typical features of deficits of spatial awareness, both visuomotor and topographic, following brain damage have been described with reference to the important body of knowledge relative to space representation in the animal and neurologically intact human brain. From this it may be concluded that space representation is a complex neurological function relying on a multicomponent neural network. In particular, different structures control spatial awareness for near versus far or bodily versus extrapersonal space representation, reaching towards visual objects and spatial localization and navigation through familiar or novel environments, allowing our daily complex and efficient interactions with the external world.

References

Aglioti, S., Smania, N., Manfredi, M., and Berlucchi, G. (1996). Disownership of left hand and objects related to it in a patient with right brain damage. *Neuroreport* **8** (1), 293–6.

Aglioti, S., Smania, N., and Peru, A. (1999). Frames of reference for mapping tactile stimuli in brain-damaged patients. *J. Cogn. Neurosci.* **11** (1), 67–79.

Aguirre, G.K., Detre, J.A., Alsop, D.C., and D'Esposito, M. (1996). The parahippocampus subserves topographical learning in man. *Cereb. Cortex* **6** (6), 823–9.

Albert, M.L. (1973). A simple test for visual neglect. *Neurology* **23**, 658–64.

Andersen, R.A., Snyder, L.H., Bradley, D.C., and Xing, J. (1997). Multimodal representation of space in the posterior parietal cortex and its use in planning movements. *Annu. Rev. Neurosci.* **20**, 303–30.

Andre, J.M., Beis, J.M., Morin, N., and Paysant, J. (2000). Buccal hemineglect. *Arch. Neurol.* **57** (12), 1734–41.

Babinski, J. (1914). Contribution à l'étude des troubles mentaux dans l'hémiplégie organique cérébrale (anosognosie). *Rev. Neurol. (Paris)* **27**, 845–8.

Balint, R. (1909). Seelenlahmung des 'schauens', optische atazie, raumliche storung der aufmerksamleit. *Monatsschr. Psychiatrie Neurol.* **25**, 51–81.

Bartolomeo, P., Dalla Barba, G., Boisse, M.F., Bachoud-Levi, A.C., Degos, J.D., and Boller, F. (1998). Right-side neglect in Alzheimer's disease. *Neurology* **51** (4), 1207–9.

Bartolomeo, P., Perri, R., and Gainotti, G. (2004). The influence of limb crossing on left tactile extinction. *J. Neurol. Neurosurg. Psychiatry* **75** (1), 49–55.

Bellas, D.N., Novelly, R.A., Eskenazi, B., and Wasserstein, J. (1988*a*). The nature of unilateral neglect in the olfactory sensory system. *Neuropsychologia* **26** (1), 45–52.

Bellas, D.N., Novelly, R.A., Eskenazi, B., and Wasserstein, J. (1988*b*). Unilateral displacement in the olfactory sense: a manifestation of the unilateral neglect syndrome. *Cortex* **24** (2), 267–75.

Bellas, D.N., Novelly, R.A., and Eskenazi, B. (1989). Olfactory lateralization and identification in right hemisphere lesion and control patients. *Neuropsychologia* **27** (9), 1187–91.

Bellmann, A., Meuli, R., and Clarke, S. (2001). Two types of auditory neglect. *Brain* **124** (4), 676–87.

Bender, M. (1945). Extinction and precipitation of cutaneous sensations. *Arch. Neurol. Psychiatry* **54**, 1–9.

Bender, M.B. (1970). Perceptual interactions. In *Modern trends in neurology* (ed. D. Williams), Vol. 5, pp. 1–28. Butterworths, London.

Bender, M.B. and Feldman, D.S. (1952). Extinction of taste sensation on double simultaneous stimulation. *Neurology* **2**(3), 195–202.

Bender, M.B. and Teuber, H.L. (1947). Spatial organization of visual perception following injury to the brain. *Arch. Neurol. Psychiatry* **58**, 721–38.

Berlucchi, G., Moro, V., Guerrini, C., and Aglioti, S.M. (2004). Dissociation between taste and tactile extinction on the tongue after right brain damage. *Neuropsychologia* **42** (8), 1007–16.

Berti, A. (2002). Unconscious processing in neglect. In *The cognitive and neural bases of spatial neglect* (ed. H.O. Karnath, A.D. Milner, and G. Vallar), pp. 313–26. Oxford University Press, New York.

Berti, A. and Frassinetti, F. (2000). When far becomes near: re-mapping of space by tool use. *J. Cogn. Neurosci.* **12** (3), 415–20.

Berti, A. and Rizzolatti, G. (1992). Visual processing without awareness: evidence from unilateral neglect. *J. Cogn. Neurosci.* **4**, 345–51.

Berti, A., Allport, A., Driver, J., Dienes, Z., Oxbury, J., and Oxbury, S. (1992). Levels of processing for visual stimuli in an extinguished field. *Neuropsychologia* **30** (5), 403–15.

Berti, A., Frassinetti, F., and Umiltà, C. (1994). Nonconscious reading? Evidence from neglect dyslexia. *Cortex* **30** (2), 181–97.

Berti, A., Làdavas, E., and Della, C.M. (1996). Anosognosia for hemiplegia, neglect dyslexia, and drawing neglect: clinical findings and theoretical considerations. *J. Int. Neuropsychol. Soc.* **2** (5), 426–40.

Berti, A., Oxbury, S., Oxbury, J., Affanni, P., Umiltà, C., and Orlandi, L. (1999). Somatosensory extinction for meaningful objects in a patient with right hemispheric stroke. *Neuropsychologia* **37** (3), 333–43.

Binkofski, F., Buccino, G., Dohle, C., Seitz, R.J., and Freund, H.J. (1999). Mirror agnosia and mirror ataxia constitute different parietal lobe disorders. *Ann. Neurol.* **46** (1), 51–61.

Bisiach, E. (1991). Extinction and neglect: same or different? In *Brain and space* (ed. J. Paillard), pp. 251–7. Oxford University Press, Oxford.

Bisiach, E. and Geminiani, G. (1991). Anosognosia related to hemiplegia and hemianopia. In *Awareness of deficit after brain injury* (ed. G.P. Prigatano and D. Shacter), pp. 17–39. Oxford University Press, New York.

Bisiach, E. and Luzzatti, C. (1978). Neglect of representational space. *Cortex* **14**, 129–33.

Bisiach, E. and Vallar, G. (2000). Unilateral neglect in humans. In *Handbook of neuropsychology*, 2nd edn (ed. F. Boller and J. Grafman), pp. 459–502. Elsevier, Amsterdam.

Bisiach, E., Cornacchia, L., Sterzi, R., and Vallar, G. (1984). Disorders of perceived auditory lateralization after lesions of the right hemisphere. *Brain* **107** (1), 37–52.

Bisiach, E., Perani, D., Vallar, G., and Berti, A. (1986*a*). Unilateral neglect: personal and extra-personal. *Neuropsychologia* **24** (6), 759–67.

Bisiach, E., Vallar, G., Perani, D., Papagno, C., and Berti, A. (1986*b*). Unawareness of disease following lesions of the right hemisphere: anosognosia for hemiplegia and anosognosia for hemianopia. *Neuropsychologia* **24**, 471–82.

Bisiach, E., Geminiani, G., Berti, A., and Rusconi, M.L. (1990). Perceptual and premotor factors of unilateral neglect. *Neurology* **40** (8), 1278–81.

Bisiach, E., Rusconi, M.L., and Vallar, G. (1991). Remission of somatoparaphrenic delusion through vestibular stimulation. *Neuropsychologia* **29** (10), 1029–31.

Bisiach, E., Brouchon, M., Poncet, M., and Rusconi, M.L. (1993). Unilateral neglect in route description. *Neuropsychologia* **31** (11), 1255–62.

Bisiach, E., Ricci, R., Berruti, G., Genero, R., Pepi, R., and Fumelli, T. (1999). Two-dimensional distortion of space representation in unilateral neglect: perceptual and response-related factors. *Neuropsychologia* **37** (13), 1491–8.

Bottini, G., Cappa, S., Geminiani, G., and Sterzi, R. (1990). Topographic disorientation—a case report. *Neuropsychologia* **28** (3), 309–12.

Bottini, G., Bisiach, E., Sterzi, R., and Vallar, G. (2002). Feeling touches in someone else's hand. *Neuroreport* **13** (2), 249–52.

Bottini, G., Paulesu, E., Gandola, M., Loffredo, S., Scarpa, P., Sterzi, R., *et al.* (2005). Left caloric vestibular stimulation ameliorates right hemianesthesia. *Neurology* **65** (8), 1278–83.

Bundesen, C. (1990). A theory of visual attention. *Psychol. Rev.* **97**, 523–47.

Burgess, N., Jeffery, K.J., and O'Keefe, J. (Eds.) (1999). *The hippocampal and parietal foundations of spatial cognition*. Oxford University Press, Oxford.

Calvert, G.A., Campbell, R., and Brammer, M.J. (2000). Evidence from functional magnetic resonance imaging of crossmodal binding in the human heteromodal cortex. *Curr. Biol.* **10** (11), 649–57.

Calvert, G.A., Spence, C., and Stein, B.E. (Eds.) (2004). *The handbook of multisensory processes*. MIT Press, Cambridge, Massachusetts.

Caramazza, A. and Hillis, A.E. (1990). Spatial representation of words in the brain implied by studies of a unilateral neglect patient. *Nature* **346** (6281), 267–9.

Castaigne, P., Laplane, D., and Degos, J. (1972). [3 cases of motor neglect due to prerolandic frontal lesion]. *Rev. Neurol. (Paris)* **126** (1), 5–15.

Chatterjee, A. (1995). Cross-over, completion and confabulation in unilateral spatial neglect. *Brain* **118** (2), 455–65.

Clarke, S. and Thiran, A.B. (2004). Auditory neglect: what and where in auditory space. *Cortex* **40** (2), 291–300.

Cocchini, G., Beschin, N., and Jehkonen, M. (2001). The fluff test: a simple task to assess body representation neglect. *Neuropsycho. Rehabil.* **11** (1), 17–31.

Colby, C.L., Duhamel, J.-R., and Goldberg, M.E. (1993). Ventral intraparietal area of the macaque: anatomic location and visual response properties. *J. Neurophysiol.* **69** (3), 902–14.

Corbetta, M. and Shulman, G.L. (2002). Control of goal-directed and stimulus-driven attention in the brain. *Nature Rev. Neurosci.* **3** (3), 201–15.

Corbetta, M., Kincade, J.M., Ollinger, J.M., McAvoy, M.P., and Shulman, G.L. (2000). Voluntary orienting is dissociated from target detection in human posterior parietal cortex. *Nature Neurosci.* **3** (3), 292–297.

Cowey, A., Small, M., and Ellis, S. (1994). Left visuo-spatial neglect can be worse in far than in near space. *Neuropsychologia* **32** (9), 1059–66.

Cowey, A., Small, M., and Ellis, S. (1999). No abrupt change in visual hemineglect from near to far space. *Neuropsychologia* **37** (1), 1–6.

Daini, R., Angelelli, P., Antonucci, G., Cappa, S.F., and Vallar, G. (2002). Exploring the syndrome of spatial unilateral neglect through an illusion of length. *Exp. Brain Res.* **144** (2), 224–37.

Denny-Brown, D., Meyer, J.S., and Horenstein, S. (1952). The significance of perceptual rivalry resulting from parietal lesion. *Brain* **75** (4), 433–71.

Deouell, L.Y., Bentin, S., and Soroker, N. (2000*a*). Electrophysiological evidence for an early(pre-attentive) information processing deficit in patients with right hemisphere damage and unilateral neglect. *Brain* **123**, 353–65.

Deouell, L.Y., Hamalainen, H., and Bentin, S. (2000*b*). Unilateral neglect after right-hemisphere damage: contributions from event-related potentials. *Audiol. Neurootol.* **5** (3–4), 225–34.

De Renzi, E., Faglioni, P., and Scotti, G. (1971). Judgment of spatial orientation in patients with focal brain damage. *J. Neurol. Neurosurg. Psychiatry* **34**, 489–95.

De Renzi, E., Gentilini, M., and Pattacini, F. (1984). Auditory extinction following hemisphere damage. *Neuropsychologia* **22** (6), 733–44.

Desimone, R. and Duncan, J. (1995). Neural mechanisms of selective visual attention. *Annu. Rev. Neurosci.* **18**, 193–222.

di Pellegrino, G. and De Renzi, E. (1995). An experimental investigation on the nature of extinction. *Neuropsychologia* **33**, 153–70.

di Pellegrino, G., Basso, G., and Frassinetti, F. (1997*a*). Spatial extinction on double asynchronous stimulation. *Neuropsychologia* **35**(9), 1215–23.

di Pellegrino, G., L‡davas, E., and FarnÈ, A. (1997*b*). Seeing where your hands are. *Nature* **388** (6644), 730.

Driver, J., Baylis, G., and Rafal, R. (1993). Preserved figure–ground segmentation and symmetry perception in a patient with neglect. *Nature* **360**, 73–5.

Driver, J., Mattingley, J.B., Rorden, C., and Davis, G. (1997). Extinction as a paradigm measure of attentional bias and restricted capacity following brain injury. In *Parietal lobe contributions to orientation in 3D space* (ed. P. Thier and H.-O. Karnath), pp. 401–29. Springer Verlag, Heidelberg.

Driver, J., Vuilleumier, P., Eimer, M., and Rees, G. (2001). Functional magnetic resonance imaging and evoked potential correlates of conscious and unconscious vision in parietal extinction patients. *Neuroimage* **14** (2), S68–75.

Duhamel, J.-R., Bremmer, F., BenHamed, S., and Graf, W. (1997). Spatial invariance of visual receptive fields in parietal cortex neurons. *Nature* **389** (23), 845–8.

Duhamel, J.-R., Colby, C.L., and Goldberg, M.E. (1998). Ventral intraparietal area of the macaque: Congruent visual and somatic response properties. *J. Neurophysiol.* **79** (1), 126–36.

Eimer, M., Maravita, A., Van Velzen, J., Husain, M., and Driver, J. (2002). The electrophysiology of tactile extinction: ERP correlates of unconscious somatosensory processing. *Neuropsychologia* **40** (13), 2438–47.

Faglioni, P., Scotti, G., and Spinnler, H. (1971). The performance of brain-damaged patients in spatial localization of vuisual and tactile stimuli. *Brain* **94**, 443–54.

Farnè, A. and Làdavas, E. (2000). Dynamic size-change of hand peripersonal space following tool use. *Neuroreport* **11** (8), 1645–9.

Farnè, A. and Ladàvas, E. (2002). Auditory peripersonal space in humans. *J. Cogn. Neurosci.* **14** (7), 1030–43.

Fiorelli, M., Blin, J., Bakchine, S., Laplane, D., and Baron, J.C. (1991). Pet studies of cortical diaschisis in patients with motor hemi-neglect. *J Neurol Sci* **104** (2), 135–42.

Fogassi, L., Gallese, V., Fadiga, L., Luppino, G., Matelli, M., and Rizzolatti, G. (1996). Coding of peripersonal space in inferior premotor cortex (area F4). *J. Neurophysiol.* **76** (1), 141–57.

Frassinetti, F., Bolognini, N., and Ladàvas, E. (2002). Enhancement of visual perception by crossmodal visuo-auditory interaction. *Exp. Brain Res.* **147** (3), 332–43.

Galati, G., Lobel, E., Vallar, G., Berthoz, A., Pizzamiglio, L., and Le Bihan, D. (2000). The neural basis of egocentric and allocentric coding of space in humans: a functional magnetic resonance study. *Exp. Brain Res.* **133** (2), 156–64.

Gialanella, B., Monguzzi, V., Santoro, R., and Rocchi, S. (2005). Functional recovery after hemiplegia in patients with neglect: the rehabilitative role of anosognosia. *Stroke* **36** (12), 2687–90.

Graziano, M.S.A. and Botvinick, M.M. (2002). How the brain represents the body: insights into neurophysiology and psychology. In *Common mechanisms in perception and action: attention and performance XIX* (ed. W. Prinz and B. Hommel), pp. 136–57. Oxford University Press, Oxford.

Graziano, M.S. and Gross, C.G. (1994). The representation of extrapersonal space: a possible role for bimodal, visual–tactile neurons. In *The cognitive neurosciences* (ed. M.S. Gazzaniga), pp. 1021–34. MIT Press, Cambridge, Massachusetts.

Graziano, M.S., Reiss, L.A., and Gross, C.G. (1999). A neuronal representation of the location of nearby sounds. *Nature* **397** (6718), 428–30.

Graziano, M.S., Taylor, C.S., Moore, T., and Cooke, D.F. (2002). The cortical control of movement revisited. *Neuron* **36** (3), 349–62.

Guariglia, C., Padovani, A., Pantano, P., and Pizzamiglio, L. (1993). Unilateral neglect restricted to visual imagery. *Nature* **364** (6434), 235–7.

Habib, M. and Sirigu, A. (1987). Pure topographical disorientation: a definition and anatomical basis. *Cortex* **23**, 73–85.

Halligan, P. and Marshall, J. (1988). How long is a piece of string? A study of line bisection in a case of visual neglect. *Cortex* **24** (2), 321–8.

Halligan, P.W. and Marshall, J.C. (1991). Left neglect for near but not far space in man. *Nature* **350** (6318), 498–500.

Halligan, P.W. and Marshall, J.C. (1995). Lateral and radial neglect as a function of spatial position: a case study. *Neuropsychologia* **33** (12), 1697–702.

Halligan, P.W., Marshall, J.C., and Wade, D.T. (1995). Unilateral somatoparaphrenia after right hemisphere stroke: a case description. *Cortex* **31** (1), 173–82.

Heilman, K. and Valenstein, E. (1972). Auditory neglect in man. *Arch. Neurol.* **26**, 32–5.

Heilman, K. and Valenstein, E. (1979). Mechanisms underlying hemispatial neglect. *Ann. Neurol.* **5** (2), 166– 70.

Heilman, K.M. and Valenstein, E. (2003). *Clinical neuropsychology*, 4th edn. Oxford University Press, Oxford.

Heilman, K., Bowers, D., Coslett, H., Whelan, H., and Watson, R. (1985). Directional hypokinesia: prolonged reaction times for leftward movements in patients with right hemisphere lesions and neglect. *Neurology* **35** (6), 855–9.

Husain, M. and Rorden, C. (2003). Non-spatially lateralized mechanisms in hemispatial neglect. *Nature Rev. Neurosci.* **4**, 26–36.

Husain, M., Shapiro, K., Martin, J., and Kennard, C. (1997). Abnormal temporal dynamics of visual attention in spatial neglect patients. *Nature* **385**, 154–6.

Husain, M., Mattingley, J.B., Rorden, C., Kennard, C., and Driver, J. (2000). Distinguishing sensory and motor biases in parietal and frontal neglect. *Brain* **123** (8), 1643–59.

Inhoff, A.W., Rafal, R.D., and Posner, M.J. (1992). Bimodal extinction without cross-modal extinction. *J. Neurol. Neurosurg. Psychiatry* **55** (1), 36–9.

Jehkonen, M., Laihosalo, M., and Kettunen, J.E. (2006). Impact of neglect on functional outcome after stroke: a review of methodological issues and recent research findings. *Restor. Neurol. Neurosci.* **24** (4–6), 209–15.

Karnath, H.O., Ferber, S., and Himmelbach, M. (2001). Spatial awareness is a function of the temporal not the posterior parietal lobe. *Nature* **411** (6840), 950–3.

Karnath, H.O., Milner, A.D., and Vallar, G. (2002). *The cognitive and neural bases of spatial neglect.* Oxford University Press, New York.

Karnath, H.O., Himmelbach, M., and Kuker, W. (2003). The cortical substrate of visual extinction. *Neuroreport* **14** (3), 437–42.

Kinsbourne, M. (1977). Hemi-neglect and hemisphere rivalry. *Adv. Neurol.* **18**, 41–9.

Kooistra, C.A. and Heilman, K.M. (1989). Hemispatial visual inattention masquerading as hemianopia. *Neurology* **39** (8), 1125–7.

Làdavas, E. (2002). Functional and dynamic properties of visual peripersonal space. *Trends Cogn. Sci.* **6** (1), 17–22.

Laplane, D. and Degos, J. (1983). Motor neglect. *J. Neurol. Neurosurg. Psychiatry* **46** (2), 152–8.

Liu, G., Bolton, A., Price, B., and Weintraub, S. (1992). Dissociated perceptual-sensory and exploratory-motor neglect. *J. Neurol. Neurosurg. Psychiatry* **55** (8), 701–6.

Macaluso, E. and Driver, J. (2003). Multimodal spatial representations in the human parietal cortex: evidence from functional imaging. *Adv Neurol* **93**, 219–33.

Macaluso, E., Frith, C.D., and Driver, J. (2000). Modulation of human visual cortex by crossmodal spatial attention. *Science* **289** (5482), 1206–8.

Manly, T., Woldt, K., Watson, P., and Warburton, E. (2002). Is motor perseveration in unilateral neglect 'driven' by the presence of neglected left-sided stimuli? *Neuropsychologia* **40** (11), 1794–803.

Maravita, A. (1997). Implicit processing of somatosensory stimuli disclosed by a perceptual after-effect. *Neuroreport* **8** (7), 1671–4.

Maravita, A. (2006). From 'body in the brain' to 'body in space'. Sensory and intentional components of body representation. In *Human body perception from the inside out* (ed. G. Knoblich, I. Thornton, M. Grosjean, and M. Shiffrar), pp. 65–88. Oxford University Press, New York.

Maravita, A. and Iriki, A. (2004). Tools for the body (schema). *Trends Cogn. Sci.* **8** (2), 79–86.

Maravita, A., Husain, M., Clarke, K., and Driver, J. (2001). Reaching with a tool extends visual–tactile interactions into far space: evidence from cross-modal extinction. *Neuropsychologia* **39** (6), 580–5.

Maravita, A., Clarke, K., Husain, M., and Driver, J. (2002). Active tool-use with contralesional hand can reduce crossmodal extinction of touch on that hand. *Neurocase* **8**, 411–16.

Maravita, A., McNeil, J., Malhotra, P., Greenwood, R., Husain, M., and Driver, J. (2003*a*). Prism adaptation can improve contralesional tactile perception in neglect. *Neurology* **60** (11), 1829–31.

Maravita, A., Spence, C., and Driver, J. (2003*b*). Multisensory integration and the body schema: Close to hand and within reach. *Curr. Biol.* **13** (13), 531–9.

Marshall, J. and Halligan, P. (1988). Blindsight and insight in visuo-spatial neglect. *Nature* **336** (6201), 766–7.

Marshall, J.C. and Halligan, P.W. (1993). Visuo-spatial neglect: a new copying test to assess perceptual parsing. *J. Neurol.* **240** (1), 37–40.

Marzi, C.A., Smania, N., Martini, M.C., Gambina, G., Tomelleri, G., Palamara, A., *et al.* (1996). Implicit redundant target-effects in visual extinction. *Neuropsychologia* **34**, 9–22.

Marzi, C.A., Girelli, M., Miniussi, C., Smania, N., and Maravita, A. (2000). Electrophysiological correlates of conscious vision: evidence from unilateral extinction. *J.Cogn. Neurosci.* **12** (5), 869–77.

Mattingley, J.B., Davis, G., and Driver, J. (1997*a*). Preattentive filling-in of visual surfaces in parietal extinction. *Science* **275**, 671–4.

Mattingley, J.B., Driver, J., Beschin, N., and Robertson, I. H. (1997*b*). Attentional competition between modalities: extinction between touch and vision after right hemisphere damage. *Neuropsychologia* **35** (6), 867–80.

Mattingley, J.B., Husain, M., Rorden, C., Kennard, C., and Driver, J. (1998). Motor role of human inferior parietal lobe revealed in unilateral neglect patients. *Nature* **392** (6672), 179–82.

Meador, K.J., Allen, M.E., Adams, R.J., and Loring, D.W. (1991). Allochiria vs allesthesia. Is there a misperception? *Arch. Neurol.* **48** (5), 546–9.

Mesulam, M.M. (1985). *Principles of behavioral neurology*. F.A. Davis, Philadelphia.

Milner, A. D. (1997). Neglect, extinction and the cortical streams of visual processing. In *Parietal lobe contributions to orientation in 3D space* (ed. P. Thier and H.-O. Karnath), pp. 3–22. Springer-Verlag, Heidelberg.

Milner, A., Harvey, M., Roberts, R., and Forster, S. (1993). Line bisection errors in visual neglect: Misguided action or size distortion? *Neuropsychologia* **31** (1), 39–49.

Mort, D.J., Malhotra, P., Mannan, S.K., Rorden, C., Pambakian, A., Kennard, C., *et al.* (2003). The anatomy of visual neglect. *Brain* **126** (9), 1986–97.

Moschowitch, M. and Behrmann, M. (1994). Coding of spatial information in the somatosensory system: evidence from patients with neglect following parietal lobe damage. *J. Cogn. Neurosci.* **6** (2), 151–5.

Ogden, J. A. (1985). Anterior-posterior interhemispheric differences in the loci of lesions. *Brain Cogn.* **4**, 59–75.

Pavani, F., Meneghello, F., and Làdavas, E. (2001). Deficit of auditory space perception in patients with visuospatial neglect. *Neuropsychologia* **39** (13), 1401–9.

Pavani, F., Làdavas, E., and Driver, J. (2002). Selective deficit of auditory localisation in patients with visuospatial neglect. *Neuropsychologia* **40** (3), 291–301.

Pavani, F., Làdavas, E., and Driver, J. (2003). Auditory and multisensory aspects of visuospatial neglect. *Trends Cogn. Sci.* **7** (9), 407–14.

Pavani, F., Husain, M., Làdavas, E., and Driver, J. (2004). Auditory deficits in visuospatial neglect patients. *Cortex* **40** (2), 347–65.

Perenin, M.T. (1997). Clinical evidence for dissociable spatial functions. In *Parietal lobe contributions to orientation in 3d space* (ed. P. Thier and H.-O. Karnath), pp. 289–308. Springer Verlag, Heidelberg.

Perenin, M.T. and Vighetto, A. (1988). Optic ataxia: a specific disorder in visuomotor coordination. In *Visually oriented behavior* (ed. A. Hein and M. Jeannerod), pp. 305–26. Springer, Heidelberg.

Pisella, L., Binkofski, F., Lasek, K., Toni, I., and Rossetti, Y. (2006). No double-dissociation between optic ataxia and visual agnosia: multiple sub-streams for multiple visuo-manual integrations. *Neuropsychologia* **44** (13), 2734–48.

Pizzamiglio, L., Cappa, S., Vallar, G., Zoccolotti, P., Bottini, G., Ciurli, P., *et al.* (1989). Visual neglect for far and near extra-personal space in humans. *Cortex* **25** (3), 471–7.

Rafal, R.D. (1994). Neglect. *Curr. Opin. Neurobiol.* **4**, 2312–16.

Rafal, R. (1997). Balint syndrome. In *Behavioral neurology and neuropsychology* (ed. T.E. Feinberg and M.J. Farah), pp. 337–56. Mc Graw-Hill, New York.

Rapcsak, S.Z., Watson, R.T., and Heilman, K.M. (1987). Hemispace–visual field interactions in visual extinction. *J. Neurol. Neurosurg. Psychiatry* **50** (9), 1117–24.

Rees, G., Wojciulik, E., Clarke, K., Husain, M., Frith, C., and Driver, J. (2000). Unconscious activation of visual cortex in the damaged right hemisphere of a parietal patient with extinction. *Brain* **123** (8), 1624–33.

Ringman, J.M., Saver, J.L., Woolson, R.F., Clarke, W.R., and Adams, H.P. (2004). Frequency, risk factors, anatomy, and course of unilateral neglect in an acute stroke cohort. *Neurology* **63** (3), 468–74.

Rizzolatti, G. and Berti, A. (1990). Neglect as a neural representation deficit. *Rev. Neurol. (Paris)* **146** (10), 626–34.

Rizzolatti, G., Scandolara, C., Matelli, M., and Gentilucci, M. (1981). Afferent properties of periarcuate neurons in macaque monkeys. II. Visual responses. *Behav. Brain Res.* **2** (2), 147–63.

Rizzolatti, G., Matelli, M., and Pavesi, G. (1983). Deficits in attention and movement following the removal of postarcuate (area 6) and prearcuate (area 8) cortex in macaque monkeys. *Brain* **106** (3), 655–73.

Rizzolatti, G., Fadiga, L., Fogassi, L., and Gallese, V. (1997). The space around us. *Science* **277** (5323), 190–1.

Rizzolatti, G., Luppino, G., and Matelli, M. (1998). The organization of the cortical motor system: New concepts. *Electroencephalogr. Clin. Neurophysiol.* **106** (4), 283–96.

Robertson, I., Mattingley, J.B., Rorden, C., and Driver, J. (1998). Phasic alerting of neglect patients overcomes their spatial deficit in visual awareness. *Nature* **395**, 169–72.

Robertson, L.C. and Rafal, R. (2000). Disorders of visual attention. In *The cognitive neurosciences*, 2nd edn (ed. M.S. Gazzaniga), pp. 633–49. MIT Press, Cambridge, Massachusetts.

Robertson, L.C., Treisman, A., and Friedman-Hill, S. (1997). The interaction of spatial and object pathways: evidence from the Balint syndrome. *J. Cogn. Neurosci.* **9**, 295–317.

Rorden, C., Mattingley, J.B., Karnath, H.O., and Driver, J. (1997). Visual extinction and prior entry: impaired perception of temporal order with intact motion perception after unilateral parietal damage. *Neuropsychologia* **35** (4), 421–33.

Rossetti, Y., Pisella, L., and Vighetto, A. (2003). Optic ataxia revisited: visually guided action versus immediate visuomotor control. *Exp. Brain Res.* **153** (2), 171–9.

Rusconi, M.L., Maravita, A., Bottini, G., and Vallar, G. (2002). Is the intact side really intact? Perseverative responses in patients with unilateral neglect: a productive manifestation. *Neuropsychologia* **40** (6), 594–604.

Sarri, M., Balnkenburg, F., and Driver, J. (2006). Neural correlates of crossmodal visual-tactile extinction and of tactile awareness revealed by fMRI in a right-hemisphere stroke patient. *Neuropsychologia* **44**, 2398–410.

Semmes, J., Weinstein, S., Ghent, L., and Teuber, H.L. (1955). Spatial orientation in man after cerebral injury. 1: Analysis by locus of lesion. *J. Psychol.* **39**, 227–44.

Semmes, J., Weinstein, S., Ghent, L., and Teuber, H.L. (1963). Correlate of impaired orientation in personal and extra-personal space. *Brain* **86**, 747–72.

Soroker, N., Calamaro, N., and Myslobodsky, M.S. (1995). Ventriloquist effect reinstates responsiveness to auditory stimuli in the 'ignored' space in patients with hemispatial neglect. *J. Clin. Exp. Neuropsychol.* **17** (2), 243–55.

Spence, C. and Driver, J. (2004). *Crossmodal space and crossmodal attention.* Oxford University Press, Oxford.

Spence, C., Pavani, F., Maravita, A., and Holmes, N. (2004). Multisensory contributions to the 3-D representation of visuotactile peripersonal space in humans: evidence from the crossmodal congruency task. *J. Physiol. Paris* **98** (1–3), 171–89.

Stein, B.E. (2005). The development of a dialogue between cortex and midbrain to integrate multisensory information. *Exp. Brain Res.* **166** (3–4), 305–15.

Stein, B.E. and Meredith, M.A. (1993). *The merging of the senses.* MIT Press, Cambridge, Massachusetts.

Sterzi, R., Bottini, G., Celani, M.G., Righetti, E., Lamassa, M., Ricci, S., *et al.* (1993). Hemianopia, hemi-anaesthesia, and hemiplegia after right and left hemisphere damage. A hemispheric difference. *J. Neurol. Neurosurg. Psychiatry* **56** (3), 308–10.

Takahashi, N., Kawamura, M., Shiota, J., Kasahata, N., and Hirayama, K. (1997). Pure topographic disorientation due to right retrosplenial lesion. *Neurology* **49** (2), 464–9.

Tanaka, H., Hachisuka, K., and Ogata, H. (1999). Sound lateralisation in patients with left or right cerebral hemispheric lesions: relation with unilateral visuospatial neglect. *J. Neurol. Neurosurg. Psychiatry* **67** (4), 481–6.

Tegner, R. and Levander, M. (1991). Through a looking glass. A new technique to demonstrate directional hypokinesia in unilateral neglect. *Brain* **114** (4), 1943–51.

Tinazzi, M., Ferrari, G., Zampini, M., and Aglioti, S.M. (2000). Neuropsychological evidence that somatic stimuli are spatially coded according to multiple frames of reference in a stroke patient with tactile extinction. *Neurosci. Lett.* **287** (2), 133–6.

Ungerleider, L.G. and Mishkin, M. (1982). The two cortical systems. In *Analysis of visual behaviour* (ed. D.I. Ingle, M.A. Goodale, and R.J.W. Mansfield), pp. 549–86. MIT Press, Cambridge, Massachusetts.

Valenza, N., Murray, M.M., Ptak, R., and Vuilleumier, P. (2004*a*). The space of senses: impaired crossmodal interactions in a patient with Balint syndrome after bilateral parietal damage. *Neuropsychologia* **42** (13), 1737–48.

Valenza, N., Seghier, M.L., Schwartz, S., Lazeyras, F., and Vuilleumier, P. (2004*b*). Tactile awareness and limb position in neglect: functional magnetic resonance imaging. *Ann. Neurol.* **55** (1), 139–43.

Vallar, G. and Perani, D. (1986). The anatomy of unilateral neglect after right-hemisphere stroke lesions. A clinical/CT-scan correlation study in man. *Neuropsychologia* **24** (5), 609–22.

Vallar, G. and Ronchi, R. (2006). Anosognosia for motor and sensory deficits after unilateral brain damage: a review. *Restor. Neurol. Neurosci.* **24** (4–6), 247–57.

Vallar, G., Sterzi, R., Bottini, G., Cappa, S., and Rusconi, M. (1990). Temporary remission of left hemianes-thesia after vestibular stimulation. A sensory neglect phenomenon. *Cortex* **26** (1), 123–31.

Vallar, G., Bottini, G., Sterzi, R., Passerini, D., and Rusconi, M. (1991*a*). Hemianesthesia, sensory neglect, and defective access to conscious experience. *Neurology* **41** (5), 650–2.

Vallar, G., Sandroni, P., Rusconi, M.L., and Barbieri, S. (1991*b*). Hemianopia, hemianesthesia, and spatial neglect: a study with evoked potentials. *Neurology* **41** (12), 1918–22.

Vallar, G., Antonucci, G., Guariglia, C., and Pizzamiglio, L. (1993*a*). Deficits of position sense, unilateral neglect and optokinetic stimulation. *Neuropsychologia* **31** (11), 1191–200.

Vallar, G., Bottini, G., Rusconi, M., and Sterzi, R. (1993*b*). Exploring somatosensory hemineglect by vestibular stimulation. *Brain* **116**, 71–86.

Vallar, G., Rusconi, M.L., Bignamini, L., Geminiani, G., and Perani, D. (1994). Anatomical correlates of visual and tactile extinction in humans: a clinical CT scan study. *J. Neurol. Neurosurg. Psychiatry* **57** (4), 464–70.

Vallar, G., Guariglia, C., Nico, D., and Bisiach, E. (1995*a*). Spatial hemineglect in back space. *Brain* **118** (2), 467–72.

Vallar, G., Rusconi, M.L., Barozzi, S., Bernardini, B., Ovadia, D., Papagno, C., *et al.* (1995*b*). Improvement of left visuo-spatial hemineglect by left-sided transcutaneous electrical stimulation. *Neuropsychologia* **33** (1), 73–82.

Vallar, G., Lobel, E., Galati, G., Berthoz, A., Pizzamiglio, L., and Le Bihan, D. (1999). A fronto-parietal system for computing the egocentric spatial frame of reference in humans. *Exp. Brain Res.* **124** (3), 281–6.

Vallar, G., Bottini, G., and Paulesu, E. (2003*a*). Neglect syndromes: The role of the parietal cortex. *Adv. Neurol.* **93**, 293–319.

Vallar, G., Bottini, G., and Sterzi, R. (2003*b*). Anosognosia for left-sided motor and sensory deficits, motor neglect, and sensory hemiinattention: is there a relationship? *Prog. Brain Res.* **142**, 289–301.

von Giesen, H.J., Schlaug, G., Steinmetz, H., Benecke, R., Freund, H.J., and Seitz, R.J. (1994). Cerebral network underlying unilateral motor neglect: evidence from positron emission tomography. *J. Neurol. Sci.* **125** (1), 29–38.

Vuilleumier, P. (2002). Perceived gaze direction in faces and spatial attention: a study in patients with parietal damage and unilateral neglect. *Neuropsychologia* **40** (7), 1013–26.

Vuilleumier, P., Valenza, N., Mayer, E., Reverdin, A., and Landis, T. (1998). Near and far visual space in unilateral neglect. *Ann. Neurol.* **43** (3), 406–10.

Vuilleumier, P., Valenza, N., Mayer, E., Perrig, S., and Landis, T. (1999). To see better to the left when looking more to the right: effects of gaze direction and frames of spatial coordinates in unilateral neglect. *J. Int. Neuropsychol. Soc.* **5** (1), 75–82.

Vuilleumier, P., Sagiv, N., Hazeltine, E., Poldrack, R.A., Swick, D., Rafal, R.D., *et al.* (2001). Neural fate of seen and unseen faces in visuospatial neglect: a combined event-related functional MRI and event-related potential study. *Proc. Natl. Acad. Sci. USA* **98** (6), 3495–500.

Wallace, M.T. and Stein, B.E. (1994). Cross-modal synthesis in the midbrain depends on input from cortex. *J. Neurophysiol.* **71** (1), 429–32.

Walsh, K.W. and Darby, D. (1999). *Neuropsychology: a clinical approach*, 4th edn. Churchill Livingstone, Edinburgh.

Ward, R., Goodrich, S., and Driver, J. (1994). Grouping reduces visual extinction: neuropsychological evidence for weight-linkage in visual attention. *Visual Cogn.* **1**, 101–29.

Wilson, B., Cockbourn, J., and Halligan, P. (1987). *Behavioural inattention test*. Thames Valley, Titchfield, England.

Chapter 7

Memory disorders

Sandra Lehmann and Armin Schnider

7.1 Introduction

Memory is the capacity to acquire, store, and retrieve information. It is composed of multiple systems and processes, with different functional roles and anatomical substrates (Table 7.1). One of the main dissociations in memory concerns the duration of storage systems. Short-term memory holds information active in the mind over limited time periods, while long-term memory stores information durably (Hebb 1949). Dissociation of these systems is common in amnesia. Amnesic patients tend to show relatively preserved short-term memory, but fail to encode information into a more durable and stable trace. A second distinction concerns declarative and non-declarative memory systems (Squire 1987). Declarative memory defines the capacity to learn, store, and recall information explicitly; non-declarative memory refers to the capacity to learn information implicitly, mainly through repeated exposure to a stimulus or task. Declarative memory is divided into an episodic component that stores information about events together with their spatio-temporal context, and a semantic component devoted to storing general knowledge about words, objects, and concepts (Tulving 1972). Declarative memory is impaired in amnesia, in particular, the capacity to encode and retrieve new episodic information. Brain lesions can cause anterograde amnesia, which denotes the difficulty to form new memories. They can also induce retrograde amnesia, i.e. an incapacity to retrieve memories that were formed before the injury. Semantic memory is comparatively less vulnerable, but may be impaired through lesions to distinct anatomical structures. Non-declarative memory functions comprise a variety of effects: (1) priming is the enhanced information processing that can occur through repeated exposure to a stimulus; (2) procedural learning denotes the capacity to develop new skills by repeatedly executing a series of actions and organized procedures; and (3) automatic stimulus–response associations can be formed through conditioning. Implicit forms of memory depend on brain areas that are involved in the sensory and perceptual processing of information, and are relatively preserved in amnesia.

> Memory is composed of multiple dissociable systems, varying according to the length of retention interval, level of consciousness, and modality of information to be learned. Memory systems are differentially affected in amnesia, depending from localization and aetiology of brain lesions.

7.2 Short-term and working memory

Short-term memory is an explicit form of memory. It allows a limited amount of information to be kept active in the mind during brief time intervals. The definition of short-term memory

Table 7.1 Memory systems

Short-term memory	
Working memory	
Long-term memory	
Declarative	*Non-declarative*
Episodic memory	Priming
Autobiographical memory	Procedural learning
Semantic memory	Conditioning
	Habit learning

progressively evolved into a more dynamic concept, called working memory, composed of three subsystems (Baddeley 1992, 2003). There are two short-term storage 'slave' systems: the phonological loop, devoted to verbal information; and the visuospatial sketchpad, which keeps visual and spatial information active in the mind. The third component, the central executive, is an attentional system responsible for selecting, controlling, and coordinating strategies. Complex processing tasks, which require coordination of verbal and visuospatial short-term stores, updating of information, inhibition, and selective attention, depend on this system. The central executive is also involved in activating and manipulating information stored in long-term memory (Baddeley 1996). Working memory has a highly functional role in everyday life, for instance, when information must be briefly kept in mind, while dialling a phone number, writing under dictation, understanding and producing speech, and manipulating mental images.

The phonological loop stores verbal information (words or sounds). It is composed of a short-term store and an articulatory rehearsal process that keeps information active by refreshing their traces. Verbal span is tested by presenting progressively longer sequences of digits, letters, or words, which the subject has to recall. The number of items that can be held in working memory depends on their similarity, i.e. recall of phonologically dissimilar words is easier, and on their length, i.e. more short than long words can be rehearsed before the trace of the first word begins to decay (Baddeley 2003). Selective impairments of verbal short-term memory are rare and may occur through lesions to the auditory association cortex in the left temporal convexity or the left parietal cortex (Vallar and Papagnano 1995). Verbal short-term memory impairments most often appear in the context of aphasia (Vallar *et al.* 1992). Aphasic patients present speech perception and production deficits, which interfere with repetition of short word or digit sequences. Verbal span deficits may interfere with abilities that set high demands on this system, e.g. sentence comprehension (Wilson and Baddeley 1993).

The visuospatial sketchpad is the non-verbal homologue of the phonological loop. It stores visual information about object features or patterns and spatial information concerning locations or spatial sequences independently (Della Sala *et al.* 1999). Non-verbal span, in particular the spatial component, is classically measured by means of the Corsi Block Tapping Test (Milner 1971). Pattern Span was subsequently developed to test the visual component (Della Sala *et al.* 1999). In these tasks, subjects reproduce progressively longer spatial sequences on a display of nine blocks (Corsi Block Tapping Test) or grids of black and white cells (Pattern Span); the longest correctly reproduced sequence is recorded. In most cases, non-verbal short-term memory impairments affect visual and spatial components, although dissociations have been found in a small number of patients (Warrington and Rabin 1971; Della Sala *et al.* 1999). Non-verbal short-term memory impairments are associated with lesions within parietal regions (De Renzi and Nichelli 1975) and are frequently observed in the context of spatial neglect (De Renzi *et al.* 1977). Mental imagery deficits can arise, since non-verbal short-term memory impairments interfere with the capacity to keep visuospatial information active in the mind (Hanley *et al.* 1991).

The central executive refers to a diversity of processes: the capacity to coordinate performance and divide attention when performing two tasks simultaneously; the capacity to resist interference while maintaining information active in the mind; and the capacity to manipulate and update information in memory (Baddeley 1996; Miyake *et al.* 2000). Dysfunction of the central executive has classically been associated with lesions within the dorsolateral frontal lobe (Baddeley 1986; Shallice 1988).

> Working memory is the capacity to keep information active in the mind during brief delays. It is composed of independent verbal and visuospatial storage systems, as well as an integrative component, i.e. the central executive. These systems are respectively affected by lesions to the left parieto-temporal cortex, the parietal cortex, and the dorsolateral frontal lobe.

7.3 Episodic memory

Episodic memory is the capacity to learn, store, and retrieve information about specific episodes consciously over extended periods of time (Tulving 1972, 1983). Autobiographical memory designates episodic memory for personally experienced events. Information stored in episodic memory concerns specific events set in a precise spatiotemporal context. Encoding is the process that converts a stimulus or an event into a mnesic trace. The strength of that trace depends on the depth of processing performed on the stimulus during encoding: semantic processing and cognitive elaboration of information reinforces its strength and positively influences subsequent retrieval (Craik and Lockhart 1972). Information is then consolidated and stored in long-term memory. Retrieval is the process of reactivating information from long-term memory. Several forms of retrieval can be distinguished: free recall is the ability to retrieve information actively from memory; cued recall is the retrieval of information facilitated by the presentation of clues; and recognition is the capacity to acknowledge that an information has previously been encountered.

7.3.1 The amnesic syndrome

The amnesic syndrome is characterized by an episodic memory disorder due to organic brain dysfunction in the absence of confusional state (Parkin and Leng 1993). Amnesia appears as the primary deficit and cannot be explained by other cognitive impairments. Anterograde amnesia denotes the incapacity to learn new information, starting from the time of the brain lesion. It may be associated with retrograde amnesia, a failure to recall events that occurred prior to the brain injury and that pertain to the individual's past. The capacity to recognize information is less severely affected than recall, and may be intact in some patients (Squire and Shimamura 1986; Schnider *et al.* 1996*a*). Short-term memory, semantic memory, and implicit forms of memory are usually comparatively well preserved.

Evaluation of anterograde amnesia is based on episodic memory tests. Examples of standardized episodic memory tests can be found in Lezak (1995). These tests are classically divided into encoding and recall phases (Van der Linden *et al.* 2000). During the encoding phase, patients explicitly learn new information, e.g. word lists or a series of abstract drawings. In a second phase, they are asked to retrieve the information presented during the encoding phase. Depending on the type of pathology, recall may improve when a cue is provided. Different forms of relation exist between the item and the cue: semantic (plum–apple); phonological (plum–crumb); visual (plum–baseball). During recognition, items that were presented during the encoding phase (target items) are mixed with new items (distracters), and the patient is asked to identify the target items. Episodic memory evaluation should test encoding and retrieval of verbal and non-verbal information. Amnesic patients can show different patterns of performance in episodic tests, between measures of recall and recognition (Hirst *et al.* 1986; Aggleton and Brown 1999) or verbal and non-verbal material (Tranel 1991; Morris *et al.* 1995). A large discrepancy between severe free recall impairment and relatively preserved recognition suggests that the patient may have difficulties in accessing information in long-term memory despite relatively spared encoding capacities (Swick and Knight 1999).

> Episodic memory refers to the function of encoding, storing, and retrieving information together with its precise spatiotemporal context. This system is primarily affected in the amnesic syndrome. Anterograde amnesia affects the capacity to learn new information starting at the moment of the brain lesion, whereas retrograde amnesia affects memories that were formed previously.

7.3.2 **Confabulation**

Certain amnesic patients may confuse ongoing reality and confabulate during a more or less extended period after brain injury. At least two forms of confabulation (provoked and spontaneous) can be distinguished, with different underlying mechanisms and anatomical correlates (Kopelman 1987; Schnider *et al.* 1996*a*).

Provoked confabulations occur when amnesic patients try to recall information with more details than are actually available. Typically, non-presented words (intrusions) are produced in free recall of word lists or stories. These false productions appear to be the trade-off for increased item recollection (Schnider *et al.* 1996*a*). Provoked confabulations can appear at any moment during the evolution of amnesia and have no specific anatomical meaning. A similar failure, false recognition, can be observed in recognition tests in which patients mistakenly identify novel items as repetitions. False recognition has repeatedly been associated with frontal lesions (Schacter 1996), but may also appear with non-frontal lesions (Schnider *et al.* 1996*b*; Schnider and Ptak 1999). The production of intrusions and false recognition responses is not pathological *per se*; these errors have also been observed in normal subjects (Burgess and Shallice 1996; Schacter 1996). Nonetheless, an excessive number of errors in memory tests is much more common in brain-damaged subjects (Mercer *et al.* 1977; Schnider *et al.* 1996*a*).

Behaviourally, spontaneous confabulations are observed in patients who are disoriented and suffer from severe amnesia. They spontaneously speak about matters or daily plans that do not pertain to ongoing reality and occasionally act upon such plans. For instance, a patient may leave the hospital with the idea that he/she has to attend an important meeting. Confabulations are often in relation to past habits. These patients fail to suppress the interference of memories that do not pertain to ongoing reality (Schnider *et al.* 1996*a*; Schnider and Ptak 1999). Based on studies with healthy subjects, we suggested that memories are subjected to a filter mechanism that allows them to be matched with ongoing reality, even before the content of these memories is accessible consciously (Schnider *et al.* 2002). We hypothesized that this filter mechanism may be deficient in spontaneous confabulators, which would explain why they fail to adapt their thoughts to ongoing reality and are convinced about the reality they are acting in (Schnider 2003). Spontaneous confabulation constitutes a distinct disorder, associated with lesions in the anterior limbic system, in particular the posterior orbitofrontal cortex or structures directly connected with it (Schnider 2003). Other forms–momentary and fantastic confabulations–have less pathophysiological and anatomical specificity (Schnider 2008).

Confabulations are normally associated with amnesia and can appear in several dissociable forms. Provoked confabulations are the consequence of increased item recollection and have no specific anatomical correlate, whereas behaviourally spontaneous confabulations reflect an incapacity to suppress the interference of irrelevant memories and occur after orbitofrontal lesions.

7.3.3 **Neuroanatomy of the amnesic syndrome**

Amnesia can occur as a consequence of lesions to a large variety of brain structures (Fig. 7.1). Damage to the medio-temporal lobes is a main cause of pure and severe amnesia. The description of patient HM is prototypical of amnesia following extended medio-temporal lobe lesions. This patient became deeply amnesic at age 27 after bilateral temporal lobe resection to treat pharmaco-resistant epilepsy (Scoville and Milner 1957). Medio-temporal lobes, amygdala, anterior hippocampus, and adjacent entorhinal cortex were removed bilaterally. After the operation, HM was unable to learn any new information explicitly. Retrograde amnesia covered several years preceding the operation (Corkin 1984). Implicit and procedural learning were preserved (Corkin 2002). The lesions of bilateral hippocampi and entorhinal and parahippocampal cortices appear determinant in explaining the severity of HM's amnesia has similarly severe amnesia has been observed without amygdala lesion (Schnider *et al.* 1995*a*).

Unilateral temporal lesions can give rise to less severe and material-specific amnesia: left temporal lesions primarily affect verbal memory (Tranel 1991), whereas right lesions appear to selectively affect non-verbal memory (Morris *et al.* 1995). Partial hippocampal damage can induce anterograde amnesia with primary recall deficits (Aggleton and Shaw 1996; Vargha-Khadem *et al.* 1997; Mayes *et al.* 2004). Although it has been suggested that recognition does not depend on the hippocampus (Aggleton and Brown 1999), impaired recognition has been observed in patients with selective hippocampal lesions (Reed and Squire 1997; Schnider *et al.* 1995*a*). Retrograde amnesia appears to follow a similar pattern. Lesions limited to the hippocampus can produce mild and temporally limited retrograde amnesia, while extensive retrograde amnesia is observed in medio-temporal lobe lesions that extend beyond the hippocampus (Squire 1992; Squire and Alvarez 1995). In general, patients suffering from medio-temporal lesions produce few false memories: they may occasionally confabulate in reponse to questions or produce intrusions in memory tests, but they do not act according to their confabulations (Schnider *et al.* 1995*a*).

Amnesia is also a clinical manifestation of lesions to structures that disconnect the hippocampus and the thalamus, such as the fornix, the mamillary bodies, and the anterior thalamic nucleus. Selective lesions to the fornix occur mainly as a consequence of third ventricle tumour excisions (Sweet *et al.* 1959; Gaffan and Gaffan 1991; Aggleton *et al.* 2000). Mamillary body lesions are often related to the presence of infiltrating tumours (Tanaka *et al.* 1997). Circumscribed anterior thalamic nucleus lesions are rare, but might also be responsible for anterograde amnesia (Aggleton and Sahgal 1993).

Severe amnesia can also appear as a consequence of lesions to structures within the diencephalon (Aggleton and Brown 1999). It has been suggested that lesions of the mamillo-thalamic tract that disconnect the mamillary bodies and the anterior thalamic nucleus or lesions of the lamina medullaris interna disconnecting the dorsomedian nucleus from the amygdala and the orbito-frontal cortex are necessary for amnesia to occur after paramedian thalamic damage (von Cramon *et al.* 1985; Graff-Radford *et al.* 1990). Lesions to the internal capsule resulting in a disconnection of the frontal cortex and the thalamus occasionally provoke amnesia (Tatemichi *et al.* 1992; Schnider *et al.* 1996*b*). Lesions to the cingulum and the retrosplenial cortex may also cause amnesia, as these structures participate in connecting medio-temporal structures with the anterior thalamus (Valenstein *et al.* 1987; Rudge and Warrington 1991).

Finally, lesions to structures that do not belong to the classical Papez circuit can produce severe amnesia, such as lesions to the basal forebrain and posterior orbitofrontal cortex. Structures of the

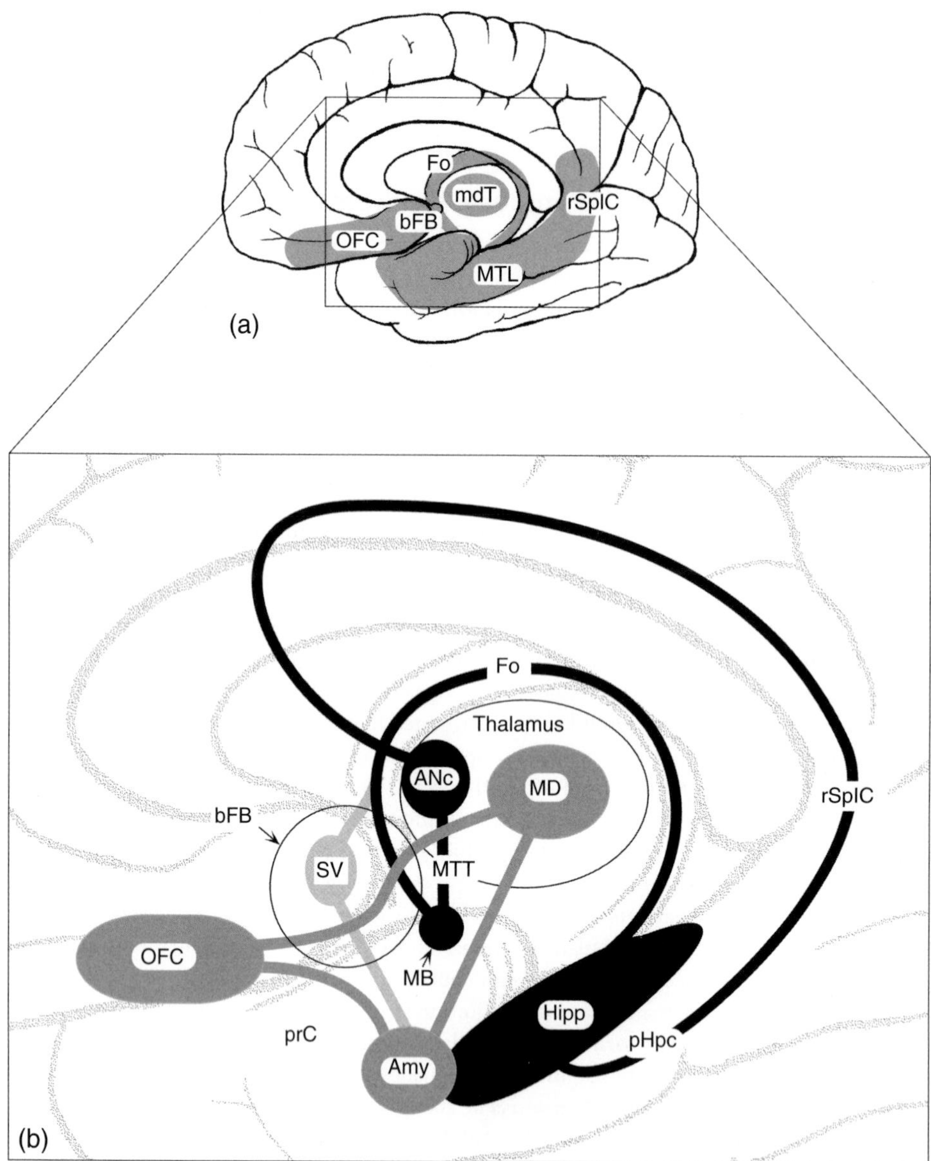

Fig. 7.1 Anatomy of anterograde amnesia. (a) Areas whose lesion is well documented to be a cause of amnesia. (b) Main connections within this area. The black loop represents the classic Papez circuit (hippocampal loop). The mid-grey loop shows the lateral limbic loop (amygdala-dorsomedial thalamus-orbitofrontal cortex). The connections of the septum verum are indicated in light-grey. Amy, Amygdala; ANc, anterior nucleus anterior of the thalamus; bFB, basal forebrain; Fo, fornix; Hipp, hippocampal formation; MB, mammillary bodies; MD, dorsomedial nucleus of the thalamus; mdT, medial thalamus; MTL, medial temporal lobe; MTT, mammillo-thalamic tract; OFC, orbitofrontal cortex; pHpc, parahippocampal gyrus; prC, perirhinal cortex; rSplC, retrosplenial cortex; SV, septum verum. Adapted, with permission, from Schnider (2004).

basal forebrain, i.e. the septal nuclei, send cholinergic projections to the hippocampus and neocortical structures, and it has been suggested that interruption of these projections may account for amnesia (Gade 1982; Damasio *et al.* 1985; Goldenberg *et al.* 1999). Orbitofrontal lesions may be more important for the occurrence of spontaneous confabulations and disorientation (Schnider 2003). Patients with lesions in the basal forebrain and orbitofrontal cortex often show relatively preserved recognition memory, but tend to be unaware of their amnesia and confabulate spontaneously for months (Damasio *et al.* 1985; DeLuca and Diamond 1995; Schnider 2001).

7.3.4 Aetiologies

Lesions in the brain regions mentioned above can be traced back to a variety of aetiologies, e.g. post-anoxic encephalopathy, herpes simplex encephalitis, Wernicke–Korsakoff syndrome, vascular diseases, traumatic brain injury, Alzheimer's disease, or epilepsy (Table 7.2).

Table 7.2 Main aetiologies of anterograde amnesia and proven or presumed lesion site*

Aetiology	Mediotemporal	Diencephalon	Basal forebrain
Transient global amnesia	×		
Transient epileptic amnesia	×		
Traumatic brain injury	×		×
Vascular aetiologies			
Bilateral hippocampal stroke	×		
Thalamic stroke (in particular, paramedian thalamic infarction)		×	
Lacunar stroke of the capsular genu		×	
Rupture of an aneurysm of the anterior communicating artery			×
Hypoxia	×		
Inflammatory, metabolic aetiologies			
Herpes simplex encephalitis	×		×
Limbic encephalitis	×		(×)
Systemic lupus erythematosus	×		
Wernicke–Korsakoff syndrome		×	
Degenerative			
Age-associated memory impairment	×		
Alzheimer's disease	×		(×)
Others			
Tumours (e.g. astrocytoma)	×	×	×
Surgery of 3rd ventricle tumours			×

* 'Mediotemporal' denotes lesions of the hippocampus and adjacent cortex. 'Diencephalon' designates lesions of the thalamus (dorsomedial nucleus, mammillo-thalamic tract, etc.). 'Basal forebrain' includes lesions of the fornix and the orbitofrontal cortex (ventromedial frontal area). (×) indicates presumed lesion sites. Adapted, with permission, from Schnider (2004).

Post-anoxic encephalopathy is the result of a severe hypoxic episode, for instance in the context of cardiac and respiratory arrest, carbon monoxide poisoning, drug overdoses, or suicide attempts (Wilson 1996). Neurons in the CA1 area of the hippocampus appear to be particularly vulnerable to hypoxia. Post-anoxic amnesia has been associated with selective hippocampal damage (Zola-Morgan 1986). However, lesions can extend to other regions. Medio-temporal atrophy (Kopelman *et al.* 2001), fornix atrophy (Kesler *et al.* 2001), and reduced glucose metabolism in thalamic structures have been observed in hypoxic patients (Reed *et al.* 1999; Markowitsch *et al.* 1997). The degree and specificity with which brain lesions involve the hippocampal formation determine the pattern and severity of cognitive deficits.

Herpes simplex encephalitis is associated with bilateral lesions in the limbic system, involving the hippocampal formation and the amygdala (Hierons *et al.* 1978; Damasio and Van Hoesen 1985). Damage often extends into the infero-temporal cortex, the anterior temporal pole, the basal forebrain, and the orbito-frontal cortex. Onset is acute; patients typically, but not always, present with high fever, confusion, and epileptic seizures. Dense amnesia can persist in the chronic phase (Kapur *et al.* 1994). Retrograde amnesia can extend over several decades (Stefanacci *et al.* 2000; McCarthy *et al.* 2005). Semantic memory is commonly affected due to the involvement of the left temporal neocortex (Wilson 1997). Both classic amnesia and spontaneous confabulation may result from herpes simplex encephalitis (Schnider and Ptak 1999). Severe and persistent amnesia has also been obseved in systemic lupus erythematosus as a consequence of autoimmune lesions in bilateral hippocampi (Schnider *et al.* 1995*a*). Paraneoplastic limbic encephalitis is associated with prominent memory disorders, as well as personality changes and epileptic seizures (Gultekin *et al.* 2000). This form of encephalitis appears to be related to an immune response (Posner and Furneaux 1990; Sutton *et al.* 2000) that causes neuronal loss in limbic regions. Neurological symptoms of paraneoplastic limbic encephalitis often precede the diagnosis of a carcinoma (Bakheit *et al.* 1990).

The classic Korsakoff syndrome is a combination of severe amnesia, disorientation, and confabulations (Korsakoff 1889). This syndrome appears in the context of Wernicke's encephalopathy, secondary to thiamine deficiency (Wernicke–Korsakoff syndrome; Victor *et al.* 1989). The neuroanatomy of lesions responsible for Wernicke–Korsakoff syndrome is subject to controversy. Lesions of the mamillary bodies are present in both amnesic and non-amnesic patients (Mayes *et al.* 1988; Victor *et al.* 1989), whereas lesions in the dorso-median thalamic nucleus (Victor *et al.* 1989) or the anterior thalamic nucleus (Harding *et al.* 2000) seem to be more specific for the presence of amnesia. Evidence of frontal damage has also been advanced (Reed *et al.* 2003). Recent studies have observed additional structural modifications and dysfunction in medio-temporal areas (Jernigan *et al.* 1991; Reed *et al.* 2003).

Severe amnesia can have a vascular origin. Amnesia has been observed after posterior cerebral artery infarcts that induce bilateral lesions of the hippocampus and adjacent cortex (Victor *et al.* 1961; Mohr *et al.* 1971; Schnider *et al.* 1994). Paramedian thalamic infarcts can provoke amnesia associated with a state of altered consciousness and eye movement disturbances (Von Cramon *et al.* 1985; Graff-Radford *et al.* 1990; Perren *et al.* 2005). Material-specific anterograde amnesia can appear in the context of unilateral thalamic infarcts, whereas bilateral infarcts are associated with severe and persistent amnesia in all modalities. In the acute phase, patients have no insight into their amnesia and may confabulate. Extensive retrograde amnesia has been reported (Stuss *et al.* 1988; Hodges and McCarthy 1993). Internal capsule infarcts are also associated with amnesia, presumably due to the disconnection of the projections between the dorsomedian thalamic nucleus and the orbitofrontal cortex (Markowitsch *et al.* 1990; Tatemichi *et al.* 1992; Schnider *et al.* 1996*b*).

Severe amnesia is frequent after rupture of anterior communicating artery aneurysms (Damasio *et al.* 1985; DeLuca and Diamond 1995). Lesions may encompass the basal forebrain, the ventral striatum, and the ventromedial frontal area, including the orbitofrontal cortex and the anterior thalamus (Alexander and Freedman 1984). Patients who have suffered a rupture of the anterior communicating artery may confabulate spontaneously for long periods after the brain lesion (Damasio *et al.* 1985; DeLuca and Diamond 1995; Schnider *et al.* 1996*a*), particularly when lesions involve both basal forebrain and orbito-frontal structures.

Traumatic brain injury causes different types of lesions in the brain, such as diffuse axonal lesions, contusions, cerebral oedema, ischaemia, and haemorrhages (Vakil 2005). Abnormalities preferentially affect the frontal and temporal poles (Russell and Smith 1961; Kesler*et al.* 2000). Post-traumatic amnesia refers to the period of confusion and disorientation that follows the injury during which patients fail to record information about daily events (Goldstein and Levin 1995). Duration of post-traumatic amnesia is an important prognostic factor and predicts the chronicity of memory impairment (Dikmen *et al.* 1995). When a chronic amnesic syndrome persists, it is mainly characterized by moderate to severe anterograde amnesia (Levin *et al.* 1988; Zec *et al.* 2001). Retrograde amnesia is usually limited in time, affecting the period immediately preceding the trauma, but can occasionally extend over longer periods (Carlesimo *et al.* 1998).

Dementia is a combined dysfunction of multiple domains (i.e. language, memory, visuospatial functions, executive functions, cognition, behaviour, and affect) that interfers with daily functioning (American Psychiatric Association 1994). In some forms of dementia, particularly in Alzheimer's disease, memory impairment is a core feature. Neuropathological changes in Alzheimer's disease, due to neurofibrillary tangles and amyloid deposits, first occur in memory-related brain areas, i.e. the hippocampal formation, before spreading to other limbic structures and neocortical association cortices (Arnold *et al.* 1991; Braak and Braak 1991). Relatively isolated episodic memory deficits appear during the early stages of this disease, before evolving into a dense amnesic syndrome and global cognitive decline (Welsh *et al.* 1992). The insidious development of memory disorders in the early stage of dementia can be difficult to differentiate from memory decline related to age. The apparition of isolated memory impairments beyond that expected for age in elderly people who do not fulfil the criteria for dementia is referred to as mild cognitive impairment (MCI; Peterson *et al.* 1999). MCI is considered to be a high-risk condition for the development of dementia, but it may also be reversible or stable (Portet *et al.* 2006). The level of cognitive impairment, in particular increased impairment of delayed free recall in episodic memory tests, appears to be predicitve of dementia (Welsh *et al.* 1992). MCI subjects who later develop dementia also tend to show larger hippocampal atrophy (Apostolova *et al.* 2006).

Transient global amnesia is characterized by an acute onset and limited duration (Hodges 1991). Patients present with severe amnesia, confusion, and disorientation. No other neurological symptoms or signs are present. Normalization of the clinical picture occurs within 24 hours. Recurrence of transient global amnesic episodes is rare. The exact aetiology remains unclear. Medication side-effects (benzodiazepine, sildenafil), CT contrast material, or stressful events can occasionally account for this syndrome (Simon and Hodges 2000). Growing evidence suggests that functional changes in the temporal region account for transient global amnesia. Although pathological changes are not evident during the acute phase, diffusion-weighted imaging studies have shown lesions in the hippocampal formation after 24 hours (Sedlaczek *et al.* 2004). High-field MRI of the hippocampus in a group of patients showed that they all had delayed neuronal loss within the CA1 area, similar to ischaemic or anoxic lesions (Nakada *et al.* 2005). Functional imaging during the amnesic episode showed decreased activation of parahippocampal and retrosplenial cortices in a memory task (LaBar *et al.* 2002). Neuropsychological evaluation in the acute phase has shown that anterograde amnesia is severe and probably related to a temporary incapacity to encode new information. Persistence of an amnesic gap for the main episode is common. Subtle amnesic symptoms can persist after the amnesic episode, but usually disappear after several days or weeks (Regard and Landis 1984). Retrograde amnesia during the acute phase is variable and can occasionally extend to several years or even decades. Recovery of retrograde memory can follow a temporal gradient, with more remote episodes reappearing first. In other patients, shrinkage of retrograde amnesia is irregular, 'spotty' (Guillery-Girard *et al.* 2004). However, limited amnesia persists for the minutes or hours preceding the episode and for the episode itself.

Unlike transient global amnesia, transient epileptic amnesia is associated with abnormal electroencephalographic activity, episodes of shorter duration (several minutes to an hour), and frequent recurrence (Hodges and Warlow 1990). Anterograde amnesia during episodes is often incomplete and patients can later 'remember not being able to remember' (Zeman *et al.* 1998). The extent of the retrograde amnesia during attacks varies from days to years. Aspects of anterograde and retrograde amnesia may persist between epileptic attacks (Kopelman *et al.* 1994; Zeman *et al.* 1998).

> Lesions to different parts of the limbic system and connected regions are responsible for the occurrence of the amnesic syndrome. Most frequent aetiologies are post-anoxic encephalopathy, herpes simplex encephalitis, the Wernicke–Korsakoff syndrome, vascular diseases, traumatic brain injury, Alzheimer's disease, and epilepsy.

7.4 **Retrograde memory**

Retrograde amnesia is the loss of information that was encoded before the onset of brain lesions. It is a frequent characteristic of the amnesic syndrome. Its severity correlates with the severity of anterograde amnesia (Schmidtke and Vollmer 1997). Different types of retrograde amnesia can occur, according to the episodic, autobiographical, or semantic nature of memories. The episodic component of retrograde memory concerns contextually and temporally defined events of the past. Retrograde memory is generally tested with news events and famous people from different periods. Standardized tests have been developed, but require constant updating and re-standardization and are culturally bound (Hodges 1995). Evaluation of memory for autobiographical knowledge or personal events is difficult, as every subject has his/her own personal experiences. Collecting information from the patient's relatives allows the examiner to verify the responses provided by patients on such tests. Investigations should cover different life periods, as well as the recent past. The autobiographical memory interview (Kopelman *et al.* 1989) is a frequently used semi-structured interview that was designed to evaluate autobiographical and personal semantic memory. This test covers three different periods of life, i.e. childhood, early adulthood, and recent past.

Classically, patients with selective hippocampal damage are described as showing mild retrograde amnesia, extending back only a few years (Squire and Alvarez 1995). In large medio-temporal lesions involving the hippocampus and the entorhinal cortex, retrograde amnesia appears to be longer and temporally graded, with recent memories more severely affected than remote memories (Schnider *et al.* 1995*a*; Rempel-Clower *et al.* 1996; Corkin 2002). Extensive retrograde amnesia, equally distributed over time, occurs as a consequence of damage extending beyond the medio-temporal lobes (Schnider *et al.* 1994; Squire and Alvarez 1995; Bayley *et al.* 2005). On the basis of these observations, classical models suggested that remote memories lose their episodic characteristics and become semantic over time (Cermak 1984). Repeated reactivation of hippocampal–cortical networks allows consolidation of cortical representations, which progressively become independent from the hippocampus (Squire and Alvarez 1995; McClelland *et al.* 1995). Recent models propose that only semantic memory impairments follow a temporal gradient, whereas episodic memories are impaired uniformly over time (Nadel and Moscovitch 1997; Moscovitch *et al.* 2006). They postulate that retrieval of detailed episodic and spatial remote memories always involves hippocampo-cortical networks, whereas retrieval of semantic memories depends only on cortical areas and is possible without hippocampal involvement.

Rare patients show severe and persistent retrograde amnesia, despite recovery from anterograde amnesia. These cases of 'isolated' retrograde amnesia have been largely described in psychogenic disorders (Schacter *et al.* 1982). Neurological patients can present similar symptoms. Different aetiologies can account for this phenomenon, such as traumatic brain injury, temporal lobe epilepsy, and herpes simplex encephalitis (Goldberg *et al.* 1981; Kapur *et al.* 1989, 1992; O'Connor *et al.* 1992; Markowitsch *et al.* 1993). 'Isolated' retrograde amnesia appears to depend on neocortical lesions, in particular in the anterior temporal lobe (Kapur *et al.* 1992; Markowitsch *et al.* 1993).

> Retrograde amnesia denotes the incapacity to retrieve memories that were formed before brain injury. It can cover time periods of variable length and often follows a temporal gradient. Storage of memories depends on hippocampal–cortical networks. There is a current controversy over the involvement of the hippocampus during retrieval of remote episodic and semantic memories.

7.5 **Semantic memory**

Semantic memory is considered an independent system in models of memory (Tulving 1972). It processes, stores, and retrieves information about the meaning of things, without any reference to a specific temporal and spatial context. However, observations of anterograde amnesia have brought some authors to consider that episodic and semantic memory systems may not be completely independent. First, patients with anterograde amnesia are often impaired in learning new semantic knowledge (Gabrieli *et al.* 1988; Corkin 2002; Bayley and Squire 2005). Contrasting data has been advanced on the basis of hypoxic ischaemia sustained perinatally or during early childhood (Vargha-Khadem *et al.* 2001). These patients develop relatively normal semantic memory, despite severe episodic memory deficits, suggesting that different neural networks sustain episodic and semantic memory.

Semantic memory is a system that receives information from sensory, perceptual, and language systems and determines different forms of production. Activities such as denominating a picture, defining a word, sorting pictures into categories, or pointing out pictures among a set of distracters require intact access to representations in semantic memory (Patterson and Hodges 1995). Organization of knowledge within semantic memory is subject to many controversies. Several models consider that there is a unique semantic system in which all concepts are represented equally (Tyler and Moss 2001; Caramazza *et al.* 1990). Other models suggest that there are multiple semantic systems, organized according to concept properties (visual versus verbal) or categories (living versus non-living concepts; Warrington and Shallice 1984; Tranel *et al.* 1997).

Evaluation combines different modalities (visual, verbal, etc.) in order to determine semantic memory loss and to investigate access deficits limited to specific input or output modalities. It also comprises items from a large variety of semantic categories, such as animals, manufactured objects, concrete concepts, and abstract concepts (e.g. Warrington and Shallice 1984). Evaluation also investigates knowledge about an item's sensory properties (a chair has four legs) and function (a chair is made for sitting on). Standardized material is used to test differences between semantic categories, avoiding variations due to item familiarity and frequency. Associated deficits in peripheral and language systems should not account for semantic errors.

Semantic memory deficits are associated with different neurological entities. They are the key feature of several degenerative diseases, in particular semantic dementia and advanced stages of Alzheimer's disease (Hodges *et al.* 1992; Daum *et al.* 1996). The region commonly affected in these pathologies is the anterolateral temporal neocortex (Patterson and Hodges 1995). Semantic impairments may also result from focal damage, e.g. herpes simplex encephalitis, in which medio-temporal lesions extend to temporal and frontal neocortex (Pietrini *et al.* 1988). Semantic memory deficits have also been reported in the context of cerebrovascular accidents, particularly when the middle and posterior arteries are involved (Patterson and Hodges 1995), and after traumatic brain injury (Wilson 1997; Rosazza *et al.* 2003).

Semantic memory impairments can affect categories differentially. The most common dissociation reported in the literature concerns memory for living (biological entities) and non-living (artefacts) categories. A selective impairment for living things, such as animals, vegetables, fruit, and flowers, has frequently been observed (Warrington and Shallice 1984; Sartori *et al.* 1993). In rare cases, the semantic deficit disproportionately affects one category within the living domain, e.g. fruit and vegetables (Samson and Pillon 2003) or plants (Pietrini *et al.* 1988). The opposite dissociation, a selective impairment of semantic knowledge for non-living things with relative preservation of knowledge for living things, is less common (Warrington and McCarthy 1987; Moss and Tyler 2000). Neuroanatomical studies suggest that different brain regions may be involved in category-specific semantic deficits. Bilateral temporo-limbic structures and inferior temporal lobes are preferentially involved in cases of selective impairment for biological entities, whereas left fronto-parietal areas are involved in selective impairment for artefacts (Gainotti *et al.* 1995). Warrington and Shallice (1984) proposed that identification of living things relies mainly on perceptual features, and that identification of non-living things is based on functional attributes. The living versus non-living dissociation is thus explained by a differential weighting of sensory and functional features in both categories. Alternatively, Caramazza and Shelton (1998) claim that living things (potential predators, food, and medicine) and artefacts are domains with different evolutionary importance, subserved by distinct neural mechanisms.

> Semantic memory stores and retrieves information about the meaning of things. Impairments can affect categories differentially. Dissociations between living and non-living entities are frequently reported. Semantic memory is impaired through lesions to temporal neocortex.

7.6 **Non-declarative forms of memory**

Interest in non-declarative memory developed with the observation that severely amnesic patients can improve their performance on motor and cognitive tasks through repeated exposure to stimuli (Milner 1962; Milner *et al.* 1968; Warrington and Weiskrantz 1968; Squire 1992; Stefanacci *et al.* 2000). Non-declarative memory is implicit and incidental and does not rely on episodic memory (Squire 1992). In comparison with explicit forms of memory, implicit memory is expressed mostly through action. Evaluation of implicit memory is not systematic in clinical settings and standardized tasks are rare.

7.6.1 **Priming**

Priming is the effect of prior exposure to a specific stimulus on subsequent ability to identify that stimulus. Priming generally results in improved performance on a task, with higher response accuracy and faster response time. Different types of priming have been distinguished: (1) perceptual priming is based on physical or perceptual features and operates at a pre-semantic level, and (2) semantic priming is based on semantic or associative resemblances between stimuli and is mediated by semantic memory (Tulving and Schacter 1990). Priming is direct when the benefit is obtained through presentation of the same stimulus. Indirect priming is obtained through presentation of different stimuli that share perceptual, associative, or semantic features.

Evaluation of priming is performed in two phases. During the study phase, a set of stimuli, e.g. comprising words or drawings, is presented to the subject. After a delay, a test phase is performed, in which another set of items is presented. This set comprises target items that are identical or connected to the items viewed during the study phase, as well as distracters that were not presented previously. The priming effect is the difference between performance in response to target items and distracters in the test phase. Stem completion is a task used to measure perceptual or semantic priming (Warrington and Weiskrantz 1974). During the study phase, the subject executes a task on a set of stimuli (count the vowels of words in the perceptual version or make a sentence with the words in the semantic version). In the test phase, the subject is asked to complete a list of word stems with the first word that comes to mind. Priming is the tendency to complete the stems with the words presented in the study phase. Perceptual priming can also be measured by presenting items, usually drawings, with progressive degrees of perceptual degradation or masking. In such tasks, subjects will tend to identify the items at a higher degree of degradation or masking in the test phase than in the study phase (Tulving and Schacter 1990).

Studies on healthy subjects have indicated that priming depends on neocortical regions. Perceptual priming has often been related to activation modulations in the visual cortex (Wiggs and Martin 1998) and semantic priming appears to preferentially involve the left inferior frontal cortex and the anterior temporal lobe (Henson 2003). These regions are distinct from the medio-temporal and diencephalic regions affected in the amnesic syndrome. In fact, preserved priming effects have repeatedly been observed in amnesic patients (Tulving and Schacter 1990; Squire 1992; Curran and Schacter 1997; Stefanacci *et al.* 2000). However, the medial temporal lobes and the diencephalic structures are responsible for the formation of associations between stimuli, which may explain why many amnesic patients fail on the priming tasks that require complex associations (Paller and Mayes 1994; Gooding *et al.* 2000).

Patients suffering from Alzheimer's disease also show preservation of perceptual priming (Deweer *et al.* 1994; Postle *et al.* 1996), but they tend to develop semantic priming deficits (Brandt *et al.* 1988; Fleischman *et al.* 2005). These deficits have been associated with degeneration of the temporo-parietal association cortex (Gabrieli *et al.* 1994).

Perceptual priming is vulnerable to lesions in the visual cortex. Keane *et al.* (1995) reported a patient with bilateral occipital lobe lesions who was impaired on perceptual priming for visually presented material, despite normal recognition memory. He also showed preserved semantic priming.

7.6.2 **Procedural learning**

Procedural learning refers to the capacity to progressively and automatically acquire motor, verbal, or cognitive skills (Cohen and Squire 1980). New skills are acquired by optimally executing a series of actions and organized procedures (Beaunieux *et al.* 2003). Experimental tasks are composed of several invariable learning sessions, in order to train the subjects on repetitive tasks. Improvement of performance over training sessions (faster performance and less errors) is the expression of procedural memory. Procedural memory is largely intact in amnesia (Cohen and Squire 1980; Deweer *et al.* 1994).

Motor learning is evaluated with many different tasks. Tasks often used are the pursuit rotor test, the serial reaction-time test, and mirror drawing. In the pursuit rotor test, the subject learns to maintain contact between a stylus and a circular spot located on a rotating disk (Ammons 1947). In the serial reaction-time test, subjects improve their speed at pressing buttons in different locations on a keyboard, according to an implicit sequence (Nissen and Bullemer 1987). In mirror drawing, subjects draw the outline of a form, when all visual input is mirror-reversed (Milner 1962). Motor learning is affected by basal ganglia dysfunction in the context of Parkinson's disease (Pascual-Leone *et al.* 1993; Schnider *et al.* 1995*b*) and Huntington's disease (Heindel *et al.* 1989). Lesions within the supplementary motor area, the adjacent anterior cingulate, and the anterior insular region also disrupt motor learning (Kornhuber *et al.* 1995). Patients with cerebellar lesions are selectively impaired in learning motor sequences (Pascual-Leone *et al.* 1993; Molinari *et al.* 1997). These patients fail the motor learning tasks, despite relatively preserved recognition of the task. In the amnesic syndrome, motor learning is preserved, despite poor explicit recall or recognition of the task procedure (Deweer *et al.* 1994; Heindel *et al.* 1989).

Verbal perceptual learning is tested with mirror reading, in which subjects improve their speed at reading mirror-reversed words. On the basis of this task Cohen and Squire (1980) showed that amnesic patients were able to normally improve their performance through repeated execution of the task. Patients with Alzheimer's disease fail to acquire mirror-reading skills, suggesting that the temporo-parietal association cortex is involved in verbal skill learning (Heindel *et al.* 1989; Grober *et al.* 1992). Demented Huntington patients are also impaired at acquiring skills. However, they normally recognize the stimuli, showing a clear dissociation with amnesic patients (Martone *et al.* 1984).

Cognitive learning is the capacity to improve strategies in cognitive tasks through repetition. The Tower of Hanoi, London, or Toronto tests are classically used to test cognitive learning (Simon 1975; Shallice 1982; Saint-Cyr *et al.* 1988). For instance, the tower of Hanoi is a tower of eight disks piled on one of three pegs placed in front of the subject. The objective is to transfer the tower to another peg, with a minimum number of moves and respecting several rules, such as to move only one disk at a time and to never place a large disk on a small disk. With repetition of the task, there is a decrease in the number of moves, errors, and time needed for executing the task. Controversial accounts of cognitive learning capacities have been reported in amnesia (Cohen *et al.* 1985; Butters *et al.* 1985). Xu and Corkin (2001) suggested that cognitive learning is not a pure form of implicit memory and that episodic memory plays a role in the acquisition of strategies in the Tower of Hanoi problem. However, Beaunieux *et al.* (1998) demonstrated that an amnesic patient showed cognitive learning on the Tower of Hanoi when the examiner provided compensation for declarative memory difficulties, by repeating the rules during the test and showing pictures of the initial and final position of the disks.

7.6.3 Conditioning

Conditioning encompasses the association between two stimuli, an unconditioned stimulus that elicits an automatic response (e.g. blink response to an air puff in the eye), and a conditioned stimulus that does not (e.g. a sound; Thompson *et al.* 2000). When these two stimuli are presented together repeatedly, they become associated and the subject blinks on presentation of the sound only. This effect is absent in patients with cerebellar lesions, who fail to acquire new conditioned responses (Daum *et al.* 1993; Bracha *et al.* 1997; Woodruff-Pak 1997). Patients with amygdala lesions are unable to acquire fear conditioning, in which a neutral (conditioned) stimulus is paired with an unpleasant (unconditioned) stimulus, although they can explicitly recall the stimuli that are associated (Bechara *et al.* 1995). The opposite effect is observed in amnesic patients with hippocampal lesions. They fail to recall the associations; however, they show normal conditioning when both stimuli are presented within short delays (Bechara *et al.* 1995; Clark and Squire 1998). This is not the case when an interval separates the presentation of the conditioned and unconditioned stimuli, as in trace conditioning. The hippocampus is involved in the formation of trace conditioning (Clark and Squire 1998; Knight *et al.* 2004). Amnesic patients, with lesions to this structure, have been shown to fail trace conditioning (McGlinchey-Berroth *et al.* 1997).

> Non-declarative forms of memory are based on improvement of perceptual or cognitive skills through repeated exposure. They depend on brain areas that are involved in the sensory and perceptual processing of information and are relatively preserved in amnesia.

References

Aggleton, J.P. and Brown, M.W. (1999). Episodic memory, amnesia, and the hippocampal-anterior thalamic axis. *Behav. Brain Sci.* **22** (3), 425–44.

Aggleton, J.P. and Sahgal, A. (1993). The contribution of the anterior thalamic nuclei to anterograde amnesia. *Neuropsychologia* **31** (10), 1001–19.

Aggleton, J.P. and Shaw, C. (1996). Amnesia and recognition memory: a re-analysis of psychometric data. *Neuropsychologia* **34** (1), 51–62.

Aggleton, J.P., McMackin, D., Carpenter, K., Hornak, J., Kapur, N., Halpin, S., *et al.* (2000). Differential cognitive effects of colloid cysts in the third ventricle that spare or compromise the fornix. *Brain* **123** (4), 800–15.

Alexander, M.P. and Freedman, M. (1984). Amnesia after anterior communicating artery aneurysm rupture. *Neurology* **34** (6), 752–7.

American Psychiatric Association (1994). *Diagnostic and statistical manual of mental disorders*, 4th edn. American Psychiatric Association, Washington, DC.

Ammons, R.B. (1947). Acquisition of motor skills: II. Rotary pursuit performance with continuous practice before and after a single rest. *J. Exp. Psychol.* **37**, 393–411.

Apostolova, L.G., Dutton, R.A., Dinov, I.D., Hayashi, K.M., Toga, A.W., Cummings, J.L., *et al.* (2006). Conversion of mild cognitive impairment to Alzheimer disease predicted by hippocampal atrophy maps. *Arch. Neurol.* **63** (5), 693–9.

Arnold, S.E., Hyman, B.T., Flory, J., Damasio, A.R., and Van Hoesen, G.W. (1991). The topographical and neuroanatomical distribution of neurofibrillary tangles and neuritic plaques in the cerebral cortex of patients with Alzheimer's disease. *Cereb. Cortex* **1** (1), 103–16.

Baddeley, A. (1986). *Working memory*. Clarendon Press, Oxford.

Baddeley, A. (1992). Working memory. *Science* **255** (5044), 556–9.

Baddeley, A. (1996). Exploring the central executive. *Quart. J. Exp. Psychol. A* **49** (1), 5–28.

Baddeley, A. (2003). Working memory: looking back and looking forward. *Nature Rev. Neurosci.* **4** (10), 829–39.

Bakheit, A.M., Kennedy, P.G., and Behan, P.O. (1990). Paraneoplastic limbic encephalitis: clinico-pathological correlations. *J. Neurol. Neurosurg. Psychiatry* **53** (12), 1084–8.

Bayley, P.J. and Squire, L.R. (2005). Failure to acquire new semantic knowledge in patients with large medial temporal lobe lesions. *Hippocampus* **15** (2), 273–80.

Bayley, P.J., Gold, J.J., Hopkins, R.O., and Squire, L.R. (2005). The neuroanatomy of remote memory. *Neuron* **46** (5), 799–810.

Beaunieux, H., Desgranges, B., Lalevee, C., de la Sayette, V., Lechevalier, B., and Eustache, F. (1998). Preservation of cognitive procedural memory in a case of Korsakoff's syndrome: methodological and theoretical insights. *Percept. Mot. Skills* **86** (3), 1267–87.

Beaunieux, H., Lebreton, K., and Giffard, B. (2003). Evaluation des capacités de mémoire implicite: enjeux et limites. In *Evaluation et prise en charge des troubles mnésiques* (ed. T. Meulemans, B. Desgranges, S. Adam, and F. Eustache), pp. 223–48. Solal, Marseille.

Bechara, A., Tranel, D., Damasio, H., Adolphs, R., Rockland, C., and Damasio, A.R. (1995). Double dissociation of conditioning and declarative knowledge relative to the amygdala and hippocampus in humans. *Science* **269** (5227), 1115–18.

Braak, H. and Braak, E. (1991). Alzheimer's disease affects limbic nuclei of the thalamus. *Acta Neuropathol. (Berl.)* **81** (3), 261–8.

Bracha, V., Zhao, L., Wunderlich, D.A., Morrissy, S.J., and Bloedel, J. R. (1997). Patients with cerebellar lesions cannot acquire but are able to retain conditioned eyeblink reflexes. *Brain* **120** (8), 1401–13.

Brandt, J., Spencer, M., McSorley, P., and Folstein, M.F. (1988). Semantic activation and implicit memory in Alzheimer disease. *Alzheimer Dis. Assoc. Disord.* **2** (2), 112–19.

Burgess, P.W. and Shallice, T. (1996). Confabulation and the control of recollection. *Memory* **4** (4), 359–411.

Butters, N., Wolfe, J., Martone, M., Granholm, E., and Cermak, L.S. (1985). Memory disorders associated with Huntington's disease: verbal recall, verbal recognition, and procedural memory. *Neuropsychologia* **6**, 729–44.

Caramazza, A. and Shelton, R.S. (1998). Domain-specific knowledge systems in the brain: the animate–inanimate distinction. *J. Cogn. Neurosci.* **10**, 1–34.

Caramazza, A., Hillis, A.E., Rapp, B.C., and Romani, C. (1990). The multiple semantics hypothesis: multiple confusions? *Cogn. Neuropsychol.* **7**, 161–89.

Carlesimo, G.A., Sabbadini, M., Bombardi, P., Di Porto, E., Loasses, A., and Caltagirone, C. (1998). Retrograde memory deficits in severe closed-head injury patients. *Cortex* **34** (1), 1–23.

Cermak, L. S. (1984). The episodic/semantic distinction in amnesia. In *The neuropsychology of memory* (ed. L.R. Squire and N. Butters), pp. 55–62. Guilford Press, New York.

Clark, R.E. and Squire, L.R. (1998). Classical conditioning and brain systems: the role of awareness. *Science* **280** (5360), 77–81.

Cohen, N.J. and Squire, L.R. (1980). Preserved learning and retention of pattern-analyzing skill in amnesia: dissociation of knowing how and knowing that. *Science* **210** (4466) 207–10.

Cohen, N.J., Eichenbaum, H., DeAcedo, B.S., and Corkin, S. (1985). Different memory systems underlying acquisition of procedural and declarative knowledge. *Ann. NY Acad. Sci.* **444**, 54–71.

Corkin, S. (1984). Lasting consequences of bilateral medial temporal lobectomy: clinical course and experimental findings in H.M. *Semin. Neurol.* **4**, 249–59.

Corkin, S. (2002). What's new with the amnesic patient H.M.? *Nature Rev. Neurosci.* **3** (2), 153–60.

Craik, F.I.M., and Lockhart, R.S. (1972). Levels of processing. A framework for memory research. *J. Verb. Learn. Verb. Behav.* **11**, 671–84.

Curran, T. and Schacter, D.L. (1997). Implicit memory: what must theories of amnesia explain? *Memory* **5** (1–2), 37–47.

Damasio, A.R. and Van Hoesen, G.W. (1985). The limbic system and the localisation of herpes simplex encephalitis. *J. Neurol. Neurosurg. Psychiatry* **48** (4), 297–301.

Damasio, A.R., Graff-Radford, N.R., Eslinger, P.J., Damasio, H., and Kassell, N. (1985). Amnesia following basal forebrain lesions. *Arch. Neurol.* **42** (3), 263–71.

Daum, I., Schugens, M.M., Ackermann, H., Lutzenberger, W., Dichgans, J., and Birbaumer, N. (1993). Classical conditioning after cerebellar lesions in humans. *Behav. Neurosci.* **107** (5), 748–56.

Daum, I., Riesch, G., Sartori, G., and Birbaumer, N. (1996). Semantic memory impairment in Alzheimer's disease. *J. Clin. Exp. Neuropsychol.* **18** (5), 648–65.

Della Sala, S., Gray, C., Baddeley, A., Allamano, N., and Wilson, L. (1999). Pattern span: a tool for unwelding visuo-spatial memory. *Neuropsychologia* **37** (10), 1189–99.

DeLuca, J., and Diamond, B. J. (1995). Aneurysm of the anterior communicating artery: a review of neuroanatomical and neuropsychological sequelae. *J. Clin. Exp. Neuropsychol.* **17** (1), 100–21.

De Renzi, E. and Nichelli, P. (1975). Verbal and non-verbal short-term memory impairment following hemispheric damage. *Cortex* **11** (4), 341–54.

De Renzi, E., Faglioni, P., and Previdi, P. (1977). Spatial memory and hemispheric locus of lesion. *Cortex* **13** (4), 424–33.

Deweer, B., Ergis, A.M., Fossati, P., Pillon, B., Boller, F., Agid, Y., *et al.* (1994). Explicit memory, procedural learning and lexical priming in Alzheimer's disease. *Cortex* **30** (1), 113–26.

Dikmen, S.S., Ross, B.L., Machamer, J.E., and Temkin, N.R. (1995). One year psychosocial outcome in head injury. *J. Int. Neuropsychol. Soc.* **1** (1), 67–77.

Fleischman, D.A., Wilson, R.S., Gabrieli, J.D., Schneider, J.A., Bienias, J.L., and Bennett, D.A. (2005). Implicit memory and Alzheimer's disease neuropathology. *Brain* **128** (9) 2006–15.

Gabrieli, J.D., Cohen, N.J., and Corkin, S. (1988). The impaired learning of semantic knowledge following bilateral medial temporal-lobe resection. *Brain Cogn.* **7** (2), 157–77.

Gabrieli, J.D., Keane, M.M., Stanger, B.Z., Kjelgaard, M.M., Corkin, S., and Growdon, J. H. (1994). Dissociations among structural–perceptual, lexical–semantic, and event–fact memory systems in Alzheimer, amnesic, and normal subjects. *Cortex* **30** (1), 75–103.

Gade, A. (1982). Amnesia after operations on aneurysms of the anterior communicating artery. *Surg. Neurol.* **18** (1), 46–9.

Gaffan, D. and Gaffan, E.A. (1991). Amnesia in man following transection of the fornix. A review. *Brain* **114** (6), 2611–18.

Gainotti, G., Silveri, M.C., Daniele, A., and Giustolisi, L. (1995). Neuroanatomical correlates of category-specific semantic disorders: a critical survey. *Memory* **3** (3–4), 247–64.

Goldberg, E., Antin, S.P., Bilder, R.M., Jr., Gerstman, L.J., Hughes, J.E., and Mattis, S. (1981). Retrograde amnesia: possible role of mesencephalic reticular activation in long-term memory. *Science* **213** (4514), 1392–4.

Goldenberg, G., Schuri, U., Gromminger, O., and Arnold, U. (1999). Basal forebrain amnesia: does the nucleus accumbens contribute to human memory? *J. Neurol. Neurosurg. Psychiatry* **67** (2), 163–8.

Goldstein, F.C. and Levin, H.S. (1995). Post-traumatic and anterograde amnesia following closed head injury. In *Handbook of memory disorders* (ed. A.D. Baddeley, B. Wilson, and F.N. Watts), pp. 187–209. Wiley, Chichester.

Gooding, P.A., Mayes, A.R., and van Eijk, R. (2000). A meta-analysis of indirect memory tests for novel material in organic amnesics. *Neuropsychologia* **38** (5), 666–76.

Graff-Radford, N.R., Tranel, D., Van Hoesen, G.W., and Brandt, J.P. (1990). Diencephalic amnesia. *Brain* **113** (1), 1–25.

Grober, E., Ausubel, R., Sliwinski, M., and Gordon, B. (1992). Skill learning and repetition priming in Alzheimer's disease. *Neuropsychologia* **30** (10), 849–58.

Guillery-Girard, B., Desgranges, B., Urban, C., Piolino, P., de la Sayette, V., and Eustache, F. (2004). The dynamic time course of memory recovery in transient global amnesia. *J. Neurol. Neurosurg. Psychiatry* **75** (11), 1532–40.

Gultekin, S.H., Rosenfeld, M.R., Voltz, R., Eichen, J., Posner, J.B., and Dalmau, J. (2000). Paraneoplastic limbic encephalitis: neurological symptoms, immunological findings and tumour association in 50 patients. *Brain* **123** (7), 1481–94.

Hanley, J.R., Young, A.W., and Pearson, N.A. (1991). Impairment of the visuo-spatial sketch pad. *Quart. J. Exp. Psychol.* A, **43** (1), 101–25.

Harding, A., Halliday, G., Caine, D., and Kril, J. (2000). Degeneration of anterior thalamic nuclei differentiates alcoholics with amnesia. *Brain* **123** (1), 141–54.

Hebb, D.O. (1949). *Organization of behavior*. Wiley, New York.

Heindel, W.C., Salmon, D.P., Shults, C.W., Walicke, P.A., and Butters, N. (1989). Neuropsychological evidence for multiple implicit memory systems: a comparison of Alzheimer's, Huntington's, and Parkinson's disease patients. *J. Neurosci.* **9** (2), 582–7.

Henson, R.N. (2003). Neuroimaging studies of priming. *Prog. Neurobiol.* **70** (1), 53–81.

Hierons, R., Janota, I., and Corsellis, J.A. (1978). The late effects of necrotizing encephalitis of the temporal lobes and limbic areas: a clinico-pathological study of 10 cases. *Psychol. Med.* **8** (1), 21–42.

Hirst, W., Johnson, M.K., Kim, J.K., Phelps, E.A., Risse, G., and Volpe, B.T. (1986). Recognition and recall in amnesics. *J. Exp. Psychol. Learn. Mem.Cogn.* **12** (3), 445–51.

Hodges, J.R. (1991). Transient amnesia: clinical and neuropsychological aspects. W.B. Saunders, London.

Hodges, J.R. (1995). Retrograde amnesia. In *Handbook of memory disorders* (ed. A.D. Baddeley, B.A. Wilson, and F.N. Watts), pp. 81–107. Wiley, Chichester.

Hodges, J.R. and McCarthy, R.A. (1993). Autobiographical amnesia resulting from bilateral paramedian thalamic infarction. A case study in cognitive neurobiology *Brain* **116** (4), 921–40.

Hodges, J.R. and Warlow, C.P. (1990). The aetiology of transient global amnesia. A case-control study of 114 cases with prospective follow-up. *Brain* **113** (3), 639–57.

Hodges, J.R., Patterson, K., Oxbury, S., and Funnell, E. (1992). Semantic dementia. Progressive fluent aphasia with temporal lobe atrophy. *Brain* **115** (6), 1783–806.

Jernigan, T.L., Schafer, K., Butters, N., and Cermak, L.S. (1991). Magnetic resonance imaging of alcoholic Korsakoff patients. *Neuropsychopharmacology* **4** (3), 175–86.

Kapur, N., Young, A., Bateman, D., and Kennedy, P. (1989). Focal retrograde amnesia: a long term clinical and neuropsychological follow-up. *Cortex* **25** (3), 387–402.

Kapur, N., Ellison, D., Smith, M.P., McLellan, D.L., and Burrows, E.H. (1992). Focal retrograde amnesia following bilateral temporal lobe pathology. A neuropsychological and magnetic resonance study. *Brain* **115** (1), 73–85.

Kapur, N., Barker, S., Burrows, E.H., Ellison, D., Brice, J., Illis, L.S., *et al.* (1994). Herpes simplex encephalitis: long term magnetic resonance imaging and neuropsychological profile. *J. Neurol. Neurosurg. Psychiatry* **57** (11), 1334–42.

Keane, M.M., Gabrieli, J.D., Mapstone, H.C., Johnson, K.A., and Corkin, S. (1995). Double dissociation of memory capacities after bilateral occipital-lobe or medial temporal-lobe lesions. *Brain* **118** (5), 1129–48.

Kesler, S.R., Adams, H.F., and Bigler, E.D. (2000). SPECT, MR and quantitative MR imaging: correlates with neuropsychological and psychological outcome in traumatic brain injury. *Brain Inj.* **14** (10), 851–7.

Kesler, S.R., Hopkins, R.O., Blatter, D.D., Edge-Booth, H., and Bigler, E.D. (2001). Verbal memory deficits associated with fornix atrophy in carbon monoxide poisoning. *J. Int. Neuropsychol. Soc.* **7** (5), 640–6.

Knight, D.C., Cheng, D.T., Smith, C.N., Stein, E.A., and Helmstetter, F.J. (2004). Neural substrates mediating human delay and trace fear conditioning. *J. Neurosci.* **24** (1), 218–28.

Kopelman, M.D. (1987). Two types of confabulation. *J. Neurol. Neurosurg. Psychiatry* **50** (11), 1482–7.

Kopelman, M.D., Wilson, B.A., and Baddeley, A.D. (1989). The autobiographical memory interview: a new assessment of autobiographical and personal semantic memory in amnesic patients. *J. Clin. Exp. Neuropsychol.* **11** (5), 724–44.

Kopelman, M.D., Panayiotopoulos, C.P., and Lewis, P. (1994). Transient epileptic amnesia differentiated from psychogenic 'fugue': neuropsychological, EEG, and PET findings. *J. Neurol. Neurosurg. Psychiatry* **57** (8), 1002–4.

Kopelman, M.D., Lasserson, D., Kingsley, D., Bello, F., Rush, C., Stanhope, N., *et al.* (2001). Structural MRI volumetric analysis in patients with organic amnesia, 2: correlations with anterograde memory and executive tests in 40 patients. *J. Neurol. Neurosurg. Psychiatry* **71** (1), 23–8.

Kornhuber, A.W., Lang, W., Becker, M., Uhl, F., Goldenberg, G., and Lang, M. (1995). Unimanual motor learning impaired by frontomedial and insular lesions in man. *J. Neurol.* **242** (9), 568–78.

Korsakoff, S. S. (1889). *Psychic disorder in conjunction with peripheral neuritis.* [Translated and republished by Victor, M., Yakovlev, P.I. (1955). *Neurology* **5**, 394–406.]

LaBar, K.S., Gitelman, D.R., Parrish, T.B., and Mesulam, M.M. (2002). Functional changes in temporal lobe activity during transient global amnesia. *Neurology* **58** (4), 638–41.

Levin, H.S., Goldstein, F.C., High, W.M., Jr., and Eisenberg, H.M. (1988). Disproportionately severe memory deficit in relation to normal intellectual functioning after closed head injury. *J. Neurol. Neurosurg. Psychiatry* **51** (10), 1294–301.

Lezak, M. (1995). *Neuropsychological assessment*, 3rd edn. Oxford University Press, New York.

Markowitsch, H.J., von Cramon, D.Y., Hofmann, E., Sick, C.D., and Kinzler, P. (1990). Verbal memory deterioration after unilateral infarct of the internal capsule in an adolescent. *Cortex* **26** (4), 597–609.

Markowitsch, H.J., Calabrese, P., Haupts, M., Durwen, H.F., Liess, J., and Gehlen, W. (1993). Searching for the anatomical basis of retrograde amnesia. *J. Clin. Exp. Neuropsychol.* **15** (6), 947–67.

Markowitsch, H.J., Weber-Luxenburger, G., Ewald, K., Kessler, J., and Heiss, W.-D. (1997). Patients with heart attacks are not valid models for medial temporal lobe amnesia. A neuropsychological and FDG-PET study with consequences for memory research. *Eur. J. Neurol.* **4**, 178–84.

Martone, M., Butters, N., Payne, M., Becker, J.T., and Sax, D.S. (1984). Dissociations between skill learning and verbal recognition in amnesia and dementia. *Arch. Neurol.* **41** (9), 965–70.

Mayes, A.R., Meudell, P.R., Mann, D., and Pickering, A. (1988). Location of lesions in Korsakoff's syndrome: neuropsychological and neuropathological data on two patients. *Cortex* **24** (3), 367–88.

Mayes, A.R., Holdstock, J.S., Isaac, C.L., Montaldi, D., Grigor, J., Gummer, A., *et al.* (2004). Associative recognition in a patient with selective hippocampal lesions and relatively normal item recognition. *Hippocampus* **14** (6), 763–84.

McCarthy, R.A., Kopelman, M.D., and Warrington, E.K. (2005). Remembering and forgetting of semantic knowledge in amnesia: a 16-year follow-up investigation of RFR. *Neuropsychologia* **43** (3), 356–72.

McClelland, J.L., McNaughton, B.L., and O'Reilly, R.C. (1995). Why there are complementary learning systems in the hippocampus and neocortex: insights from the successes and failures of connectionist models of learning and memory. *Psychol. Rev.* **102** (3), 419–57.

McGlinchey-Berroth, R., Carrillo, M.C., Gabrieli, J.D., Brawn, C.M., and Disterhoft, J.F. (1997). Impaired trace eyeblink conditioning in bilateral, medial-temporal lobe amnesia. *Behav. Neurosci.* **111** (5), 873–82.

Mercer, B., Wapner, W., Gardner, H., and Benson, D.F. (1977). A study of confabulation. *Arch. Neurol.* **34** (7), 429–33.

Milner, B. (1962). Les troubles de la mémoire accompagnant les lésions hippocampiques bilatérales. In *Physiologie de l'hippocampe*, Colloques Internationaux No. 107, pp. 257–72. CNRS, Paris.

Milner, B. (1971). Interhemispheric differences in the localization of psychological processes in man. *Br. Med. Bull.* **27** (3), 272–7.

Milner, B., Corkin, S., and Teuber, H.-L. (1968). Further analyses of the hippocampal amnesic syndrome: 14-year follow up study of H.M. *Neuropsychologia* **6**, 215–34.

Miyake, A., Friedman, N.P., Emerson, M.J., Witzki, A.H., Howerter, A., and Wager, T.D. (2000). The unity and diversity of executive functions and their contributions to complex 'Frontal Lobe' tasks: a latent variable analysis. *Cogn. Psychol.* **41** (1), 49–100.

Mohr, J.P., Leicester, J., Stoddard, L.T., and Sidman, M. (1971). Right hemianopia with memory and color deficits in circumscribed left posterior cerebral artery territory infarction. *Neurology* **21** (11), 1104–13.

Molinari, M., Leggio, M.G., Solida, A., Ciorra, R., Misciagna, S., Silveri, M.C., *et al.* (1997). Cerebellum and procedural learning: evidence from focal cerebellar lesions. *Brain* **120** (10), 1753–62.

Morris, R.G., Abrahams, S., and Polkey, C.E. (1995). Recognition memory for words and faces following unilateral temporal lobectomy. *Br. J. Clin. Psychol.* **34** (4), 571–6.

Moscovitch, M., Nadel, L., Winocur, G., Gilboa, A., and Rosenbaum, R.S. (2006). The cognitive neuroscience of remote episodic, semantic and spatial memory. *Curr. Opin. Neurobiol.* **16** (2), 179–90.

Moss, H.E. and Tyler, L.K. (2000). A progressive category-specific semantic deficit for non-living things., *Neuropsychologia* **38**, 60–82.

Nadel, L. and Moscovitch, M. (1997). Memory consolidation, retrograde amnesia and the hippocampal complex. *Curr. Opin. Neurobiol.* **7** (2), 217–27.

Nakada, T., Kwee, I.L., Fujii, Y., and Knight, R.T. (2005). High-field, T2 reversed MRI of the hippocampus in transient global amnesia. *Neurology* **64** (7), 1170–4.

Nissen, M.J. and Bullemer, P. (1987). Attentional requirements of learning: evidence from performance measures. *Cogn. Psychol.* **19**, 1–32.

O'Connor, M., Butters, N., Miliotis, P., Eslinger, P., and Cermak, L.S. (1992). The dissociation of anterograde and retrograde amnesia in a patient with herpes encephalitis. *J. Clin. Exp. Neuropsychol.* **14** (2), 159–78.

Paller, K.A. and Mayes, A.R. (1994). New-association priming of word identification in normal and amnesic subjects. *Cortex* **30** (1), 53–73.

Parkin, A.J., and Leng, N.R.C. (1993). *Neuropsychology of the amnesic syndrome.* Lawrence Erlbaum Associates Ltd, Hove.

Pascual-Leone, A., Grafman, J., Clark, K., Stewart, M., Massaquoi, S., Lou, J.S., *et al.* (1993). Procedural learning in Parkinson's disease and cerebellar degeneration. *Ann. Neurol.* **34** (4), 594–602.

Patterson, K. and Hodges, J.R. (1995). Disorders of semantic memory. In *Handbook of memory disorders* (ed. A.D. Baddeley, B. Wilson, and F.N. Watts), pp. 167–86. Wiley, Chichester.

Perren, F., Clarke, S., and Bogousslavsky, J. (2005). The syndrome of combined polar and paramedian thalamic infarction. *Arch. Neurol.* **62** (8), 1212–16.

Petersen, R.C., Smith, G.E., Waring, S.C., Ivnik, R.J., Tangalos, E.G., and Kokmen, E. (1999). Mild cognitive impairment: clinical characterization and outcome. *Arch. Neurol.* **56** (3), 303–8.

Pietrini, V., Nertempi, P., Vaglia, A., Revello, M.G., Pinna, V., and Ferro-Milone, F. (1988). Recovery from herpes simplex encephalitis: selective impairment of specific semantic categories with neuroradiological correlation. *J. Neurol. Neurosurg. Psychiatry* **51** (10), 1284–93.

Portet, F., Ousset, P.J., Visser, P.J., Frisoni, G.B., Nobili, F., Scheltens, P., *et al.* (2006). Mild cognitive impairment (MCI) in medical practice: a critical review of the concept and new diagnostic procedure. Report of the MCI Working Group of the European Consortium on Alzheimer's Disease. *J. Neurol. Neurosurg. Psychiatry* **77** (6), 714–18.

Posner, J.B. and Furneaux, H.M. (1990). Paraneoplastic syndromes. In *Immunologic mechanisms in neurologic and psychiatric disease* (ed. B.H. Waksman), pp. 187–219. Raven, New York.

Postle, B.R., Corkin, S., and Growdon, J.H. (1996). Intact implicit memory for novel patterns in Alzheimer's disease. *Learn. Mem.* **3** (4), 305–12.

Reed, J.M. and Squire, L.R. (1997). Impaired recognition memory in patients with lesions limited to the hippocampal formation. *Behav. Neurosci.* **111** (4), 667–75.

Reed, L.J., Marsden, P., Lasserson, D., Sheldon, N., Lewis, P., Stanhope, N., *et al.* (1999). FDG-PET analysis and findings in amnesia resulting from hypoxia. *Memory* **7** (5–6), 599–612.

Reed, L.J., Lasserson, D., Marsden, P., Stanhope, N., Stevens, T., Bello, F., *et al.* (2003). FDG-PET findings in the Wernicke–Korsakoff syndrome. *Cortex* **39** (4–5), 1027–45.

Regard, M. and Landis, T. (1984). Transient global amnesia: neuropsychological dysfunction during attack and recovery in two 'pure' cases. *J. Neurol. Neurosurg. Psychiatry* **47** (7), 668–72.

Rempel-Clower, N.L., Zola, S.M., Squire, L.R., and Amaral, D.G. (1996). Three cases of enduring memory impairment after bilateral damage limited to the hippocampal formation. *J. Neurosci.* **16** (16), 5233–55.

Rosazza, C., Imbornone, E., Zorzi, M., Farina, E., Chiavari, L., and Cappa, S.F. (2003). The heterogeneity of category-specific semantic disorders: evidence from a new case. *Neurocase* **9** (3), 189–202.

Rudge, P. and Warrington, E.K. (1991). Selective impairment of memory and visual perception in splenial tumours. *Brain* **114** (1B), 349–60.

Russell, W.R. and Smith, A. (1961). Post-traumatic amnesia in closed head injury. *Arch. Neurol.* **5**, 4–17.

Saint-Cyr, J.A., Taylor, A.E., and Lang, A.E. (1988). Procedural learning and neostriatal dysfunction in man. *Brain* **111**, 941–59.

Samson, D. and Pillon, A. (2003). A case of impaired knowledge for fruit and vegetables. *Cogn. Neuropsychol.* **20** (3–6), 373–400.

Sartori, G., Miozzo, M., and Job, R. (1993). Category-specific naming impairments? Yes. *Quart. J. Exp. Psychol. A* **46** (3), 489–509.

Schacter, D.L. (1996). Illusory memories: a cognitive neuroscience analysis. *Proc. Natl. Acad. Sci. USA* **93** (24), 13527–33.

Schacter, D.L., Wang, P.L., Tulving, E., and Freedman, M. (1982). Functional retrograde amnesia: a quantitative case study. *Neuropsychologia* **20** (5), 523–32.

Schmidtke, K. and Vollmer, H. (1997). Retrograde amnesia: a study of its relation to anterograde amnesia and semantic memory deficits. *Neuropsychologia* **35** (4), 505–18.

Schnider, A. (2001). Spontaneous confabulation, reality monitoring, and the limbic system—a review. *Brain Res. Rev.* **36** (2–3), 150–60.

Schnider, A. (2003). Spontaneous confabulation and the adaptation of thought to ongoing reality. *Nature Rev. Neurosci.* **4** (8), 662–71.

Schnider, A. (2004). *Verhaltensneurologie. Die neurologische Seite der Neuropsychologie.* 2nd ed, Thieme, Stuttgart.

Schnider, A. (2008). *The confabulating mind. How the brain creates reality.* Oxford University Press, Oxford.

Schnider, A. and Ptak, R. (1999). Spontaneous confabulators fail to suppress currently irrelevant memory traces. *Nature Neurosci.* **2** (7), 677–81.

Schnider, A., Regard, M., and Landis, T. (1994). Anterograde and retrograde amnesia following bitemporal infarction. *Behav. Neurol.* **7**, 87–92.

Schnider, A., Bassetti, C., Schnider, A., Gutbrod, K., and Ozdoba, C. (1995*a*). Very severe amnesia with acute onset after isolated hippocampal damage due to systemic lupus erythematosus. *J. Neurol. Neurosurg. Psychiatry* **59** (6), 644–6.

Schnider, A., Gutbrod, K., and Hess, C.W. (1995*b*). Motion imagery in Parkinson's disease. *Brain* **118** (2), 485–93.

Schnider, A., von Daniken, C., and Gutbrod, K. (1996*a*). The mechanisms of spontaneous and provoked confabulations. *Brain* **119** (4), 1365–75.

Schnider, A., Gutbrod, K., Hess, C.W., and Schroth, G. (1996*b*). Memory without context: amnesia with confabulations after infarction of the right capsular genu. *J. Neurol. Neurosurg. Psychiatry* **61** (2), 186–93.

Schnider, A., Valenza, N., Morand, S., and Michel, C.M. (2002). Early cortical distinction between memories that pertain to ongoing reality and memories that don't. *Cereb. Cortex* **12** (1), 54–61.

Scoville, W.B. and Milner, B. (1957). Loss of recent memory after bilateral hippocampal lesions. *J. Neurol. Neurosurg. Psychiatry* **20** (1), 11–21.

Sedlaczek, O., Hirsch, J.G., Grips, E., Peters, C.N., Gass, A., Wohrle, J., *et al.* (2004). Detection of delayed focal MR changes in the lateral hippocampus in transient global amnesia. *Neurology* **62** (12), 2165–70.

Shallice, T. (1982). Specific impairments of planning. *Phil. Trans. R. Soc. Lond. B* **298**, 199–209.

Shallice, T. (1988). *From neuropsychology to mental structures.* Cambridge University Press, Cambridge.

Simon, H.A. (1975). The functional equivalence of problem solving skills. *Cogn. Psychol.* **7**, 268–88.

Simon, J.S. and Hodges, J.R. (2000). Transient global amnesia. *Neurocase* **6**, 211–30.

Squire, L.R. (1987). The organization and neural substrates of human memory. *Int. J. Neurol.* **21–22**, 218–22.

Squire, L.R. (1992). Memory and the hippocampus: a synthesis from findings with rats, monkeys, and humans. *Psychol. Rev.* **99** (2) 195–231.

Squire, L.R. and Alvarez, P. (1995). Retrograde amnesia and memory consolidation: a neurobiological perspective. *Curr. Opin. Neurobiol.* **5** (2), 169–77.

Squire, L.R. and Shimamura, A.P. (1986). Characterizing amnesic patients for neurobehavioral study. *Behav. Neurosci.* **100** (6), 866–77.

Stefanacci, L., Buffalo, E.A., Schmolck, H., and Squire, L.R. (2000). Profound amnesia after damage to the medial temporal lobe: a neuroanatomical and neuropsychological profile of patient E. P. *J. Neurosci.* **20** (18), 7024–36.

Stuss, D.T., Guberman, A., Nelson, R., and Larochelle, S. (1988). The neuropsychology of paramedian thalamic infarction. *Brain Cogn.* **8** (3), 348–78.

Sutton, I., Winer, J., Rowlands, D., and Dalmau, J. (2000). Limbic encephalitis and antibodies to Ma2: a paraneoplastic presentation of breast cancer. *J. Neurol. Neurosurg. Psychiatry* **69** (2), 266–8.

Sweet, W.H., Talland, G.A., and Ervin, F.R. (1959). Loss of recent memory following section of fornix. *Trans. Am. Neurol. Assoc.* **84**, 76–82.

Swick, D. and Knight, R.T. (1999). Contributions of prefrontal cortex to recognition memory: electrophysiological and behavioral evidence. *Neuropsychology* **13** (2), 155–70.

Tanaka, Y., Miyazawa, Y., Akaoka, F., and Yamada, T. (1997). Amnesia following damage to the mammillary bodies. *Neurology* **48** (1), 160–5.

Tatemichi, T.K., Desmond, D.W., Prohovnik, I., Cross, D.T., Gropen, T.I., Mohr, J.P., *et al.* (1992). Confusion and memory loss from capsular genu infarction: a thalamocortical disconnection syndrome? *Neurology* **42** (10) 1966–79.

Thompson, R.F., Swain, R., Clark, R., and Shinkman, P. (2000). Intracerebellar conditioning—Brogden and Gantt revisited. *Behav. Brain Res.* **110** (1–2), 3–11.

Tranel, D. (1991). Dissociated verbal and nonverbal retrieval and learning following left anterior temporal damage. *Brain Cogn.* **15** (2), 187–200.

Tranel, D., Damasio, H., and Damasio, A.R. (1997). A neural basis for the retrieval of conceptual knowledge. *Neuropsychologia* **35** (10), 1319–27.

Tulving, E. (1972). Episodic and semantic memory. In *Organization of memory* (ed. E. Tulving and W. Donaldson), pp. 381–403. Academic Press, New York.

Tulving, E. (1983). *Elements of episodic memory*. Oxford University Press, New York.

Tulving, E. and Schacter, D.L. (1990). Priming and human memory systems. *Science* **247** (4940), 301–6.

Tyler, L.K. and Moss, H.E. (2001). Towards a distributed account of conceptual knowledge. *Trends Cogn. Sci.* **5** (6), 244–52.

Vakil, E. (2005). The effect of moderate to severe traumatic brain injury (TBI) on different aspects of memory: a selective review. *J. Clin. Exp. Neuropsychol.* **27** (8), 977–1021.

Valenstein, E., Bowers, D., Verfaellie, M., Heilman, K.M., Day, A., and Watson, R.T. (1987). Retrosplenial amnesia. *Brain* **110** (6), 1631–46.

Vallar, G. and Papagno, C. (1995). Neuropsychological impairments of short-term memory. In *Handbook of memory disorders* (ed. A.D. Baddeley, B.A. Wilson, and F.N. Watts), pp. 135–66. Wiley, Chichester.

Vallar, G., Corno, M., and Basso, A. (1992). Auditory and visual verbal short-term memory in aphasia. *Cortex* **28** (3), 383–9.

Van der Linden, M., Meulemans, T., Belleville, S., and Collette, F. (2000). L'évaluation des troubles de la mémoire. In *Traité de neuropsychologie clinique* (ed. X. Seron and M. Van der Linden), pp. 115–55. Solal, Marseille.

Vargha-Khadem, F., Gadian, D.G., Watkins, K.E., Connelly, A., Van Paesschen, W., and Mishkin, M. (1997). Differential effects of early hippocampal pathology on episodic and semantic memory. *Science* **277** (5324), 376–80.

Vargha-Khadem, F., Gadian, D.G., and Mishkin, M. (2001). Dissociations in cognitive memory: the syndrome of developmental amnesia. *Phil. Trans. R. Soc. Lond. B: Biol. Sci.* **356** (1413), 1435–40.

Victor, M., Angevine, J.B., Mancall, E.L., and Fisher, C.M. (1961). Memory loss with lesions of hippocampal formation. *Arch. Neurol.* **5**, 26–45.

Victor, M., Adams, R.D., and Collins, G.H. (1989). *The Wernicke–Korsakoff syndrome and related neurological disorders due to alcoholism and malnutrition*, 2nd edn. F.A. Davis, Philadelphia.

von Cramon, D.Y., Hebel, N., and Schuri, U. (1985). A contribution to the anatomical basis of thalamic amnesia. *Brain* **108** (4), 993–1008.

Warrington, E.K. and McCarthy, R. (1987). Categories of knowledge. Further fractionations and an attempted integration. *Brain* **110**, 1273–96.

Warrington, E.K. and Rabin, P. (1971). Visual span of apprehension in patients with unilateral cerebral lesions. Quarterly *J. Exp. Psychol.* **23** (4), 423–31.

Warrington, E.K. and Shallice, T. (1984). Category specific semantic impairments. *Brain* **107** (3), 829–54.

Warrington, E.K. and Weiskrantz, L. (1968). New method of testing long-term retention with special reference to amnesic patients. *Nature* **217** (132), 972–4.

Warrington, E.K. and Weiskrantz, L. (1974). The effect of prior learning on subsequent retention in amnesic patients. *Neuropsychologia* **12** (4), 419–28.

Welsh, K.A., Butters, N., Hughes, J.P., Mohs, R.C., and Heyman, A. (1992). Detection and staging of dementia in Alzheimer's disease. Use of the neuropsychological measures developed for the Consortium to Establish a Registry for Alzheimer's Disease. *Arch. Neurol.* **49** (5), 448–52.

Wiggs, C.L. and Martin, A. (1998). Properties and mechanisms of perceptual priming. *Curr. Opin. Neurobiol.* **8** (2), 227–33.

Wilson, B.A. (1996). Cognitive functioning of adult survivors of cerebral hypoxia. *Brain Inj.* **10** (12), 863–74.

Wilson, B.A. (1997). Semantic memory impairments following non-progressive brain injury: a study of four cases. *Brain Inj.* **11** (4), 259–69.

Wilson, B.A. and Baddeley, A. (1993). Spontaneous recovery of impaired memory span: does comprehension recover? *Cortex* **29** (1), 153–9.

Woodruff-Pak, D.S. (1997). Classical conditioning. *Int. Rev. Neurobiol.* **41**, 341–66.

Xu, Y. and Corkin, S. (2001). H.M. revisits the Tower of Hanoi Puzzle. *Neuropsychology* **15** (1), 69–79.

Zec, R.F., Zellers, D., Belman, J., Miller, J., Matthews, J., Femeau-Belman, D., *et al.* (2001). Long-term consequences of severe closed head injury on episodic memory. *J. Clin. Exp. Neuropsychol.* **23** (5), 671–91.

Zeman, A.Z., Boniface, S.J., and Hodges, J.R. (1998). Transient epileptic amnesia: a description of the clinical and neuropsychological features in 10 cases and a review of the literature. *J. Neurol. Neurosurg. Psychiatry* **64** (4), 435–43.

Zola-Morgan, S., Squire, L.R., and Amaral, D.G. (1986). Human amnesia and the medial temporal region: enduring memory impairment following a bilateral lesion limited to field CA1 of the hippocampus. *J. Neurosci.* **6** (10), 2950–67.

Chapter 8

Neurobehavioural disorders after stroke

Jean-Marie Annoni

8.1 Introduction

The term 'behavioural' is often used in neurology to denote non-cognitive mental symptoms or disorders, thus including many psychiatric symptoms such as mood and psychotic disorders but also abnormal personality traits such as impulsivity and aggression or even social isolation. However, in this chapter we will focus on a more operational and restricted definition of this term. In psychology, the notion of behaviour includes the responses or reactions of an individual in front of a stimulus or in a given environment. Thus, behaviour reflects a phenomenon of adaptation that allows fulfilling and/or satisfying biological and social necessities of life, such as food, reproduction, optimal survival in a given social surround, etc. Some behaviours are *innate*: these innate behaviours are 'instinctive' and genetically driven individual responses already present at birth. One example could be the grasping and sucking reflexes in babies, which are necessary for survival. After different experiences, persons can modify and adapt their manners to act in a stable way and can develop *learned behaviours* (e.g. development of eating habits, how to be dressed, adaptation to the laws dictated by a human group, etc.). The behaviour of a person reflects therefore the integration of a genetic set for survival and the individual modifications of this set, which depend on the person's learning and experiences.

In the clinical setting, behaviour often has an interpersonal or a social connotation, and usually means the manner in which a subject acts in a specific situation, according to the patient's internal mood and goals and those of the persons or resources around him. For example, what will the subject do if he/she wants to rent a movie at the shop, but the car does not start? An implicit or explicit evaluation of the situation will be needed in order to choose one answer between many possible ones. The evaluation criteria of the patient's choice will depend on his/her perceptive, cognitive, and emotional state, moral principles, the expected immediate or future satisfactions brought by one or another decision (e.g. call a taxi, ask a friend, postpone the movie, set fire to the car, cry ...), etc. Our behaviour will therefore in the first place be induced by our subjective preferences, our experiences, and our knowledge (semantic memory and social cognition), as well as our moral values, which can influence our judgement of the situation and our priorities. Moreover, the intensity of this reaction can be modulated by our 'striving' state: either strong (aggressiveness) or weak (athymhormia, apathy). Sometimes, the behavioural choice does not follow logically on initial analysis, but is replaced by another automated and involuntary behaviour (e.g. addictive or compulsive conduct, immediate reward) that will replace the initially foreseen action.

Brain lesions, particularly in prefrontal and limbic areas, can modify the standard coordinates that determine a patient's decision or impair his/her ability to integrate these data and orient his/her action. Studies have recently started to focus on personality, but also on behavioural changes (e.g. in independence, patience, energy, enthusiasm, etc.) after strokes (Stone *et al.* 2004). However, descriptions of modifications of behaviour have been known for a long time in neurological pathology. General palsy, for example, induces not only disturbances in language and memory, but also irritability, antisocial reactions, and megalomania and has been regarded since the nineteenth century as a classical cause of behavioural modification. Post-traumatic encephalopathies frequently cause behavioural problems such as aggression and emotional incontinence, often as handicapping as classical frontal cognitive disturbances such as planning impairment (Merrit *et al.* 1946). Such observations have also been done in paediatric pathology. It has been reported that children with hemiplegic cerebral palsy have an increased incidence of psychiatric problems: approximately 50% of a cohort of hemiplegic children were found during psychiatric interviews to have behavioural or psychiatric problems, including hyperactivity, conduct disorders, aggression, and oppositional behaviours (Goodman and Graham 1997) The behavioural disturbances are influenced by the site of the cerebral dysfunction. For example, patients suffering from frontotemporal dementia (Miller *et al.* 1997) who have increased behavioural and antisocial disturbances present right frontal hypometabolism. Increasing number of cohort studies and single case observations bring evidence that cerebrovascular accidents can intervene at different steps involved in a behaviour. The different alterations that we will report (see the following box) are: (1) behavioural changes related to *perceptual or mental alterations*, particularly present in the acute phase of stroke; (2) *qualitative modifications* of the semantic knowledge and individual preferences (food or sexual preferences, moral and social knowledge, as well as religious values); (3) *quantitative modifications* of the reactivity in a given situation (athymhormia, apathy, or, in contrast, hyperactivity and impulsiveness); (4) *behavioural deviances* (compulsive disturbances); and (5) the *loss of the perception* of the patient's own behaviour (decreased self-awareness, anosognosia) or of the behaviour of others ('theory of mind').

Neurological modifications acting on different steps of a behavioural response

- Perceptual and mental impairment
- Modifications of preferences and semantic knowledge
- Decreased or increased intensity of the reaction
- Decreased self-awareness or awareness of others

8.2 Behavioural changes in acute stroke related to perceptual and mental alterations

Misperception of what happens during the acute phase can explain maladapted behaviours that are particularly frequent in the acute phase. Patients' attitudes towards their stroke and the resulting symptoms are distorted by false beliefs (Croquelois *et al.* 2005). More than half of patients do not initially recognize their symptoms as a stroke (Meijer *et al.* 2003). Defective cognitive–emotional integration is what can be called 'acute memory or acute remembering impairment' in patients with acute stroke. Acute stroke is an active injury to the 'self' that makes the patient underestimate the ongoing changes in his/her sensorimotor interactions with both the internal and external world, independently of classical anosognosia (Bogousslavsky 2003*a*), and consequently leads to an underestimation of cognitive impairments by the emergency caregivers. An analysis of a cohort of acute patients reported that behaviours such as disinhibition (56%), lack of adaptation (44%), environmental withdrawal (40%), passivity (24%), and aggressiveness (11%) occur quite often in the first days after strokes, independently of specific cognitive deficits (Ghika-Schmidt *et al.* 1999; see Table 8.1). With regard to the importance of the mental alterations that

Table 8.1 Behavioural changes after acute stroke (adapted from Ghika-Schmidt *et al.* 1999)

Behavioural symptoms	Percentage
Disinhibition	56
Lack of adaptation	44
Environmental withdrawal	40
Passivity	24
Aggressiveness	11

can occur during the acute phase of the stroke, up to one-third of stroke patients have no, or only a poor, memory of what actually happened during the acute phase. The interesting aspect is that this usually occurs without specific damage to the classic anatomical structures known to be involved in learning (Grotta and Bratina 1995). Whether this is a very acute phenomenon, perhaps linked to some kind of 'sideration' of brain function, or to the natural difficulty that the brain has in recognizing a neurological impairment is not always clear. In making therapeutic decisions, this point must be carefully examined in order to determine whether or not the patient's judgement and decision-making capacities are altered (Hacke *et al.* 2000).

Misperception of mechanism can explain defective cognitive–emotional integration. Low *et al.* (1999) describe a poststroke patient whose behaviour was altered (agitation; restless and noisy behaviour—shouting) after an infarct in the territory of the left posterior cerebral artery. The behaviour of Low *et al.*'s patient also showed signs of a confusional state. Changes in perception of the interpersonal environment and psychotic symptoms have been associated with acute temporal dysfunction in neurological illnesses. Bouvier-Peyrou *et al.* (2000) considered the implication of paralimbic structures in delusional misindentification syndrome (DMS). However, in all these cases temporal dysfunction seems to be associated to a more generalized brain dysfunction, with associated brain injury, of more general cognitive impairment although right hemispheric lesions seem to preferentially induce DMS-like phenomena (Brugger *et al.* 1997).

8.3 **Qualitative modifications of knowledge and preferences**

8.3.1 **An example: food habits**

Brain lesions can modify the preferences and the subjective necessities that determine our eating behaviour. Hyperphagia has been reported with a variety of lesions in the thalamus, hypothalamus, and frontal lobe (see Dusoir *et al.* 2005). Quantitative or qualitative eating disorders can arise after a cerebrovascular accident (CVA) and are frequent in diencephalic strokes. Bulimia is described in five out of eight cases of paramedian thalamic infarcts (Gentilini *et al.* 1987) or in temporal lesion (Barbizet and Poirier 1982; associated with other characteristics of Kluver–Bucy syndrome). Along the same lines, stereotactic thalamotomy has sometimes been used as a treatment for anorexia nervosa. Recently a case of spontaneous recovery from anorexia after left posterolateral thalamus and posterior temporal lobe CVA (left inferolateral artery territory) was reported (Dusoir *et al.* 2005). Organic bulimia has sometimes been controlled with opiates. In contrast, isolated loss of interest for food such as in anorexia has also been associated with dorsomedial thalamic infarction and studies coming from the field of dementia suggest that anorexia may be linked to the extent of temporal atrophy.

The 'gourmand syndrome' (Regard and Landis 1997), a passion for eating associated with right frontal lesions and characterized by a new and irresistible desire for refined cooking, is a typical example of change in the eating pleasures and gastronomic preferences of these patients.[1] The discovery of the gourmand syndrome is quite interesting. Regard examined a 48-year-old businessman with a left hemiparesis. The patient didn't complain about walking difficulties, but he griped about hospital meals. When she asked him to keep a diary of his thoughts, the man exhibited an inordinate preoccupation with food. Before the stroke, he had an interest in politics and had shown no particular food preferences. Afterwards, he lived for food and, as soon as he resumed work, he left his former job to become a columnist on fine dining. Then, in a prospective study, among 723 neurological patients, 34 showed features of gourmand syndrome. Such patients usually had right frontal strokes, spatial memory problems, and diminished control over impulsive behaviours, but did not become overweight.

8.3.2 Modifications of moral, social, or religious principles

Focal brain lesions may modify a person's moral values and social reasoning. Difficulties in developing an acceptable form of moral reasoning were described in patients with early damage in the prefrontal cortex, suggesting in these cases an absence of 'adequate' explicit or implicit learning and not a change of preferences during life, particularly after adolescence (Anderson *et al.* 1999). It is possible that a deficit in probabilistic learning, i.e learning to make a decision by estimating the probability of a certain outcome contingent on a given behaviour, could play a role in this acquisition deficit (Ptak 1999). Price and colleagues described two adults who had severely aberrant behaviour and had suffered bilateral prefrontal damage early in life. Neuropsychological testing in these patients suggested that social and moral development was arrested at an immature stage. Deficits were found in the areas of insight, social judgement, empathy, and complex reasoning (Price *et al.* 1990). Lesions of orbital or mesial prefrontal cortex have often been associated with such deficits (for discussion see Trauner *et al.* 2001). Some other unpublished descriptions mention a change of moral values developing after acquired frontal lesions. Despite the fact that no evidence of specific and significant behavioural problems with increasing age could prospectively be demonstrated in children with focal perinatal lesions, Trauner *et al.* (2001) report some behavioural deviances on the social problems and attention problems scales. Such results could suggest that social knowledge should be more regularly paid attention to in patients with early strokes.

Hyperreligiosity is defined as a pathological interest in religions or divinity. It can present itself as a psychotic disturbance taking religious beliefs as the main subject of potential delirium, thus leading to auto-mutilation or misidentifications (patients taking themselves to be mythological or well known religious persons), or it can take the form of a religious adopted posture such as crucifixion. The neurological patients can present modifications of religious behaviour, notably in the form of a religious delirium or auditory hallucinations (e.g. the voice of God ordering the patient to leave the family), that persist for several years after brain injury (Assal and Bindschaedler 1992). Hyperreligiosity has usually been associated with brain trauma and epilepsy, but seldom with stroke.

1 Although eating disorders represent a classic example of preference modification, other interests can be modified. For example, we followed a young epileptic who, after a left amygdalo-hippocampectomy, lost his interest in old buildings and started visiting cities, looking at and admiring modern architectural complexes.

8.3.3 Sexual and loving preferences

Modifications of sexual interest or interpersonal love interests are rarely described after focal brain lesions, probably because of infrequent questioning. They are generally described as a pronounced sexual decline (Giaquinto *et al.* 2003). They can take the form of enigmatic changes in interest for a person in right temporal syndromes (Bogousslavsky 2003*b*) or for a gender and are rarely considered as 'pathological' because of the lack of social implications. They may, however, be an example of modification in mental and affective functioning induced by organic brain changes.

Hyposexuality is a decrease of libido and of sexual drive, impotence, or a decline in erotic thinking and discourse. This is a common phenomenon after a CVA and seems especially present after strokes involving inferior and medial frontal structures and median areas, although these areas seem to be more specifically involved after brain injury (Boller and Frank 1982) than after a cerebrovascular event. This decline has multiple origins, including organic, psychological, and social factors. Important explanatory factors may be general attitude toward sexuality, fear of impotence, inability to discuss sexuality, unwillingness to participate in sexual activity, and the degree of functional disability (Korpelainen *et al.* 1999). In fact, it can sometimes be explained by the fear of a new CVA, related to perceptive deficits such as post-stroke hypoaesthesia, or to more cognitive or even emotional changes linked to the CVA.

Hypersexuality is a less frequent abnormal sexual behaviour than hyposexuality. It has been described after temporal or diencephalic dysfunctions and is characterized by inappropriate social behaviour such as masturbation in the presence of other persons or by persistent deviating verbal comments with explicit or implicit sexual connotation (Spinella 2004). Some more qualitative aspects include changes of sexual preferences. Recently, Cheasty *et al.* (2002) described a heterosexual man in his seventies who developed transvestite urges and homosexual thoughts, fantasies, and activity after minor ischaemic lesions in the left thalamus and temporal lobe. The authors question the role of such structures in sexual preferences (Cheasty *et al.* 2002). Unusual and inappropriate erotic conducts (paraphilia) have been described more in epileptic patients but not yet after focal strokes. Concerning potential therapy, hypersexuality has been successfully treated with medroxyprogesterone acetate. Other treatments include behavioural therapies and selective serotonin inhibitors, particularly when compulsive aspects are observed.

8.3.4 Artistic preferences and creativity

Creativity refers to the ability to produce original, new material that responds to a motivational drive, or to a need, or is useful in the broader sense of this term. Creativity is not limited to art, and there are daily examples of creativity in virtually all domains, including economics, cooking, and science. However, art is a particularly good example of human creativity. Creative painting is a complex behaviour, relying on multiple brain areas. It may, for example, be modulated by the way we

Table 8.2 Modulation of artistic creativity

Perceptual abilities	Executive abilities
Scan objects or scenes	Drawing abilities
Aesthetic analysis of stimuli and faces	Decision-taking abilities: colour attribution
Mental imagery	Personality Emotional state

recognize and scan objects or scenes (Smith *et al.* 2003). It necessitates aesthetic analysis of stimuli and faces (Zaidel *et al.* 1995), mental imagery, and drawing abilities (Jeziernicka and Turowski 1978). Most of these processes are sensitive to right parieto-occipital damage, although left posterior lesions may specifically alter mental imagery of shape (Goldenberg 1992). Besides perceptive manipulations, creativity is also modulated by decision-taking abilities, such as deciding the attribution of real or factitious colour (Zeki and Marini 1998). Artists could be more creative through being receptive to stimuli generally neglected in quotidian themes in non-artistic contexts, a feature that could resemble certain mild dysexecutive syndromes (Carson *et al.* 2003). Finally, creativity has been also linked to the artist's personality and emotional state (Heilman *et al.* 2003).

Some reports concern artistic changes after focal brain lesions and focus on the effect of visuospatial disturbances (i.e. hemispatial neglect) on drawing (Vigouroux e*t al.* 1990), as well as the effect of important emotional and personality changes on artistic production (Bogousslavsky 2003*b*). The effect of lesions within fronto-subcortical networks subserving executive functions might be more subtle, intervening in the process of screening the figurative relevance of stimuli or in expressing novel order-relationships between concepts (Heilman *et al.* 2003). Limited subcortical and posterior strokes with no residual sensorimotor deficits have been reported to modify artistic style in painters, independently of any other personality change (Heilman *et al.* 2003; Annoni *et al.* 2005). These changes, of which patients may be unaware, have been associated with mild changes in executive abilities and emotional regulation. Aphasia is not an obstacle for successful development and evolution of artistic painting after stroke (Boller 2005). In such patients, facilitation of creativity has been attributed to a mechanism called 'paradoxical functional facilitation' (Kapur 1996), corresponding to a shift from a left to a right hemisphere mode of functioning. Table 8.2 summarizes the abilities involved in artistic creativity that may be affected by stroke.

8.4 **Quantitative dysregulation of behavioural reaction**

8.4.1 Apathy and athymhormia

Apathy is a specific neuropsychiatric syndrome, arising without other depressive signs. It consists of a loss of interest and of drive, decreased motivation, reduction in artlessness, sometimes associated with emotional flattening and lack of interest for new projects (Marin 1991). It is thus characterized by a decrease of goal-directed activities due to reduced motivation. According to this definition, it is not the direct consequence of more general intellectual impairment, mood disorder, or diminished level of consciousness (Marin 1993). In order to make such a diagnosis, one should be sure that apathy constitutes a significant change from the subject's personality before stroke and that it has significant consequences on his/her activities of daily living. It is also important to differentiate apathy from similar associated symptoms occurring in poststroke depression. The intensity of apathy is variable. Extreme states of apathy are called abulia and, at the most extreme, akinetic mutism. Patients with these symptoms may be unable to begin a motor act and to communicate or such a behaviour can necessitate a long delay (of the order of seconds or even minutes) to be initiated. They may eat and drink only when presented with food and speak only if questioned.

Apathy has cognitive and emotional components. The cognitive dimension is related to loss of motivation or interest in engaging in activities and the emotional dimension corresponds to emotional flattening and decreased emotional experience (Schmahmann and Sherman 1998). This type of emotional flattening seems to be associated with impaired response of the autonomic system to the emotional valence of stimuli (Annoni *et al.* 2003). Clinical tools include the apathy evaluation scale ((Brodaty *et al.* 2005) or subscales adapted from the neuropsychiatric inventory. Such scales include items concerning spontaneity, initiation, emotionality, activity level, and interest in hobbies, which are scored by the patient's caregiver. Data on stroke patients show an incidence varying between 20% and 50% in the acute phases (Okada 1997). However, these scales, if used in isolation, do not always differentiate apathy from depression (Levy 1998).

Apathy is classically associated with frontal lesions, particularly including the dorsolateral prefrontal convexity, as well as the basal ganglia, thalamus, and related networks. Functional imaging has suggested that apathy is also favoured by cortical hypometabolism in frontal and temporal areas, more particularly right dorsolateral and left basal frontal and anterior temporal (Okada 1997). Such studies underline the contribution of frontal subcortical cingular loops. Apathy is common (26%) following a cerebrovascular event (Brodaty *et al.* 2005). According to the authors, the presence of apathy may be related to older age and right fronto-subcortical pathway pathology, rather than stroke severity. It is associated with functional impairment and cognitive deficits. A core neurophysiological component of apathy is an impaired neural processing of novel events within the frontal subcortical system; according to Yamagata *et al.* (2004) novelty P3 is a useful physiological measure for assessing apathy after stroke.The apathy is also accompained by a reduction of verbal spontaneity (long latencies, short sentences, or even monosyllabic responses), motor inertia, a decrease of fields of interest, and emotional indifference. Dopaminergic agonists seem to have an effect on the apathy, in particular, bromocriptin (5–20 mg/day) and amantadin. The few descriptions of therapy after stroke have focused notably on akinetic mutism, frontal syndrome, and motor transcortical aphasia (Albert *et al.* 1988). Emotional flattening is the frequent consequence of amygdala or medio-ventral frontal cortex damage and can be associated with impaired autonomic reactivity (Bechara *et al.* 1999). However, blunting of affect or disinhibited and inappropriate behaviours can be observed—together with executive and other cognitive dysfunction— in patients with lesions involving the posterior lobe of the cerebellum and the vermis, or even the floccular nucleus (Schmahmann and Sherman 1998; Annoni *et al.* 2003).

Athymhormia is a specific 'amotivational' syndrome. It is essentially a lack of motivation, and vital strength, with apathetic, aspontaneous, and indifferent behaviour, combined with motor and affective drive loss but without anxiety. It was first reported in some schizophrenic patients but has also been described in cases of striatal lesions (Habib and Poncet 1988; Laplane *et al.* 1989). Clinically, it is characterized by mental emptiness without cognitive impairment. The main difference from apathy is that adequate activity can be obtained upon stimulation, underlying the contrast between impaired self-activation and intact hetero-activation that is found in this syndrome. Moreover, unlike patients with apathy, poststroke athymormic patients do not necessarily present dysexecutive symptoms (perseverations, grasping, utilization behaviour, memory and attention deficits). They also do not present with sadness or the usual signs of depression. In contrast to apathy, athymhormia is environment-dependent and, when they are stimulated, athymhormic patients can normalize their initiation and cognitive capacities (Bellmann and Assal 1996).

As regards the causes, athymormia has been reported in several patients after focal ischaemic lesions or carbon monoxide poisoning. In such cases, lesions were generally multiple and bilateral and included basal ganglia (head of caudate nuclei, putamen, and gobus pallidum), medial thalamus (Laplane *et al.* 1989), internal capsules, or other subcortical structures (corona radiata and semiovale centres). Based on the analysis of case reports and theoretical knowledge, Habib and Poncet (1988) suggested that converting motivation into effective conduct is subserved by specific frontal, striatal thalamic fronto-subcortical circuits. In this circuit, the caudate and globus pallidum have a central role in coupling the valence or the reward nature of stimuli with cognitive process, emotional expressiveness, and motor activity within frontal lobe systems. In such a model, selective lesions disconnecting among them the different relay-nuclei of frontal systems are responsible for a pure dysfunction in initiation, while motor and mental activity are spared (Bellmann and Assal 1996).

8.4.2 Impulsiveness, irritability, and aggressiveness

The reasons why borderline-like (Van Reekum *et al.* 1996) and acquired antisocial personalities are often described after brain lesion are linked to the concepts of impulsiveness and aggression (Weiger and Bear 1988). Both traits are often linked to some kind of disinhibition but they are in fact quite different. Impulsiveness is defined as the impossibility of withstanding an impulse or temptation that can have dangerous consequences for oneself or others. This characteristic, associated with disinhibition (Blumer and Benson 1975) or with irritability (a condition where the patient is reported to be easily angered), reflects difficulties in emotional control. Aggressiveness is considered to be a defect of emotional regulation and induces predetermined acts of violence towards others. In an interesting and terrible case Sweet (1969) drew attention to the neurological component of aggression by illustrating the behaviour of CW, who killed his mother and wife, climbed on a tower, and directed his gun at many unknowns, shot them, and then killed himself. He had written in his memories that he wanted his brain autopsied after his death, because he was feeling 'strange and uncontrolled impulses...'. A tumour compressing the temporal amygdala was discovered. In general, non-directed aggressiveness arises without being released at an object. These behaviours may be reinforced by anger, a basic emotion characterized by indignation, and by a more cognitive component, hostility.

As with many behaviours, there are many factors involved in development of impulsivity and aggression (social factors, prior exposure to violence, presence of mood disorders, medication, and history of alcoholism). Anger-trait after stroke probably also has a premorbid component, since anger may be a risk factor for stroke. There seems to be an association between post-stroke irritability, younger age left hemisphere lesions, and aphasia (Angelelli *et al.* 2004). Moreover, among the 127 patients studied, irritability was one of the most frequent symptoms during the first year after stroke (33%). It was characterized by impatience with little events (such as waiting) and less frequently by flashes of anger, rapid mood changes, and quarrelling. Moreover, according to the authors, irritability remained present also in the post-acute phase (at 1 year). Using the 10-item Spielberger Trait Anger Scale (see box), Kim *et al.* (2002) interviewed 145 stroke patients. Inability to control anger or aggression was described in 47 (32%) of stroke patients. Such inability was more present in patients with motor impairment, dysarthria, and emotional incontinence, particularly after subcortical lesions (Kim *et al.* 2002).

The 10-item Spielberger trait anger scale (after Kim *et al.* 2002)

1 I am quick-tempered
2 I have a fiery temper
3 I am a hotheaded person
4 I get angry when I am slowed down by others' mistakes
5 I feel annoyed when I am not given recognition for doing good work
6 I fly off the handle
7 When I get angry, I say nasty things
8 It makes me furious when I am criticized in front of others
9 When I get frustrated, I feel like hitting someone
10 I feel infuriated when I do a good job and get a poor evaluation

A related behaviour, the 'catastrophic reaction' (CR) has been described as an outburst of frustration, depression, and anger that start suddenly and goes on to a paroxysm, with sobbing and accompanying gestures. The patient may refuse to carry on with any language procedure. The sobbing may last many minutes and the negativism for considerably longer. CR is probably multicomponent but has been described in 12/326 (3.7%) patients with first-ever acute stroke (Carota *et al.* 2001), All such patients had left hemisphere—particularly insular—lesions and aphasia. According to the authors, the stereotypical and intense character of CR appeared to correspond more to a reflex behaviour than to a psychological reaction. The fact that a tendency to impulsiveness is frequently also found in other basal ganglia dysfunctions, such as attention deficit/hyperactivity disorder or Tourette's syndrome, also suggests a role of basal ganglia in control of behavioural reaction (The Tourette's Syndrome Study Group 2002). Concerning possible therapies (Table 8.3), a line of approach consists of cognitive and behavioural methods, in which patients have to recognize initial symptoms of aggression, as well as relaxation methods. However, since brain lesion patients may have cognitive difficulties, pharmacological therapies are often necessary to control such symptoms, for example, beta blockers, neuroleptics, or buspirone (Steven 1994). Mood stabilizers such as carbamazepine had equally good results (Azouvi *et al.* 1999). Interestingly, some functional neurosurgical operations, such as amygdalo-hippocampectomy for intractable epilepsies, have been observed to reduce aggression (Sachdev *et al.* 1992). Whether this is an effect of the surgery or of seizure control is unclear at the moment.

8.5 Stereotyped deviances in behavioural response

8.5.1 Addictive conducts and obsessive compulsive disorders

Addictions have been described in many neurological pathologies including Parkinson's disease (Houeto 2002). The classical examples are pathological gambling (Regard *et al.* 2003) and alcohol.

Table 8.3 Modification of intensity of behavioural reaction and recommended pharmacological therapies

Clinical picture	Brain structures involved	Suggested therapies in the literature*
Decreased behavioural reaction		
Apathy	Frontal dorsolateral Basal ganglia	Dopamine agonists
Athymormia	Basal ganglia Subcortical structures	Change environment
Increased behavioural reaction		
Impulsivity		SSRIs
Irritability	Little specificity	Control fatigue
	Left hemisphere lesion	
Aggression	Diffuse subcortical	Neuroleptics, AEDs, buspirone
Catastrophic reaction	Insula	Beta-blockers, buspirone, neuroleptics, AEDs

* SSRI, Selective serotonin re-uptake inhibitor; AED, anti-epileptic drug.

This phenomenon has only recently interested neurologists and the rare studies that have tried to describe it have suggested a relationship between development of addiction and dysfunction of subcortical prefrontal structures or basal nuclei (Lim *et al.* 2002). There are very few reports of pathological gambling after stroke, suggesting that such changes are rarely induced by focal lesions, and that the specific mechanisms that underlie these changes have still to be made precise.

Obsessive compulsive disorders (OCDs) have also been described in several neurological pathologies involving the basal ganglia. It is important to remember that the principal characteristic of OCD is the presence of obsessions and/or intrusive thoughts that will generate stereotyped and repeated conduct. This compulsive behaviour differs from other perseverative behaviour induced by frontal lesions both in the 'auto-induced' aspect, which is independent of the context, and in the anxiety that is related to the eventual attempts to inhibit such a behaviour. This type of repeated activity was also observed in patients with vascular lesions of basal ganglia, particularly of putamen and pallidum. For example, some patients with athymormia induced by bilateral strokes of the basal ganglia show, besides mental inertia, stereotypical activities with compulsive and obsessive motor, verbal, or cognitive behaviours. On the basis of a frontal-associated hypometabolism, Laplane *et al.* (1989) suggested that disconnections between cortical and frontal systems could have certain behavioural consequences such as a loss of the capacity to inhibit ongoing motor or verbal partially activated programmes.

A similar difficulty in inhibiting certain intruding processes has been also evoked in the persistence of post-traumatic stress manifestations 1 year after stroke (Bruggimann *et al.* 2006). Not only are such manifestations not rare (one-third of patients have significant scores on a validated impact of event scale) but intrusive symptoms are also more frequent after basal ganglia stroke, suggesting that the phenomenon of re-experiencing may be modulated by thalamo-subcortical pathways. This result is in agreement with some of studies indicating a possible role for basal ganglia and thalamic dysfunction in flashbacks (Liberzon *et al.* 1996). Basal ganglia lesions seem thus to be involved in situations where the obsessive or intrusive and repetitive cannot be inhibited. These observations are complementary to those found in psychiatric research in which hypometabolism has been described in functional OCD (McGuire 1995). Therapies of post-stroke OCD include medication, but cognitive behaviour therapy—in the form of exposure and response prevention—also seems to be potentially effective (Carmin *et al.* 2002).

8.5.2 Altered decision-making and myopia for the future

In his book *Descarte's error: emotion, reason and the human brain*, Damasio (1994) describes the case of an intelligent patient without cognitive disturbance, who, after removal of a frontomedial meningioma, no longer succeeded in taking coherent decisions in his daily life, although he successfully performed all the possible tests of executive function (Eslinger and Damasio 1985). Other similar patients have described, especially after amygdala or fronto-basal lesions, an inability to feel the emotion linked to a similar previous experience (Bechara *et al.* 1999). Altered decision-making is a known cause of functional impairment in the social environment (Bar-On *et al.* 2003), since this is one of the constant challenges in daily life. This behavioural process depends on the individual's situational cognitive analysis and emotional state, and can be impaired in spite of normal cognitive capacity. Patients presenting with altered decision-making ability thus cannot experience and use emotions effectively. Decision-making capacity can be measured using the gambling task (GT), a task that models real-life decisions (Bechara *et al.* 1996). In this task, subjects have to make a long series of decisions, picking cards from four decks (Fig. 8.1) that are either advantageous (i.e. small immediate gain, but also smaller loss) or disadvantageous (i.e. large immediate gain, but even larger loss). Over a hundred trials, healthy subjects typically learn to avoid disadvantageous decks. This adaptive decision-taking ability requires

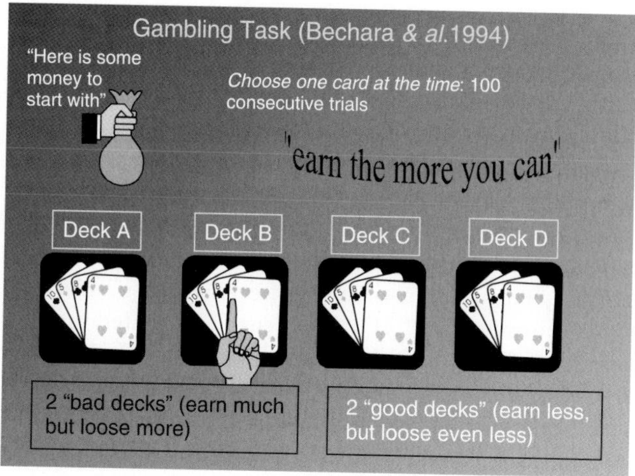

Fig. 8.1 Illustration of the gambling task (see text for explanation).

both an adequate analysis of the situation and an effective emotional regulation, since the subject must be able to delay immediate reward to ensure a final favourable issue. Patients with ventromedial lesions, for example, are insensitive to future consequences, positive or negative, and are primarily guided by immediate prospects. This 'myopia towards the future' seems to persist in the face of severe adverse consequences, i.e. rising future punishment or declining future reward (Bechara *et al.* 2000). This concept tends to overlap with the concept of emotional intelligence regarding the use of emotions to guide human behaviour (Bar On *et al.* 2003; see box). During GT, such a physiological correlate of decision-making consists in the development of an anticipatory skin conductance response (SCR) prior to card selection from the disadvantageous decks, which normally functions as a covert or overt signpost for helping with the process of making advantageous choices for the organism (Bechara *et al.* 1996). However, decision-making in social interaction can also be altered by more perceptive emotional deficits, such as impaired recognition of emotions in facial expressions, especially fear, after temporal amygdalar lesions (Adolphs *et al.* 1999). Moreover, there is evidence that high-level emotions such as regret, which depends on the integrity of the orbito-frontal cortex, strongly influence decision-making (Coricelli *et al.* 2005).

Different concepts used in the literature related to decision-making (see Bar-On *et al.* 2003)

What protects from myopia towards the future?

Emotional and social intelligence provide valuable approaches to understanding why some people behave more intelligently than others. Related concepts include the following.

- Emotional awareness (Lane and Schwartz 1987)
- Empathy (Brothers 1990; Preston and de Waal 2002)
- Psychological mindedness (McCallum 1989)
- Practical intelligence (Sternberg 1985)
- Successful intelligence (Sternberg 1997)

8.5.3 Post-stroke fatigue

Fatigue is a complex, subjective experience that is among the most significant complaints made by stroke patients (Glader *et al.* 2002; Staub *et al.* 2005). It can be defined as a reversible decrease or loss of abilities associated with a heightened sensation of physical or mental strain, even without conspicuous effort, due to an overwhelming feeling of exhaustion, which leads to an inability to sustain, or a difficulty in sustaining, even routine activities. It is associated with young age, neurological impairment, and anxiety level, and, for cortical lesions, with attentional performances (Staub *et al.* 2005). There was no significant association with laboratory work-up (cortisol, thryoxin (T4) free, thyroid stimulating hormone (TSH), adrenocorticotrophic hormone (ACTH)). The neurological literature suggests that there is a large variety of types of tiredness, whose characteristics depend on the pathology of the disease, the cerebral location of the lesions, and mood aspects such as depression (Choi-Kwon *et al.* 2005). Data show that patients with fatigue can be depressed, but that a large cohort (20–50%) of patients who have post-stroke fatigue do not show either severe neurological disturbance or functional impairment. Our preliminary findings emphasize that patients with so-called primary post-stroke fatigue at 1 year may have mainly brainstem lesions (Staub *et al.* 2005).

8.6 Altered judgement about one's own state or that of another

8.6.1 Impairment of self: anosognosia

There are commonly said to be two types of anosognosia: a 'perceptive' anosognosia, characterized by the decreased awareness of impairment, and a second more 'behavioural' type, where the patients do not perceive their own behaviour (if it is adequate or not in respect to a position or to a person). Anosognosia following severe left hemiplegia, exemplified in the Anton–Babinski syndrome, reflects an ill-understood type of brain damage, where patients may remain unaware of their handicap and deny it. Whether this is a very acute phenomenon, perhaps linked to some kind of 'sideration' of brain function (Grotta and Bratina 1995), or is linked to the natural difficulty experienced by the brain in recognizing neurological impairment (Safran *et al.* 1999) is not always clear. According to Vuilleumier (2004), appreciation, belief, and check operations may contribute to abnormal cognitive and affective appraisal of a deficit. In acute cases, the patient is convinced that he or she is not ill, does not have motor impairment, does not have a potentially severe medical condition, or does not have a brain problem. The particularity of these impairments during the acute phase can explain why immediate post-stroke emotional changes are different from those in the more chronic stages. If such symptoms are longlasting, they are particularly predictive of decreased outcome (Gialanella *et al.* 2005). In the other form (a more 'behavioural anosognosia'), which often is observed in the later phase of recovery when the patient has reached independence again, the clinical characteristics are related to the non-perception of the behaviour by the patient themselves (Prigatano *et al.* 1997). Such loss of self-awareness is often described after frontal brain lesion and is particularly frequent after brain injuries. Such anosognosia is potentiated by executive dysfunction, independently of lateralization of the lesion. The following box summarizes the classical anosognosic syndromes.

Classical anosognosic syndromes

- Anton's syndrome (cortical blindness)
- Anton–Babinski's syndrome (non-perception of hemiplegia)
- Callosal syndrome
- Loss of self-awareness ('frontal anosognosia')
- Decreased perception of other people's mental state: impairment in 'theory of mind'

The ability to attribute mental states to others (to form a 'theory of mind' or ToM) is necessary in order to understand the complex social interactions that we encounter in our everyday life and allows us to react adequately in a certain situation (Frith and Frith 1999). This ability does not concern only cognitive states, but also desires and beliefs (Baron-Cohen 1995; Baron-Cohen *et al.* 1994). Evidence from neuroimaging and neuropsychological studies has led researchers to conclude that ToM is subserved by dedicated brain systems, including the amygdala, temporoparietal junction, orbital frontal cortex, and, in particular, the medial frontal lobes (Siegal and Varley 2002; Frith and Frith 2003). Recently, however, the role of the medial frontal cortex in such processing has been questioned, on the basis of a careful cognitive and anatomical assessment in a patient with bilateral stroke of the anterior cerebral arteries, including regions identified as critical for 'theory of mind' by functional neuroimaging of healthy subjects. Despite dysexecutive syndrome and tendency to confabulate, this patient had no significant impairment on tasks probing her ability to construct a 'theory of mind', suggesting that medial frontal regions were not necessary for this function (Bird *et al.* 2004).

Another group of patients who has been suggested to have ToM impairment is right hemisphere stroke patients. Such patients have difficulty deriving implicit meaning from the relevant context (Kaplan *et al.* 1990) or attributing internal emotional states (Cicone *et* al. 1980). Surian and Siegal (2001) tested patients with right (RHD) and left (LHD) sylvian unilateral stroke on ToM tasks presented with visual aids that illustrated the relevant premises. Both RHD and LHD patients performed well on the ToM tasks presented with visual aids, but RHD patients displayed difficulty when the same tasks were presented only verbally (Surian and Siegal 2001). Since these patients also had pragmatic difficulties, the authors suggested that their difficulties on tasks devised to test ToM understanding may stem from impaired visuospatial buffers and working memory processes required for pragmatic competence rather than a fundamental representational deficit. Mental state understanding also necessitates making sense of non-literal utterances that can also give insight into the other's physical state. Such an ability has also been shown to be sensitive to the effects of right hemisphere stroke (Happé *et al.* 1999).

8.7 **Conclusion**

Behaviour refers in the clinical situation to the manner in which a person acts in a given situation, depending on the environment and the persons with whom he/she interacts at that moment. It is intimately related to the person's cognitive and affective status, thus being affected by brain pathology. The mechanisms by which brain lesions can affect a patient's behaviour depend on the pathogeny of lesions but also on their localization. In the acute case, altered perceptual and mental states can mimic confusional states and delusional symptoms. In the more chronic states, different deficits can modify behavioural response after stroke, and these causes correspond to the different steps that will lead to the patient's reaction. First, a neurological disease can alter a patient's values and preferences, as in the case of taste modifications and religious and moral changes after brain lesions, or even alteration of sexual habits. Changes in such values can lead to a different response or even an absence of response for a stimulus that produced attraction or repulsion before the disease. Second, the intensity of the reaction can be flattened (apathy, athymormia) or abnormally strong (impulsivity, aggression), leading to acquired sociopathy, for example. Third, a normal expected reaction could be disturbed by an overwhelming 'stereotyped' reaction, which at the same time prevents any constructed and adapted behaviour. This is the case for addiction and obsessive compulsive disorders or myopia towards the future. Finally, the monitoring system for behaviour can be impaired, as in the case of anosognosia or theory of mind impairment. Thus, it is quite understandable that behaviour can be altered in any kind of neuropsychological modification, thus in any kind of brain lesion. However, right and anterior lesions seem to give the most noticeable changes.

Acknowledgements

This work has been partly supported by a Swiss National Science Foundation, grant no. 3151AO-102271. Acknowledgements to: Antonio Carota, Julien Bogousslavsky, and Theodor Landis, all from the Department of Neurology, Lausanne, Switzerland, for their advice in the construction of the chapter and for their help in the literature review.

References

Adolphs, R., Tranel, D., Hamann, S., Young, A.W., Calder, A.J., Phelps, E.A., Anderson, A., Lee, G.P., and Damasio. A.R. (1999). Recognition of facial emotion in nine individuals with bilateral amygdala damage. *Neuropsychologia* **37** (10), 1111–17.

Albert, M., Bachman, D., Morgan, A., and Helm-Estabrooks, N. (1988). Pharmacotherapy for aphasia. *Neurology* **38**, 877–9.

Anderson, S., Bechara, A., Damasio, H., Tranel, D., and Damasio, A. (1999). Impairment of social and moral behaviour related to early damage in human prefrontal cortex. *Nature Neurosci.* **2**, 1032–7.

Angelelli, P., Paolucci, S., Bivona, U., Piccardi, L., Ciurli, P., Cantagallo, A., Antonucci, G., Fasotti, L., Di Santantonio, A., Grasso, M.G., and Pizzamiglio, L. (2004). Development of neuropsychiatric symptoms in poststroke patients: a cross-sectional study. *Acta Psychiatrica Scand.* **110** (1), 55–63.

Annoni, J.M., Ptak, R., Caldara-Schnetzer, A.S., Khateb, A., and Pollermann, B.Z. (2003). Decoupling of autonomic and cognitive emotional reactions after cerebellar stroke. *Ann. Neurol.* **53** (5), 654–8.

Annoni, J.M., Devuyst, G., Carota, A., Bruggimann, L., and Bogousslavsky, J. (2005). Changes in artistic style after minor posterior stroke. *J. Neurol. Neurosurg. Psychiatry* **76**, 797–803.

Assal, G. and Bindschaedler, C. (1992). Délire mystique 13 ans aprés un traumatisme cranio-cérébral. *Neurochirurgie* **38**, 381–4.

Azouvi, P., Jokic, C., Attal, N., Denys, P., Marcabi, S., and Bussel, B. (1999). Carbamazepine in agitation and aggressive behavior following severe closed-head injury. Results of an open trial. *J. Head Trauma Rehabil.* **14**, 567–80.

Barbizet, J. and Poirier, J. (1982). Astrocytome fronto-temporal. Etude anatomo-clinique et discussion des troubles comportementaux. *Ann. Méd. Psychol. (Paris)* **140**, 1015–22.

Bar-On, R., Tranel, D., Denburg, N.L., and Bechara, A. (2003). Exploring the neurological substrate of emotional and social intelligence. *Brain* **126**, 1790–800.

Baron-Cohen, S. (1995). *Mindblindness: an essay on autism and theory of mind.* MIT Press, Cambridge, Massachusetts.

Baron-Cohen, S., Ring, H., Moriarty, J., Schmitz, B., Costa, D., and Ell, P. (1994). Recognition of mental state terms. Clinical findings in children with autism and a functional neuroimaging study of normal adults. *Br. J. Psychiatry* **165** (5), 640–9.

Bechara, A., Tranel, D., Damasio, H., and Damasio, A.R. (1996). Failure to respond automatically to anticipated future outcomes following damage to prefrontal cortex. *Cereb. Cortex* **6**, 215–25.

Bechara, A., Damasio, H., and Damasio, A. (1999). Different contributions of the human amygdala and ventromedial prefrontal cortex to decision-making. *J. Neurosci.* **19**, 5473–81.

Bechara, A., Tranel, D., and Damasio, H. (2000). Characterization of the decision-making deficit of patients with ventromedial prefrontal cortex lesions. *Brain* **123** (11), 2189–202.

Bellmann, A. and Assal, G. (1996). Les multiples propos d'une athymhormique. *Rev. Neuropsychol.* **6**, 101–2.

Bird, C.M., Castelli, F., Malik, O., Frith, U., and Husain, M. (2004). The impact of extensive medial frontal lobe damage on 'theory of mind' and cognition *Brain* **127** (4), 914–28.

Blumer, D. and Benson, D. (1975). Personality changes with frontal and temporal lobe lesions. In *Psychiatric aspects of neurologic diseases* (ed. D. Benson and D. Blumer), pp. 497–522. Grune and Stratton, New York.

Bogousslavsky, J. (2003*a*). Emotions, mood, and behavior after stroke, William Feinberg Lecture 2002. *Stroke* **34** (4), 1046–50.

Bogousslavsky, J. (2003*b*). L'amour perdu de Gui et Madeleine. Le syndrome émotionnel et comportemental temporal de Guillaume Apollinaire. *Rev. Neurol. (Paris)* **15**, 171–9.

Bogousslavsky, J. (2005). Artistic creativity, style and brain disorders *Eur. Neurol.* **54**, 103–11.

Boller, F. (2005). Alajouanine's painter: Paul-Elie Gernez. In *Neurological disorders in famous artists* (ed. J. Bogousslavsky and F. Boller), pp. 92–100, Frontiers in Neurology and Neuroscience, Vol. 19. Karger, Basel.

Boller, F. and Frank, E. (1982). *Sexual dysfunction in neurological disorders: diagnosis, management and rehabilitation.* Raven Press, New York.

Bouvier-Peyrou, M., Landis, T., and Annoni, J.M. (2000). Self-duplication shifted in time: a particular form of delusional misidentification syndrome. *Neurocase* **6**, 57–63.

Brodaty, H., Sachdev, P.S., Withall, A., Altendorf, A., Valenzuela, M.J., and Lorentz. L. (2005). Frequency and clinical, neuropsychological and neuroimaging correlates of apathy following stroke—the Sydney Stroke Study. *Psychol. Med.* **35** (12), 1707–16.

Brothers, L. (1990). The neural basis of primate social communication. *Motivation Emotion* **14**, 81–91.

Brugger, P., Regard, M., and Landis, T. (1997). Illusory reduplication of one's own body: phenomenology and classification of autoscopic phenomena. *Cogn, Neuropsychiatry* **2**, 19–38.

Bruggimann, L., Annoni, J.M., Staub, F., von Steinbüchel, N., Van der Linden, M., and Bogousslavsky, J. (2006). Chronic post-traumatic stress symptoms after non-severe stroke. *Neurology* **66**, 513–16.

Carmin, C.N., Wiegartz, P.S., Yunus, U., and Gillock, K.L. (2002). Treatment of late-onset OCD following basal ganglia infarct. *Depress. Anxiety* **15** (2), 87–90.

Carota, A., Rossetti, A.O., Karapanayiotides, T., and Bogousslavsky, J. (2001). Catastrophic reaction in acute stroke: a reflex behavior in aphasic patients. *Neurology* **57** (10), 1902–5.

Carson, S., Peterson, J., and Higgins, D. (2003). Decreased latent inhibition is associated with increased creative achievement in high-functioning individuals. *J. Pers. Soc. Psychol.* **85**, 499–506.

Cheasty, M., Condren, R., and Cooney, C. (2002). Altered sexual preference and behaviour in a man with vascular ischaemic lesions in the temporal lobe. *Int. J. Geriatr. Psychiatry* **17** (1), 87–8.

Choi-Kwon, S., Han, S.W., Kwon, S.U., and Kim, J.S. (2005). Poststroke fatigue: characteristics and related factors. *Cerebrovasc Dis.* **19** (2), 84–90.

Cicone, M., Wapner, W., and Gardner, H. (1980). Sensitivity to emotional expressions and situations in organic patients. *Cortex* **16**, 145–58.

Coricelli, G., Critchley, H.D., Joffily, M., O'Doherty, J., Sirigu, A., and Dolan, R.J. (2005). Regret and its avoidance: a neuroimaging study of choice behavior. *Nature Neurosci.* **8**, 1255–62.

Croquelois, A., Assal, G., JM Annoni, J.M., and Bogousslavsky, J. (2005). Diseases of the nervous system: patients' etiological beliefs. *J. Neurol. Neurosurg. Psychiatry* **76** (4), 582–4.

Damasio, A.R. (1994). *Descarte's error: emotion, reason and the human brain.* Grosset Putman, New York.

Dusoir, H., Owens, C., Forbes, R.B., Morrow, J.I., Flynn, P.A., and McCarron, M.O. (2005). Anorexia nervosa remission following left thalamic stroke. *J. Neurol. Neurosurg. Psychiatry* **76**, 144–5.

Eslinger, P.J. and Damasio, A.R. (1985). Severe disturbance of higher cognition after bilateral frontal lobe ablation: patient EVR. *Neurology* **35**, 1731–41.

Frith, C.D. and Frith, U. (1999). Interacting minds: a biological basis. *Science* **286**, 1692–5.

Frith, U. and Frith, C.D. (2003). Development and neurophysiology of mentalizing. *Phil. Trans. R. Soc. Lond. B Biol. Sci.* **358**, 459–73.

Gentilini, M., De Renzi, E., and Crisi, G. (1987). Bilateral paramedian thalamic artery infarcts: report of eight cases. *J. Neurol. Neurosurg. Psychiatry* **50** (7), 900–9.

Ghika-Schmid, F., van Melle, G., Guex, P., and Bogousslavsky, J. (1999). Subjective experience and behavior in acute stroke: the Lausanne Emotion in Acute Stroke Study. *Neurology* **52**, 22–8.

Gialanella, B., Monguzzi, V., Santoro, R., and Rocchi, S. (2005). Functional recovery after hemiplegia in patients with neglect: the rehabilitative role of anosognosia. *Stroke* **36** (12), 2687–90.

Giaquinto, S., Buzzelli, S., Di Francesco, L., and Nolfe, G. (2003). Evaluation of sexual changes after stroke. *J. Clin. Psychiatry* **64** (3), 302–7.

Glader, E.L., Stegmayr, B., and Asplund, K. (2002). Poststroke fatigue: a 2-year follow-up study of stroke patients in Sweden. *Stroke* **33** (5), 1327–33.

Goldenberg, G. (1992). Loss of visual imagery and loss of visual knowledge—a case study. *Neuropsychologia* **30**, 1081–99.

Goodman, R. and Graham, P. (1996). Psychiatric problems in children with hemiplegia: cross-sectional epidemiological survey. *Br. Med. J.* **312**, 1065–9.

Grotta, J. and Bratina, P. (1995). Subjective experiences of 24 patients dramatically recovering from stroke. *Stroke* **26**, 1285–8.

Habib, M. and Poncet, M. (1988). Perte de l'élan vital, de l'intérêt et de l'affectivité (syndrome athymormique) au cours de lésions lacunaires des corps strié. *Rev. Neurol. (Paris)* **144**, 571–7.

Hacke, W., Kaste, M., Skyhoj Olsen, T., Orgogozo, J.M., and Bogousslavsky, J. (2000). European Stroke Initiative (EUSI) recommendations for stroke management. The European Stroke Initiative Writing Committee. *Eur. J. Neurol.* **7**, 607–23.

Hall, K., Karzmark, P., Stevens, M., Englander, J., O'Hare, P., and Wright, J. (1994). Family stressors in traumatic brain injury: a two-year follow-up. *Arch. Physical Med. Rehabil.* **75**, 876–84.

Happé, F., Brownell, H., and Winner, E. (1999). Acquired 'theory of mind' impairments following stroke. *Cognition* **70**, 211–40.

Heilman, K., Nadeau, S., and Beversdorf. D. (2003). Creative innovation. Possible brain mechanisms. *Neurocase* **9**, 369–79.

Houeto, J.L., Mesnage, V., Mallet, L., *et al.* (2002). Behavioural disorders, Parkinson's disease and subthalamic stimulation. *J. Neurol. Neurosurg. Psychiatry* **72**, 701–7.

Jeziernicka, B. and Turowski, K. (1978). [Drawings by patients with unilateral visuospatial agnosia]. *Neurol. Neurochir. Pol.* **12**, 595–601.

Kaplan, J.A., Brownell, H.H., Jacobs, J.R., and Gardner, H. (1990). The effects of right hemisphere damage on the pragmatic interpretation of conversational remarks. *Brain Lang.* **38**, 315– 33.

Kapur, N. (1996). Paradoxical functional facilitation in brain–behavior research. A critical review. *Brain* **119**, 1775–90.

Kim, J.S., Choi, S., Kwon, S.U., and Seo, Y.S. (2002). Inability to control anger or aggression after stroke. *Neurology* **58** (7), 1106–8.

Korpelainen, J.T., Nieminen, P., and Myllyla, V.V. (1999). Sexual functioning among stroke patients and their spouses. *Stroke* **30** (4), 715–19.

Lane, R.D. and Schwartz, G.E. (1987). Levels of emotional awareness: a cognitive developmental theory and its application to psychopathology. *Am. J. Psychiatry* **144**, 133–43.

Laplane, D., Levasseur, M., Pillon, B., Dubois, B., Baulac, M., Mazoyer, B., Tran Kinh, S., Sette, G., Danze, F., and Baron, J. (1989). Obsessive-compulsive disorder and other behavioural changes with bilateral basal gangia lesions. *Brain* **112**, 699–725.

Levy, M.L. (1998). Apathy is not depression. *J. Neuropsychiatry Clin. Neurosci.* **10**, 314–19.

Liberzon, I., Taylor, S.F., Fig, L.M., and Koeppe, R.A. (1996). Alteration of corticothalamic perfusion ratios during a PTSD flashback. *Depress Anxiety* **4**, 146–50.

Lim, K.O., Choi, S.J., Pomara, N., Wolkin, A., and Rotrosen, J.P. (2002). Reduced frontal white matter integrity in cocaine dependence: a controlled diffusion tensor imaging study. *Biol. Psychiatry* **51** (11), 890–5.

Low, J.A., Yap, K.B., and Chan, K.M. (1999). Posterior cerebral artery territory infarct presenting as acute psychosis. *Singapore Med. J.* **40**, 702–3.

Marin, R.S. (1991). Apathy: a neuropsychiatric syndrome. *J. Neuropsychiatry Clin. Neurosci.* **3**, 243–54.

Marin, R.S. (1993). The sources of convergence between measures of apathy and depression. *J. Affective Dis.* **28**, 117–24.

McCallum, M. (1989). A controlled study of effectiveness and patient suitability for short-term group psychotherapy [doctoral dissertation]. McGill University, Montreal.

McGuire, P. (1995). The brain in obsessive compulsive disorder. *J. Neurol. Neurosurg. Psychiatry* **59**, 457–9.

Meijer, R., Ihnenfeldt, D.S., van Limbeek, J., Vermeulen, M., and de Haan, R.J. (2003). Prognostic factors in the subacute phase after stroke for the future residence after six months to one year. A systematic review of the literature. *Clin. Rehabil.* **17** (5), 512–20.

Merrit, H., Adams, R., and Solomon, H. (1946). *Neurosyphilis*. Oxford University Press, Oxford.

Miller, B., Darby, A., Benson, D., Cummings, J., and Miller, M. (1997). Aggressive, socially disruptive and antisocial behaviour associated with fronto-temporal dementia. *Br. J. Psychiatry* **170**, 150–4.

Okada, K. (1997). Poststroke apathy and regional cerebral blood flow. *Stroke* **28**, 2437–41.

Preston, S. and de Waal, F. (2002). Empathy: its ultimate and proximate bases. *Behav. Brain Sci.* **25**, 1–71.

Price, B.H., Daffner, K.R., Stowe, R.M., and Mesulam, M.M. (1990). The comportmental learning disabilities of early frontal lobe damage. *Brain* **113**, 1383–93.

Prigatano, G., Ogano, M., and Amakusa, B. (1997). A cross-cultural study on impaired self-awareness in Japanese patients with brain dysfunction. *Neuropsychiatry Neuropsychol. Behav. Neurol.* **10**, 135–43.

Ptak, R. (1999). Probabilistisches Lernen bei Amnestikern und Patienten mit frontalen Dysfunktionen [PhD thesis]. University of Berne, Berne.

Regard, M. and Landis, T. (1997). 'Gourmand syndrome': eating passion associated with right anterior lesions. *Neurology* **48**, 1185–90.

Regard, M., Knoch, D., Gutling, E., and Landis, T. (2003). Brain damage and addictive behavior: a neuropsychological and electroencephalogram investigation with pathologic gamblers. *Cogn. Behav. Neurol.* **16** (1), 47–53.

Sachdev, P., Smith, J., Matheson, J., Last, P., and Blumberg, P. (1992). Amygdalo-hippocampectomy for pathological aggression. *Aust. NZ J. Psychiatry* **26**, 671–6.

Safran, A., Achard, O., Duret, F., and Landis, T. (1999). The 'thin man' phenomenon: a sign of cortical plasticity following inferior homonymous paracentral scotomas. *Br. J. Ophthalmol.* **83**, 137–42.

Schmahmann, J. and Sherman, J. (1998). The cerebellar cognitive affective syndrome. *Brain* **121**, 561–79.

Siegal, M. and Varley, R. (2002). Neural systems involved in 'theory of mind'. *Nature Rev. Neurosci.* **3**, 463–71

Smith, W., Mindelzun, R., and Miller, B. (2003). Simultanagnosia through the eyes of an artist. *Neurology* **60**, 1832–4.

Spinella, M. (2004). Hypersexuality and dysexecutive syndrome after a thalamic infarct. *Int. J. Neurosci.* **114** (12), 1581–90.

Starkstein, S. and Robinson, R. (1997). Mechanism of disinhibition after brain lesions. *J. Nerv. Mental Dis.* **114**, 108.

Staub, F., Annoni, J.M., Gramigna, S., and Bogousslavsky, J. (2005). The 'post-stroke fatigue' prospective study: final results. 14th European Stroke Conference Bologna, Italy 25–28 May, 2005.

Sternberg, R.J. (1985). *Beyond IQ: a triarchic theory on human intelligence*. Cambridge University Press, New York.

Sternberg, R.J. (1997). *Successful intelligence.* Plume, New York.

Steven, W.S. (1994). Buspirone efficacy in organic-induced aggression. *J. Clin. Psychopharmacol.* **14**, 126–30.

Stone, J., Townend, E., Kwan, J., Haga, K., Denni, M.S., and Sharpe, M. (2004). Personality change after stroke: some preliminary observations *J. Neurol. Neurosurg. Psychiatry* **75**, 1708–13.

Surian, L. and Siegal, M. (2001). Sources of performance on theory of mind tasks in right hemisphere-damaged patients. *Brain Lang.* **78**, 224–32.

Sweet, W. (1969). The relationship of violent behavior to focal cerebral disease. In *Aggressive behavior* (ed. S. Garattini and E. Sigg), pp. 161–71. Excerpta Medica, Amsterdam.

Tourette's syndrome study group (2002). Treatment of ADHD in children with tics: a randomized controlled trial. *Neurology* **58**, 527–36.

Trauner, D.A., Nass, R., and Ballantyne, A. (2001). Behavioural profiles of children and adolescents after pre- or perinatal unilateral brain damage. *Brain* **124** (5), 995–1002.

Van Reekum, R., Links, P., Finlayson, M., Boyle, M., Boiago, I., Ostrander, L., and Moustacalis, E. (1996). Repeat neurobehavioral study of borderline personality disorder. *Psychiatry Neurosci.* **21**, 13–20.

Vigouroux, R., Bonnefoi, B., and Khalil, R. (1990). [Pictorial creations of a painter presenting with left-sided neglect]. *Rev. Neurol. (Paris)* **146**, 665–70.

Vuilleumier, P. (2004). Anosognosia: the neurology of beliefs and uncertainties. *Cortex* **40** (1):9–17.

Weiger, W. and Bear, D. (1988). An approach to the neurology of aggression. *J. Psychiatr. Res.* **22**, 85–98.

Yamagata, S., Yamaguchi, S., and Kobayashi, S. (2004). Impaired novelty processing in apathy after subcortical stroke. *Stroke* **35** (8), 1935–40.

Zaidel, D., Chen, A., and German, C. (1995). She is not a beauty even when she smiles: possible evolutionary basis for a relationship between facial attractiveness and hemispheric specialization. *Neuropsychologia* **33**, 649–55.

Zeki, S. and Marini, L. (1998). Three cortical stages of colour processing in the human brain. *Brain* **121**, 1669–85.

Chapter 9

Cognitive and behavioural disorders associated with space-occupying lesions

Stefano F. Cappa and Lisa Cipolotti

9.1 Introduction

Space-occupying lesions (tumours, abscesses, and post-traumatic haematomas) affecting different brain areas are associated with clinical presentations in which cognitive and/or behavioural manifestations are the predominant, or even the only, feature. These syndromes are not only clinically relevant, but also provide a source of unique evidence about brain and cognition.

With regard to the first aspect, it is clear that in current neurological practice, which is characterized, at least in affluent societies, by easy access to imaging investigations, the relevance of a careful mental state evaluation as a tool for the early diagnosis of an insidious neurological condition, such as a brain tumour, is necessarily decreased. At the earliest suspicion of a brain disorder, a computerized tomographic (CT) or magnetic resonance (MR) scan is ordered and the diagnosis is easily made (for a review of MR in brain tumours see Rees 2003). The 'earliest suspicion', however, continues to depend on the clinical acumen of the neurologist (or psychiatrist). Even in these days, it is not unheard of for there to be a significant diagnostic delay because the clinician was not fully familiar with the subtle changes in personality or social behaviour associated with dysfunction of the frontobasal region, or with the possibility that mild memory disturbances are not due to stress or overwork but to compression of the diencephalic region.

Regarding the contribution to cognitive neuroscience research, it must be underlined that vascular lesions of the brain have historically played a major role in the investigation of the neurological foundation of language, praxis, and other cognitive functions. Strokes, however, do not represent a random sampling of lesion location, since they are obviously constrained by the vascular anatomy and by the predilection sites of vascular pathology. These other pathological conditions are thus a precious source of information about the participation in cognitive function of brain regions that are infrequently affected by vascular pathology. Needless to say, a space-occupying lesion interferes with brain function in ways that are extremely different from those associated with stroke. In the first instance, tumours develop gradually, with a time course that is dependent upon their biological features (for a review of neurological oncology see Rees 2004). Tumours of the meninges, as well as extracerebral haemorrhages, affect the brain by compression; intrinsic processes, such as the glial tumours, give rise to neural dysfunction by infiltration as well as by indirect effects, such as oedema. A large amount of information is derived from the investigation of the consequences of the surgical removal of tumours: in this case we have a situation that is in principle closer to the stroke model, or in general to the ablation model of experimental neuropsychology. It is not unusual to perform group studies that include patients affected by brain lesions that are defined on the basis of the topography and include not only infarcts or haemorrhages, but also surgical resections of meningiomas and gliomas (usually low-grade;

see Peers *et al.* 2005; Reverberi *et al.* 2005). This approach appears to be entirely legitimate, when all potential confounding factors such as medication, or associated disorders, are considered.

In this chapter, we describe the main syndromes characterized by prominent cognitive and behavioural disorders that are associated with commonly observed space-occupying lesions in clinical practice.

9.2 **Frontal tumours**

Much of what we know about the role of the prefrontal cortex in human cognition and behaviour has been learned from the effects of brain tumours, or from the consequences of selective frontal ablations following their surgical removal. As outlined above, an early diagnosis still depends very much upon an adequate consideration of cognitive and behavioural symptoms. These symptoms can be rather subtle and misleading, especially in the case of slowly growing tumours, such as meningiomas.

> A useful clinical rule is to obtain a neuroimaging investigation in any patient who develops psychological and behavioural symptoms that cannot be explained by a previous psychiatric history.

A strict application of this rule would imply that one should perform a CT or MRI at the onset of any psychiatric condition, which may not be too inconsistent with current practice in most academic psychiatric institutions.

The developments in our understanding of the function of the frontal lobe in recent years have been remarkable and have resulted from the convergence of research results from animal studies and functional neuroimaging in humans. The literature in this area is very extensive (for selected recent reviews see Duncan and Owen 2000; Miller and Cohen 2001; Wood and Grafman 2003). The traditional distinction between the primary motor cortex, the premotor cortex, which is responsible for motor control, and the prefrontal (granular) cortex, associated with the control of cognition and behaviour, has been substantially revised in recent years. In particular, a very influential line of investigation on the anatomical and functional complexity of the 'premotor' areas (Rizzolatti and Luppino 2001) has blurred this distinction (Fig. 9.1). This has suggested that high order processes related to space representation, action recognition, and learning are crucially dependent on neural activity characterized by complex patterns of responses, such as in the case of canonical neurons and mirror neurons. The situation appears to be similar in monkeys and humans, as indicated by the results of imaging studies (Rizzolatti and Craighero 2004).

> The traditional distinction between 'premotor' and 'prefrontal' cortex has been challenged by recent evidence of the participation of premotor areas in high-order cognitive functions.

The evidence from lesion studies is, of course, compatible with the evidence for functional heterogeneity in the frontal cortex, even if there has been a clear lag between the research advances and the tools applied to the neurological and neuropsychological evaluation of patients with frontal damage. The clinical evaluation is based on the so-called 'frontal lobe' tests, an array of empirically based tasks that explore a variety of complex performances requiring problem-solving, decision-making, and performance monitoring. Besides the cognitive aspects, frontal lobe lesions are associated with modifications that are apparent at the behavioural level and that may mimic

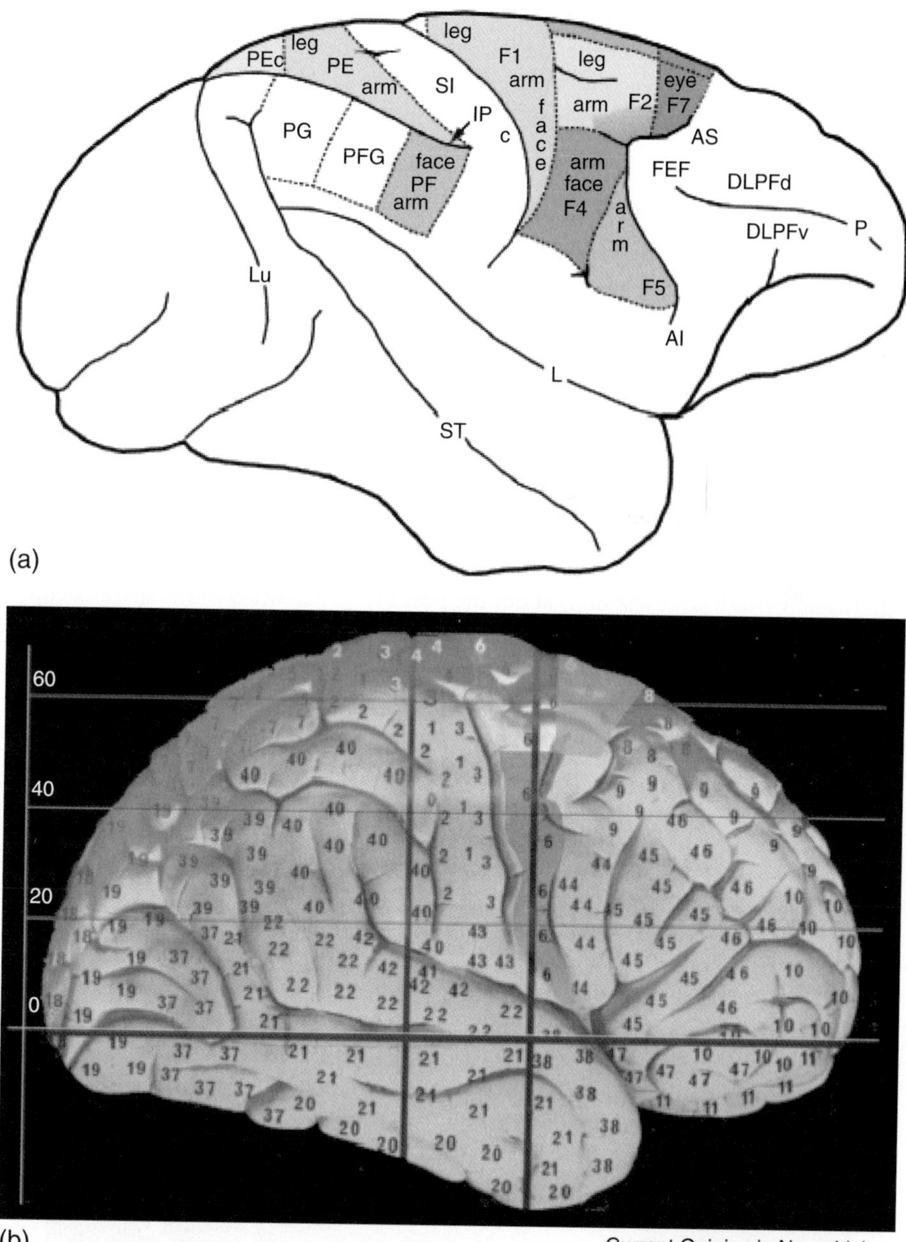

Fig. 9.1 The cortical motor system in monkey and man. (Taken with permission from Rizzolatti *et al.* 2002.) This is a black and white version of Plate 6.

all the aspects of psychiatric psychopathology, from depression to agitation to personality changes. On the basis of the combination of cognitive and behavioural disturbances a classical distinction can be made between the clinical syndromes associated with space-occupying lesions involving the lateral frontal cortex, the medial frontal areas, and the orbital (or ventromedian) cortex, respectively.

9.2.1 Tumours involving the lateral frontal cortex

The most common neoplasms affecting the frontal lobe are malignant gliomas and meningiomas (Fig. 9.2). The former are associated with cognitive and behavioural disturbances that, due to the rapid rate of growth and the frequent multifocality, are usually severe. A number of studies have been devoted to the cognitive consequences of radiotherapy and chemotherapy in patients with malignant gliomas (Taphoorn and Klein 2004). The problem of cognitive sequelae is particularly relevant in the case of low-grade gliomas (astrocytomas, oligodendrogliomas), in which long-term survival can be expected. Conversely, frontal meningiomas of the convexity are characterized by the slow growth and the frequent absence of focal signs. They are often associated with subtle cognitive and behavioural modifications, which may escape detection for a long time. This results in a delayed diagnosis. It is actually not uncommon to detect the presence of a frontal meningioma in an elderly patient submitted to CT or MR for the evaluation of dementia, giving rise to (usually fruitless) discussions about the possible contribution of the space-occupying lesions to the clinical picture.

> Tumours affecting the lateral frontal cortex are associated with the insidious onset of the classical 'frontal lobe syndrome' characterized by perseverative behaviours, easy distractibility, and disinhibition.

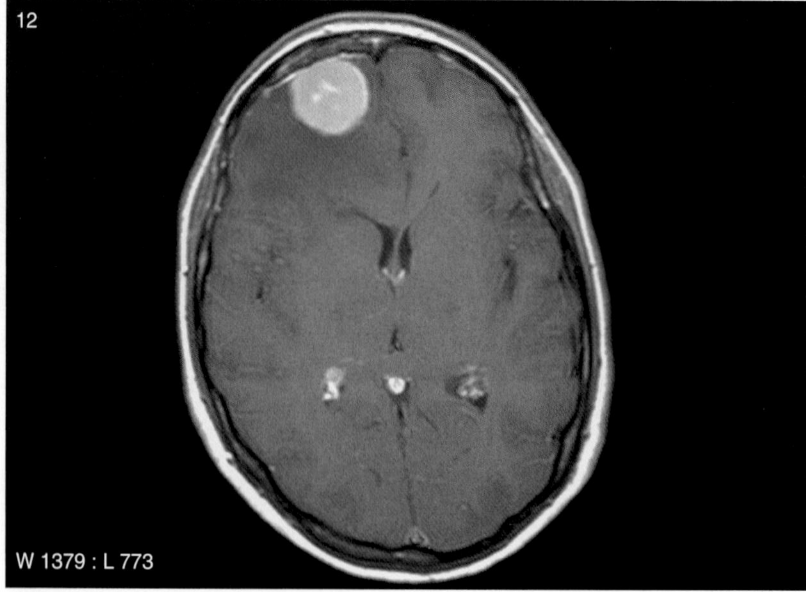

Fig. 9.2 MR image of prefrontal meningioma. (Courtesy of Dr Andrea Falini.)

The subtle changes in cognition and behaviour reflect some of the basic aspects of the classical 'frontal syndrome'. These are: (1) perseverative responses, which indicate difficulty in shifting between responses; (2) difficulties in concentration and in the ability to ignore distractions; and (3) defective inhibition of behaviours that are routinely triggered by cues in the external environment. These modifications may create the impression that the patient's personality has changed. Often (but by no ways invariably) these cognitive and behavioural changes, which are observed by co-workers and relatives in the complex activities of daily life, are reflected in an impaired performance in tests of working memory that require the maintenance and monitoring of external information and in other 'frontal lobe' tests that tap the ability to divide attention and to change in a flexible way an ongoing problem-solving behaviour, such as, for example, the Wisconsin Card Sorting Test.

The idea that the lateral frontal cortex plays a crucial role in the control of behaviour is well established and can be traced back to authors such as Bianchi, Goldstein, and Luria. In more recent years, one of the most successful attempts to define this concept has been the proposal that the frontal lobe is the neural machinery responsible for the operation of the 'supervisory attentional system' (Norman and Shallice 1986) or the 'central executive' (Baddeley 1996). These cognitive components were postulated on the basis of experimental evidence and are responsible for the allocation of processing resources and for the organization of plans of willed action.

While these broad concepts can be relatively satisfactory at the functional level, it is clearly disappointing to relate these complex functions to the lateral frontal cortex as a whole, as this is a very large region of the brain that is highly heterogeneous at the anatomical and physiological level. The traditional distinction between premotor and prefrontal areas has been mentioned above. Another important subdivision is that between the ventrolateral and the dorsolateral region. There is considerable evidence, based largely on primate studies and neuroimaging investigations in humans, that supports the functional heterogeneity between these two regions. Using a very gross distinction, the dorsolateral prefrontal cortex (DLPFC) includes areas 9 and 46, while the ventrolateral prefrontal cortex (VLPFC) corresponds to areas 44, 45, and 47. In the case of working memory, the ventral part seems to be responsible for the storage of information, while the dorsal part plays a crucial role in the manipulation and monitoring of information (Fletcher and Henson 2001). The ventrolateral area on the left side includes Broca's area, which plays a crucial role in language, as well as in a number of extralinguistic functions.

9.2.1.1 Impairments following lesions in the inferior frontal gyrus (BA 44 and 45)

Patients with malignant tumours in the left frontal lobe have allowed the characterization of the neurocognitive underpinnings of dynamic aphasia. Dynamic aphasia is a severe impairment in propositional language characterized by a marked reduction of speech production. Patients with dynamic aphasia very rarely initiate spontaneous speech. They are unable to provide a narrative or story when elaboration or formulation of thought is required. However, they can answer, albeit on occasion rather telegraphically, direct questions and describe complex pictures (Luria 1966, 1970). This severe reduction of spontaneous speech occurs in the context of well preserved nominal, transcoding, repetition, reading and comprehension skills.

> The language disorder typically associated with slowly progressive damage to the left ventrolateral frontal cortex is characterized by a severe reduction of spontaneous speech production (dynamic aphasia).

On the basis of the language profile it has been suggested that dynamic aphasia can be subdivided into two forms: *pure* and *mixed* (Robinson *et al.* 2005). Patients with pure dynamic aphasia present with severely reduced spontaneous speech without other language impairments (e.g. Costello and Warrington 1989; Gold *et al.* 1997; Luria 1970, Robinson *et al.* 1998), whereas patients with mixed dynamic aphasia present with severely reduced spontaneous speech as well as additional phonological, lexical, syntactical, and articulatory impairments (e.g. Esmonde *et al.* 1996; Luria 1970; Raymer *et al.* 2002; Robinson *et al.* 2005; Snowden *et al.* 1996; Warren *et al.* 2003).

Recently, it has been suggested that there may be a further subdivision within dynamic aphasia (Robinson *et al.* 2006). The majority of dynamic aphasia patients have been shown to have difficulty completing experimental tasks requiring them to generate a word (e.g. generate a word to complete the sentence *he posted the letter without a* ...) or a sentence level response (e.g. generate a sentence with the word *table*). Interestingly, when closely analysed, the impairment of these dynamic aphasia patients on word and sentence level generation tasks is only present when a stimulus activates many response options (Robinson *et al.* 1998, 2005). However, the impairment was absent for tests involving stimuli that activate few or single dominant response options. To illustrate, these patients had significant difficulty generating a sentence from common nouns that have many potential response options (e.g. table). By contrast, they are able to generate a sentence from proper nouns that activate few or single dominant response options (e.g. London, Hitler). This type of impairment appeared to be specific to the language production domain. A detailed investigation using non-verbal generation tests indicated that one of these patients with dynamic aphasia performed normally on non-verbal generation tests (Robinson *et al.* 2005). Patients with this type of dynamic aphasia present with unilateral posterior left frontal lesions. For example, the patient described by Robinson *et al.* (1998) had a malignant meningioma that specifically impinged on BA45 and on BA44 to a lesser extent (for a review see Robinson *et al.* 2006).

Interestingly, there is a second group of patients with dynamic aphasia who presented with a preserved performance on word and sentence level generation tasks (e.g. Snowden *et al.* 1996; Esmonde *et al.* 1996). For example, Robinson *et al.* (2006) described a dynamic aphasic patient who performed virtually at ceiling on verbal generation tasks. For example, when given the word 'phone' she had no difficulty in generating the sentence '*I was talking on the phone*', despite her dynamic aphasia being as severe as that of the previously discussed patients. For example, when she was asked to talk about her favourite actress, she was only able to produce the response '*Vanessa Redgrave*', after a 15 second pause. When invited again to say why she liked this actress she added after another 20 second pause '*she makes everything believable*'. Notably all patients with this second subtype of dynamic aphasia have bilateral frontal (and possibly subcortical) involvement. The existence of these two different subtypes of dynamic aphasia allows one to hypothesize that two sets of functionally independent mechanisms may be involved in the generation of conceptual structures. One set of mechanisms is involved in the selection of a verbal response option among competitors. A second set of mechanisms is involved in the generation of a fluent sequence of novel thought. Damage to the first set of mechanisms causes a verbal generation impairment characterized by an inability to select a single response option from among competitors. Damage to the second set of mechanisms causes a verbal generation impairment characterised by an inability to generate novel concepts.

9.2.1.2 Impairments following lesions in the rostral frontal region (BA 10)

Relatively little is known about the anterior prefrontal cortex, or frontal pole (Ramnani and Owen 2004). This is remarkable, since this is the only part of the frontal lobe that is significantly larger in humans than in other primates (for a novel view of this traditional concept see Semendeferi *et al.* 2002). Hypotheses regarding the function of this area have been put forward on the basis of functional imaging as opposed to lesion studies. It has been suggested that this region is involved in the integration of different subprocesses in order to achieve a higher order goal. An elegant experiment by Koechlin *et al.* (2003) supports the idea of a caudal to rostral hierarchy in the level of cognitive control operated by the frontal cortex; the most anterior part appears responsible for the highest level of control of plans involving specific behavioural rules. An impairment of this mechanism may thus be proposed to be responsible for some typical behavioural modifications observed in patients affected by space-occupying lesions affecting this part of the cortex.

Slowly progressive damage to the anterior frontal lobe is compatible with preserved performance on 'frontal lobe tests', and is associated with increasing difficulties in everyday life, due to defective coordination among the multiple demands of the environment.

Typically, patients with lesions in BA10 perform well on standard neuropsychological measures of intellectual functioning, memory, and perception and even on traditional tests of executive functions. Their most noticeable impairment manifests itself in everyday life as a marked multi-tasking problem (e.g. Shallice and Burgess 1991). Two recent human lesion group studies have documented this type of impairment. Burgess *et al.* (2000) examined a series of 60 acute neurological patients (approximately three-quarters of whom were suffering from brain tumours) and 60 healthy controls matched for age and IQ on a multi-task test called the Greenwich test. In this test subjects are presented with three different simple tasks and told that they have to attempt at least some of each of the tasks in 10 minutes while following a set of rules. Despite being able to learn the task rules, form a plan, remember their actions, and say what they should have done, patients with left hemisphere rostral lesions showed a significant multi-tasking impairment. These patients were able to perform the individual subtasks perfectly well but tended not to switch tasks. When they did switch tasks they showed a problem following the rules of the other tasks. A further recent group study supported these results (Burgess *et al.*, submitted). On the basis of these data the author hypothesized that the rostral prefrontal cortex is subserving a system that biases the relative influence of stimulus-oriented and stimulus-independent thought (the gateway hypothesis of rostral prefrontal function, Burgess *et al.* 2005). This cognitive control function is used in a wide range of situations critical to competent human behaviour in everyday life such as, for example, remembering to carry out intended actions after a delay and multi-tasking. According to the author, such activities require one to be particularly alert to the environment, to concentrate on one's thought, and to be able to consciously switch between these states.

9.2.2 Mesial frontal tumours

The typical mesial frontal tumour is the meningioma of the falx, which can be associated with a rather distinctive clinical syndrome characterized by a progressive reduction of initiative in the motor and verbal domain.

The syndrome of akinetic mutism has been observed as a consequence of progressive dysfunction of the mesial prefrontal areas, such as in the case of meningioma of the falx.

As in the case of the lateral frontal cortex, the convergent results of animal studies and functional neuroimaging have led to considerable insights into the complex structure and function of the medial frontal cortex (Fig. 9.3). Medial area 6 can subdivided in the supplementary motor area proper (SMA) and a preSMA, connected to motor and to prefrontal regions respectively. Anteriorly, lies the mesial part of area 9. The cingulate sulcus divides this region from the anterior cingulate cortex (ACC). It has been proposed that, while the preSMA plays a crucial role in the selection of action plans, the fundamental contribution of the ACC lies in relating actions to their consequences (both in term of error detection and positive reinforcement). This is a crucial step required before making decision about future actions (Rushworth *et al.* 2004). The output of this process is then relayed to the lateral prefrontal cortex for the adjustment of performance (Ridderinkhof *et al.* 2004).

9.2.2.1 Cognitive impairments

A relatively small number of patients with ACC lesions have been described with cognitive impairments, including deficits in executive tasks requiring conflict monitoring, such as the Stroop test, and sustained attention tasks necessitating allocation of attentional resources, such as the 6-elements test (Wilson *et al.* 1996) and the SART test (Robertson *et al.* 1997) which requires patients to name digits on a computer screen except for a target digit (e.g. Stemmer *et al.* 2003; Swick and colleagues 2002*a*, *b*). The data from these patients are thought to

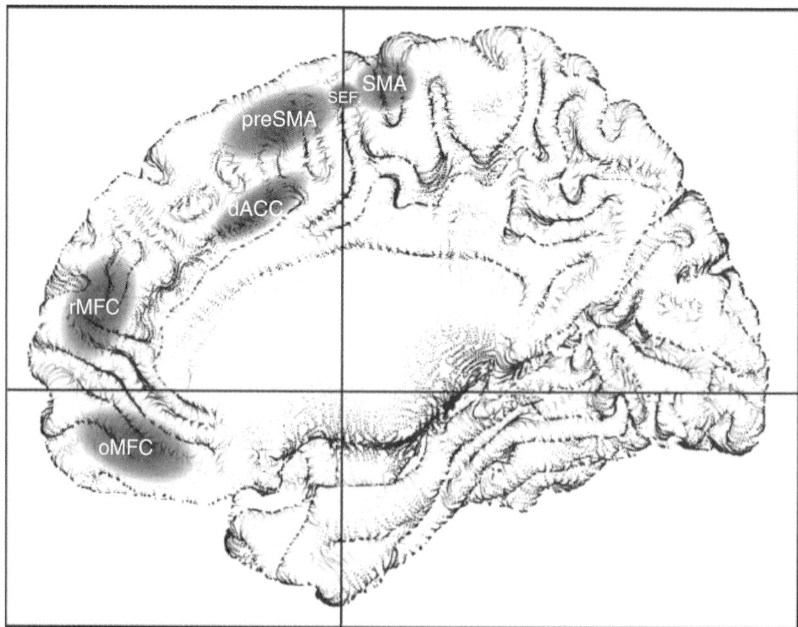

Fig. 9.3 Sketch of the approximate locations of medial frontal areas as referred to in the text, superimposed on a single individual template brain normalized into standard stereotactic space (colin brain, http://brainmap.wustl.edu/resources/caretnew.html) and rendered using non-photorealistic techniques (http://www.opennpar.org). SMA, Supplementary motor area; SEF, supplementary eye field; dACC, dorsal anterior cingulate; oMFC, orbitofrontal ventromedial cortex; rMFC, rostral ventromedial cortex. (Taken with permission from Nachev 2006).

support two main theories of the role of the ACC in cognition based on neuroimaging findings: the conflict monitoring and the anterior attention theory. The notion of conflict monitoring assumes that the ACC monitors the attentional requirements by evaluating conflict between the current and desired responses, and engages other systems to modulate cognitive processing appropriately (e.g. Botvinick *et al.* 2001; Carter *et al.* 1998, 2000). The anterior attention account of ACC functions suggest that the ACC directly allocates attentional resources to implement cognitive control (e.g. Posner and Digirolamo 1998; Posner and Petersen 1990). However, some of the patients described above had lesions extending well beyond the ACC; therefore it remains unclear whether their impairment could be attributed solely to the ACC lesions. Interestingly, two recent studies involving patients with ACC damage question the two theories suggesting that ACC plays a role in conflict monitoring and anterior attention. Fellows and Farah (2005) described four patients with an intact performance on two tasks of cognitive control such as the Stroop Test and the Go-No-Go task. Furthermore, Baird *et al.* (2006) described two patients with tumoural lesions involving the ACC who performed satisfactorily on very demanding anterior attention tasks such as the SART and the 6-elements test. In general, both patients did not show any significant generalized cognitive impairment. Interestingly, both patients showed abnormalities in autonomic cardiovascular responses, with blunted autonomic arousal to mental stress during performance of cognitive tasks (mental arithmetic and motor tasks; Critchley *et al.* 2003). This suggests that in these two patients the ACC lesions are associated with abnormalities in behaviourally integrated autonomic responses. This finding supports a hypothesis suggesting that the ACC is involved in the generation of preparatory and facilitatory bodily arousal states during volitional behaviours, rather than having a primary role in associated cognitive computations (e.g. Critchley *et al.* 2003, 2005).

9.2.2.2 Social cognition[1] impairments after medial frontal lobe damage

On the basis of imaging studies the medial prefrontal cortex has also been implicated in the network of areas engaged by tasks that tap the human ability to predict and explain the behaviours of co-specifics on the basis of an attribution of mental states, such as beliefs and desires (Gallagher *et al.* 2000). It is thus remarkable that a recent study of a patient with extensive damage to the medial prefrontal cortex failed to produce any impairment on theory of mind tests (Bird *et al.* 2004).[2] Abnormal autistic behaviour is often interpreted in terms of 'theory of mind' (ToM) or mentalizing impairment. In this patient the damage included the rostral and ventral areas of ACC but spared the dorsal regions bilaterally. This raises the possibility that different parts of the ACC may be differentially involved in ToM tasks. Consistent with this, Baird *et al.* (2006) recently reported three patients with medial prefrontal cortex lesions including the ACC. In one patient the ACC damage was bilateral but more prominent on the left. The remaining two patients had unilateral right ACC lesions. The nature of the lesions in two of these three patients was tumoural. Only the patient with bilateral ACC damage more prominent on the left showed a deficit in two ToM tasks. The two patients with a selective right ACC damage performed as well as controls on these two tasks. These data suggest that the left ACC may be more critical than the right in mentalizing. However, this conclusion can be regarded as tentative as the current neuroimaging and neuropsychological literature regarding a possible laterality effect in theory of

1 Knowledge about the social appropriateness of action and inference regarding the thoughts of others.

2 The term 'theory of mind' (ToM) refers to the human ability to attribute mental states such as belief, intention, and desire to others (e.g. Frith and Frith 2003).

mind is inconclusive. For example, Calarge *et al.* (2003) found greater activation in the left frontal lobe, including the left ACC, in a positron emission tomographic (PET) study of theory of mind function, whereas Vogeley *et al.* (2001) emphasized the role of the right ACC and Gallagher *et al.* (2002) found bilateral anterior para-cingulate activation. Some neuropsychological studies have emphasized the role of the left frontal lobe in mentalizing (e.g. Channon and Crawford 2000); others have found greater ToM impairment in patients with right frontal lesions (e.g. Stuss *et al.* 2001; Shamay-Tsoory *et al.* 2003) or no laterality effect (e.g. Rowe *et al.* 2001). None of these studies made specific reference to the ACC. Clearly, further research is required to explore a potential laterality effect in the mediation of theory of mind.

> The complex cognitive functions that have been attributed to the anterior cingulate region, mostly on the basis of functional imaging results, are only partially supported by clinical findings.

9.2.3 Tumours involving the orbito-frontal cortex

The orbito-frontal syndrome can be observed as a consequence of extracerebral compression by a slowly developing mengioma of the olfactory grove (Fig. 9.4). The syndrome is usually characterized by headache and what are generally described as 'personality changes'. Occasionally the patient comes to clinical observation because of the onset of epileptic seizures.

The orbito-frontal cortex is a paralimbic region, with extensive connection to sensory areas, lateral prefrontal cortex, amygdala, and other limbic structures (Fig. 9.5). Its postulated function is the integration of cognitive and emotional information about external stimuli and the computation of their motivational value on the basis of potential reward. Thus, it is not surprising that lesions in this region of the frontal lobe have traditionally been associated with the most

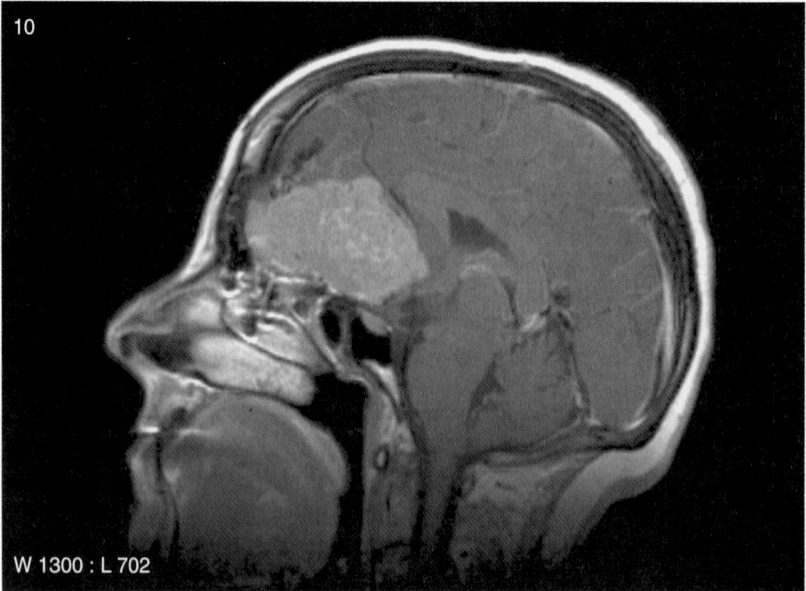

Fig. 9.4 MR image of olfactory grove meningioma. (Courtesy of Dr Andrea Falini.)

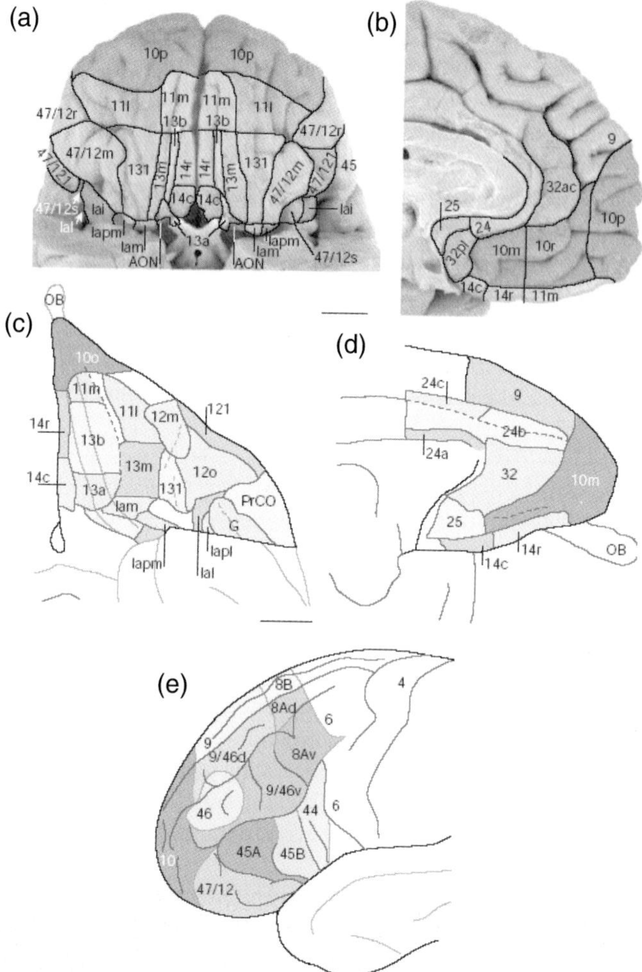

Fig. 9.5 The orbitofrontal cortex in (a), (b) man and (c), (d) monkey, (e) human lateral prefrontal cortex. (Taken with permission from Petrides and Pandya 1994.) This is a black and white version of Plate 7.

disruptive behavioural disturbances. Typically, patients with orbito-frontal cortex damage score normally on standard neuropsychometry testing (including tests of executive function), yet exhibit marked motivational, emotional, and social dysfunction in daily life. For example, they may exhibit deficits in motivational decision-making tasks, demonstrating that they are unable to develop risk-contemplating responses and do not learn to adapt their decisions advantageously. Deficits in emotional processing and social cognition have also been observed in patients with both orbito-frontal cortex and amygdala lesions. For instance, patients with orbito-frontal damage have often been described as presenting diminished social awareness and a lack of concern for social rules (e.g. Stuss *et al.* 1992; Damasio *et al.* 1994). Frequently, increased levels of aggression and aberrant behaviour are reported both when the lesions are acquired early in life and when they are acquired in adulthood (e.g. Grafman *et al.* 1996; Price *et al.* 1990). These emotional and behavioural changes following lesions to the orbito-frontal cortex have also been classed with the term 'acquired sociopathy' (Damasio *et al.* 1990) since some patients can fulfil the DSM-III (*Diagnostic and Statistical Manual of Mental Disorders*; American Psychiatric Association 1980) criteria for 'sociopathic disorder'. For example, Damasio and colleagues described patient EVR who prior to his orbitofrontal meningioma was a happily married, successful professional. Subsequent to his surgery he divorced twice and was eventually declared bankrupt. Blair and Cipolotti (2000) described patient JS who, following orbito-frontal damage, failed to conform to social norms, was irritable and aggressive, and demonstrated to be reckless regarding the personal safety of others. For example, he could quite easily beat the nurses on the basis that they were 'slow in doing their job' or continue to push around a wheelchair-bound patient despite her screams of terror.

> Lesions involving the orbito-frontal cortex are often associated with severe behavioural disturbances, disrupting social behaviours, which may mimic personality disorders (acquired sociopathy).

One of the most influential models of human rationality and decision-making, the 'somatic marker hypothesis' (Damasio *et al.* 1991; Damasio 1994), assigns a crucial role to the ventromedial (VM) orbital cortex. Together with the amygdala, the VM cortex is thought to be involved in the integration of external information with information about emotional states, as well as internal body states. In particular, the amygdala seems to be concerned with responding to primary inducers of pleasurable or aversive experiences, while the VM cortex is responsible for induction of similar experiences by thoughts and memories about the same inducers (Bechara *et al.* 2003). This interplay between body responses and information-processing is the main determinant of appropriate decision-making for the individual operating in a social context. Thus, the dysfunction of the system, which can be due to multiple mechanisms, including an acquired lesion of the orbitofrontal cortex, may be responsible for the inappropriate social behaviour that is one of the hallmarks of the frontal lobe syndrome.

Central to the notion of the somatic marker hypothesis is the idea that autonomically generated bodily arousal responses feed back to guide motivational decision-making, emotional processing, and social cognition. This hypothesis predicts that absent bodily arousal responses will be associated with behavioural deficits (e.g. Bechara *et al.* 2003; Tranel 2000) and perhaps influence emotional processing and social cognition (e.g. Damasio 1994). However, a study investigating motivational decision-making, emotional processing, and social cognition in patients with pure autonomic failure who cannot generate (or feed back) integrated peripheral autonomic responses reported unimpaired motivational decision-making, emotional processing, and social cognition (Heims *et al.* 2004). This suggests that autonomic responses (such as electrodermal activity) do not represent the principal avenue of bodily feedback for behavioural guidance. Emotional and social functioning are not critically dependent on an ongoing experience of autonomic arousal state. This leaves open the possibility that feedback of 'somatic markers' may alternatively or primarily draw on somatomotor responses to guide and influence behaviour.

The therapy and prognosis of cognitive and behavioural disturbances due to brain tumours depend upon the pathological nature of the lesion. A recent investigation has shown a postoperative improvement in attentional and executive functions in a relatively large sample of patients with frontobasal, convexity, sphenoid wing, and falx meningiomas (Tucha *et al.* 2003).The improvement was most marked in the case of removal of right hemispheric meningiomas.

9.3 Memory disorders due to brain tumours

While the hallmark of frontal tumours is behavioural disturbances, tumours involving the structures that are considered to be part of the limbic network are typically associated with memory disorders. The difference is not absolute, but rather a matter of degree, as memory disorders are a part of the frontal syndrome, and executive dysfunction is often observed in amnesia.

> Memory disorders are a frequent consequence of brain tumours. The classical amnesic syndrome, characterized by anterograde and retrograde memory impairment, is a consequence of lesions involving temporo-limbic structures.

Amnesia is a memory impairment that usually occurs in the absence of clear intellectual dysfunction and/or loss of general knowledge. We are going to discuss the pattern of memory impairments associated with temporo-limbic lesions and those associated with frontal lesions separately. The material-specific memory impairments (e.g. topographical memory, memory for human faces) will not be considered here.

9.3.1 Memory deficits following temporal lesions

The memory impairment is usually global, e.g. both anterograde and retrograde. Both impairments cover a complex set of phenomena whose extent, nature, and anatomical basis are still relatively poorly understood. Further, different, often contrasting cognitive theories have been proposed to account for the pattern of retrograde and anterograde memory loss. It is generally accepted that severe amnesic states are only observed in patients with bilateral damage. However, there is considerable debate concerning the role played in amnesia by several critical structures within the medial temporal lobe (hippocampus, entorhinal, perirhinal, parahippocampal cortices) and the related diencephalic midline structures (mamillary bodies, anterior thalamic nuclei, medial dorsal thalamic nuclei, thalamic nucleus, mamillary thalamic tract). Most of the current debate is primarily concerned with the role of the hippocampus and related structure in retrograde and anterograde amnesia.

9.3.1.1 Retrograde amnesia

In terms of the role of the hippocampus in retrograde amnesia different theories have been suggested regarding its function and its interaction with the neocortex (e.g. McClelland *et al.* 1992; 1995; Treves and Rolls 1992, 1994; Murre 1992). Central to most theories is the view that the hippocampus is important in memory consolidation and providing extra learning opportunities for the neocortical permanent memory store. This view predicts that, following damage to the medial temporal lobe, only recent retrograde memory should be impaired in neurological patients. Loss of both recent and remote retrograde memories implies additional damage in the neocortex. Compelling evidence for this view comes from studies that report that hippocampal amnesics show a selective memory deficit for material acquired shortly before their lesion occurred. Retrieval of more remote memories appears to be relatively preserved (e.g. Reed and Squire 1998; Manns *et al.* 2003; Bayley *et al.* 2003, 2005). However, patients have also been reported who had lesions restricted to the medial temporal lobe and who exhibited loss of remote memories extending for decades (e.g. Sanders and Warrington 1971; Fuji 2002; Cipolotti *et al.* 2001; see for further discussion Nadel *et al.* 2000; Cipolotti and Moscovitch 2005). Differences in the severity of the amnesia, the methodology employed for testing remote memory, and the extent of the hippocampal lesion may play a crucial role in determining the reported differences in the extent of the patients' retrograde amnesia. Therefore, the question regarding the neuroanatomy of remote memory and in particular the role of the medial temporal lobe and hippocampus is far from being resolved.

9.3.1.2 Anterograde amnesia

Regarding the role of the hippocampus in anterograde amnesia, disagreement exists in the literature over whether anterograde amnesia involves the recollective-based recognition processes[3] and/or the familiarity processes[4], depending on whether the anatomical damage is restricted to the hippocampus or also involves adjacent areas, particularly the entorhinal and perirhinal cortices (e.g. Aggleton and Brown 1999; Brown and Aggleton 2001; Mishkin *et al.* 1997; Squire 1992). So far only very few patients have been described with severe anterograde amnesia for whom detailed neuroanatomical and neuropsychological data are available. In these few hippocampal amnesic patients important differences in their anterograde memory profile have been documented. On the one hand, patients have been reported with intact recognition but impaired recall memory (e.g. Hodlstock *et al.* 2002; Mayes *et al.* 2002; Vargha-Khadem *et al.* 1997; Bastin *et al.* 2004; Aggleton *et al.* 2005; Yonelinas *et al.* 2002). On the other hand, patients have been described with equally impaired recognition and recall memory (e.g. Reed and Squire 1997; Cipolotti *et al.* 2006; Manns *et al.* 2003; Wais *et al.* 2006). Thus, at present it remains difficult to make direct comparisons between these patients. Certainly, factors such as the possible functionality of residual hippocampal tissue and the possibility of functional reorganization may play a critical role for these differences. For example, two recent fMRI studies reported strikingly different patterns of activation in the brain of an adult acquired anoxic hippocampal pathology compared with those of perinatally acquired anoxic hippocampal damage (Maguire *et al.* 2001, 2005). The adult acquired hippocampal patient with a memory profile characterized by recall and recognition impairment was effectively ahippocampal. In contrast, the perinatally acquired hippocampal patient with a memory profile characterized by impaired recall and spared recognition was still able to activate the residual hippocampal tissue. This suggests that the age at which the hippocampal damage occurs may have implications for the subsequent functionality of residual hippocampal tissue.

9.3.2 Memory deficits following frontal lesions

Damage to the frontal lobes does not result in the amnesic syndrome typical of lesions to the temporal encephalic structures. There is a large body of evidence suggesting that it may lead to a range of more subtle impairments of memory, particularly in recall tasks (e.g. Dimitrov *et al.* 1999; Janowsky *et al.* 1989; Wheeler *et al.* 1995).

> Memory disorders can also be present in the case of frontal tumours, as one of the aspects of the dysexecutive syndrome.

Recall tasks are relatively effortful compared with recognition tasks, as they require the participant both to initiate an effective search in memory and to evaluate the products of research.

[3] Recollection: items are recalled with associated phenomenological aspects of an encoded event.

[4] Familiarity: items are recognized without retrieval of other details (e.g. Jacoby and Dallas 1981; Mandler 1980; Tulving 1985).

Consequently, recall memory deficits are thought to be secondary to impairment in frontally located supervisory processes, rather than being pure memory deficits. Studies using functional lesion localization techniques to assess the contribution of different subregions of the frontal lobes to memory processes have reported that left frontal (particularly left dorsal lateral) damage impaired recall in a list-learning task (e.g. Stuss *et al.* 1994). In keeping with this, Alexander *et al.* (2003) reported marked free recall deficits in patients with posterior left dorsal lateral lesions but also in those with posterior medial frontal lesions. In addition to a poor performance in recall memory tasks, patients with frontal damage, in particular with right lateral frontal lesions, have been reported to produce excess repetitions in their recall (e.g. Stuss *et al.* 1994). This pattern of responses was attributed to impairment in monitoring the output of recall, which prevented the editing of words already recalled.

Confabulation has been defined as a falsification of memory occurring in clear consciousness in association with an organically derived amnesia (Berlyne 1972). It involves the production of false beliefs that the patient believes to be true and involves no intent to deceive the listener. These false beliefs may either be provoked in response to a memory test or questioning or be spontaneous, in which case there is an unprovoked outpouring of erroneous memory (e.g. Kopelman 1987). The context of spontaneous confabulations may range from subtle alterations of true events to bizarre and implausible stories. Patients with frontal damage, in particular patients with damage involving the inferior medial prefrontal cortex, are known to produce confabulations. Confabulations are often observed following rupture and repair of an anterior communicating artery aneurysm, which tends to result in ventral medial and basal forebrain lesions. However, confabulations are also common following frontal tumours. The critical cognitive deficit underlying confabulation remains unclear. Several authors have proposed that they result from amnesia overlaid with a frontal dysexecutive syndrome (e.g. Baddeley and Wilson 1988; Kapur and Coughlan 1980; Fisher *et al.* 1995; Cunningham *et al.* 1997). Other authors have suggested that confabulations result from a selective impairment in a control system involved in memory (e.g. Damasio *et al.* 1985; Schnider *et al.* 2000, 2003).

9.3.3 **Memory deficits following lesions in other locations**

Several tumours affecting the diencephalic region can be associated with a clinical picture of relatively pure amnesia. The most common are pituitary tumours and craniopharingiomas. Other tumours of the third ventricle that can result in memory disturbances are ependimomas, germinomas, colloid cyst, and gliomas. The amnesia is considered to follow from damage to several structures, which include the dorsomedial and anterior thalamic nuclei, fornix, septal nuclei, and mamillary bodies. There is evidence that damage restricted to the mamillary bodies is sufficient to produce severe anterograde amnesia, which can be fully reversed by tumour removal (Kupers *et al.* 2004).

Pituitary tumours are frequent (10% of intracranial tumours) and are usually benign. Memory disorders can result from compression by the tumour itself or (nowadays more frequently) from the effects of surgical or radiation therapy. It is also possible that hormonal dysfunction due to secreting adenomas may affect memory functions. On the basis of a retrospective study with 90 treated patients, Guinan *et al.* (1998) argued for a major role of treatment in producing the selective memory disorder observed in these patients. No difference was found between surgical removal and radiotherapy from the point of view of the severity of post-treatment amnesia.

Splenial tumours (Rudge and Warrington 1991), usually gliomas, have been associated with pure amnesia and disorders of visual perception. This clinical observation, which was relatively unexpected at the time, is fully convergent with the results of functional imaging studies, which have indicated an important role of the retrosplenial region in memory function (Fletcher *et al.* 1995).

Notably, in recent years it has been shown that radiotherapy for several brain, head, and neck tumours involving the medial temporal lobe region is associated with memory dysfunction. This effect has been attributed to depressed neurogenesis, which in animal models is linked to the formation of memory traces (Byrne 2005).

9.4 Cerebellar tumours

The cerebellum is frequently affected by tumours including meningioma, low grade glioma, and metastasis.

> The cerebellum is now considered to be involved not only in motor control, but in a wide range of cognitive functions.

It is well-known that the cerebellum plays an important role in motor control. However, the notion of whether the cerebellum may also be involved in other functions is controversial (e.g. Glickstein 2006; Schmahmann and Caplan 2006). In the past decade a growing body of evidence derived largely from functional neuroimaging studies has implicated the cerebellum in higher cognitive functions. However, the documentation of cognitive deficits in patients with cerebellar lesions has been somewhat less convincing. A notable exception is represented by the study of Schmahmann and Sherman (1998). This study documented clear-cut cognitive deficits in patients with cerebellar lesions with or without motor deficits. The authors introduced the concept of the 'cerebellar cognitive affective syndrome' (CCAS). According to the authors this syndrome manifests with four cardinal symptoms including impairments in: (1) executive functions (planning, set shifting, verbal fluency, abstract reasoning, working memory); (2) spatial cognition (visual memory and visuospatial organization); (3) linguistic processing (dysprosodia and agrammatism); and (4) personality change/disregulation of affect. A relatively small number of lesion studies support the existence of this syndrome. For example, Gottwald *et al.* (2004) found that the cognitive impairments were particularly severe in patients with right cerebellar tumours and appeared to be partially independent from motor dysfunction and that this reflects a planning function of the cerebellum that goes beyond the action domain. Ravizza and colleagues (2006) reported reduced verbal but not spatial forward and backward span in patients with unilateral cerebellar lesions. There are also a small number of studies suggesting that the cerebellum may play a role in social cognition. Interestingly, there is neuropathological and structural MRI evidence implicating the cerebellum in autism (e.g. Bauman and Kemper 1990; Salmond *et al.* 2003; Fatemi *et al.* 2002). In this context two recent studies have reported cognitive and social cognition impairments in patients with three neurological syndromes involving primarily the cerebellum: superficial siderosis and spinocerebellar ataxia types 3 and 6. In all three conditions patients presented with dysprosodia and frontal 'executive' and visual recall memory impairments. In addition, patients presented with a selective deficit in theory of mind tasks (e.g. Van Harskamp *et al.* 2005; Martin *et al.* submitted). These data suggest that the cerebellum may play a role in both cognition and social cognition.

References

Aggleton, J.P. and Brown, M.W. (1999). Episodic memory, amnesia and the hippocampal–anterior thalamic axis. *Behav. Brain Sci.* **22**, 425–44.

Aggleton, J.P., Vann, S.D., Denby, C., Dix, S., Mayes, A.R., Roberts, N. *et al.* (2005). Sparing of the familiarity component of recognition memory in a patient with hippocampal pathology. *Neuropsychologia* **43**, 1810–23.

Alexander, M.P., Stuss, D.T., and Fansabedian, N. (2003). California Verbal Learning Test: performance by patients with focal frontal and non-frontal lesions. *Brain* **126**, 1493–503.

American Psychiatric Association (1980). *Diagnostic and statistical manual of mental disorders*, 3rd edn, DSM-III. American Psychiatric Association, Washington DC.

Baddeley, A. (1996). Exploring the central executive. *Quart. J. Exp. Psychol.* **49A**, 5–28.

Baddley, A.D. and Wilson, B. (1988). Frontal amnesia and the dysexecutive syndrome. *Brain Cogn.* **7**, 212–30.

Baird, A., Dewar, B.K., Critchley, H., Dolan, R., Shallice, T., and Cipolotti, L. (2006). Cognitive functioning after medial frontal lobe damage including the anterior cingulate cortex: a preliminary investigation. *Cogn. Neuropsychiatry* **60** (2), 166–75.

Bastin, C., Van der Linden, M., Charnallet, A., Denby, C., Montaldi, D., Roberts, N., *et al.* (2004). Dissociation between recall and recognition memory performance in an amnesic patient with hippocampal damage following carbon monoxide poisoning. *Neurocase* **10**, 330–44.

Bauman, M.L. and Kemper, T.L. (1990). Limbic and cerebellar abnormalities are also present in an autistic child of normal intelligence. *Neurology* **40**, 307.

Bayley, P.J., Hopkins, R.O., and Squire, L.R. (2003). Successful recollection of remote autobiographical memories by amnesic patients with medial temporal lobe lesions. *Neuron* **38**, 135–44.

Bayley, P.J., Gold, J.J., Hopkins, R.O., and Squire, L.R. (2005). The neuroanatomy of remote memory. *Neuron* **46**, 799–810.

Bechara, A., Damasio, H., and Damasio, A.R. (2003). Role of the amygdala in decision-making. *Ann. NY Acad. Sci.* **985**, 356–69.

Berlyne, N. (1972). Confabulation. *Br. J. Psychiatry* **120**, 31–9.

Bird, C.M., Castelli, F., Malik, O., Frith, U., and Husain, M. (2004). The impact of extensive medial frontal lobe damage on 'theory of mind' and cognition. *Brain* **127**, 914–28.

Blair, R.J. and Cipolotti, L. (2000). Impaired social response reversal. A case of 'acquired sociopathy'. *Brain* **123**, 1122–41.

Botvinick, N.M., Braver, T.S., Barch, D.M., Carter, C.S., and Cohen, J.D. (2001). Conflict monitoring and cognitive control. *Psychol. Rev.* **108**, 624–52.

Brown, M.W. and Aggleton, J.P. (2001). Recognition memory: what are the roles of the perirhinal cortex and hippocampus. *Nature Rev. Neurosci.* **2**, 51–61.

Burgess, P.W., Veitch, E., de Lacy, A., and Shallice, T. (2000). The cognitive and neuroanatomical correlates of multitasking. *Neuropsychologia* **38**, 848–63.

Burgess, P.W., Simons, J.S., Dumontheil, I., and Gilbert, S.J. (2005). The gateway hypothesis of rostral prefrontal cortex (area 10) function. In *Measuring the mind: speed, control and age* (ed. J. Duncan, L. Philips, and P. McLeod), pp. 217–48. Oxford University Press, Oxford.

Byrne, T.N. (2005). Cognitive sequelae of brain tumour treatment. *Curr. Opin. Neurol.* **18**, 662–6.

Calarge, C., Andreasen, N.C., and O'Leary, D.S. (2003). Visualising how one brain understands another: a PET study of theory of mind. *Am. J. Psychiatry* **160**, 1954–64.

Carter, C.S., Braver, T.S., Barch, D.M., Botvinick, N.M., Noll, D., and Cohen, J.D. (1998). Anterior cingulate cortex, error detection and the online monitoring of performance. *Science* **280**, 747–9.

Carter, C.S., MacDonald, A.M., Botvinick, M., Ross, L.L., Stenger, V.A., Noll, D.D., *et al.* (2000). Parsing executive processes: strategic vs. evaluative functions of the anterior cingulate cortex. *Proc. Natl. Acad. Sci. USA* **97**, 1944–8.

Channon, S. and Crawford, A. (2000). The effects of anterior lesions on performance on a story comprehension test. Left anterior impairment on a theory of mind-type task. *Neuropsychologia* **38**, 1006–17.

Cipolotti, L. and Moscovitch, M. (2005). The hippocampus and remote autobiographical memory. *Lancet Neurol.* **4**, 792–3.

Cipolotti, L., Shallice, T., Chan, D., Fox, N., Scahill, R., Harrison, G., Stevens, J., and Rudge, P. (2001). Long-term retrograde amnesia: the crucial role of the hippocampus. *Neuropsychologia* **39**, 151–72.

Cipolotti, L., Bird, C., Good, T., MacManus, D., Rudge, P, and Shallice, T. (2006). Recollection and familiarity in dense hippocampal amnesia: a case study. *Neuropsychologia* **44**, 489–506.

Costello de, L. and Warrington, E.K. (1989). Dynamic aphasia. The selective impairment of verbal planning. *Cortex* **25**, 103–14.

Critchley, H.D., Mathias, C.J., Josephs, O., O'Doherty, J., Zanini, S., Dewar, B.K., *et al.* (2003). Human cingulate cortex and autonomic cardiovascular control: converging neuroimaging and clinical evidence. *Brain* **126**, 2139–52.

Critchley, H.D., Rotshtein, P., Nagai, Y., O'Doherty, J., Mathias, C.J., and Dolan, R.J. (2005). Activity in the human brain predicting differential heart rate responses to emotional facial expressions. *Neuroimage* **24**, 751–62.

Cunningham, J.M., Pliskin, N.H., Cassisi, J.E., Tsang, B., and Rao, S.M. (1997). Relationship between confabulation and measures of memory and executive function. *J. Clin. Exp. Neuropsychol.* **19**, 867–77.

Damasio, A.R. (1994). *Descartes' error. Emotion, reason and the human brain.* Avon Books, New York.

Damasio, A.R., Eslinger, P.J., Damasio, H., Van Hoesen, G.W., and Cornell, S. (1985). Multimodal amnesic syndrome following bilateral temporal and basal forebrain damage. *Arch. Neurol.* **42**, 252–9.

Damasio, A.R., Tranel, D., and Damasio, H. (1990). Individuals with sociopathic behaviour caused by frontal damage fail to respond autonomically to social stimuli. *Behav. Brain Res.* **41**, 81–94.

Damasio, A.R., Tranel, D., and Damasio, H. (1991). *Somatic markers and the guidance of behaviour: theory and preliminary testing.* Oxford University Press, New York.

Dimitrov, M., Phipps, M., Zahn, T.P., and Grafman, J. (1999). A thoroughly modern Gage. *Neurocase* **5**, 345–54.

Duncan, J. and Owen, A.M. (2000). Common regions of the human frontal lobe recruited by diverse cognitive demands. *Trends Neurosci.* **23**, 475–83.

Esmonde, T., Giles, E., Xuereb, J., and Hodges, J. (1996). Progressive supranuclear palsy presenting with dynamic aphasia. *J. Neurol. Neurosurg. Psychiatry* **60**, 403–10.

Fatemi, S.H., Halt, A.R., Realmuto, G., Earle, J., Kist, D.A., Thuras, P., and Merz, A. (2002). Purkinje cell size is reduced in cerebellum of patients with autism. *Cell Mol. Neurobiol.* **22**, 171–5.

Fellows, L.K. and Farah, M.J. (2005). Is anterior cingulate cortex necessary for cognitive control? *Brain* **128**, 788–96.

Fischer, R.S., Alexander, M.P., D'Esposito, M., and Otto, R.R. (1995). Neuropsychological and neuroanatomical correlates of confabulation. *J. Clin. Exp. Neuropsychol.* **17**, 20–8.

Fletcher, P.C. and Henson, R.N.A. (2001). Frontal lobes and human memory. Insights from functional neuroimaging. *Brain* **124**, 849–81.

Fletcher, P.C., Frith, C.D., Baker, S.C., Shallice, T., Frackowiak, R.S.J., and Dolan, R.J. (1995). The mind's eye: precuneus activation in memory-related imagery. *Neuroimage* **2**, 195–200.

Frith, U. and Frith, C.D. (2003). Development and neurophysiology of mentalising. *Phil. Trans. R. Soc. Lond. B Biol. Sci.* **358**, 459–73.

Fujii, T., Okuda, J., Tsukiura, T., Ohtake, H., Miura, R., Fukatsu, R. *et al.* (2002). The role of the basal forebrain in episodic memory retrieval: a positron emission tomography study. *Neuroimage* **15**, 501–8.

Gallagher, H.L., Happé, F., Brunswick, N., Fletcher, P.C., Frith, U., and Frith, C.D. (2000). Reading the mind in cartoons and stories: an fMRI study of 'theory of mind' in verbal and nonverbal tasks. *Neuropsychologia* **38**, 11–21.

Gallagher, H., Jack, A.I., Roepstorff, A., and Frith, C.D. (2002). Imaging the intentional stance in a competitive games. *Neuroimage* **16**, 814–21.

Glickstein, M. (2006). Thinking about the cerebellum. *Brain* **129**, 288–90.

Gold, M., Nadeau, S.E., Jacobs, D.H., Adair, J.C., Rothi, L.J.G., and Heilman, K.M. (1997). Adynamic aphasia: a transcortical motor aphasia with defective semantic strategy information. *Brain Lang.* **57**, 374–93.

Gottwald, B., Wilde, B., Mihajlovic, Z., and Mehdorn, H.M. (2004). Evidence for distinct cognitive deficits after focal cerebellar lesions. *J. Neurol. Neurosurg. Psychiatry* **75**, 1524–31.

Grafman, J., Schwab, K., Warden, D., Pridgen, B.S., Brown, H.R., and Salazar, A.M. (1996). Frontal lobe injuries, violence and aggression: a report of the Vietnam Head Injury Study. *Neurology* **46**, 1231–8.

Guinan, E.M., Lowy, C., Stanhope, N., Lewis, P.D., and Kopelman, M.D. (1998). Cognitive effects of pituitary tumours and their treatments: two case studies and an investigation of 90 patients. *J. Neurol. Neurosurg. Psychiatry* **65**, 870–6.

Heims, H.C., Critchley, H.D., Dolan, R., Mathias, C.J., and Cipolotti, L. (2004). Social and motivational functioning is not critically dependent on feedback of autonomic responses: neuropsychological evidence from patients with pure autonomic failure. *Neuropsychologia* **42**, 1979–88,

Holdstock, J.S., Mayes, A.R., Roberts, N., Cezayirli, E., Isaac, C.L., O'Reilly, R.C., *et al.* (2002). Under what conditions is recognition spread relative to recall after selective hippocampal damage in humans? *Hippocampus* **12**, 341–51.

Jacoby, L.L. and Dallas, M. (1981). On the relationship between autobiographical memory and perceptual learning. *J. Exp. Psychol. Gen.* **110**, 306–40.

Janowsky, J.S., Shimamura, A.P., and Squire, L.R. (1989). Source memory impairment in patients with frontal lobe lesions. *Neuropsychologia* **27**, 1043–56.

Kapur, N. and Coughlan, A.K. (1980). Confabulation and frontal lobe dysfunction. *J. Neurol. Neurosurg. Psychiatry* **43**, 461–3.

Koechlin, E., Ody, C., and Kouneiher, F. (2003). The architecture of cognitive control in the human prefrontal cortex. *Science* **302**, 1181–5.

Kopelman, M.D. (1987). Two types of confabulation. *J. Neurol. Neurosurg. Psychiatry* **50**, 1482–7.

Kupers, R.C., Fortin, A., Astrup, J., Gjedde, A., and Ptito, M. (2004). Recovery of anterograde amnesia in a case of craniopharyngioma. *Arch. Neurol.* **61**, 1948–52.

Luria, A.R. (1966). *Human brain and psychological processes.* Harper and Row Publishers, New York.

Luria, A.R. (1970). *The working brain: an introduction to neuropsychology.* Penguin Books.

Maguire, E.A., Vargha-Khadem, F., and Mishkin, M. (2001). The effects of bilateral hippocampal damage on fMRI regional activations and interactions during memory retrieval. *Brain* **124**, 1156–70.

Maguire, E.A., Frith, C.D., Rudge, P., and Cipolotti, L. (2005). The effect of adult-acquired hippocampal damage on memory retrieval: an fMRI study. *Neuroimage* **27**, 146–52.

Mandler, G. (1980). Recognising: the judgment of previous occurrence. *Psychol. Rev.* **87**, 252–71.

Manns, J.R., Hopkins, R.O., Reed, J.M., Kitchener, E.G., and Squire, L.R. (2003). Recognition memory and the human hippocampus. *Neuron* **37**, 171–80.

Mayes, A.R., Holdstock, J.S., Issac, C.L., Hunkin, N.M., and Roberts, N. (2002). Relative sparing of item recognition memory in a patient with adult-onset damage limited to the hippocampus. *Hippocampus* **12**, 325–40.

McClelland, J.L., McNaughton, B.L., O'Reilly, R.C., and Nadel, L. (1992). Complementary learning systems in the hippocampus and neocortex in learning and memory. Society for Neuroscience Abstracts, 18: 1216,

McClelland, J.L., McNaughton, B.L., and O'Reilly, R.C. (1995). Why there are complementary learning systems in the hippocampus and neocortex: insights from the success and failures of connectionist models of learning and memory. *Psychol. Rev.* **102**, 419–57.

Miller, E.K. and Cohen, J.D. (2001). An integrative theory of prefrontal cortex function. *Ann. Rev. Neurosci.* **24**, 167–202.

Mishkin, M., Suzuki, W.A., Gadian, D.G., and Vargha-Khadem, F. (1997). Hierarchical organisation of cognitive memory. *Phil.Trans. R. Soc. Lond. B Biol. Sci.* **352**, 1461–7.

Murre, J.M.J. (1992). *Categorisation and learning in modular neural networks.* Lawrence Erlbaum, Hillsdale, New Jersey.

Nachev, P. (2006). Cognition and medial frontal cortex in health and disease. *Curr. Opin. Neurol.* **19**, 586-92.

Nadel, L., Samsonovich, A., Ryan, L., and Moscovitch, M. (2000). Multiple trace theory of human memory: computational, neuroimaging and neuropsychological results. *Hippocampus* **10**, 352–68.

Norman, D.A. and Shallice, T. (1986). Attention to action: willed and automatic control of behaviour. In *Consciousness and self-regulation: advances in research and theory* (ed. R.J. Davidson, G.E. Schwartz, and D. Shapiro), Vol. 4, pp. 1–18. Plenum Press, New York.

Peers, P.V., Ludwig, C.J., Rorden, C., Cusack, R., Bonfiglioli, C., Bundesen, C., Driver, J., Antoun, N., and Duncan, J. (2005). Attentional functions of parietal and frontal cortex. *Cereb. Cortex* **15**, 1469–84.

Petrides, M. and Pandya, D.N. (1994). Comparative architectonic analysis of the human and the macaque frontal cortex. In *Handbook of neuropsychology*, Vol. 9 (ed. J. Grafman), pp. 17–58. Elsevier, Amsterdam.

Posner, M.I. and Digirolamo, G.J. (1998). Executive attention: conflict, target detection and cognitive control. In *The attentive brain* (ed. R. Parasuraman), pp. 401–23. MIT Press, Cambridge, Massachusetts.

Posner, M.I. and Petersen, S.E. (1990). The attention system of the human brain. *Ann. Rev. Neurosci.* **13**, 25–42.

Price, B.H., Daffner, K.R., Stowe, R.M., and Mesulam, M.M. (1990). The compartmental learning disabilities of early frontal lobe damage. *Brain* **113**, 1383–98.

Ramnani, N. and Owen, A.M. (2004). Anterior prefrontal cortex. Insights into function from anatomy and neuroimaging. *Nature Rev. Neurosci.* **5**, 184–94.

Ravizza, S.M., McCormick, C.A., Schlerf, J.E., Justus, T., Ivry, R.B., and Fiez, J.A. (2006). Cerebellar damage produces selective deficits in verbal working memory. *Brain* **129**, 306–20.

Raymer, A.M., Rowland, L., Haley, M., and Crosson, B. (2002). Nonsymbolic movement training to improve sentence generation in transcortical motor aphasia: a case study. *Aphasiology* **16**, 493–506.

Reed, J.M. and Squire, L.R. (1997). Impaired recognition memory in patients with lesions limited to the hippocampal formation. *Behav. Neurosci.* **1111**, 667–75.

Reed, J.M. and Squire, L.R. (1998). Retrograde amnesia for facts and events: findings from four new cases. *J. Neurosci.* **18**, 3943–54.

Rees, J. (2003). Advances in magnetic resonance imaging of brain tumours. *Curr. Opin. Neurol.* **16**, 643–50.

Rees, J. (2004). Paraneoplastic syndromes—when to suspect, how to confirm and how to manage. *J. Neurol. Neurosurg. Psychiatry* **75**, 43–50.

Reverberi, C., Lavaroni, A., Gigli, G.L., Skrap, M., and Shallice, T. (2005). Specific impairments of rule induction in different frontal lobe subgroups. *Neuropsychologia* **43**, 460–72.

Ridderinkhof, K.R., Ullsperger, M., Crone, E.A., and Nieuwenhuis, S. (2004). The role of the medial frontal cortex in cognitive control. *Science* **306**, 443–7.

Rizzolatti, G. and Craighero, L. (2004). The mirror-neuron system. *Annu. Rev. Neurosci.* **27**, 169–92.

Rizzolatti, G. and Luppino, G. (2001). The cortical motor system. *Neuron* **31**, 889–901.

Rizzolatti, G., Fogassi, L., and Gallese, V. (2002). Motor and cognitive functions of the ventral premotor cortex. *Curr. Opin. Neurobiol.* **12**, 149–54.

Robertson, I.H., Manly, T., Andrade, J., Baddeley, B.T., and Yiend, J. (1997). 'Oops!': performance correlates of everyday attentional failures in traumatic brain injured and normal subjects. *Neuropsychologia* **35**, 747–58.

Robinson, G., Blair, J., and Cipolotti, L. (1998). Dynamic aphasia: an inability to select between competing verbal responses? *Brain* **121**, 77–89.

Robinson, G., Shallice, T., and Cipolotti, L. (2005). A failure of high level verbal response selection in progressive dynamic aphasia. *Cogn. Neuropsychol.* **22**, 661–94.

Robinson, G., Shallice, T., and Cipolotti, L. (2006). Dynamic aphasia in progressive supranuclear palsy: A deficit in generating a fluent sequence of novel thought. *Neuropsychologia* **44** (8), 1344–60.

Rowe, A., Bullock, P.R., Polkey, C.E., and Morris, R.G. (2001). 'Theory of mind' impairments and their relationship to executive functioning following frontal lobe excisions. *Brain* **124**, 600–16.

Rudge, P. and Warrington, E.K. (1991). Selective impairment of memory and visual perception in splenial tumours. *Brain* **114**, 349–60.

Rushworth, M.F., Walton, M.E., Kennerley, S.W., and Bannerman, D.M. (2004). Action sets and decisions in the medial frontal cortex. *Trends Cogn. Sci.* **8**, 410–17.

Salmond, C.H., de Haan, M., Friston, K.J., Gadian, D.G., and Varga-Khadem, F. (2003). Investigating individual differences in brain abnormalities in autism. *Phil. Trans. R. Soc. Lond. B* **358**, 405–13.

Sanders, H.I. and Warrington, E.K. (1971). Memory for remote events in amnesic patients. *Brain* **94**, 661–8.

Schmahmann, J.D. and Caplan, D. (2006). Cognition, emotion and the cerebellum. *Brain* **129**, 290–2.

Schmahmann, J.D. and Sherman, J.C. (1998). The cerebellar cognitive affective syndrome. *Brain* **121** (4), 561–79.

Schnider, A. (2003). Spontaneous confabulation and the adaptation of thought to ongoing reality. *Nature Rev. Neurosci.* **4**, 662–71.

Schnider, A., Treyer, V., and Buck, A.A. (2000). Selection of currently relevant memories by the human posterior medial orbitofrontal cortex. *J. Neurosci.* **20**, 5880–4.

Semendeferi, K., Lu, A., Schenker, N., and Damasio, H. (2002). Humans and great apes share a large frontal cortex. *Nature Neurosci.* **5**, 272–6.

Shallice, T. and Burgess, P.W. (1991). Deficits in strategy application following frontal lobe damage in man. *Brain* **114**, 727–41.

Shamay-Tsoory, S., Tomet, R., Berger, B.D., and Aharon-Peretz, J. (2003). Characterisation of empathy deficits following prefrontal brain damage: the role of the right ventromedial prefrontal cortex. *J. Cogn. Neurosci.* **15**, 324–37.

Singer, T., Seymour, B., O'Doherty, J., Kaube, H., Dolan, R.J., and Frith, C.D. (2004). Empathy for pain involves the affective but not sensory components of pain. *Science* **303**, 1157–62.

Snowden, J.S., Griffiths, H.L., and Neeary, D. (1996). Progressive language disorder associated with frontal lobe degeneration. *Neurocase* **2**, 429–40.

Squire, R.L. (1992). Memory and the hippocampus: a synthesis from findings with rats, monkeys and humans. *Psychol. Rev.* **99**, 195–231.

Stemmer, B., Segalowitz, S.J., Witzke, W., and Schoenle, P.W. (2003). Error detection in patients with lesions to the medial prefrontal cortex: an ERP study. *Neuropsychologia* **42**, 118–30.

Stuss, D.T, Gow, C.A., and Hetherington, C.R. (1992). 'No longer Gage': frontal lobe dysfunction and emotional changes. *J. Consult. Clin. Psychol.* **60**, 349–59.

Stuss, D.T, Alexander, M.P., Palumbo, C.L., Buckle, L., Sayer, L., and Pogue, J. (1994). Organisational strategies of patients with unilateral or bilateral frontal lobe injury in word list learning tasks. *Neuropsychology* **8**, 355–73.

Stuss, D.T, Gallup, G.G. Jr. and Alexander, M.P. (2001). The frontal lobes are necessary for 'theory of mind'. *Brain* **124**, 279–86.

Swick, D. and Jovanovic, J. (2002). Anterior cingulate cortex and the Stroop task: neuropsychological evidence for topographic specificity. *Neuropsychologia* **40**, 1240–53.

Swick, D. and Turken, U. (2002). Dissociation between conflict detection and error monitoring in the human anterior cingulate cortex. *Proc. Natl. Acad. Sci. USA* **99**, 16354–9.

Taphoorn, M.J. and Klein, M. (2004). Cognitive deficits in adult patients with brain tumours. *Lancet Neurol.* **3**, 159–168.

Tranel, D. (2000). Electrodermal activity in cognitive neuroscience: neuroanatomical and neuropsychological correlates. In *Cognitive neuroscience of emotion* (ed. R.D. Lane and L. Nadel), pp. 192–224. Oxford University Press, New York.

Treves, A. and Rolls, E.T. (1992). Computational constraints suggest the need for two distinct input systems to the hippocampal CA3 network. *Hippocampus* **2**, 189–99.

Treves, A. and Rolls, E.T. (1994). Computational analysis of the role of the hippocampus in memory. *Hippocampus* **4**, 374–91.

Tucha, O., Smely, C., Preier, M., Becker, G., Paul, G.M., and Lange, K.W. (2003). Preoperative and postoperative cognitive functioning in patients with frontal meningiomas. *J. Neurosurg.* **98**, 21–31.

Tulving, E. (1985). Memory and consciousness. *Can. J. Exp. Psychol.* **26**, 1–12.

Van Harskamp, N.J., Rudge, P., and Cipolotti, L. (2005). Cognitive and social impairments in patients with superficial siderosis. *Brain* **128**, 1082–92.

Vargha-Khadem, F., Gadian, D.G., Watkins, K.E., Connelly, A., Van Paesschen, W., and Mishkin, M. (1997). Differential effects of early hippocampal pathology on episodic and semantic memory. *Science* **277**, 376–80.

Vogeley, K., Bussfeld, S.P., Newen, A., Herrmann, S., Happé, F., Falkai, P., Maier, W., Shah, N.J., Fink, G.R., and Zilles, K. (2001). Mind reading: neural mechanisms of theory of mind and self-perspective. *Neuroimage* **14**, 170–81.

Wais, P.E., Wixted, J.T., Hopkins, R.O., and Squire, L.R. (2006). The hippocampus supports both the recollection and the familiarity components of recognition memory. *Neuron* **49**, 459–66.

Warren, J.D., Warren, J.E., Fox, N.C., and Warrington, E.K. (2003). Nothing to say, something to sing: primary progressive dynamic aphasia. *Neurocase* **9**, 140–55.

Wheeler, M.A., Stuss, D.T., and Tulving, E. (1995). Frontal lobe damage produces episodic memory impairment. *J. Int. Neuropsychol. Soc.* **1**, 525–36.

Wilson, B.A., Alderman, N., Burgess, P.W., Emslie, H., and Evans, J.J. (1996). *Behavioural assessment of the dysexecutive syndrome* (*BADS*). Thames Valley Tests, Bury St Edmunds.

Wood, J.N. and Grafman, J. (2003). Human prefrontal cortex: processing and representational perspectives. *Nature Rev. Neurosci.* **4**, 139–47.

Yonelinas, A.P., Kroll, N.E., Quamme, J.R., Lazzara, M.M., Sauve, M.J., Widaman, K.F., *et al.* (2002). Effects of extensive temporal lobe damage or mild hypoxia on recollection and familiarity. *Nature Neurosci.* **5**, 1236–41.

Part 3

Dementias

Chapter 10

Differential diagnosis in dementia

Peter Garrard

10.1 Introduction

- The neurodegenerative dementias incorporate a range of pathological processes, many of which show distinctive clinical signatures.
- Although neurodegenerative processes are irreversible and difficult to modify pharmacologically, careful evaluation is an important part of the clinician's role, a major objective being to exclude alternative, potentially treatable causes of cognitive decline.

The dramatic technical innovations of the last two decades have generated enthusiasm, hypotheses, and a deeper theoretical understanding of the principles of neural science, which in turn has given rise to a revolution in the clinical concept of dementia. It seems incredible that, as recently as the 1970s, the (now doctrinal) view that neurodegenerative dementia might encompass a range of processes whose clinical expression depends on their nature and distribution was restricted to a heretical minority (Schwartz 1990). Likewise, that case reports documenting noteworthy patterns of progressive cognitive deficit referred to diagnostic categories such as 'progressive cerebral atrophy' or 'general dementia', terms that would nowadays be considered inadmissibly vague. Even the status of senile dementia as a clinical entity distinct from Alzheimer's disease continued to be actively debated until relatively recently (Katzman 1976).

The clinical categories that have emerged to classify the common causes of late-onset neurodegenerative dementia capture a range of clinically and pathologically distinct entities, each of which forms the basis of a chapter in the remainder of this section. The cardinal clinical and neuropsychological features of these conditions are summarized in Table 10.1.

A major theme in the understanding of dementia, however, is the extent to which more fine-grained distinctions contribute to the understanding of this overarching classification. Larner (Chapter 11) contrasts early and late onset, familial and sporadic, typical and atypical Alzheimer's disease (AD), while Narvid and Gorno-Tempini (Chapter 12) examine the fundamental distinction between frontal and aphasic variants of frontotemporal lobar degeneration (FTLD) and draw attention to the clinically disparate group of conditions that have begun to be united under the banner of 'tauopathies'. In each case, there is emerging evidence that these clinical categories map on to differences at the pathological or molecular level. Duda and McKeith (Chapter 14) consider the relationship between dementia with Lewy bodies (DLB) and Parkinson's disease with dementia (PDD), conditions that are now recognized to have close pathological links, while Bowler (Chapter 13) discusses the variety of processes that result in cognitive impairment in the context of vascular damage. Many of these clinico-pathological correlations have been shown to have either a genetic basis or a strong genetic contribution, while the identification of gene products and their functions continue to provide insights into their pathophysiological origins.

Table 10.1 Summary of cardinal clinical features of the common neurodegenerative dementias

Executive & attentional dysfunction	Amnesia	Aphasia	Visuospatial disturbance	Behavioural disturbance
Alzheimer's disease				
Often present, but rarely prominent in history in early stages	Common at presentation; manifests as forgetfulness; may remain isolated	Common at presentation; typically fluent & anomic	Often present at presentation; may not be prominent in history	Uncommon
Frontotemporal lobar degeneration				
Common at presentation; usually overshadowed by language/behaviour	Uncommon at presentation; usually overshadowed by language/ behaviour	Seen in 50% of cases at presentation; fluent or non-fluent syndromes; latter may evolve to become consistent with AD or CBD	Uncommon	Seen in 50% of cases at presentation; protean manifestations include disinhibition, obsessionality, aboulia
Vascular cognitive impairment				
Prominent early feature; manifests as general slowing of cognition	Mild: usually due to attentional/ executive factors	Uncommon	Uncommon	Uncommon
Cortical Lewy body disease				
Present & may be prominent in history	Not prominent; may reflect dual pathology if present	Uncommon	Common & prominent in history at presentation	Fluctuating cognitive state and hallucinosis common; personality change rare

The great and growing importance of this field is comprehensively reviewed by Brooks, Loy, Kwok, and Schofield in Chapter 15.

Medical experience suggests that an improved understanding of the mechanisms by which these various pathologies are produced will in future give rise to the identification of therapeutic targets, and hence disease-specific treatments. In future, therefore, recognition of the clinical range of neurodegenerative dementia will become increasingly important. Currently, however, the foremost practical consideration in the differential diagnosis of dementia is the need to identify those few cases in whom progressive cognitive dysfunction is a symptom of some more generalized (and possibly treatable) underlying condition, rather than secondary to a neurodegenerative process. In this chapter, therefore, I will outline a clinical approach to the cognitively impaired patient, aimed at distinguishing between these two broad groups.

10.2 **Clinical approach**

- Patients with cognitive complaints tend to use the word 'memory' to stand for cognitive function in a more general sense, so this word should never be taken at face value, but explored in greater detail.
- Historical evaluation should pursue the area or areas of cognition with which the patient reports difficulty.
- Alzheimer's disease is the commonest neurodegenerative pathology over the age of 65; below this age, frontotemporal lobar degeneration is equally common.
- A history of fluctuating cognitive performance early on suggests an underlying pathology of Lewy body dementia.

The application of a few core principles can turn clinical cognitive evaluation from a frustratingly time-consuming exercise into a diagnostically rewarding and time-efficient process. Perhaps the most important of these is the need to gather clinical data not only from the patient, but also from a close associate (typically partner or spouse). The possibility of conflict or unwelcome feelings of disloyalty may inhibit the latter from disclosing diagnostically important details when in the patient's presence, so it is preferable to interview each party separately. Secondly, the use of the word 'memory' by those unacquainted with the minutiae of cognition should be taken, in the first instance, to be synonymous with practically any aspect of higher mental function and explored accordingly. (The dangers of automatically imposing a specific meaning will be familiar to those who see patients who say that they are 'dizzy'.) Thirdly, rather than attempting to quantify function in all domains of cognition individually (a difficult task even for the most skilled neuropsychologist), bedside cognitive evaluation is best focused on the principal area or areas of complaint. Finally, when considering a differential diagnosis in a patient with cognitive complaints, it is essential to realize that the range and relative likelihood of different aetiologies varies according to: (1) the patient's age; and (2) the pattern and rate of progression of the symptoms (sometimes referred to as the 'tempo of the illness').

The incidence of Alzheimer's disease increases exponentially with age, such that around one in five of over 80s are clinically affected, and an even higher number harbour presymptomatic plaque and tangle pathology (Ohm *et al.* 1995). In common with all biological processes, higher brain function declines with normal ageing, leaving the principal diagnostic dilemma in an elderly patient with cognitive dysfunction one of distinguishing incipient AD from age-related decline (or 'benign senescent forgetfulness'). In such borderline cases, the diagnostic category of mild cognitive impairment (MCI) proves to be a useful compromise: patients with cognitive complaints but defective performance on only a single domain of performance are put into this category, in the knowledge that, after a year, as many as 50% will have deteriorated to a condition consistent with early AD (Golomb *et al.* 2001). While a history of insidious cognitive decline in a patient over 65 is more likely to represent the onset of AD than any other pathological process, below this cut-off, AD and FTLD are approximately equally common (Ratnavalli *et al.* 2002). The onset of vascular dementia (VaD) is also more common in late middle than old age, and particularly likely in those with one or more vascular risk factors.

With the exception of a few atypical cases, the primary neurodegenerative dementias progress gradually and at a fairly constant rate over a period of years. Fluctuations in cognitive performance or behaviour may become a feature in the later stages of AD and FTLD, and probably reflect, in the former, variations in the maintenance of attention and in the latter loss of insight. By contrast, true fluctuations in the earlier stages appear to be a clinical marker for DLB, while an abrupt rather than gradual onset of cognitive difficulties should raise the possibility of either a vascular (including vasculitic), autoimmune, or paraneoplastic process. Survival from diagnosis is, on average, marginally shorter in FTLD than AD, though pathologically proven atypically rapid or indolent cases of both diseases have been described. Rate of progression and age at onset are important factors when considering the possibility of prion disease and other rare causes of dementia, and these conditions will be discussed in detail at the end of this chapter.

10.2.1 **History**

'It's my (his / her) memory, doctor' is usually the first piece of information to be offered in a cognitive neurology consultation. Rather than assuming that the speaker is familiar with the complex array of psychological constructs into which this overarching term is divided (Fig. 10.1; for a review see Baddeley 2004), the clinician's enquiries should focus initially on the type of information (words, names, faces, information, appointments, messages, routes, etc.) that presents the greatest difficulty. Having established whether or not the deficit is selective, the next question concerns the stage of processing at which the problem lies: decreased concentration skills ('attention span') restrict the quality and quantity of encoding of information; defective storage ('forgetfulness') restricts the permanent acquisition of new memories; impaired retrieval ('blockage') suggests difficulties at the organizational level.

Impaired concentration often accompanies—or may be a somatic manifestation of—depression and, in the absence of any other significant findings, depressive pseudodementia must be regarded as a potentially treatable (and therefore leading) diagnosis. The complaint may also,

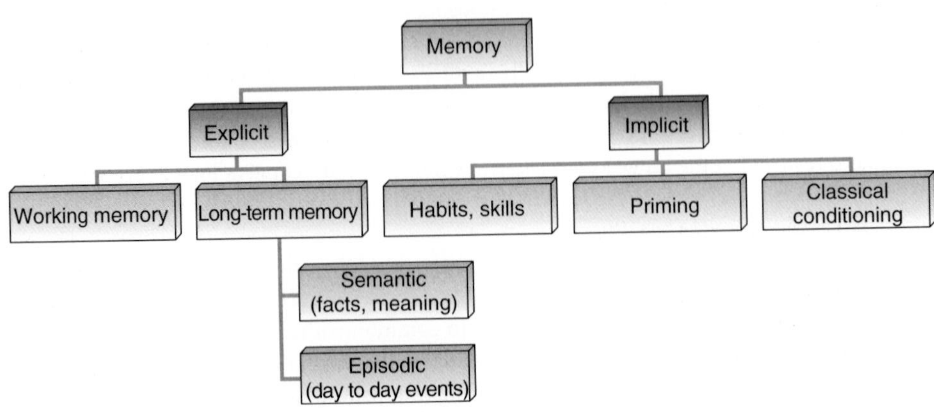

Fig. 10.1 Classification of human memory systems.

however, be accompanied by reports of more general behavioural alteration in the form of loss of interest ('aboulia'), personal neglect, or unusual obsessional traits (such as collecting or purposelessly organizing objects). Such information is rarely obtained directly from the patient, and may be withheld if the informant is not interviewed separately (as noted above), but is nonetheless critical, as it raises the possibility that the patient may be in the early stages of an organic neurodegenerative condition such as frontal variant FTLD.

Problems with memory retrieval may be accompanied by a claim that the difficulty is temporally graded (with memories from the distant past apparently much clearer than those of more recent events). Both phenomena raise the possibility that the problem originates at the level of cognitive organization or 'executive function'—a set of processes that are believed to depend largely on frontal and/or subcortical circuitry. In a patient over 70 this may turn out to be an early indicator of sporadic AD (in which early involvement of frontal regions has recently been demonstrated *in vivo*; Klunk *et al.* 2004), while in middle-aged subjects, particularly those with appropriate risk factors, the pattern of complaint raises the possibility of vascular cognitive impairment (VCI). An isolated disturbance of executive function is the most commonly identified neuropsychological deficit in the context of other chronic CNS illnesses, including multiple sclerosis, Parkinson's disease, acquired brain injury, and inherited neurodegenerative conditions. Exceptionally, progressive executive dysfunction may turn out to be a presenting feature of one of these conditions, though emotional factors, including anxiety and depression, are more often the sole determining factor in younger age-groups.

In contrast, a clear history of a progressive inability to learn new information may be regarded (with only rare exceptions—e.g. see Galton *et al.* 2000) as one of the hallmarks of AD, particularly when buttressed by collateral descriptions of uncharacteristic repetitiveness in conversation, a recent change in reliability, or topographical confusion in novel environments (e.g. while on holiday). This typical clinical pattern sits comfortably with what is known about the progression of pathology in AD, which involves structures such as the hippocampus, parahippocampal gyrus, or other components of the limbic circuitry concerned with episodic memory formation(Nestor *et al.* 2003), before spreading to other temporal and isocortical regions (Braak and Braak 1996).

Memory disturbance often turns out, after further enquiry, to refer to language (or 'memory of words') and, if this is the case, the balance of probabilities favours FTLD rather than AD, particularly if the patient is under 60. A full description of the range of aphasic subtypes in FTLD is provided by Narvid and Gorno-Tempini in Chapter 12, and shows that the relative likelihood of FTLD and AD varies depending on which of these standard clinical patterns best describes the disorder. Non-fluent speech output, characterized by hesitancy and/or phonological and grammatical irregularities, has been described as a presenting feature of sporadic and familial AD (Godbolt *et al.* 2004), Corticobasal degeneration (Graham *et al.* 2003) and Creutzfeldt–Jakob disease (Mandell *et al.* 1989), as well as FTLD, and the additional features associated with these alternative diagnoses should be specifically sought (see below). In contrast, progressive fluent aphasia, particularly when accompanied by clear evidence of single word comprehension difficulties (semantic dementia (SD)), is more often associated with focal atrophy in temporofrontal regions and non-Alzheimer pathology (Garrard and Hodges 2000), usually with histological features characterized by either tau or ubiquitin deposition (Davies *et al.* 2005). Although the latter is the pathological hallmark of amyotrophic lateral sclerosis, clinical evidence of this condition is not typically seen in the context of SD.

Dyspraxia and visuospatial disturbance (difficulty using tools/implements; loss of visual discrimination in the presence of normal acuity; hallucinations) are more uncommon presenting complaints, though the latter represents a well-recognized clinical variant of AD (see Chapter 11). Both deficits should, however, be thoroughly explored in the history, as their presence, even to a subtle degree, in association with early memory or language difficulties, raises the possibility of alternative pathological substrates. Hallucinations typically occur earlier and visuospatial difficulties are more profound with cortical Lewy body disease (CLBD) than with AD (see Chapter 14), while a dyspraxic deficit is one of the cardinal clinical manifestations of CBD (Jacobs *et al.* 1999).

Background medical details can also be diagnostically helpful. Previous psychiatric illness (particularly if treated with electroconvulsive therapy (ECT)), a history of major head trauma, and alcohol or drug abuse all have long-term (though at present rather poorly characterized) cognitive sequelae. A past history of malignancy raises the possibility that the cognitive symptoms may be mediated either by a paraneoplastic autoimmune process or a late complication of chemo- or radiotherapy. Finally, the presence of vascular risk factors may weight the diagnosis in favour of VCI, as well as offering a potential target for treatment, which may modify the clinical course even when there is additional or coexistent degenerative pathology.

10.3 **Clinical examination**

- Multiple cognitive domains can be examined simultaneously by observing the patient performing a few tasks with multiple cognitive demands (e.g. recalling recent news events or phonological fluency).
- General neurological examination can detect early extrapyramidal motor dysfunction, myoclonic jerks, and primitive reflexes.

Adequate bedside or office-based cognitive evaluation can be achieved using a minimum of equipment. The most effective and time-efficient tools are those that rely on more than one cognitive domain, but produce differential patterns of performance depending on the nature of the deficit. Spontaneous speech, for instance, which contains myriad clues to the integrity of the language system (rate of production, phonological and syntactic integrity, vocabulary) can be examined while the patient is prompted to recall recent notable news items.

Similarly, both working and verbal episodic memory can be evaluated by asking a patient to repeat and, after a delay, recall a word list or name and address. Immediate recall is impaired by working memory dysfunction, while problems with delayed recall would implicate learning and storage. An analogous test of non-verbal memory (particularly useful when evaluating a patient with an aphasic disorder) consists of asking the patient to copy and later reproduce from memory three simple geometric designs (e.g. a wire cube, a five-pointed star, and intersecting pentagons), a task that makes concurrent demands on visuospatial and constructional skills. Non-verbal memory may, in any case, be impaired independently of memory for verbal material.

Verbal fluency, using both initial letter and semantic category as a cue, is another clinical technique with compound utility: patients with executive deficits characteristically experience greater difficulty searching for words beginning with a particular letter than they do for words belonging to the same semantic category (essentially an exaggeration of normal performance, presumably due to the fact that neural states corresponding to semantically related items are mutually activating). In sharp contrast (and for similar reasons) patients with SD often produce more words per minute in the letter than category condition. Patients suffering from frontal variant frontotemporal dementia (FTD) may involuntarily perseverate on a single word, and are often unable to inhibit a tendency to produce obscenities or words with sexual connotations. Those with AD often repeat the same word several times during the course of the test due to their defective memories.

Naming errors are a further source of diagnostically important information. A series of relatively low frequency but visually distinct pictures can elicit several kinds of highly informative error patterns: phonological errors (i.e. distortions of the correct phonological form of the word) suggest that the patient has a problem in the verbal output system; circumlocutions ('a beautiful creature that jumps'), semantic errors, and overuse of category, generic, or highly prototypical terms (such as 'animal', 'dog', 'item' or 'thing') imply a breakdown at the level of meaning, or semantic memory; the patient who scrutinizes a line drawing or traces the outline with his finger before producing the name of something conceptually distinct but vaguely visually similar (e.g. 'ball' in response to a picture of an apple) is likely to be suffering from profound visuospatial impairment. These distinct patterns point clearly to dysfunction in left inferior frontal, bilateral anterior temporal, and posterior occipitoparietal regions, respectively.

Single word comprehension (impaired in fluent, preserved in non-fluent aphasia) can be tested using the same material, by asking the subject to pick out an item in response to its spoken name (e.g. 'which one is the helicopter?' or 'which ones are carnivorous?'). Occasionally this technique elicits the strikingly grammatical and insightful response 'What is [a helicopter/carnivorous]? If I knew what [a helicopter/carnivorous] was I might be able to say'. This is practically pathognomonic of SD. It is worth pointing out that word and concept knowledge in SD is highly dependent on how common or familiar the item is—even in the more advanced stages, patients retain the verbal labels 'dog', 'cat', 'horse', and 'animal' (Hodges *et al.* 1995). A set of pictures of relatively unusual items (to enhance the likelihood of informative errors) is therefore as important a piece of neurological equipment as the tendon hammer (for a suggested selection see Mathuranath *et al.* 2000).

General neurological evaluation may reveal abnormal movements or subtle motor, sensory, or coordination deficits, all of which can contribute to diagnostic decision-making. The presence of unilateral pyramidal dysfunction accompanying cognitive decline suggests that imaging should be arranged to exclude a space-occupying lesion sooner rather than at leisure. The clinical importance of primitive reflexes continues to be debated (van Boxtel *et al.* 2006), but the author's experience has been that their presence or absence can usually be predicted on the basis of the degree of cognitive dysfunction alone.

Two of the most common neurodegenerative pathologies (AD and FTLD) are only rarely associated with motor findings in the earliest stages (though myoclonic jerks are a common feature of more advanced AD, and parkinsonism may supervene with progression of FTLD). By contrast, any suggestion of parkinsonism in the context of mild cognitive deficits raises the likelihood of underlying Lewy body pathology, while myoclonic jerks may accompany the early stages of CBD. These phenomena are dealt with more fully in the Chapters 14 and 12, respectively.

10.4 **Investigation**

- Serum should be sent to exclude treatable conditions causing cognitive dysfunction, including:
  - anaemia;
  - hypothyroidism;
  - vitamin B_{12} deficiency;
  - tertiary syphilis.
- A computerized tomography (CT) or magnetic resonance imaging (MRI) brain scan can exclude a space-occupying lesion or hydrocephalus and should be performed in all cases.
- Psychometric evaluation is essential in quantifying the degree of cognitive dysfunction in each domain.

In a small proportion of cases, a definitive diagnosis of AD or FTLD can be made by demonstrating the presence of genetic mutations. Although located at distinct sites across the genome many of these mutations give rise to similar pathological phenotypes, suggesting that the pathological markers in question represent endpoints on which a variety of disrupted biological processes eventually converge. In contrast, the search for abnormalities (in blood or cerebrospinal fluid (CSF) or on structural and functional brain imaging) that correlate reliably with the much larger group of sporadic neurodegenerative pathologies and might therefore be used to support a particular diagnosis during life (often referred to as disease 'biomarkers') has so far proved disappointing (see Chapter 11, Section 11.7 of this volume for a more detailed discussion). An initial set of 'routine' blood tests is, however, essential. The aim of such tests is, first and most importantly, to exclude the presence of reversible systemic conditions manifesting as cognitive disturbance and, secondly, to identify systemic disorders that impact on diagnosis and treatment.

The potentially reversible causes of cognitive dysfunction include anaemia, uraemia, hypothyroidism, vitamin B_{12} or folate deficiency, tertiary syphilis, and giant-cell arteritis. The possibility of toxic damage due to heavy metal (lead, mercury, manganese) or solvent poisoning should be considered in those with a suggestive occupational or social history. Fluctuating patterns of disturbance raise the additional possibilities of porphyria, subclinical seizure activity ('transient epileptic amnesia'), paraneoplastic limbic encephalitis, or autoimmune mediated processes such as Hashimoto's encephalitis (Garrard *et al.* 2000) or the more recently described potassium channel antibody-associated limbic encephalitis (Vincent *et al.* 2004). The more extensive and time-consuming forms of investigation that are required to diagnose these conditions (including electroencephalography (EEG), CSF analysis, and specialist antibody assays) should therefore be reserved for cases in whom fluctuation is clearly a feature. Finally, chronic cerebral hypoxia and hypercapnia caused by obstructive sleep apnoea, a common and and treatable condition and a recognized cause of cognitive dysfunction (Foley *et al.* 1999), deserve consideration and investigation in cases where the obese physical phenotype or history of snoring with prolonged apnoeic episodes suggest it.

In the absence of evidence that cognitive decline is secondary to any of the above processes, structural magnetic resonance neuroimaging is the most informative further source of diagnostic information. In most of the primary neurodegenerative dementias, generalized shrinkage of brain substance is the most salient abnormality, though there is evidence to suggest that the distribution of such atrophic change may be different in established cases of AD and FTLD (Galton *et al.* 2001). In the absence of diagnostic clinical information, however, it is rarely possible to make a diagnosis on imaging grounds: subtle degrees of atrophy, particularly in temporal regions, may be difficult to detect using even high resolution MR images, let alone standard clinical acquisition protocols. Moreover, the degree of atrophy present in the brains of unaffected individuals overlaps with the appearances in early dementia.

Longitudinal comparison of structural scans from a single individual using high resolution images acquired 6 to 12 months apart is one possible solution to these dilemmas—on the assumption that continuous volume loss should at some point give rise to an observable difference. Such measurements have been automated and carefully quantified in some centres, and correlations demonstrated between regional change and clinical diagnosis (Whitwell *et al.* 2005). The obvious disadvantage of relying on such an approach is that diagnosis, and therefore treatment, is necessarily delayed. On the other hand, such a robust method for quantifying change following diagnosis will undoubtedly provide an invaluable tool for monitoring and comparing treatment modalities during clinical trials. For diagnostic purposes, metabolic imaging modalities such as single photon emission computed tomography (SPECT) or positron emission tomography (PET) using radiolabelled ligands with affinity to pathological substrates (e.g. Pittsburgh compound B, (PIB) which binds selectively to beta-amyloid) probably offer the best prospect for reliably differentiating degenerative pathologies during life (Klunk *et al.* 2004). There may also be a diagnostic role for magnetic resonance spectroscopy (Garrard *et al.* 2006).

Formal neuropsychometric evaluation is an essential adjunct to diagnosis in dementia. A trained neuropsychologist can detect and quantify performance deficits across the entire spectrum of cognitive function, using batteries of robustly replicable tests, many of them associated with age-specific ranges for normal performance. A neuropsychologist may identify patterns of higher functional impairment that provide localizing, and therefore diagnostically valuable, information. Dysfunction in domains that depend on posterior cortex, especially when accompanied by impoverished memory, suggests AD, whereas an anterior and asymmetric pattern is more typical of FTLD. Moreover, some patterns of deficit (e.g. a failure to demonstrate implicit learning in patients with apparent episodic memory dysfunction) may be suggestive of depressive or factitious aetiologies (Lezak 1995). Re-evaluation after an interval, to look for deterioration (or more rarely improvement), can be helpful in diagnostically difficult cases.

Brain biopsy should be considered an investigation of last resort. The possibility of discovering a potentially modifiable or reversible condition, such as isolated CNS vasculitis or chronic infection, typically considered in younger patients with an unusual or rapidly progressive pattern of cognitive dysfunction that has evaded diagnosis by less invasive methods (see below), is really the only justification for undertaking this procedure. Even among cases selected according to such stringent criteria, the incidence of modifiable pathology is rare (10% in a recent survey of 90 procedures over a 14 year period in a tertiary level service; Warren *et al.* 2005). The commonest diagnoses in this and the majority of similar series have been those of AD or non-specific cerebral gliosis.

10.5 **Factors influencing diagnosis**

> Dementia in the young (< 40 years) and a picture of rapidly progressive cognitive decline represent special situations in which different collections of possible diagnoses need to be considered.

I observed at the beginning of this chapter that the relative likelihood of the common degenerative and other underlying aetiologies in the demented patient is influenced by the patient's age and the rate of onset of the problem. Although the subsequent discussion included a number of illustrative examples, I will conclude by discussing more thoroughly the specific importance of these factors in two unusual but important clinical situations.

10.5.1 **Dementia in the young** (see Table 10.2)

The overwhelming majority of incident cases of dementia occurs in the over-60 age group, in whom the primary sporadic neurodegenerative pathologies are by far the commonest underlying causes. Although these processes may on occasion show onset before the age of 40, such diseases are more likely to be genetically determined in younger patients. As a general rule, therefore, the genetic mutations known to be responsible for AD should be looked for in all those from whom a family history of early onset dementia is obtained, as well as cases with the onset of AD-like features before the age of 60. Additional clinical observation may suggest alternative genetic diagnoses. Linguistic or behavioural features raise the possibility of mutations in the tau or progranulin genes. The presence of a movement disorder in association with cognitive decline in a young

Table 10.2 Possible causes of dementia in a patient under 40 years old

Condition	Suggestive clinical features	Diagnostic test(s)*
Infective causes		
Whipple's disease	Hypersomnia; hyperphagia; ophthalmoplegia; nystagmus; oculomasticatory myorhythmia; ataxia	Small bowel biopsy
Neurosyphilis	Delusions of grandeur; disinhibition; tremor; hyperreflexia; pupillary abnormalities	Serum and CSF VDRL
Subacute sclerosing panencephalitis	Myoclonus; absence seizures; tics; tremor; dyspraxia; choreoathetosis	Serum and CSF measles virus antibodies
Progressive multifocal leucoencephalopathy	Immunosuppressed state	JC virus
HIV dementia/AIDS dementia complex	Psychiatric symptoms; spasticity; extensor plantar responses	HIV-1 serology; exclusion of associated cerebral infection (toxoplasmosis; cryptococcosis;CMV; PML), or lymphoma
Variant Creutzfeldt–Jakob disease	Psychiatric symptoms; myoclonus; ataxia	Histology
Genetic causes		
Huntington's disease	Chorea; extrapyramidal motor deficits; psychiatric features	Genetic
Neuroacanthocytosis	Involuntary orofacial & limb movements; tics; psychiatric features	Excess acanthocytes on a peripheral blood film
Cerebrotendinous xanthomatosis	Ataxia; peripheral neuropathy; cataracts; tendon xanthomas	Serum cholestanol
Adult GM2 gangliosidosis	Amyotrophy; cerebellar ataxia	Hexosaminidase A activity
Hallervorden–Spatz disease	Extrapyramidal motor deficit; dystonia; involuntary movements; myoclonus	MRI; electron microscopy of circulating lymphocytes; genetic
Kuf's disease	Myoclonus; dysarthria; cerebellar ataxia	Skin biopsy
Wilson's disease	Dystonia; chorea; Kayser–Fleischer rings	Serum copper and caeruloplasmin
Niemann–Pick disease type C	Organomegaly; supranuclear ophthalmoplegia; dystonia	Skin biopsy; bone marrow aspiration
Metachromatic leucodystrophy	Spasticity; involuntary movements; peripheral neuropathy	Arylsulphatase A activity
Mitochondrial disease	Ataxia; pigmentary retinopathy; deafness; myopathy	Serum lactate; muscle biopsy
Adrenoleucodystrophy	Peripheral neuropathy; spastic paraparesis; adrenal insufficiency	Very long chain fatty acids

Inflammatory causes		
Neuro-Behçet's	Orogenital ulceration; ocular inflammation; skin lesions; arthralgia; meningoencephalitis; dural sinus thrombosis	Clinical only
Neurosarcoidosis	Cranial neuropathies; ocular inflammation; hypopituitarism; neuropathy/mononeuritis multiplex	Biopsy of nerve, muscle, skin; gallium scan
Multiple sclerosis	Optic atrophy; cerebellar dysarthria & ataxia; disinhibition	MRI; delayed evoked responses; CSF oligoclonal bands
Cerebral vasculitis, including: Primary CNS angiitis Giant cell arteritis Sjögren's syndrome Polyarteritis nodosa/SLE	Headache; focal neurological deficits; multisystem involvement; CSF pleocytosis	Autoimmune serology; temporal artery biopsy; cerebral angiography; cerebral biopsy
Malignant cause		
Cerebral lymphoma	Progressive white-matter disease; CSF cytology	Cerebral biopsy

* VDRL, Viral and Rickettsial Disease Laboratory (test); CMV, cytomegalovirus; PML, progressive multifocal leucoencephalopathy.

patient should prompt exclusion of the gene mutations responsible for Huntington's disease (HD) and, if onset is rapid, for prion disease. A more detailed discussion of the diagnostic properties of genetic tests in dementia is found in Chapter 15.

In a younger age group the possibility of variant Creutzfeldt–Jakob disease (see below) and of rarer causes, such as subacute sclerosing panencephalitis (a rare post-infectious sequela of measles virus infection), Whipple's disease, systemic or CNS vasculitis, and other inflammatory encephalopathies, should also be raised. Although typically considered to be disorders of childhood, the mitochondrial encephalomyopathies and inherited metabolic and leucodystrophic disorders (e.g. Wilson's disease, metachromatic leucodystrophy and adrenoleucodystrophy, and Niemann–Pick disease type C) may all show delayed onset, and should be considered in the differential diagnosis of dementia and neuropsychiatric disorders in the early decades of adulthood. All of these conditions can be definitively diagnosed on histological and/or biochemical grounds and most are associated with additional clinical markers, such as peripheral nerve involvement in leucodystrophy, ocular changes in Wilson's disease, organomegaly in the storage disorders, and supranuclear gaze paresis in Niemann–Pick disease, all of which should be specifically sought during clinical evaluation of patients in this age group.

10.5.2 **Rapidly progressive dementia**

Progression in AD and FTLD is, as a rule, imperceptibly slow, with average life expectancies from diagnosis of the order of 6 and 4 years, respectively (Rascovsky *et al.* 2005). A picture of rapid cognitive decline, in which the patient progresses from the earliest stages to a state of established dementia over weeks rather than months, and when brain imaging has excluded the presence of a space-occupying or diffuse infiltrative lesion, shifts the diagnostic spotlight to a different set of disorders.

The group of conditions known as transmissible spongiform encephalopathies (TSEs) were, until recently, regarded as unusual causes of human morbidity. Sporadic Creutzfeldt–Jakob disease (sCJD) remains a rare cause of late onset dementia, with an incidence of around 1 per million. An accelerated onset of cognitive problems, in association with ataxia, myoclonus, and periodic bi- or triphasic sharp wave complexes on EEG, is highly suggestive of this rapidly progressive and invariably fatal condition.

The mechanism of pathogenesis in TSEs appears to be driven by conformational change in the structure of a normal cell membrane glycoprotein component (prion protein, or PrP) from a soluble state (PrP_c) into an insoluble form (PrP_{sc}). In the latter conformation the protein becomes highly pathogenic, forming stable aggregates that not only cause neuronal dysfunction and death, but also promote similar changes in remaining PrP_c, setting up an inrreversible feed-forward pathological cascade. The trigger for the formation of a critical mass of PrP_{sc} can, in a small proportion of cases, be traced to a mutation in the gene (on chromosome 20) that codes for the prion protein (*PRNP*) and, in others, to the introduction of foreign PrP_{sc} aggregates (e.g. via corneal grafts, contaminated neurosurgical instruments, or treatment with human growth hormone in childhood). The cause of sCJD, however, remains unknown.

Rapid onset of cognitive decline in a younger patient raises the possibility of a more recently described form of prion disease—variant CJD (vCJD). The recognition of vCJD as a separate pathological entity was first documented in 1996, following a number of reports of CJD cases occurring well before the typical age of onset (Will *et al.* 1996). This early onset, with cognitive decline often preceded by depressive or other psychiatric features and a subjective disturbance of sensation, absence of the EEG changes typical of sporadic CJD, slightly longer average survival, and novel neuropathological appearances (Ironside *et al.* 2002), points to a distinct process of prion protein aggregation.

As well as the clinical and neurophysiological features, the differentiation of sCJD from vCJD may be helped by MR appearances (hyperintensity in the anterior basal ganglia in sCJD, and in the posterior nuclei of the thalamus ('pulvinar sign') in vCJD; Schrorter *et al.* 2000) or by tonsil biopsy, which exploits the tendency of vCJD pathology to affect lymphoreticular as well as neural tissue (Hill *et al.* 1997).

Many of the clinical features of the prion diseases (rapid onset, associated myoclonus and ataxia, and EEG changes) can be mimicked by other processes, some of which are potentially treatable. A rapidly progressive cognitive and behavioural syndrome with myoclonus and other motor features is seen in SSPE. Subacute encephalitis may be mediated by infection with herpes simplex virus (HSV), human immunodeficiency virus (HIV), fungi, or *Borrelia*, or by toxic, granulomatous, autoimmune, paraneoplastic, malignant, or inflammatory mechanisms. In such cases, blood and/or CSF should be examined for diagnostic markers of infection, and for autoantibodies, particularly those directed against thyroid (Hashimoto's encephalitis), neural tissue, and voltage-gated potassium channels. Heavy metal assays should be considered in cases with historical clues to a toxic aetiology. Cerebral lymphoma may present with dementia of rapid onset, and in its intravascular form may be associated with normal MR imaging. An aggressive inflammatory encephalopathy may be caused by a vasculitic process, which may either be associated with systemic markers or confined to the CNS. In the latter case, diagnosis often necessitates the more invasive procedures of angiography or, if all else fails, cerebral biopsy.

References

Baddeley, A.D. (2004). The psychology of memory. In *The essential handbook of memory disorders* (ed. A.D. Baddeley, M.D. Kopelman, and B.A.Wilson), pp. 3–15. John Wiley and Sons, Ltd, New York.

Braak, H. and Braak, E. (1996). Evolution of the neuropathology of Alzheimer's disease. *Acta Neurol. Scand. Suppl.* **165**, 3–12.

Davies, R.R., Hodges, J.R., Kril, J.J., Patterson, K., Halliday, G.M., and Xuereb, J.H. (2005). The pathological basis of semantic dementia. *Brain* **128**, 1984–95.

Foley, D.J., Monjan, A.A., Masaki, K.H., Enright, P.L., Quan, S.F., and White, L.R. (1999). Associations of symptoms of sleep apnea with cardiovascular disease, cognitive impairment, and mortality among older Japanese-American men. *J. Am. Geriatr. Soc.* **47**, 524–8.

Galton, C.J., Patterson, K., Xuereb, J.H., and Hodges, J.R. (2000). Atypical and typical presentations of Alzheimer's disease: a clinical, neuropsychological, neuroimaging and pathological study of 13 cases. *Brain* **123** (3), 484–98.

Galton, C.J., Patterson, K., Graham, K., Lambon-Ralph, M.A., Williams, G., Antoun, N., Sahakian, B.J., and Hodges, J.R. (2001). Differing patterns of temporal atrophy in Alzheimer's disease and semantic dementia. *Neurology* **57**, 216–25.

Garrard, P. and Hodges, J.R. (2000). Semantic dementia: clinical, radiological and pathological perspectives. *J. Neurol.* **247**, 409–22.

Garrard, P., Hodges, J.R., De Vries, P.J., Hunt, N., Crawford, A., Hodges, J.R., and Balan, K. (2000). Hashimoto's encephalopathy presenting as 'myxodematous madness'. *J. Neurol. Neurosurg. Psychiatry* **68**, 102–3.

Garrard, P., Schott, J.M., McManus, D., Hodges, J.R., Fox, N.C., and Waldman, A. (2006). Posterior cingulate neurometabolite profiles and clinical phenotype in frontotemporal dementia. *Cogn. Behav. Neurol.* **19** (4), 185–9.

Godbolt, A.K., Beck, J.A., Collinge, J., Garrard, P., Warren, J.D., Fox, N.C., and Rossor, M.N. (2004). A presenilin 1 R278I mutation presenting with language impairment. *Neurology* **63**, 1702–4.

Golomb, J., Kluger, A., Garrard, P., and Ferris, S.H. (2001). *Physician's manual on mild cognitive impairment.* Science Press Ltd, London.

Graham, N.L., Bak, T., Patterson, K., and Hodges, J.R. (2003). Language function and dysfunction in corticobasal degeneration. *Neurology* **61**, 493–9.

Hill, A.F., Butterworth, R.J., Joiner, S., Jackson, G., Rossor, M.N., Thomas, D.J., Frosh, A., Tolley, N., Bell, J.E., Spencer, M., King, A., Al-Sarraj, S., Ironside, J.W., Lantos, P.L., and Collinge, J. (1997). Investigation of variant Creutzfeldt–Jakob disease and other human prion diseases with tonsil biopsy samples. *Lancet* **353**, 183–9.

Hodges, J.R., Graham, N., and Patterson, K. (1995). Charting the progression in semantic dementia: implications for the organisation of semantic memory. *Memory* **3**, 463–95.

Ironside, J.W., Head, M.W., McCardle, L., and Knight, R. (2002). Neuropathology of variant Creutzfeldt-Jakob disease. *Acta Neurobiol. Exp.* **62**, 175–82.

Jacobs, D.H., Adair, J.C., Macauley, B., Gold, M., Gonzalez Rothi, L.J., and Heilman, K.M. (1999). Apraxia in corticobasal degeneration. *Brain Cogn.* **40**, 336–54.

Katzman, R. (1976). The prevalence and malignancy of Alzheime'rs disease. *Arch. Neurol.* **33**, 217–18.

Klunk, W. E.E., H., Nordberg, A., Wang, Y., Blomqvist, G., Hot, D.P., Bergstrom, M., Savitcheva, I., Huang, G-F., Estrada, S., Ausen, B., Debnath, M.L., Barletta, J., Price, J.C., Sandell, J., Lopresti, B.J., Wall, A., Koivisto, P., Antoni, G., Mathis, C.A., and Langstrom, B. (2004). Imaging brain amyloid in Alzheimer's disease with Pittsburgh Compound-B. *Ann. Neurol.* **55**, 306–19.

Lezak, M.D. (1995). *Neuropsychological assessment.* Oxford University Press, New York.

Mandell, A.M., Alexander, M.P., and Carpenter, S. (1989). Creutzfeldt–Jakob disease presenting as isolated aphasia. *Neurology* **39**, 55–8.

Mathuranath, P.S., Nestor, P.J., Berrios, G.E., Rakowicz, W., and Hodges, J.R. (2000). A brief cognitive test battery to differentiate Alzheimer's disease and frontotemporal dementia. *Neurology* **55**, 1613–20.

Nestor, P.J., Fryer, T.D., Smielewski, P., and Hodges, J.R. (2003). Limbic hypometabolism in Alzheimer's disease and mild cognitive impairment. *Ann. Neurol.* **54**, 343–51.

Ohm, T.G., Müller, H., Braak, H., and Bohl, J. (1995). Close-meshed prevalence rates of different stages as a tool to uncover the rate of Alzheimer's disease-related neurofibrillary changes. *Neuroscience* **64**, 209–17.

Rascovsky, K., Salmon, D.P., Lipton, A.M., Leverenz, J.B., DeCarli, C., Jagust, W.J., Clark, C.M., Mendez, M.F., Tang-Wai, D.F., Graff-Radford, N.R., and Galasko, D. (2005). Rate of progression differs in frontotemporal dementia and Alzheimer disease. *Neurology* **65**, 397–403.

Ratnavalli, E., Brayne, C., Dawson, K., and Hodges, J.R. (2002). The prevalence of frontotemporal dementia. *Neurology* **58**, 1615–21.

Schrorter, A., Zerr, I., Henkel, K., Tschampa, H.J., Finkenstaedt, M., and Poser, S. (2000). Magnetic resonance imaging in the clinical diagnosis of Creutzfeldt–Jakob disease. *Arch. Neurol.* **57**, 1751–1757.

Schwartz, M.F. (1990). *Modular deficits in Alzheimer-type dementia.* MIT Press, Cambridge, Massachusetts.

Van Boxtel, M.P., Bosma, H., Jolles, J., and Vreeling, F.W. (2006). Prevalence of primitive reflexes and the relationship with cognitive change in healthy adults: a report from the Maastricht Aging Study. *J. Neurol.* **253**, 935–41.

Vincent, A., Buckley, C., Schott, J.M., Baker, I., Dewar, B.K., Detert, N., Clover, L., Parkinson, A., Bien, C.G., Omer, S., Lang, B., Rossor, M.N., and Palace, J. (2004). Potassium channel antibody-associated encephalopathy: a potentially immunotherapy-responsive form of limbic encephalitis. *Brain* **127**, 701–12.

Warren, J.D., Schott, J.M., Fox, N.C., Thom, M., Revesz, T., Holton, J.L., Scaravilli, F., Thomas, D.G.T., Plant, G.T., Rudge, P., and Rossor, M.N. (2005). Brain biopsy in dementia. *Brain* **128**, 2016–25.

Whitwell, J.L., Josephs, K.A., Rossor, M.N., Stevens, J.M., Revesz, T., Holton, J.L., Al-Sarraj, S., Godbolt, A.K., Fox, N.C., and Warren, J.D. (2005). Magnetic resonance imaging signatures of tissue pathology in frontotemporal dementia. *Arch. Neurol.* **62**, 1402–8.

Will, R.G., Ironside, J.W., Zeidler, M., Cousens, S.N., Estibeiro, K., Alperovitch, A., Poser, S., Pocchiari, M., Hofman, A., and Smith, P.G. (1996). new variant of Creutzfeldt–Jakob disease in the UK. *Lancet* **347**, 921–5.

Chapter 11

Alzheimer's disease

Andrew J. Larner

11.1 Definition

- Current diagnostic criteria are associated with high sensitivity and specificity.
- Alzheimer's disease (AD) may be considered as a possible, probable, or definite diagnosis.
- Patients with mild cognitive impairment (MCI) complain of memory impairment without meeting clinical criteria for AD and may represent a 'prediagnostic' state.

The development of clinical diagnostic criteria for AD under the auspices of the National Institute of Neurological and Communicative Disorders and Stroke–Alzheimer's Disease and Related Disorders Association (NINCDS-ADRDA; McKhann *et al.* 1984) has rightly been hailed as a major landmark in dementia research. These criteria have become widely accepted because of their validity, reliability, and utility to research. Although the sensitivity and specificity of the criteria for a diagnosis of AD are good (e.g. 87% and 83%, respectively; McKeith *et al.* 2000), likelihood ratios (the comparison of post-test odds to pre-test odds, and hence a measure of 'diagnostic gain') are only modest (Chui and Lee 2002). Guidelines to assist clinicians in making the diagnosis of AD have been issued by both European and North American neurological societies (Waldemar *et al.* 2000; Knopman *et al.* 2001). The criteria are relatively easy to use, being clinically based, and do not require expensive investigations.

The diagnosis of AD may be *possible*, *probable*, or *definite*. In clinical practice, most diagnoses are of *probable* AD: dementia is established on the basis of clinical examination and neuropsychological testing, and there is evidence of progressive worsening of memory and other cognitive functions without disturbance of consciousness. Supportive features include impaired activities of daily living (ADL), behavioural changes, and a positive family history of similar disease, particularly if confirmed by neuropathology. Supportive investigations include a normal cerebrospinal fluid (CSF), normal or non-specific electroencephalographic (EEG) changes, and cerebral atrophy on computerized tomography (CT) with progression documented by serial observation. Other features deemed consistent with probable AD include plateaus in the course of the illness, various associated behavioural features, and certain neurological signs including myoclonus and seizures. Features that make the diagnosis uncertain or unlikely include sudden onset, focal neurological findings, or seizures early in the course, though none of these excludes the diagnosis.

A diagnosis of *possible* AD may be made when the onset, presentation, or clinical course is atypical, or when a second pathology—sufficient to cause dementia but which is not considered to be the cause of dementia—is present. A diagnosis of *definite* AD may be made when the clinical criteria for probable AD are met and when histological criteria are seen on a biopsy or autopsy specimen. Agreement between *ante-mortem* clinical and *post-mortem* neuropathological diagnosis is usually 80% or better, though lower when considering mild or early stage disease.

Cases with age at onset ≤ 65 years may be labelled as early-onset AD (EOAD), and those with age of onset > 65 years as late-onset AD (LOAD) (McKhann *et al.* 1984). Whilst this is probably an arbitrary distinction, the differentiation of sporadic (i.e. no family history of the condition) from familial AD (one or more similarly affected first-degree relatives) is of crucial biological significance (see Section 11.3.1). Moreover, the reliability of such labels depends on the available information. Family pedigrees in a late-onset disease such as AD may be censored by early death from other causes.

A Lewy body variant of Alzheimer's disease (LBVAD) has been proposed (Hansen *et al.* 1990) based on the finding of neuropathological changes sufficient to meet criteria for AD together with Lewy body pathology (Mirra *et al.* 1991). Whether this represents a variant of AD or a separate disorder is debated, but most authorities would probably now label this as the 'common form' of dementia with Lewy bodies (DLB).

Individuals who have mild memory difficulties but are not functionally impaired have been recognized clinically for many years. Since their deficits are insufficient to fulfil the clinical diagnostic criteria for AD, various other terms have been used to describe them, with recent consensus developing around the idea of mild cognitive impairment (MCI; Petersen 2003, 2004), though this may simply represent 'prodromal AD'. The identification of such patients is important since 10–15% of them progress to AD per year and most, though not all, will ultimately convert. Therapeutic intervention at the MCI stage may therefore prevent or retard the onset of AD.

11.2 **Epidemiology**

Numerous studies of the epidemiology of AD have been undertaken, with the dual aims of social planning and identifying potentially modifiable risk factors for the development of the disease (Jorm 1990). The most important risk factor for AD is increasing age, with incidence rising exponentially at least up to the age of 90 years (Jorm and Jolley 1998), by which time as many as one in four individuals may be affected. The hypothetical issue of whether everyone would develop AD if they lived long enough remains unresolved. There is a higher prevalence of AD among women than men, due either to a higher incidence or to longer survival after development of the disease (Launer *et al.* 1999). Studying disease prevalence and incidence across national and racial boundaries poses difficult methodological issues, but there is some evidence that AD has a higher incidence in developed compared to developing nations (Hendrie *et al.* 2001). Epidemiological studies have also identified other possible risk factors and also protective factors for AD (see below).

11.3 **Aetiological factors**

- AD is usually sporadic, though in around 5% of cases (mostly in younger age-groups) the disease is inherited in an autosomal dominant fashion.
- Mutations in genes coding for amyloid precursor protein (APP) and presenilin (PS1 and PS2) produce a clinical picture of Alzheimer's disease in all carriers.
- Mechanisms leading to the commoner (sporadic) form of AD are incompletely understood.

11.3.1 **Genetic**

Alzheimer's disease with a familial component was recognized as early as the 1920s, but Lowenberg and Waggoner (1934) were the first to report in detail an autosomal dominant pedigree with neuropathological confirmation. Elucidation of the kindred of Alzheimer's second patient, Johann F., suggests an autosomal dominant disorder with variable penetrance and age of onset between the 30s and mid 60s (Klünemann *et al.* 2002), though the index case showed only plaques and was negative for APP gene mutations (Graeber *et al.* 1997). To date, three genes have been described in which mutations may be deterministic for AD, usually of early-onset. These mutations, namely, amyloid precursor protein (APP) presenilin-1 (PS1) and presenilin-2 (PS2), are discussed in more detail in Chapter 15.

The only genetically determined risk factor to have been demonstrated relates to allelic variation in the apolipoprotein E (ApoE) gene (Roses 1996; Saunders 2001). Other genetic loci of possible interest have been identified, particularly those on chromosomes 12 and 10, the former possibly associated with genes encoding α_2-macroglobulin and low-density lipoprotein receptor (Bertram and Tanzi 2005). Rarely, kindreds with tau gene mutations, which typically present with fronto-temporal dementia (FTD), may have an AD-like presentation (Doran *et al.* in preparation).

11.3.1.1 Amyloid precursor protein (APP)

The first APP mutation, V717I, was identified in 1991 (Goate *et al.* 1991). Around 20 further genomic mutations have since been reported, an up-to-date record of which is held on the Alzheimer Disease and Frontotemporal Dementia Mutation Database (*www.molgen.ua.ac.be/Admutations*). Mutations are located in proximity to the α-, β-, and γ-secretase cleavage sites of APP, and many have been shown to increase production of amyloid β-peptides (Aβ or βA4) in stably transfected cell lines (Scheuner *et al.* 1996), particularly of the longer variant (Aβ42), which has a particular propensity to aggregate and is more toxic to neurons (Jarrett *et al.* 1993). Mutations in the APP gene have also been found in hereditary cerebral haemorrhage with amyloidosis Dutch type (HCHWA-D), a rare familial form of cerebral amyloid angiopathy whose chief clinical features are recurrent cerebral haemorrhages and early death, with dementia occurring in only a minority of patients.

11.3.1.2 Presenilin 1 and presenilin 2 (PS1, PS2)

A missense mutation in a gene on chromosome 14 that was deterministic for autosomal dominant EOAD was reported in 1995 (Sherrington *et al.* 1995). A homologous gene was identifed on chromosome 1, and found to bear mutations in the Volga–German AD kindred (Levy-Lahad *et al.* 1995; Rogaev *et al.* 1995). The two genes were named presenilin-1 and presenilin-2.

PS1 mutations are the commonest identified genetic cause of AD, with well over 100 different genomic mutations reported to date (Larner and Doran 2006; *www.molgen.ua.ac.be/Admutations*). In a study of 31 families fulfilling strict criteria for autosomal dominant EOAD, the PS1 mutation frequency for probable and definite AD was 77% and 82%, respectively (Janssen *et al.* 2003). PS2 mutations are less common, with only 10 mutations and 18 families reported at the time of writing.

As with APP, most PS mutations are associated with increased production of Aβ42 both *in vitro* and *in vivo* (Scheuner *et al.* 1996; Mehta *et al.* 1998). Although these findings bear out the predictions of the amyloid hypothesis, the mechanism(s) by which Aβ causes AD remains a subject of debate. Certainly Aβ is toxic to neurons in high concentration, possibly through enhanced levels of oxidative stress and deregulation of intracellular calcium ion concentrations (Iversen *et al.* 1995), but Aβ is also found in tissue fluids of normal individuals, suggesting a physiological role, perhaps as an inhibitor of neurite growth (Larner 1995*a*, 1997*a*), which becomes dystrophic with abnormal Aβ levels, leading to synaptic alterations, neuronal degeneration, and clinical dementia (Larner 1997*b*).

11.3.1.3 Apolipoprotein E (ApoE)

Apolipoprotein E, a lipid transport molecule, has been identified as a genetically determined risk factor for the development of AD (Roses 1996; Saunders 2001). The protein has three isoforms, E2, E3, and E4, encoded by alleles ε2, ε3, and ε4. In patients with late-onset AD the ε4 allele is found with much greater frequency than in controls (e.g. 52% versus 16%; Saunders 2001). Hence, possession of an ε4 allele, though neither necessary nor sufficient for the development of AD, increases the risk. This increase is of the order of twofold in heterozygotes, and between six- and eightfold in homozygotes (Corder *et al.* 1993). ApoE genotype also appears to modulate the age of onset in patients with EOAD related to APP mutations (Saunders *et al.* 1993), but not PS (van Broeckhoven *et al.* 1994, though see Larner and Doran 2006 for some possible exceptions).

The mechanism by which the ApoE ε4 genotype increases risk is uncertain. A number of possibilities exist, of which increase in amyloid deposition may be the most important (Polvikoski *et al.* 1995), though ApoE also has roles in synaptogenesis and neurite growth (Poirier 1994; Roses 1996; Saunders 2001).

11.3.2 Acquired

Epidemiological studies have suggested a number of possible risk factors for the development of AD. In terms of the potential for modification, perhaps the most important of these are hypertension and hypercholesterolaemia in mid-life (Kivipelto *et al.* 2001). Vascular risk factors, once thought of greater importance in vascular dementia (VaD), are now widely acknowledged to be risk factors for AD (Shobab *et al.* 2005; Stewart 2005) and there is often significant cerebrovascular disease in addition to typical AD pathology in the brains of elderly demented individuals (see Section 11.8). A number of studies have suggested that treatment of hypertension may reduce the risk of dementia in general, including AD (Forette *et al.* 1998, 2002; Lithell *et al.* 2003; Tzourio *et al.* 2003), but in none of these studies was cognition the primary outcome measure.

The possible roles of education and recreation in the pathogenesis of AD are subjects of much current interest. Low levels of education seem to be a risk factor for AD (Launer *et al.* 1999). In the religious orders ('nun') study, verbal ability in young adulthood, as evidenced by idea density and grammatical complexity in written work, correlated with cognitive function in old age, low verbal ability being related to AD pathology (Snowdon *et al.* 1996). There is some evidence that AD patients engage in fewer physical and recreational activities in midlife (Friedland *et al.* 2001), and regular recreational activities, both physical and intellectual, may be protective (Wilson *et al.* 2002; Verghese *et al.* 2003).

Diet has also been investigated. In view of the possible importance of oxidative stress in neurodegenerative pathogenesis, use of vitamin supplements has been studied, with the finding that combined use of vitamin E and vitamin C (ascorbic acid) was associated with reduced prevalence and incidence of AD. However, the effect was not observed for either vitamin in isolation nor for multivitamin supplements (Zandi *et al.* 2004). Data on smoking have been inconsistent, with both increased and decreased risk reported (Launer *et al.* 1999). Alcohol in moderate amounts may be protective (Huang *et al.* 2002).

Epidemiological studies have suggested possible beneficial effects of a number of drug classes in preventing AD, including: nonsteroidal anti-inflammatory drugs (NSAIDs); lipid-lowering agents, particularly statins (HMG CoA reductase inhibitors); and oestrogens, all of which are associated with biologically plausible explanations. In several cases, however, controlled clinical trials of these agents have proved negative. NSAID use has repeatedly been found to offer a protective effect (McGeer *et al.* 1996; In't Veld *et al.* 2001; Etminan *et al.* 2003), a finding buttressed by the observation of an inflammatory response in AD brain tissue. However, clinical trials of NSAIDs in established AD have been repeatedly disappointing, though there may be valid reasons for the failure to observe any benefit (van Gool *et al.* 2003). Likewise, observational studies have suggested that statin therapy is associated with a lower prevalence of AD (Wolozin *et al.* 2000; Rockwood *et al.* 2002) and may slow progress of established disease (Masse *et al.* 2005), while others have found no association between statin use and subsequent AD (Zandi *et al.* 2005). A brief trial of the HMG CoA reductase inhibitor simvastatin in AD patients had no effect on CSF Aβ levels and, although there was a favourable difference between the Mini-Mental State Examination (MMSE) scores of treated and placebo groups, this was not reflected in the functional outcome (Simons *et al.* 2002). Epidemiological evidence suggesting a protective effect of hormone replacement therapy in postmenopausal women (Henderson 1997; Zandi *et al.* 2002) prompted a clinical trial, but this was stopped because of excess dementia in the treatment group (Shumaker *et al.* 2003). Hence, to date, none of these agents can be recommended in established disease, though a role in primary prevention remains possible (Doraiswamy and Xiong 2006).

Exposure to metals, particularly aluminium, was once believed to be relevant (Doll 1993), in part because of the phenomenon of 'dialysis dementia' that occurred in renal patients exposed to dialysate with high concentrations of aluminium. Although these patients have neurofibrillary pathology typical of AD (Harrington *et al.* 1994), aluminium is no longer perceived as aetiologically important. Likewise zinc can induce Aβ aggregation *in vitro* (Bush *et al.* 1994), but evidence for a role of zinc in AD is equivocal (Nachev and Larner 1996). In an intriguing contrast to the trial data discussed above, however, the metal chelator clioquinol has produced encouraging results in a preliminary trial in AD (Ritchie *et al.* 2003).

Head injury with loss of consciousness has been found to increase Aβ expression in the brain (Roberts *et al.* 1991,1994), and boxers are at risk of *dementia pugilistica*, which shares some neuropathological features with AD. The results of epidemiological studies on the risks of AD after head injury are equivocal, largely because of methodological difficulties (Launer *et al.* 1999; Fleminger *et al.* 2003), though there is an interaction between head injury and ApoE genotype in increasing risk of developing AD pathology (Nicoll *et al.* 1995).

11.4 **Clinical features**

Forgetfulness is the cardinal clinical presentation in AD, though 'atypical' clinical patterns are seen, probably indicating variation in the distribution of the degenerative lesion.

11.4.1 **Typical presentations**

Forgetfulness is usually the earliest symptom of AD, commonly manifesting as repetitive questioning. Day-to-day, events or appointments may also be forgotten, pointing to a problem with the episodic or autobiographical component of memory. Difficulty in mastering new routines or household appliances (i.e. acquisition and retention of new information) is another reflection of this anterograde amnesic syndrome. In contrast, personal events of long ago may be readily recalled, indicating a temporal gradient of memory impairment. These remote memories are assumed to have become part of the semantic component of declarative memory which, though not normal (Garrard *et al.* 2004), is rarely as profoundly impaired as new learning. Difficulty with the production of names (of both people and objects) is probably an early reflection of semantic memory impairment (Garrard *et al.* 2005), while aspects of implicit (non-declarative) memory function are relatively preserved.

11.4.2 Atypical presentations

Although slowly progressive anterograde amnesia is the commonest clinical presentation of AD, 'variant' presentations in which cognitive symptoms other than amnesia are prominent or even isolated (e.g. agnosia, aphasia, apraxia, or behavioural and psychological features) are well recognized. These are not 'subtypes', a term that implies a different causative factor (Jorm 1985), but simply reflections of the clinical heterogeneity of AD, due to variation in the distribution of pathology. Such variants are not uncommon, accounting for just under 10% of AD presentations over a 6-year period in the author's cognitive function clinic (though specialist clinics are subject to selection bias in favour of atypical cases).

11.4.2.1 Visual disruption

Posterior cortical atrophy (PCA; Benson *et al.* 1988) and visual variant of AD (Levine *et al.* 1993) are names given to AD with predominantly visuospatial dysfunction as the presenting feature, such as visual agnosia, alexia, and Balint's syndrome. Diagnostic criteria for PCA have been proposed (Mendez *et al.* 2002), and most cases presenting in this way turn out to have AD as their neuropathological substrate, though other disorders are occasionally encountered (Pantel and Schröder 1996). The heterogeneity of clinical features reflects the different ways in which visual processing may be disrupted in both sporadic and familial AD (Cronin-Golomb and Hof 2004), though it should be noted that visual agnosia is an uncommon feature in AD due to PS1 mutations (Larner and Doran 2006).

11.4.2.2 Progressive apraxia

Slowly progressive apraxia with the neuropathological substrate of AD has been described, as a unilateral or bilateral parietal lobe syndrome (Crystal *et al.* 1982; Mackenzie Ross *et al.* 1996; Galton *et al.* 2000). Difficulty with manual tasks and apraxic agraphia may be accompanied with visuospatial difficulties akin to those of Balint's syndrome, hence prompting the suggestion that this disorder reflects disconnection of the parietal ('where') visual pathway, whereas PCA affects the occipitotemporal ('what') visual pathway (Mackenzie Ross *et al.* 1996; Galton *et al.* 2000). AD cases have also been described that overlap clinically with, and may be mistaken for, corticobasal degeneration (Boeve *et al.* 1999; Doran *et al.* 2003), sometimes with the alien limb phenomenon (Ball *et al.* 1993). AD with progressive frontal gait disturbance (gait apraxia) has also been reported (Rossor *et al.* 1999).

11.4.2.3 Progressive aphasia

Slowly progressive aphasia is recognized to be a presenting feature of neurodegenerative disease, and may either remain focal, as in primary progressive aphasia (Mesulam 2001), or presage a more generalized dementia (Pogacar and Williams 1984; Mendez and Zander 1991; Galton *et al.* 2000). Non-fluent aphasia has been described as the presenting feature of AD due to PS1 gene mutation (Godbolt *et al.* 2004). Fluent aphasia with characteristics more in keeping with transcortical sensory aphasia may also occur in AD (Galton *et al.* 2000). Occasionally aphasia of acute onset, mimicking cerebrovascular disease, may be the first sign of AD (Larner 2005*a*).

11.4.2.4 Frontal AD

A frontal variant of AD (fvAD) was described by Johnson *et al.* (1999). Among 63 patients with pathologically confirmed AD, 19 had greater neurofibrillary pathology in frontal as compared to entorhinal cortex, and 3 had disproportionately severe impairment on two neuropsychological tests of frontal executive function. The term fvAD may also be used for inherited AD cases with a clinical phenotype reminiscent of the behavioural or frontal variant of frontotemporal dementia (fvFTD), sometimes even fulfilling suggested clinical diagnostic criteria for FTD, and is seen in association with certain mutations in the PS1 gene (Larner and Doran 2006). Rarely, sporadic early-onset AD may present with a behavioural phenotype suggestive of FTD (Larner 2006*a*). Evidence from neuropsychological assessments of a subgroup of AD patients with executive dysfunction early in the disease and apparently without behavioural dysfunction has been reported (Binetti *et al.* 1996; Royall 2000).

11.4.2.5 Psychiatric presentations

Behavioural and psychological symptoms of dementia (BPSD)—such as depression—are common in the later stages of AD (Burns *et al.* 1990; Ballard *et al.* 2001) but may sometimes be prominent presenting signs (Alzheimer 1907; Doran and Larner 2004). The difficult differential diagnosis of AD from 'depression associated with dementia' or 'depressive pseudodementia' is familiar to all who work in the field. Vigorous use of antidepressant medication with monitoring of cognitive function may be undertaken, but passage of time may be the only investigation that permits a definitive diagnosis.

AD is recognized as predisposing to an acute confusional state, and occasionally delirium may be the presenting feature. Certainly, elderly patients presenting *de novo* with delirium should be followed up since some will show evidence of progressive cognitive decline (Robertson *et al.* 1998; Rockwood *et al.* 1999). Myoclonic jerks and epileptic seizures become more prevalent with disease duration (Mendez and Lim 2003), though patients with new seizure onset and cognitive decline in whom no symptomatic cause for seizures other than AD is discovered are occasionally encountered (Lozsadi and Larner 2006). Seizures are usually of partial onset type, with or without secondary generalization, and are usually easily to control, seldom requiring more than one antiepileptic drug. A small number of cases progresss rapidly from early on and, if myoclonic jerks are present, AD may be mistaken for prion disease (Tschampa *et al.* 2001; Larner and Doran 2004). EEG periodic sharp waves and CSF 14-3-3 protein may even be present (Reinwald *et al.* 2004).

11.4.3 Examination

The general examination in patients with AD may be entirely normal, though weight loss is sometimes evident, perhaps related to inadequate food intake due to forgetfulness, apathy, or lack of initiative (Cronin-Stubbs *et al.* 1996). Patients often have a perplexed, bemused air, and there may be a lack of attention to appearance and personal hygiene.

Neurological examination may reveal primitive reflexes, such as the palmomental, grasp, and pout, though these are also seen in normal ageing (Hodges 1994; Larner 2006*c*) and may therefore be incidental to a diagnosis of AD. Testing of olfaction is seldom undertaken in the neurological examination, but hyposmia seems to be an early and consistent change in AD (Graves *et al.* 1999). The irregular shock-like jerks of myoclonus may be seen, becoming more prevalent with AD duration (Chen *et al.* 1991), and may lead to diagnostic confusion with sporadic Creutzfeldt–Jakob disease (sCJD). Extrapyramidal signs, particularly rigidity and bradykinesia, are not infrequent in AD: one study found a prevalence of 50% six years after symptom onset (Chen *et al.* 1991) though, as with frontal release signs, they may simply reflect the increased prevalence of these features with normal ageing (Bennett *et al.* 1996; Larner 2006*c*).

Neurological signs that are seen uncommonly in AD, such as cerebellar ataxia, spastic paraparesis, and slowly progressive hemiparesis, prompt a broader differential diagnosis. Although neuropathological changes may be seen in the cerebellum in AD (Larner 1997*c*), cerebellar ataxia is not generally a feature, other than in occasional pedigrees of autosomal dominant AD associated with PS1 gene mutations (Martin *et al.* 1991, Larner and Doran 2006; though see Huff *et al.* 1987 for an alternative view). Spastic paraparesis was first described in association with AD in

1913 (Barrett 1913) and is now recognized as associated with the exon 9 deletion in PS1 (Crook *et al.* 1998; Larner and Doran 2006) and with the neuropathological observation of cotton wool type amyloid plaques (Tabira *et al.* 2002). Slowly progressive hemiparesis has been reported with the pathological substrate of AD (Jagust *et al.* 1990), and may be similar to the syndrome first described by Mills (1900).

The most commonly used, brief (ca. 10 minutes), bedside test of cognitive function is the Mini-Mental State Examination (MMSE) of Folstein *et al.* (1975), a well-established instrument for testing cognitive function, with subtests of attention, memory, language, and visuospatial skills. However, there is no specific cutoff score that defines dementia in general or AD in particular. Moreover, test results are subject to educational bias. Nonetheless, MMSE scores do correlate with neuropathological markers of AD such as synaptic density (Terry *et al.* 1991). The suggestion that a subscore of the MMSE may be useful in the differential diagnosis of AD from DLB, based on the greater attentional and visuospatial deficits in DLB (Ala *et al.* 2002), has not proved specific in a prospective study (Larner 2003*a*, 2004*b*). The clock drawing test is also a popular brief screening test for AD, since it requires a mix of cognitive abilities to execute correctly (Shulman and Feinstein 2003).

Longer bedside batteries (ca. 20–45 minutes) that address some of the shortcomings of the MMSE (i.e. perfunctory testing of memory, visuospatial, and executive function) without becoming unwieldy have been developed. Of these, the Alzheimer's Disease Assessment

Typical case description: early-onset AD

A 52-year-old lady attended with her husband. The complaint was of approximately 2 years of memory difficulties, beginning around the time of the menopause, associated with feelings of anxiety. She used notes to remind herself of things to be done. Because of her forgetfulness, her husband had taken over activities such as the shopping and some of the cooking. Nonetheless, the patient was able to continue her work as a classroom assistant, helping young children with their reading. She was otherwise in good health. There was no family history of Alzheimer's disease. Anxiety improved with use of a specific serotonin reuptake inhibitor, but memory difficulties did not.

Neurological examination was normal. 'Bedside' neuropsychology testing was undertaken using the MMSE and the Addenbrooke's Cognitive Examination, on which her scores were 21/30 and 58/100, respectively; 6 months later these had declined to 18/30 and 55/100. There was disorientation in time, impairments in anterograde and retrograde memory and visuospatial skills, but relative preservation of language abilities. Formal neuropsychological assessment showed evidence of substantial generalized intellectual loss (> 30 point decline in full-scale IQ), with poor performance on all tests of verbal and visual memory for immediate and delayed recall (all measures below 1st percentile). Some difficulties were evident on the Graded Naming Test (13/30), but more severe impairments were recorded on tests of visuospatial function (copy of the Rey Figure below 1st percentile) and executive function (Benton Verbal Fluency Test below 1st percentile; Stroop Colour Test below 2nd percentile). A CT brain scan showed global cerebral atrophy greater than anticipated for age.

She was informed of the diagnosis of (probable) Alzheimer's disease and commenced treatment with a cholinesterase inhibitor. Six months later her MMSE score was 19/30 and she was able to continue with her work for a further year. Her husband reported that her condition remained much the same over the next 2 years.

Scale—Cognitive Section, ADAS-Cog (Rosen *et al.* 1984), has become widely used, including as a measure of drug efficacy in clinical trials. The Consortium to Establish a Registry for Alzheimer's Disease (CERAD) battery incorporates the MMSE and other subtests including tests of memory, naming, and verbal fluency (Morris *et al.* 1989). In the UK, the Addenbrooke's Cognitive Examination (ACE; Mathuranath *et al.* 2000) has become popular. As with the MMSE, it has good sensitivity and specificity for the diagnosis of dementia using particular cutoffs, although likelihood ratios (a measure of change in pre-test to post-test odds, hence of 'diagnostic gain') have not been overly impressive (Larner 2005*b*), but these may be improved in the revised version, ACE-R (Mioshi *et al.* 2006). ACE may be responsive to cognitive change, and hence useful in tracking progression from MCI to AD (Larner 2006*d*). The suggestion that a subscore of the ACE may be useful in the differential diagnosis of AD from frontotemporal dementia (FTD) has been largely borne out in practice (Mathuranath *et al.* 2000; Larner 2005*b*). Other widely used scales (for details see Burns *et al.* 1999), such as the Clinical Dementia Rating and the Mattis Dementia Rating Scale, are more global scales, incorporating functional (ADL) as well as cognitive assessments. Such measures, along with the Clinician's Interview-Based Impression of Change, without or with caregiver input (CIBIC, CIBIC+), are desirable in clinical trials methodology. Informant-based instruments, such as the Informant Questionnaire on Cognitive Decline in the Elderly (IQCODE) may also afford useful information. Specific assessment of behavioural features may be undertaken with instruments such as the Neuropsychiatric Inventory (NPI).

11.5 **Neuropsychology**

The battery of tests used in formal neuropsychological assessment varies from centre to centre, dependent upon local preference and familiarity with tests. Measures of IQ (verbal, performance, full scale) can be obtained with the Wechlser Adult Intelligence Scale Revised (WAIS-R). The National Adult Reading Test (NART) can be used to obtain a measure of premorbid IQ, provided there is no confounding by marked aphasia, thus allowing comparison of present and premorbid IQ to see whether there is evidence for generalized intellectual loss. Individual tests may then be used to probe specific cognitive functions, such as language (Graded Naming Test, Boston Naming Test), memory (Hopkins Verbal Learning Test, Camden Recognition Memory Tests, California Verbal Learning Test), visuoperceptual and visuospatial skills (Rey–Osterreith figure, Visual Object and Space Perception battery), and executive function (Stroop colour–word test, verbal fluency tests, Wisconsin Card Sorting test). Since affective disorders may impact on cognitive performance, some assessment of this domain is also advisable (Beck Depression Inventory, Hamilton Depression Rating Scale, Hospital Anxiety and Depression Scale). Such a battery may take 2 hours or more, and patients may become fatigued requiring a break or return on another day to complete testing.

The profile on neuropsychological assessment in AD varies according to stage, but typically there will be evidence of memory impairment, particularly learning and recalling new information (e.g. word lists). This may occur in isolation, but often by the time of presentation there will be additional language deficits, evident as word-finding and naming difficulties, sometimes with circumlocutions and sometimes phonological errors. Visuospatial and visuoperceptual difficulties may also be apparent, for example, in clock drawing or copying the Rey figure. Executive dysfunction, as evidenced by difficulties with the Stroop test or verbal fluency, may be apparent in some patients in the early stages. The neuropsychological profile is often the most helpful way to differentiate AD from other conditions such as DLB and semantic dementia. The role of computerized test batteries (e.g. CANTAB-PAL) is still being evaluated.

11.6 Imaging correlates

- Hippocampal atrophy is observed in AD, though it cannot be regarded as a necessary or sufficient feature.
- Pathology-specific functional imaging using Pittsburgh compound B (PiB), which binds with high affinity to beta-amyloid, is increasingly recognized as a potentially diagnostic investigation.

11.6.1 Structural

Guidelines for the diagnosis of AD (Waldemar *et al.* 2000; Knopman *et al.* 2001) recommend use of some form of structural brain imaging, either with CT or, preferably, magnetic resonance imaging (MRI). These modalities may display the consequences of AD: brain atrophy with an increase in CSF spaces on visual inspection of scans (Fig. 11.1). As such, these changes are rather

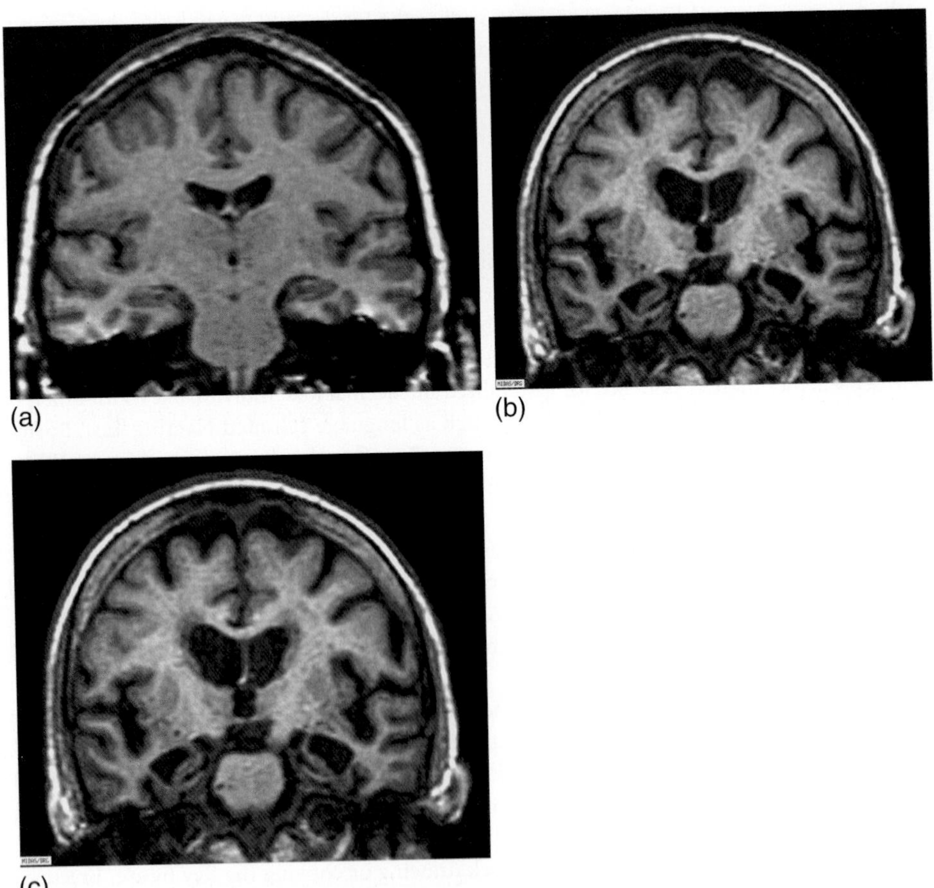

Fig. 11.1 Coronal MR images. (a) Healthy control. (b) Bilateral hippocampal atrophy in moderate AD; MMSE = 20. (c) Repeat imaging of patient in (b) at 1 year follow-up: 2% loss of brain volume. (Courtesy of Professor N.C. Fox, Dementia Research Group, Institute of Neurology Queen Square, London.)

non-specific, also occurring in normal ageing; overreliance on such features may lead to misdiagnosis (Larner 2004*a*). Moreover, in early AD scans may be judged normal for age, as acknowledged in diagnostic criteria (McKhann *et al.* 1984). Disproportionate loss of medial temporal lobe volume may be useful although this may also be seen in DLB.

Serial measurement of hippocampal volume using volumetric imaging techniques (Fig. 11.1(b), (c)) may be particularly helpful (Fox *et al.* 1996*a*). Presymptomatic individuals with deterministic AD mutations may show hippocampal volume loss before clinical deficits become apparent (Fox *et al.* 1996*b*). This imaging modality also has the capacity to be a surrogate marker for drug efficacy.

Imaging of AD pathology *per se* may become a reality in the future using ligands that bind specifically to pathological structures. One such compound, Pittsburgh compound B, is an ^{11}C-labelled positron emission tomography (PET) tracer compound that binds with high affinity to fibrillar amyloid plaques, allowing *in vivo* quantification of amyloid burden (Klunk *et al.* 2004). This compound has generated much excitement, offering the possibility not only of diagnosis of AD (and MCI) but also as a surrogate marker for monitoring the efficacy of AD disease-modifying therapies.

11.6.2 **Functional**

Single photon emission computed tomography (SPECT) is both sensitive and specific for the diagnosis of AD compared to controls, the typical signature being bilateral hypoperfusion of the temporal and parietal cortices (Dougall *et al.* 2003), although clinical variants may differ, such as the occipital hypoperfusion in PCA. SPECT may also be useful in differential diagnosis of dementia syndromes, particularly AD and FTD (Talbot *et al.* 1998; Doran *et al.* 2005).

Other functional imaging modalities include positron emission tomography (PET) and magnetic resonance spectroscopy (MRS), typically proton MRS (^{1}H-MRS), although these are not as widely available as SPECT. PET typically shows hypometabolism in those regions showing hypoperfusion on SPECT and shows a good correlation with brain pathology (Silverman *et al.* 2001). Decrease of *N*-acetyl aspartate (NAA), a neuronal marker, and elevation of myoinositol in occipital voxels, or equivalent changes in their ratios with creatine, are changes observed with ^{1}H-MRS consistent with the diagnosis of AD.

11.7 **Other investigations**

A number of other investigations may be undertaken in patients with suspected AD, as recommended by diagnostic guidelines (Waldemar *et al.* 2000; Knopman *et al.* 2001), largely to exclude other disorders rather than to confirm AD. They may be deemed unnecessary in cases where the diagnosis is established with confidence on the basis of clinical, neuropsychological, and neuroimaging information.

Blood tests may include vitamin B_{12}, thyroid function, and syphilis serology, although the pick-up rate of potentially reversible dementia syndromes is extremely low and the number that actually reverse even lower (Clarfield 2003).

Neurogenetic testing for mutations in the APP, PS1, and PS2 genes is potentially diagnostic, but cases of genetically determined AD are rare. Hence, testing, with appropriate genetic counselling to patient and family, is best reserved for those with an autosomal dominant pattern of inheritance (Cruts *et al.* 1998; Janssen *et al.* 2003). ApoE genotyping in isolation has no role as a diagnostic test.

The role of electroencephalography (EEG) in the diagnosis of AD has lessened with the advent of neuroimaging. Generally, there is a slowing of the alpha frequency, amplitude, and relative power; decrease in relative and absolute beta power; and increasing predominance of diffuse and symmetrical theta and delta waves in posterior regions (Knott *et al.* 2001). Although the EEG may be normal in the early stages of AD, it would be very unlikely to remain so throughout the course of the disease. The persistent normality of the EEG in FTD may help in differential diagnosis. Periodic sharp wave complexes, typical of sCJD, have been described on occasion in AD (Tschampa *et al.* 2001; Reinwald *et al.* 2004).

Analysis of the CSF contents is usually normal; a modest elevation of protein may be seen. An elevated white cell count would argue against a diagnosis of AD. Likewise, the finding of oligoclonal bands (OCB) would be more suggestive of an inflammatory disorder, although cases of pathologically proven AD with OCB for which no other cause could be identified have been reported (Janssen *et al.* 2004), indicating that a central immune response may occur in AD, albeit uncommonly. Measurement of CSF total tau, phospho-tau, and Aβ42 is not widely available but may help in making a diagnosis (Andreasen and Blennow 2005)

Brain biopsy for diagnostic purposes is seldom resorted to in patients with dementia, its use being largely confined to younger patients with atypical presentations, and where a suspicion of a potentially remediable inflammatory or infective aetiology is ranked high in the differential diagnosis. In reported series, where a specific diagnosis can be made, AD is one of the commonest findings (Warren *et al.* 2005), presumably reflecting the very high prevalence of AD in comparison to other dementing conditions.

11.8 **Pathology**

- The pathological hallmarks of AD are extracellular deposits of aggregated amyloid protein ('senile plaques') and intracellular accumulations of hyperphosphorylated tau-protein ('neurofibrillary tangles').

The hallmark lesions in the AD brain are amyloid (senile) plaques and neurofibrillary tangles (Fig. 11.2), although neither is unique to AD. Various other neuropathological changes have also been reported. A number of criteria have been developed to grade AD type pathology (Mirra *et al.* 1991; Braak and Braak 1991; National Institute on Aging and Reagan Institute Working Group on Diagnostic Criteria for the Neuropathological Assessment of Alzheimer Disease 1997).

11.8.1 **Macroscopic appearances**

Macroscopically there may be obvious brain atrophy, often with a frontal, temporal, and parietal bias. On brain slicing there may be obvious thinning of gyri and widening of sulci, with ventricular enlargement and sometimes visible hippocampal atrophy. Depigmentation of the locus ceruleus may be apparent.

11.8.2 **Microscopic**

11.8.2.1 Amyloid pathology: plaques and angiopathy

Amyloid plaques, originally named because of their propensity to take up stains for starch, are proteinaceous (Aβ) deposits in the extracellular space that may have various morphologies (Wisniewski *et al.* 1996). The classic neuritic or senile plaque is an amyloid core surrounded by neuritic (axonal and dendritic) processes, glial cell processes, and microglia (Fig. 11.2(a), (b)). Other proteins may co-localize with Aβ including ApoE, ubiquitin, inflammatory markers such as complement, and acute phase proteins (C-reactive protein, α_1-antichymotrypsin).

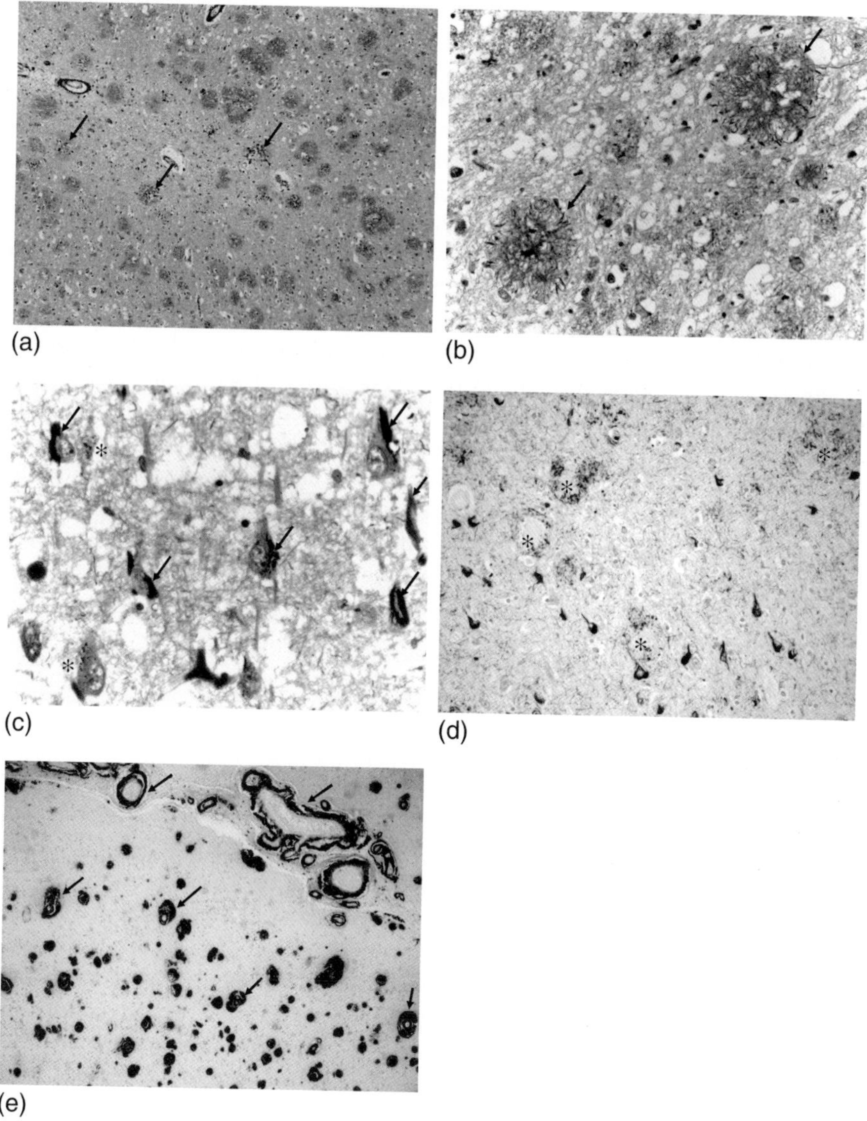

Fig. 11.2 (a) Neocortex showing a high density of silver staining amyloid plaques. Diffuse, primitive and mature/neuritic plaques (arrows) are evident. (Modified Bielchowsky stain, 100 × original magnification.) (b) Neocortex containing diffuse, primitive and mature/neuritic amyloid plaques (arrows). The neuritic plaques consist of an amyloid core surrounded by a corona of silver staining thickened, distorted dystrophic neurites. (Modified Bielchowsky stain, 400 × original magnification.) (c) Hippocampal pyramidal neurons containing silver staining neurofibrillary tangles (arrows). The neurons also show granulovacuolar degeneration. (Modified Bielchowsky stain, 630 × original magnification.) (d) Neocortex containing a high density of tau-immunopositive neurofibrillary tangles, neuropil threads, and neuritic plaques, the latter delineated by immunopositive dystrophic neurites. (Tau-immunostaining, 200 × original magnification.) (e) Cortex showing prominent leptomeningeal and intracortical amyloid angiopathy (arrows), the latter often extending into the surrounding parenchyma. Numerous dense cortical amyloid plaques, some vessel-derived. (Beta A4 amyloid immunohistochemistry, 50 × original magnification.) This is a black and white version of Plate 8. (Courtesy of Dr D.G. DuPlessis, Greater Manchester Neurosciences Centre, Salford.)

Following the characterization of Aβ from amyloid deposits, the development of Aβ antibodies permitted immunohistochemical studies of AD brain, which have revealed additional plaque morphologies. Diffuse plaques, composed mostly of Aβ42 and lacking a neuritic halo, are more widespread, and may be forerunners of neuritic plaques (Wisniewski *et al.* 1996). Cotton wool plaques are large (100–120 μm diameter) eosinophilic structures without surrounding neuritic or glial responses, first described in a Finnish pedigree with the PS1 exon 9 deletion mutation (Crook *et al.* 1998) and subsequently seen in various other PS1 mutations (Larner and Doran 2006).

Cerebral amyloid angiopathy (CAA), also known as congophilic angiopathy, is the deposition of amyloid in the walls of small parenchymal and leptomeningeal arterioles. Sometimes it extends around vessel walls into the surrounding brain parenchyma (dyshoric angiopathy).

Despite the association of APP mutations with AD, and the finding that virtually all genetic mutations deterministic for AD increase Aβ42 production, nonetheless the correlation between amyloid plaque burden and severity of cognitive impairment in AD is less impressive than for neurofibrillary tangles (McKee *et al.* 1991; Terry *et al.* 1991; Arriagada *et al.* 1992). Better correlation has been established with brain levels of soluble Aβ (Näslund *et al.* 2000). A contribution of Aβ *per se* to cognitive impairment is also suggested by the observation of dementia in some cases of HCHWA-D, independent of neurofibrillary pathology and without a clinical history of stroke or focal radiological lesions (Natté *et al.* 2001).

11.8.2.2 Neurofibrillary tangles

Neurofibrillary tangles (NFTs) are argyrophilic structures seen predominantly within the soma and apical dendrites, but not the axon, of pyramidal neurons in AD brain (Fig. 11.2(c), (d)). Extracellular or ghost tangles are occasionally seen, thought to be markers for dead neurons. Ultrastructurally, NFTs are composed of paired helical filaments (PHFs) 8–20 nm in width with a periodicity of about 80 nm (Kidd 1963; Terry 1963). Purification of the highly insoluble proteins composing PHFs revealed them to be composed of the microtubule-associated protein tau (Wischik *et al.* 1988), which is present in a hyperphosphorylated state (Goedert *et al.* 1992). Silver stains and tau immunohistochemistry also reveal dystrophic neurites as a halo around neuritic amyloid plaques and also distributed throughout the cortical neuropil (first described by Simchowicz 1911), the latter variously known as neuropil threads, curly fibres, or cortical neuritic dystrophy (Braak *et al.* 1986; Larner 1995*b*).

Neurofibrillary pathology follows a relatively stereotyped pattern of development in the AD brain, spreading from transentorhinal cortex to entorhinal cortex and hippocampus, and lastly to association cortex (Arnold *et al.* 1991; Braak and Braak 1991). This correlates with progressive cognitive decline (Braak and Braak 1991; Arriagada *et al.* 1992; Bierer *et al.* 1995; Delacourte *et al.* 1999). The presence of dystrophic neurites also correlates with cognitive decline (McKee *et al.* 1991).

11.8.2.3 Neuronal and synaptic loss

Selected populations of neurons undergo disproportionate decreases in the AD brain. Examples include pyramidal neurons in the hippocampus (Ball 1977) and neocortex, especially frontal and temporal regions (Mountjoy *et al.* 1983), and noradrenergic neurons in the locus ceruleus. However, the loss of the cholinergic forebrain projection neurons from the nucleus basalis of Meynert (Whitehouse *et al.* 1982), resulting in reduced cortical cholinergic supply and choline acetyltransferase, is perhaps of the greatest functional importance, and the stimulus for the development of cholinergic therapies in AD. Whether neuronal death is by a process of apoptosis remains unclear. Loss of neocortical neurons (Gomez-Isla *et al.* 1997) and of synaptic connections in the frontal lobe (Terry *et al.* 1991) has been shown to correlate with the severity of dementia.

11.8.2.4 Cerebrovascular disease

In addition to CAA (Fig. 11.2(e)), cerebrovascular disease is very commonly observed in the AD brain. In one community-based study, most patients with dementia coming to autopsy had mixed disease (MRC CFAS 2001) and, in a series of patients with a clinical diagnosis of VaD, most had either AD alone or mixed disease (Nolan *et al.* 1998). Considering the shared vascular risk factors of AD and VaD, this is perhaps not surprising. Moreover, double pathology may lower the threshold for clinically manifest deficits (Snowdon *et al.* 1997).

11.8.2.5 Granulovacuolar degeneration, Hirano bodies

Granulovacuolar degeneration, first described by Simchowicz (1911), is the name given to abnormal cytoplasmic structures found in hippocampal pyramidal neurons (Fig. 11.2(c)), consisting of vacuoles containing a single granule that are thought to be autophagosomes. Hirano bodies are also seen in hippocampal neurons as homogeneous, spindle-shaped inclusions that are bright pink on haematoxylin and eosin staining. Hirano bodies may also be seen in normal ageing.

11.8.2.6 Glial reaction

As mentioned, glial elements are associated with plaques. A generalized glial cell reaction, as judged by upregulation of expression of glial fibrillary acidic protein (GFAP) is found throughout the AD brain (Delacourte 1990). Activated microglia are also found in association with plaques.

11.8.2.7 Lewy bodies, Pick bodies

Although typical of other neurodegenerative disorders, the inclusion bodies of Lewy and Pick may occasionally be seen in the AD brain. Although cases labelled as the Lewy body variant of AD now fall under the rubric of DLB (McKeith *et al.* 2000), nonetheless Lewy bodies containing α-synuclein may be seen in some cases of AD with APP or PS1 mutations (Lippa *et al.* 1998). In one PS1 mutation, ΔT440, the clinical features fulfilled diagnostic criteria for DLB (Ishikawa *et al.* 2005). The precise interrelationship of AD and DLB remains to be defined.

The inclusion bodies, which are typical of tau-positive ubiquitin-positive FTD (Pick bodies), have been reported in some patients with AD associated with PS1 mutations (Larner and Doran 2006), for example M146L (Halliday *et al.* 2005), suggesting that their formation may be a downstream event of aberrant APP processing. In one family with the PS1 G183V mutation, the clinical phenotype was of FTD and the pathology was that of Pick's disease without amyloid plaques, even though cell lines transfected with this mutation did produce increased Aβ42 (Dermaut *et al.* 2004).

11.9 **Clinical course and prognosis**

- AD is relentlessly progressive, and management is mainly supportive, of both the patient and his/her carer.
- Cholinesterase inhibitors (ChEIs) are the only licensed drugs for the treatment of mild to moderate AD.
- In more advanced disease the *N*-methyl-D-aspartic acid (NMDA) receptor antagonist memantine has been shown to retard disease progression and provide clinically important benefits to patients and carers.
- Recent trials suggest that reduction of the amyloid burden using immunotherapy may be of benefit, though the approach may be associated with life-threatening complications.
- Increased understanding of disease pathobiology will undoubtedly give rise to alternative therapeutic strategies in the future.

Epidemiological studies suggest that patients destined to develop AD on long-term follow-up have poorer cognitive performance at baseline, and this may affect not only episodic memory but other cognitive domains as well (Amieva *et al.* 2005). Whether such pre-morbid individuals can be reliably identified prospectively is still open to question, but if so they would be appropriate targets for future preventive therapies. Likewise, patients with MCI.

The clinical course of established AD is one of insidious progression, but this is not necessarily linear. Following diagnosis patients may enter a prolonged plateau phase before declining once again (Stern *et al.* 1994). MMSE scores in untreated patients may decline, remain stable, or improve during the first years of follow-up (Holmes and Lovestone 2003), indicating how unreliable the use of MMSE scores may be as a method for assessing drug efficacy, and hence pointing to the need for assessment of other (functional, global) domains when making decisions about drug continuation or withdrawal (Larner and Doran 2002). AD progression over time can be modelled using a cubic or logarithmic function of MMSE score (Mendiondo *et al.* 2000).

Longitudinal studies indicate the increasing prevalence of psychiatric symptoms with disease duration (Chen *et al.* 1991). These include the misidentification syndromes—delusional conditions in which patients incorrectly identify and reduplicate people, places, objects, or events (Larner 2006*b*), for example, the belief that a close relation has been replaced by an exact alien or double (illusion of doubles) or that the house is not one's own (Capgras' syndrome, or reduplicative paramnesia). Patients may mistake their own mirror reflection for that of a stranger ('mirror sign'), leading to the belief that someone else is staying in the house ('phantom boarder sign'). This stranger may be blamed for lost items, which may in turn lead to involvement of the police. Visual hallucinations are more typical of dementia with Lewy bodies/Parkinson's disease dementia (DLB/PDD).

Other distinctive behavioural features, again commoner in the later stages of AD, include 'shadowing' (a tendency to follow the spouse or carer around the house) and 'sundowning' (increased confusion, agitation, or disorientation at the end of the day). There may be complete reversal of sleep–wake cycle with daytime somnolence and nocturnal wakefulness, resulting in getting up and dressed in the small hours, making telephone calls to relatives or walking the dog in the middle of the night. Sundowning and reversal of sleep–wake pattern may reflect a disorder of circadian rhythms related to pathology in the supraoptic nuclei (Volicer *et al.* 2001). Wandering, restlessness, abnormal vocalizations, and verbal and physical aggression may also occur (Ballard *et al.* 2001).

ADL gradually become more restricted, progressing from instrumental to basic activities. A common complication is the development of BPSD, which, along with urinary incontinence, is associated with increased likelihood of nursing home placement. Survival time from symptom onset is usually of the order of 10–15 years, but in some cases the course is more rapid.

11.10 **Management strategies**

Ideally, AD should be identified in its earliest stages. This may be facilitated through the development of the concept of MCI, or with new imaging techniques. In the absence of reliable biomarkers, however, the diagnosis remains clinical, with the risk of false negative and false positive diagnoses (Larner 2004*a*). Once established, it is now generally accepted that, unless there are exceptional reasons, patients should be told the diagnosis. Although relatives may prefer their loved ones not to be told, they themselves expect to be informed and would expect to be told if they had AD (Maguire *et al.* 1996). Knowing the diagnosis allows appropriate arrangements to be made, such as settling financial matters, allocating enduring power of attorney, applying for financial benefits, and making a living will.

Guidelines for the management of established AD have been published (Doody *et al.* 2001), encompassing both non-pharmacological and pharmacological treatments, although these predate the introduction of memantine. Certainly the age of therapeutic nihilism is over and, although curative treatment is not on the horizon, nonetheless amelioration of the lives of patients and their carers is possible.

11.10.1 Non-pharmacological management

The diagnosis of AD carries with it implications for employment and lifestyle. Employment issues are particularly relevant in younger individuals who may have young dependents and significant financial liabilities (Baldwin and Murray 2003). Advice is also required on activities such as driving: in the UK there is a statutory requirement for patients to inform the Driver and Vehicle Licensing Authority (O'Neill 2005). Appropriate restrictions to ensure safety must be counterbalanced by encouraging patients to maintain other interests and activities, if necessary with supervision, such as gardening (Larner 2005*c*) or other exercise in order to avoid any lapse into apathy, itself one of the neuropsychiatric symptoms of AD. Simple external memory aids and a regular routine may be helpful in the early stages of disease. Quality of life measures are increasingly important as outcome measures in intervention trials, although reliable measurement presents difficulties in dementia.

A multidisciplinary approach to management is advisable, including occupational therapists, social workers, and speech and language therapists, particularly as the disease progresses and problems become more prevalent. Support for patients may take various forms including assistance from a carer at home for a number of hours per week, attendance at a day care centre, and intermittent admission for respite care where resources permit. This will also impact on carers, often elderly, who are often subject to significant caregiver burden, including financial costs. Long-term nursing home care may eventually become necessary, BPSD and urinary incontinence being the symptoms that most often precipitate institutionalization. Urinary incontinence may be treated with behaviour modification, scheduled toileting, or prompted voiding (Doody *et al.* 2001). Education of caregivers is recommended (Doody *et al.* 2001), as this in itself may reduce placement of patients in nursing homes (Brodaty *et al.* 2003). Families are often keen for information, and may use telephone helplines (Harvey *et al.* 1998) or the internet (Larner 2003*b*). Alzheimer associations are active in many countries.

11.10.2 Pharmacological treatments

There are many possible pharmacological treatments for AD (Jones 2000; Larner 2002; see also the Cochrane Library for up-to-date meta-analysis), targeting both cognitive and non-cognitive (behavioural and psychological) symptoms. To date, however, the only anti-dementia drugs of proven, albeit limited, efficacy are cholinomimetics, specifically cholinesterase inhibitors (ChEI), and memantine, an uncompetitive antagonist at the NMDA subtype of ionotropic glutamate receptors.

Cholinesterase inhibitors (ChEIs), specifically donepezil, rivastigmine, and galantamine, have been the principal focus of AD treatment since their widespread licensing in the late 1990s, based on clinical trial results and subsequent meta-analyses demonstrating efficacy (e.g. Lanctôt *et al.* 2003; Ritchie *et al.* 2004), although there have been dissenting voices (AD2000 Collaborative Group 2004; Kaduszkiewicz *et al.* 2005). There seems little doubt that ChEIs as a class do produce a modest benefit in some, but not all patients, not only in terms of cognition but also for BPSD (Holmes *et al.* 2004). ChEIs do not seem to slow the rate of conversion of MCI to AD (Salloway *et al.* 2004; Petersen *et al.* 2005). Generally they are well tolerated although gastrointestinal side-effects may be limiting. In clinical practice, very high retention rate (> 90% at 1 and 2 years) may be seen (Larner 2004*c*), contrary to the expectations of the national guidelines (National Institute for Clinical Excellence 2001). Few head-to-head studies of ChEIs have been performed, showing little clinical evidence of differential efficacy (Wilcock *et al.* 2003; Bullock *et al.* 2005), despite possible differences in pharmacological actions (dual inhibition of both acetyl- and butyrylcholinesterase by rivastigmine; allosteric nicotinic receptor agonism by galantamine). Nonetheless, switching between different ChEIs when lack or loss efficacy becomes apparent may be attended with further response, albeit modest (Gauthier *et al.* 2003). The combination of ChEI and memantine ('dual therapy') may offer additional benefits over monotherapy (Tariot *et al.* 2004), in part because of memantine's different mode of action as a non-competitive NMDA receptor antagonist, which may protect against glutamate-mediated neurotoxocity (Wilcock 2003). Although trial data on memantine is sparse (Winblad and Poritis 1999; Reisberg *et al.* 2003), the reported beneficial effects in moderate to severe AD have been sufficient to gain product licence, although use of this drug is not reimbursed in some jurisdictions, leading to patchy uptake ('postcode prescribing').

A variety of other medications has been used for symptomatic treatment of AD based on limited trial data, although without being licensed for this purpose. These include anti-oxidants (vitamin E, selegiline), ginkgo, and piracetam. A controlled trial of vitamin E (α-tocopherol) in moderate to severe AD did show a delay in clinical progression to certain time points, such as institutionalization, but no effect on cognition. The monoamine oxidase-B inhibitor selegiline had a similar effect (Sano *et al.* 1997). However, a trial of vitamin E in patients with MCI showed no slowing of conversion to AD over a 3 year period (Petersen *et al.* 2005). A meta-analysis of selegiline trials suggested short term improvements in cognition and ADLs but no evidence for long term effects (Wilcock *et al.* 2002). Extracts from the leaves of the maidenhair tree, *Ginkgo biloba*, have been a popular treatment for AD. Initially these were difficult to standardize but the component EGb761 may have some effects as an anti-oxidant. One meta-analysis found ginkgo to have moderate beneficial effects, but it is telling that of 50 trials analysed only four were deemed of sufficient quality to be included (Oken *et al.* 1998). Piracetam, 2-oxo-1-pyrrolidine acetamide, a cyclic derivative of gamma aminobutyric acid (GABA), marketed as a nootropic, may have a modest impact on cognitive impairment (Waegemans *et al.* 2002).

The treatment of BPSD remains a most difficult therapeutic area (Ballard *et al.* 2001) due to a relative paucity of clinical trials, and the risk of side-effects of medications. A variety of medications may be used including typical and atypical antipsychotics, anxiolytics and sedatives, antidepressants, anticonvulsants (for their mood-stabilizing, rather than their anti-epileptic, action), and β-blockers, although options have contracted recently with the finding of an association between atypical antipsychotics and cerebrovascular events. ChEIs and memantine may also have a place in the treatment of BPSD (Holmes *et al.* 2004; Gauthier *et al.* 2005). One school of thought attempts to match the behaviour syndrome to standard therapy (the 'psychobehavioural metaphor'); hence agitation with dysphoria might be treated with an antidepressant, agitation with increased activity with a mood stabilizer, and aggression with delusions with an antipsychotic (Profenno *et al.* 2005). Another approach is case-specific, causality-targeted, largely psychosocial interventions, with or without pharmacotherapy; sometimes caregivers rather than patients may be the focus of the treatment plan (Bird 2005).

Other symptomatic features of AD may merit treatment. Seizures may be treated with standard anti-epileptic drugs, and are usually easily controlled (Mendez and Lim 2003). Myoclonus may require treatment with agents such as clonazepam, sodium valproate, or piracetam.

Many drugs are reported to cause confusion in the elderly, and hence may be best avoided in AD. It has been suggested that anticholinergic drugs accelerate cerebral amyloidosis and plaque pathology (Perry *et al.* 2003).

11.10.3 Future therapy

Although ChEIs are licensed as symptomatic treatment for mild-to-moderate AD, there is some evidence that they may have disease-modifying effects, perhaps most strikingly illustrated in an observational study suggesting reduced prevalence of institutionalization in treated patients (Lopez *et al.* 2002). Similar low levels of nursing home placement have been noted elsewhere (Larner, in preparation). However, the principal hope for future disease-modifying therapy for AD rests with agents that target the key pathophysiological pathways, specifically amyloid deposition.

The observation that transgenic mice bearing human APP mutations, animals destined to develop amyloid pathology, had a reduced burden of pathology following immunization with A peptides, in association with the production of high titres of anti-Aβ antibodies (Schenk *et al.* 1999), stimulated the development of human 'amyloid vaccines', or immunotherapy (Heppner *et al.* 2004). The pivotal clinical trial had to be halted because some patients (6%) developed meningoencephalitis. Nonetheless, trial data suggested some clinical benefit (Gilman *et al.* 2005). Perhaps surprisingly, the neuroradiological arm of the study showed evidence of increased brain shrinkage in treated as compared to placebo patients (Fox *et al.* 2005). One possible explanation of this observation is that it reflects removal of amyloid from the brain, which may correlate with limited neuropathological evidence of reduced amyloid burden in vaccine-treated patients (Nicoll *et al.* 2003). Future trials of new immunotherapeutic agents seem likely. Administration of antibodies against Aβ, which may be found in some commercially available intravenous immunoglobulin preparations, has also been suggested (Dodel *et al.* 2002).

Aβ biosynthesis from APP requires the action of β- and γ-secretase enzymes. Inhibitors of these enzymes, or modulators of α-secretase, might thus have a therapeutic role; various agents have been designed for this purpose (Larner 2004*d*). Endoproteolytic cleavage of Aβ has also been considered as a therapeutic approach, although the possibility that *N*-terminally truncated Aβ peptides may be of pathogenetic significance (Larner 1999, 2001) may limit this approach. Anti-apoptotic agents currently remain experimental (Larner 2000), as do cell transplantation and regeneration strategies (Larner and Sofroniew 2003).

Epidemiological data suggest that delaying the onset of AD by 5 years would lead to a dramatic reduction in the incidence and prevalence of AD (Jorm and Jolley 1998). The increased societal burden of AD consequent upon an ageing population demands continued efforts to define disease-modifying agents.

Acknowledgements

Thanks to my colleagues Paula Hancock, Mark Doran, and Eric Ghadiali.

References

AD2000 Collaborative Group (2004). Long-term donepezil treatment in 565 patients with Alzheimer's disease (AD2000): randomised double-blind trial. *Lancet* **363**, 2105–15.

Ala, T.A., Hughes, L.F., Kyrouac, G.A., Ghobrial, M.W., and Elble, R.J. (2002). The Mini-Mental State exam may help the differentiation of dementia with Lewy bodies and Alzheimer's disease. *Int. J. Geriatr. Psychiatry* **17**, 503–9.

Alzheimer, A. (1907). Über eine eigenartige Erkrankung der Hirnrinde. *Allg. Z. Psychiatrie Psychisch-Gerichtlich Med.* **64**, 146–8.

Amieva, H., Jacqmin-Gadda, H., Orgogozo, J-M., *et al.* (2005). The 9 year cognitive decline before dementia of the Alzheimer type: a prospective population-based study. *Brain* **128**, 1093–101.

Andreasen, N. and Blennow, K. (2005). CSF biomarkers for mild cognitive impairment and early Alzheimer's disease. *Clin. Neurol. Neurosurg.* **107**, 165–73.

Arnold, S.E., Hyman, B.T., Flory, J., Damasio, A.R. and Van Hoesen, G.W. (1991). The topographical and neuroanatomical distribution of neurofibrillary tangles and neuritic plaques in cerebral cortex of patients with Alzheimer's disease. *Cereb. Cortex* **1**, 103–16.

Arriagada, P.V., Growdon, J.H., Hedley White, E.T., and Hyman, B.T. (1992). Neurofibrillary tangles but not senile plaques parallel duration and severity of Alzheimer's disease. *Neurology* **42**, 631–9.

Baldwin, R. and Murray, M. (eds.) (2003). *Younger people with dementia: a multidisciplinary approach.* Martin Dunitz, London.

Ball, J.A., Lantos, P.L., Jackson, M., Marsden, C.D., Scadding, J.W., and Rossor, M.N. (1993). Alien hand sign in association with Alzheimer's histopathology. *J. Neurol. Neurosurg. Psychiatry* **56**, 1020–3.

Ball, M.J. (1977). Neuronal loss, neurofibrillary tangles and granulovacuolar degeneration in the hippocampus with ageing and dementia: a quantitative study. *Acta Neuropathol. (Berl.)* **37**, 111–18.

Ballard, C.G., O'Brien, J., James, I., and Swann, A. (2001). *Dementia: management of behavioural and psychological symptoms.* Oxford University Press, Oxford.

Barrett, A. (1913). A case of Alzheimer's disease with unusual neurological disturbances. *J. Nerv. Ment. Dis.* **4**, 361–74.

Bennett, D.A., Beckett, L.A., Murray, A.M., *et al.* (1996). Prevalence of parkinsonian signs and associated mortality in a community population of older people. *N. Engl. J. Med.* **334**, 71–6.

Benson, D.F., Davis, R.J., and Snyder, B.D. (1988). Posterior cortical atrophy. *Arch. Neurol.* **45**, 789–93.

Bertram, L. and Tanzi, R.E. (2005). Genetics of Alzheimer's disease. In *Neurodegenerative diseases. Neurobiology, pathogenesis and therapeutics* (ed. M.F. Beal, A.E. Lang, and A. Ludolph), pp. 441–51. Cambridge University Press, Cambridge.

Bierer, L.M., Hof, P.R., Purohit, D.P., *et al.* (1995) Neocortical neurofibrillary tangles correlate with dementia severity in Alzheimer's disease. *Arch. Neurol.* **52**, 81–8.

Binetti, G., Magni, E., Padovani, A., Cappa, S.F., Bianchetti, A., and Trabucchi, M. (1996). Executive dysfunction in early Alzheimer's disease. *J. Neurol. Neurosurg. Psychiatry* **60**, 91–3.

Bird, M. (2005). A predominantly psychosocial approach to behaviour problems in dementia: treating causality. In *Dementia*, 3rd edn (ed. A. Burns, J. O'Brien, and D. Ames), pp. 499–509. Hodder Arnold, London.

Boeve, B.F., Maraganore, M.D., Parisi, J.E., *et al.* (1999). Pathologic heterogeneity in clinically diagnosed corticobasal degeneration. *Neurology* **53**, 795–800.

Braak, H. and Braak, E. (1991). Neuropathological stageing of Alzheimer-related changes. *Acta Neuropathol. (Berl.)* **82**, 239–59.

Braak, H., Braak, E., Grundke-Iqbal, I., and Iqbal, K. (1986). Occurrence of neuropil threads in the senile human brain and in Alzheimer's disease; a third location of paired helical filaments outside the neurofibrillary tangles and neuritic plaques. *Neurosci. Lett.* **65**, 351–5.

Brodaty, H., Green, A., and Koschera, A. (2003). Meta-analysis of psychosocial interventions of caregivers of people with dementia. *J. Am. Geriatr. Soc.* **51**, 657–64.

Bullock, R., Touchon, J., Bergman, H., *et al.* (2005). Rivastigmine and donepezil treatment in moderate to moderately-severe Alzheimer's disease over a 2-year period. *Curr. Med. Res. Opin.* **21**, 1317–27.

Burns, A., Jacoby, R., and Levy, R. (1990). Psychiatric phenomena in Alzheimer's disease: IV. Disorders of behaviour. *Br. J. Psychiatry* **157**, 86–94.

Burns, A., Lawlor, B., and Craig, S. (1999). *Assessment scales in old age psychiatry.* Martin Dunitz, London.

Bush, A.I., Pettingell, W.H., Multhaup, G., *et al.* (1994). Rapid induction of Alzheimer Aβ amyloid formation by zinc. *Science* **265**, 1464–7.

Chen, J-Y., Stern, Y., Sano, M., *et al.* (1991). Cumulative risk of developing extrapyramidal signs, psychosis or myoclonus in the course of Alzheimer's disease. *Arch Neurol.* **48**, 1141–3.

Chui, H. and Lee, A-Y. (2002). Clinical criteria for dementia subtypes. In *Evidence-based dementia practice* (ed. N. Qizilbash *et al.*), pp. 106–13. Blackwell, Oxford.

Clarfield, A.M. (2003). The decreasing prevalence of reversible dementias: an updated meta-analysis. *Arch. Intern. Med.* **163**, 2219–29.

Corder, E.H., Saunders, A.M., Strittmatter, W.J., *et al.* (1993). Gene dose of apolipoprotein E type 4 allele and the risk of Alzheimer's disease in late onset families. *Science* **261**, 921–3.

Cronin-Golomb, A. and Hof, P.R. (eds.) (2004). *Vision in Alzheimer's disease.* Karger, Basel.

Cronin-Stubbs, D., Beckett, L.A., Scherr, P.A., *et al.* (1996). Weight loss in people with Alzheimer's disease: a prospective population based analysis. *Br. Med. J.* **314**, 178–9.

Crook, R., Verkkoniemi, A., Perez-Tur, J., *et al.* (1998). A variant of Alzheimer's disease with spastic paraparesis and unusual plaques due to deletion of exon 9 of presenilin 1. *Nature Med.* **4**, 452–5.

Cruts, M., van Duijn, C.M., Backhovens, H., *et al.* (1998). Estimation of the genetic contribution of presenilin-1 and -2 mutations in a population-based study of presenile Alzheimer disease. *Hum. Mol. Genet.* **7**, 43–51.

Crystal, H.A., Horoupian, D.S., Katzman, R., and Jotkowitz, S. (1982). Biopsy-proved Alzheimer disease presenting as a right parietal lobe syndrome. *Ann. Neurol.* **12**, 186–8.

Delacourte, A. (1990). General and dramatic glial reaction in Alzheimer brains. *Neurology* **40**, 33–7.

Delacourte, A., David, J.P., Sergeant, N., *et al.* (1999). The biochemical pathway of neurofibrillary degeneration in aging and Alzheimer's disease. *Neurology* **52**, 1158–65.

Dermaut, B., Kumar-Singh, S., Engelborghs, S., *et al.* (2004). A novel presenilin 1 mutation associated with Pick's disease but not β-amyloid plaques. *Ann. Neurol.* **55**, 617–25.

Dodel, R., Hampel, H., Depboylu, C., *et al.* (2002). Human antibodies against amyloid β peptide; a potential treatment for Alzheimer's disease. *Ann. Neurol.* **52**, 253–6.

Doll, R. (1993). Review: Alzheimer's disease and environmental aluminium. *Age Ageing* **22**, 138–53.

Doody, R.S., Stevens, J.C., Beck, C., *et al.* (2001). Practice parameter: management of dementia (an evidence-based review). Report of the Quality Standards Subcommittee of the American Academy of Neurology. *Neurology* **56**, 1154–66.

Doraiswamy, P.M. and Xiong, G.L. (2006). Pharmacological strategies for the prevention of Alzheimer's disease. *Expert Opin. Pharmacother.* **7**, 1–10.

Doran, M. and Larner, A.J. (2004). Prominent behavioural and psychiatric symptoms in early-onset Alzheimer's disease in a sib pair with the presenilin-1 gene R269G mutation. *Eur. Arch. Psychiatry Clin. Neurosci.* **254**, 187–9.

Doran, M., du Plessis, D.G., Enevoldson, T.P., Fletcher, N.A., Ghadiali, E., and Larner, A.J. (2003). Pathological heterogeneity of clinically diagnosed corticobasal degeneration. *J. Neurol. Sci.* **216**, 127–34.

Doran, M., Vinjamuri, S., Collins, J., Parker, D., and Larner, A.J. (2005). Single-photon emission computed tomography perfusion imaging in the differential diagnosis of dementia: a retrospective regional audit. *Int. J. Clin. Pract.* **59**, 496–500.

Dougall, N.J., Bruggink, S., and Ebmeier, K.P. (2003). The clinical use of ^{99m}Tc-HMPAO-SPECT in Alzheimer's disease. a systematic review. In *SPECT in dementia* (ed. K.P. Ebmeier), pp. 4–37. Karger, Basel.

Etminan, M., Gill, S., and Samii, A. (2003). Effect of non-steroidal anti-inflammatory drugs on risk of Alzheimer's disease: systematic review and meta-analysis of observational studies. *Br. Med. J.* **327**, 128–31.

Fleminger, S., Oliver, D.L., Lovestone, S., Rabe-Hesketh, S., and Giora, A. (2003). Head injury as a risk factor for Alzheimer's disease: the evidence 10 years on; a partial replication. *J. Neurol. Neurosurg. Psychiatry* **74**, 857–62.

Folstein, M.F., Folstein, S.E., and McHugh, P.R. (1975). 'Mini-Mental State.' A practical method for grading the cognitive state of patients for the clinician. *J. Psychiatr. Res.* **12**, 189–98.

Forette, F., Seux, M.L., Staessen, J.A., *et al.* for the Syst-Eur investigators (1998). Prevention of dementia in randomised double-blind placebo-controlled Systolic Hypertension in Europe (Syst-Eur) trial. *Lancet* **352**, 1347–51.

Forette, F., Seux, M.L., Staessen, J.A., *et al.* for the Syst-Eur investigators (2002). The prevention of dementia with anti-hypertensive treatment: new evidence from the Systolic Hypertension in Europe (Syst-Eur) study. *Arch. Intern. Med.* **162**, 2046–52.

Fox, N.C., Freeborough, P.A., and Rossor, M.N. (1996*a*). Visualisation and quantification of atrophy in Alzheimer's disease. *Lancet* **348**, 94–7.

Fox, N.C., Warrington, E.K., Freeborough, P.A., *et al.* (1996*b*). Presymptomatic hippocampal atrophy in Alzheimer's disease. A longitudinal study. *Brain* **119**, 2001–7.

Fox, N.C., Black, R.S., Gilman, S., *et al.* (2005) Effects of Abeta immunization (AN1792) on MRI measures of cerebral volume in Alzheimer disease. *Neurology* **64**, 1563–72.

Friedland, R.P., Fritsch, T., Smyth, K.A., *et al.* (2001). Patients with Alzheimer's disease have reduced activities in midlife compared with healthy control group members. *Proc. Natl. Acad. Sci. USA* **98**, 3440–5.

Galton, C.J., Patterson, K., Xuereb, J.H., and Hodges, J.R. (2000). Atypical and typical presentations of Alzheimer's disease: a clinical, neuropsychological, neuroimaging and pathological study of 13 cases. *Brain* **123**, 484–98.

Garrard, P., Patterson, K., and Hodges, J.R. (2004). Semantic processing in Alzheimer's disease. In *Cognitive neuropsychology of Alzheimer's disease*, 2nd edn (ed. R.G. Morris and J.T. Becker), pp. 179–96. Oxford University Press, Oxford.

Garrard, P., Lambon Ralph, M.A., Patterson, K., Pratt, K., and Hodges, J.R. (2005). Semantic feature knowledge and picture naming in dementia of Alzheimer's type: a new approach. *Brain Lang.* **93**, 79–94.

Gauthier, S., Emre, M., Farlow, M.R., Bullock, R., Grossberg, G.T., and Potkin, S.G. (2003). Strategies for continued successful treatment of Alzheimer's disease: switching cholinesterase inhibitors. *Curr. Med. Res. Opin.* **19**, 707–14.

Gauthier, S., Wirth, Y., and Möbius, H.J. (2005). Effects of memantine on behavioural symptoms in Alzheimer's disease patients: an analysis of the Neuropsychiatric Inventory (NPI) data of two randomised, controlled trials. *Int. J. Geriatr. Psychiatry* **20**, 459–64.

Gilman, S., Koller, M., Black, R.S., *et al.* (2005). Clinical effects of Abeta immunization (AN1792) in patients with AD in an interrupted trial. *Neurology* **64**, 1553–62.

Goate, A., Chartier, H.M., Mullan, M., *et al.* (1991). Segregation of a missense mutation in the amyloid precursor protein gene with familial Alzheimer's disease. *Nature* **349**, 704–6.

Godbolt, A.K., Beck, J.A., Collinge, J., *et al.* (2004). A presenilin 1 R278I mutation presenting with language impairment. *Neurology* **63**, 1702–4.

Goedert, M., Spillantini, M.G., Cairns, N.J., and Crowther, R.A. (1992). Tau proteins of Alzheimer paired helical filaments: abnormal phosphorylation of all six brain isoforms. *Neuron* **8**, 159–68.

Gomez-Isla, T., Hollister, R., West, H., *et al.* (1997). Neuronal loss correlates with but exceeds neurofibrillary tangles in Alzheimer's disease. *Ann. Neurol.* **41**, 17–24.

Graeber, M.B., Kösel, S., Egensperger, R., *et al.* (1997). Rediscovery of the case described by Alois Alzheimer in 1911: historical, histological and molecular genetic analysis. *Neurogenetics* **1**, 73–80.

Graves, A.B., Bowen, J.D., Rajaram, L., *et al.* (1999). Impaired olfaction as a marker for cognitive decline: interaction with apolipoprotein E epsilon 4 status. *Neurology* **53**, 1480–7.

Halliday, G.M., Song-Yun, J.C., Lepar, G., *et al.* (2005). Pick bodies in a family with presenilin-1 Alzheimer's disease. *Ann. Neurol.* **57**, 139–43.

Hansen, L.A., Salmon, D., Galasko, D., *et al.* (1990). The Lewy body variant of Alzheimer's disease: a clinical and pathological entity. *Neurology* **40**, 1–8.

Harrington, C.R., Wischik, C.M., McArthur, F.K., *et al.* (1994). Alzheimer's disease-like changes in tau protein processing: association with aluminium accumulation in brains of renal dialysis patients. *Lancet* **343**, 993–7.

Harvey, R., Roques, P.K., Fox, N.C., and Rossor, M.N. (1998). CANDID—Counselling and Diagnosis in Dementia: a national telemedicine service supporting the care of younger patients with dementia. *Int. J. Geriatr. Psychiatry* **13**, 381–8.

Henderson, V.W. (1997). The epidemiology of estrogen replacement therapy and Alzheimer's disease. *Neurology* **48** (suppl. 17), S27–35.

Hendrie, H.C., Ogunniyi, A., Hall, K.S., *et al.* (2001). Incidence of dementia and Alzheimer disease in two communities: Yoruba residing in Ibadan, Nigeria, and African Americans residing in Indianapolis, Indiana. *J. Am. Med. Assoc.* **285**, 739–47.

Heppner, F.L., Gandy, S., and McLaurin, J. (2004). Current concepts and future prospects for Alzheimer disease vaccines. *Alzheimer Dis. Assoc. Dis.* **18**, 38–43.

Hodges, J.R. (1994). Neurological aspects of dementia and normal aging. In *Dementia and normal aging* (ed. F.A. Huppert, C. Brayne, and D.W. O'Connor), pp. 118–29. Cambridge University Press, Cambridge.

Holmes, C. and Lovestone, S. (2003). Long-term cognitive and functional decline in late onset Alzheimer's disease: therapeutic implications. *Age Ageing* **32**, 200–4.

Holmes, C., Wilkinson, D., Dean, C., *et al.* (2004). The efficacy of donepezil in the treatment of neuropsychiatric symptoms in Alzheimer disease. *Neurology* **63**, 214–19.

Huang, W., Qiu, C., Winblad, B., and Fratiglioni, L. (2002). Alcohol consumption and incidence of dementia in a community sample aged 75 years and older. *J. Clin. Epidemiol.* **55**, 959–64.

Huff, F.J., Boller, F., Luchelli, F., Querriera, R., Beyer, J., and Belle, S. (1987). The neurologic examination in patients with probable Alzheimer's disease. *Arch. Neurol.* **44**, 929–32.

In't Veld, B.A., Ruitenberg, A., Hofman, A., *et al.* (2001). Nonsteroidal anti-inflammatory drugs and the risk of Alzheimer's disease. *N. Engl. J. Med.* **345**, 1515–21.

Ishikawa, A., Piao, Y.S., Miyashita, A., *et al.* (2005). A mutant PSEN1 causes dementia with Lewy bodies and variant Alzheimer's disease. *Ann. Neurol.* **57**, 429–34.

Iversen, L.L., Mortishire-Smith, R.J., Pollack, S.J., and Shearman, M.S. (1995). The toxicity *in vitro* of β-amyloid protein. *Biochem. J.* **311**, 1–16.

Jagust, W.J., Davies, P., Tiller-Borcich, J.K., and Reed, B.R. (1990). Focal Alzheimer's disease. *Neurology* **40**, 14–19.

Janssen, J.C., Beck, J.A., Campbell, T.A., *et al.* (2003). Early onset familial Alzheimer's disease. Mutation frequency in 31 families. *Neurology* **60**, 235–9.

Janssen, J.C., Godbolt, A.K., Ioannidis, P., Thompson, E.J., and Rossor, M.N. (2004). The prevalence of oligoclonal bands in the CSF of patients with primary neurodegenerative dementia. *J. Neurol.* **251**, 184–8.

Jarrett, J.T., Berger, E.P., and Lansbury, P.T. Jr. (1993). The carboxy terminus of the β amyloid protein is critical for the seeding of amyloid formation: implications for the pathogenesis of Alzheimer's disease. *Biochemistry* **32**, 4693–7.

Johnson, J.K., Head, E., Kim, R., Starr, A., and Cotman, C.W. (1999). Clinical and pathological evidence for a frontal variant of Alzheimer disease. *Arch. Neurol.* **56**, 1233–9.

Jones, R. (2000). *Drug treatment in dementia.* Blackwell Science, Oxford.

Jorm, A.F. (1985). Subtypes of Alzheimer's dementia: a conceptual analysis. *Psychol. Med.* **15**, 543–53.

Jorm, A.F. (1990). *The epidemiology of Alzheimer's disease and related disorders.* Chapman and Hall, London.

Jorm, A.F. and Jolley, D. (1998). The incidence of dementia: a meta-analysis. *Neurology* **51**, 728–33.

Kaduszkiewicz, H., Zimmermann, T., Beck-Bornholdt, H-P., and van den Bussche, H. (2005). Cholinesterase inhibitors for patients with Alzheimer's disease: systematic review of randomised clinical trials. *Br. Med. J.* **331**, 321–3.

Kidd, M. (1963). Paired helical filaments in electron microscopy of Alzheimer's disease. *Nature* **197**, 192–3.

Kivipelto, M., Helkala, E-L., Laakso, M.P., *et al.* (2001). Midlife vascular risk factors and Alzheimer's disease in later life: longitudinal, population based study. *Br. Med. J.* **322**, 1447–51.

Klünemann, H.H., Fronhöfer, W., Wurster, H., Fischer, W., Ibach, B., and Klein, H.E. (2002). Alzheimer's second patient: Johann F. and his family. *Ann. Neurol.* **52**, 520–3.

Klunk, W.E., Engler, H., Nordberg, A., *et al.* (2004). Imaging brain amyloid in Alzheimer's disease with Pittsburgh Compound-B. *Ann. Neurol.* **55**, 306–19.

Knopman, D.S., DeKosky, S.T., Cummings, J.L., *et al.* (2001). Practice parameter: diagnosis of dementia (an evidence-based review). Report of the Quality Standards Subcommittee of the American Academy of Neurology. *Neurology* **56**, 1143–53.

Knott, V., Mohr, E., Mahoney, C., and Ilivitsky, V. (2001). Quantitative electroencephalography in Alzheimer's disease: comparison with a control group, population norms and mental status. *J. Psychiatry Neurosci.* **26**, 106–16.

Lanctôt, K.L., Herrmann, N., Yau, K.K., *et al.* (2003). Efficacy and safety of cholinesterase inhibitors in Alzheimer's disease: a meta-analysis. *Can. Med. Assoc. J.* **169**, 557–64.

Larner, A.J. (1995*a*). Hypothesis: physiological and pathological interrelationships of amyloid β peptide and the amyloid precursor protein. *BioEssays* **17**, 819–24.

Larner, A.J. (1995*b*). The cortical neuritic dystrophy of Alzheimer's disease: nature, significance, and possible pathogenesis. *Dementia* **6**, 218–24.

Larner, A.J. (1997*a*). Neurite growth-inhibitory properties of amyloid β-peptides *in vitro*: Aβ25–35, but not Aβ1–40, is inhibitory. *Neurosci. Res. Commun.* **20**, 147–55.

Larner, A.J. (1997*b*). The pathogenesis of Alzheimer disease: an alternative to the amyloid hypothesis. *J. Neuropathol. Exp. Neurol.* **56**, 214–15.

Larner, A.J. (1997*c*). The cerebellum in Alzheimer's disease: a review. *Dementia Geriatr. Cogn. Dis.* **8**, 203–9.

Larner, A.J. (1999). Hypothesis: amyloid β-peptides truncated at the N-terminus contribute to the pathogenesis of Alzheimer's disease. *Neurobiol. Aging* **20**, 65–9.

Larner, A.J. (2000). Neuronal apoptosis as a therapeutic target in neurodegenerative disease. *Expert Opin. Therapeutic Patents* **10**, 1493–518.

Larner, A.J. (2001). N-terminally truncated amyloid β-peptides and Alzheimer's disease. *Neurobiol. Aging* **22**, 343.

Larner, A.J. (2002). Alzheimer's disease: targets for drug development. *Mini Rev. Medicinal Chem.* **2**, 1–9.

Larner, A.J. (2003*a*). MMSE subscores and the diagnosis of dementia with Lewy bodies. *Int. J. Geriatr. Psychiatry* **18**, 855–6.

Larner, A.J. (2003*b*). Use of the internet and of the NHS Direct telephone helpline for medical information by a cognitive function clinic population. *Int. J. Geriatr. Psychiatry* **18**, 118–22.

Larner, A.J. (2004*a*). Getting it wrong: the clinical misdiagnosis of Alzheimer's disease. *Int. J. Clin. Pract.* **58**, 1092–4.

Larner, A.J. (2004*b*). Use of MMSE to differentiate Alzheimer's disease from dementia with Lewy bodies. *Int. J. Geriatr. Psychiatry* **19**, 1209–10.

Larner, A.J. (2004*c*). Cholinesterase inhibitor use at a cognitive function clinic. *Prog. Neurol. Psychiatry* **8** (4), 14, 18, 20.

Larner, A.J. (2004*d*). Secretases as therapeutic targets in Alzheimer's disease: patents 2000–2004. *Expert Opin. Therapeutic Patents* **14**, 1403–20.

Larner, A.J. (2005*a*). 'Dementia unmasked': atypical, acute aphasic, presentations of neurodegenerative dementing disease. *Clin. Neurol. Neurosurg.* **108**, 8–10.

Larner, A.J. (2005*b*). An audit of the Addenbrooke's Cognitive Examination (ACE) in clinical practice. *Int. J. Geriatr. Psychiatry* **20**, 593–4.

Larner, A.J. (2005*c*). Gardening and dementia. *Int. J. Geriatr. Psychiatry* **20**, 796–7.

Larner, A.J. (2006*a*). 'Frontal variant Alzheimer's disease': a reappraisal. *Clin. Neurol. Neurosurg.* **108** (7), 705–8.

Larner, A.J. (2006*b*). *A dictionary of neurological signs*, 2nd edition. Springer, New York.

Larner, A.J. (2006*c*). Neurological signs of aging. In *Principles and practice of geriatric medicine*, 4th edn (ed. M.S.J. Pathy, A.J. Sinclair, and J.E. Morley), pp. 743–50. Wiley, Chichester.

Larner, A.J. (2006*d*). An audit of the Addenbrooke's Cognitive Examination (ACE) in clinical practice. 2. Longitudinal change. *Int. J. Geriatr. Psychiatry* **21** (7), 698–9.

Larner, A.J. and Doran, M. (2002). Broader assessment needed for treatment decisions in AD. *Prog. Neurol. Psychiatry* **6** (3), 5–6.

Larner, A.J. and Doran, M. (2004). Prion disease at a regional neuroscience centre: retrospective audit. *J. Neurol. Neurosurg. Psychiatry* **75**, 1789–90.

Larner, A.J. and Doran, M. (2006). Clinical phenotypic heterogeneity of Alzheimer's disease associated with mutations of the presenilin-1 gene. *J. Neurol.* **253**, 139–58.

Larner, A.J. and Sofroniew. M.V. (2003). Mechanisms of cellular damage and recovery. In *Handbook of neurological rehabilitation*, 2nd edn (ed. R.J. Greenwood, M.P. Barnes, T.M. McMillan, and C.D. Ward), pp. 71–98. Psychology Press, Hove.

Launer, L.J., Andersen, K., Dewey, M.E., *et al.* (1999). Rates and risk factors for dementia and Alzheimer's disease: results from EURODEM pooled analyses. EURODEM Incidence Research Group and Work groups. European Studies of Dementia. *Neurology* **52**, 78–84.

Levine, D.N., Lee, J.M., and Fisher, C.M. (1993). The visual variant of Alzheimer's disease: a clinicopathologic case study. *Neurology* **43**, 305–13.

Levy-Lahad, E., Wasco, W., Poorkaj, P., *et al.* (1995). Candidate gene for the chromosome 1 familial Alzheimer's disease locus. *Science* **269**, 973–7.

Lippa, C.F., Fujiwara, H., Mann, D.M.A., *et al.* (1998). Lewy bodies contain altered α-synuclein in brains of many familial Alzheimer's disease patients with mutations in presenilin and amyloid precursor protein genes. *Am. J. Pathol.* **153**, 1365–70.

Lithell, H., Hansson, L., Skoog, I., *et al.* for the SCOPE Study Group (2003). The Study on Cognition and Prognosis in the Elderly (SCOPE): principal results of a randomized double-blind intervention trial. *J. Hypertens.* **21**, 875–86.

Lopez, O.L., Becker, J.T., Wisniewski, S., Saxton, J., Kaufer, D.I., and DeKosky, S.T. (2002). Cholinesterase inhibitor treatment alters the natural history of Alzheimer's disease. *J. Neurol. Neurosurg. Psychiatry* **72**, 310–14.

Lowenberg, K. and Waggoner. R.W. (1934). Familial organic psychosis (Alzheimer's type). *Arch. Neurol. Psychiatry* **31**, 737–54.

Lozsadi, D.A. and Larner, A.J. (2006). Prevalence and causes of seizures at the time of diagnosis of probable Alzheimer's disease. *Dementia Geriatr. Cogn. Dis.* **22**, 121–4.

Mackenzie Ross, S.J., Graham, N., Stuart-Green, L., *et al.* (1996). Progressive biparietal atrophy: an atypical presentation of Alzheimer's disease. *J. Neurol. Neurosurg. Psychiatry* **61**, 388–95.

Maguire, C.P., Kirby, M., Coen, R., Coakley, D., Lawlor, B.A., and O'Neill, D. (1996). Family members' attitudes toward telling the patient with Alzheimer's disease their diagnosis. *Br. Med. J.* **313**, 529–30.

Martin, J.J., Gheuens, J., Bruyland, M., *et al.* (1991). Early-onset Alzheimer's disease in 2 large Belgian families. *Neurology* **41**, 62–8.

Masse, I., Bordet, R., Deplanque, D., *et al.* (2005). Lipid lowering agents are associated with a slower cognitive decline in Alzheimer's disease. *J. Neurol. Neurosurg. Psychiatry* **76**, 1624–9.

Mathuranath, P.S., Nestor, P.J., Berrios, G.E., Rakowicz, W., and Hodges, J.R. (2000). A brief cognitive test battery to differentiate Alzheimer's disease and frontotemporal dementia. *Neurology* **55**, 1613–20.

McGeer, P.L., Schulzer, M., and McGeer, E.G. (1996). Arthritis and anti-inflammatory agents as possible protective factors for Alzheimer's disease: a review of 17 epidemiologic studies. *Neurology* 47, 425–32.

McKee, A.C., Kosik, K.S., and Kowall, N.W. (1991). Neuritic pathology and dementia in Alzheimer's disease. *Ann. Neurol.* 30, 156–65.

McKeith, I.G., Ballard, C.G., Perry, R.H., *et al.* (2000). Prospective validation of consensus criteria for the diagnosis of dementia with Lewy bodies. *Neurology* 54, 1050–8.

McKhann, G., Drachman, D., Folstein, M., *et al.* (1984). Clinical diagnosis of Alzheimer's disease. Report of the NINCDS-ADRDA work group under the auspices of the Department of Health and Human Service Task forces on Alzheimer's disease. *Neurology* 34, 939–44.

Mehta, N.D., Refolo, L.M., Eckman, C., *et al.* (1998). Increased Aβ42(43) from cell lines expressing presenilin 1 mutations. *Ann. Neurol.* **43**, 256–8.

Mendez, M.F. and Lim, G.T.H. (2003). Seizures in elderly patients with dementia: epidemiology and management. *Drugs Aging* **20**, 791–803.

Mendez, M.F. and Zander, B.A. (1991). Dementia presenting with aphasia: clinical characteristics. *J. Neurol. Neurosurg. Psychiatry* **54**, 542–5.

Mendez, M.F., Ghajarania, M., and Perryman, K.M. (2002). Posterior cortical atrophy: clinical characteristics and differences compared to Alzheimer's disease. *Dementia Geriatr. Cogn. Dis.* **14**, 33–40.

Mendiondo, M.S., Ashford, J.W., Kryscio, R.J., and Schmitt, F.A. (2000). Modelling Mini Mental State Examination changes in Alzheimer's disease. *Statistics Med.* **19**, 1607–16.

Mesulam, M.M. (2001). Primary progressive aphasia. *Ann. Neurol.* **49**, 425–32.

Mills, C.K. (1900). A case of unilateral ascending paralysis probably presenting a new form of degenerative disease. *J. Nerv. Ment. Dis.* **27**, 195–200.

Mioshi, E., Dawson, K., Mitchell, J., Arnold, R., and Hodges, J.R. (2006). The Addenbrooke's Cognitive Examination Revised (ACE-R): a brief cognitive test battery for dementia screening. *Int. J. Geriatr. Psychiatry* **21**, 1078–85.

Mirra, S.S., Heyman, A., McKeel, D., *et al.* (1991). The Consortium to Establish a Registry for Alzheimer's Disease (CERAD). Part II. Standardization of the neuropathologic assessment of Alzheimer's disease. *Neurology* **41**, 479–86.

Morris, J., Heyman, A., Mohs, R., *et al.* (1989). The Consortium to Establish a Registry for Alzheimer's Disease (CERAD). Part I. Clinical and neuropsychological assessment of Alzheimer's disease. *Neurology* **39**, 1159–65.

Mountjoy, C.Q., Roth, M., Evans, N.J.R., and Evans, H.M. (1983). Cortical neuronal counts in normal elderly controls and demented patients. *Neurobiol. Aging* **4**, 1–11.

MRC CFAS (2001). Pathological correlates of late-onset dementia in a multicentre, community-based population in England and Wales. Neuropathology Group of the Medical Research Council Cognitive Function and Ageing Study. *Lancet* **357**, 169–75.

Nachev, P.C. and Larner, A.J. (1996). Zinc and Alzheimer's disease. *Trace Elements Electrolytes* **13**, 55–9.

Näslund, J., Haroutunian, V., Mohs, R., *et al.* (2000). Correlation between elevated levels of amyloid β-peptide in the brain and cognitive decline. *J. Am. Med. Assoc.* **283**, 1571–7.

National Institute on Aging and Reagan Institute Working Group on Diagnostic Criteria for the Neuropathological Assessment of Alzheimer Disease (1997). Consensus recommendations for the post-mortem diagnosis of Alzheimer's disease. *Neurobiol. Aging* **18** (suppl. 14), S1–2.

National Institute for Clinical Excellence (2001). *Guidance on the use of donepezil, rivastigmine and galantamine for the treatment of Alzheimer's disease*, Technology Appraisal Guidance No. 19. NICE, London.

Natté, R., Maat-Schieman, M.L.C., Haan, J., Bornebroek, M., Roos, R.A.C., and van Duinen, S.G. (2001). Dementia in hereditary cerebral hemorrhage with amyloidosis-Dutch type is associated with cerebral amyloid angiopathy but is independent of plaques and neurofibrillary tangles. *Ann. Neurol.* **50**, 765–72.

Nicoll, J.A.R., Roberts, G.W., and Graham, D.I. (1995). Apolipoprotein E epsilon-4 allele is associated with deposition of amyloid beta-protein following head injury. *Nature Med.* **1**, 135–7.

Nicoll, J.A.R., Wilkinson, D., Holmes, C., Steart, P., Markham, H., and Weller, R.O. (2003). Neuropathology of human Alzheimer disease after immunization with amyloid-beta peptide: a case report. *Nature Med.* **9**, 448–52.

Nolan, K.A., Lino, M.M., Seligmann, A.W., *et al.* (1998). Absence of vascular dementia in an autopsy series from a dementia clinic. *J. Am. Geriatr. Soc.* **46**, 597–604.

Oken, B.S., Storzbach, D.M., and Kaye, J.A. (1998). The efficacy of *Ginkgo biloba* on cognitive function in Alzheimer disease. *Arch. Neurol.* **55**, 1409–15.

O'Neill, D. (2005). Driving. In *Dementia*, 3rd edn (ed. A. Burns, J. O'Brien, and D. Ames), pp. 244–51. Hodder Arnold, London.

Pantel, J. and Schröder, J. (1996). Posterior cortical atrophy—a new dementia syndrome or a form of Alzheimer's disease? [in German]. *Fortschr. Neurol. Psychiat.* **64**, 492–508.

Perry, E.K., Kilford, L., Lees, A.J., Burn, D., and Perry, R.H. (2003). Increased Alzheimer pathology in Parkinson's disease related to antimuscarinic drugs. *Ann. Neurol.* **54**, 235–8.

Petersen, R.C. (ed.) (2003). *Mild cognitive impairment. Aging to Alzheimer's disease.* Oxford University Press, Oxford.

Petersen, R.C. (2004). Mild cognitive impairment as a diagnostic entity. *J. Intern. Med.* **256**, 183–94.

Petersen, R.C., Thomas, R.G., Grundman, M., *et al.* (2005). Vitamin E and donepezil for the treatment of mild cognitive impairment. *N. Engl. J. Med.* **352**, 2379–88.

Pogacar, S. and Williams, R.S. (1984). Alzheimer's disease presenting as slowly progressive aphasia. *R. I. Med. J.* **67**, 181–5.

Poirier, J. (1994). Apolipoprotein E in CNS models of CNS injury and in Alzheimer's disease. *Trends Neurosci.* **17**, 525–30.

Polvikoski, T., Sulkava, R., Haltia, M., *et al.* (1995). Apolipoprotein E, dementia, and cortical deposition of β-amyloid protein. *N. Engl. J. Med.* **333**, 1242–7.

Profenno, L., Tariot, P., Loy, R., and Ismail, S. (2005). Treatments for behavioural and psychological symptoms in Alzheimer's disease and other dementias. In *Dementia*, 3rd edn (ed. A. Burns, J. O'Brien, and D. Ames), pp. 482–98. Hodder Arnold, London.

Reinwald, S., Westner, I.M., and Niedermaier, N. (2004). Rapidly progressive Alzheimer's disease mimicking Creutzfeldt–Jakob disease. *J. Neurol.* **251**, 1020–2.

Reisberg, B., Doody, R., Stöffler, A., Schmitt, F., Ferris, S., Möbius, H.J. for the Memantine Study Group (2003). Memantine in moderate-to-severe Alzheimer's disease. *N. Engl. J. Med.* **348**, 1333–41.

Ritchie, C.W., Bush, A.I., Mackinnon, A., *et al.* (2003). Metal–protein attenuation with iodochlorhydroxyquin (clioquinol) targeting Aβ amyloid deposition and toxicity in Alzheimer's disease; a pilot phase 2 clinical trial. *Arch. Neurol.* **60**, 1685–91.

Ritchie, C.W., Ames, D., Clayton, T., and Lai, R. (2004). Metaanalysis of randomized trials of the efficacy and safety of donepezil, galantamine and rivastigmine for the treatment of Alzheimer disease. *Am. J. Geriatr. Psychiatry* **12**, 358–69.

Roberts, G.W., Gentlemen, S.M., Lynch, A., and Graham, D.I. (1991). βA4 amyloid protein deposition in brain after head trauma. *Lancet* **338**, 1422–3.

Roberts, G.W., Gentlemen, S.M., Lynch, A., Murray, L., Landon, M., and Graham, D.I. (1994). Beta amyloid protein deposition in the brain after severe head injury: implications for the pathogenesis of Alzheimer's disease. *J. Neurol. Neurosurg. Psychiatry* **57**, 419–25.

Robertson, B., Blennow, K., Gottfries, C.G., and Wallin, A. (1998). Delirium in dementia. *Int. J. Geriatr. Psychiatry* **13**, 49–56.

Rockwood, K., Cosway, S., Carver, D., *et al.* (1999). The risk of dementia and death following delirium. *Age Ageing* **28**, 551–6.

Rockwood, K., Kirkland, S., Hogan, D.B., *et al.* (2002). Use of lipid-lowering agents, indication bias, and the risk of dementia in community-dwelling elderly people. *Arch. Neurol.* **59**, 223–7.

Rogaev, E.I., Sherrington, R., Rogaeva, E.A., *et al.* (1995). Familial Alzheimer's disease in kindreds with missense mutations in a gene on chromosome 1 related to Alzheimer's disease type 3. *Nature* **376**, 775–8.

Rosen, W.G., Mohs, R.C., and Davis, K.L. (1984). A new rating scale for Alzheimer's disease. *Am. J. Psychiatry* **141**, 1356–64.

Roses, A.D. (1996). Apolipoprotein E alleles as risk factors in Alzheimer's disease. *Ann. Rev. Med.* **47**, 387–400.

Rossor, M.N., Tyrrell, P.J., Warrington, E.K., Thompson, P.D., Marsden, C.D., and Lantos, P. (1999). Progressive frontal gait disturbance with atypical Alzheimer's disease and corticobasal degeneration. *J. Neurol. Neurosurg. Psychiatry* **67**, 345–52.

Royall, D.R. (2000). Executive cognitive impairment: a novel perspective on dementia. *Neuroepidemiology* **19**, 293–9.

Salloway, S., Ferris, S., Kluger, A., *et al.* (2004). Efficacy of donepezil in mild cognitive impairment: a randomized placebo-controlled trial. *Neurology* **63**, 651–7.

Sano, M., Ernesto, C., Thomas, R.G., *et al.* (1997). A controlled trial of selegiline, alpha-tocopherol, or both as treatment for Alzheimer's disease. The Alzheimer's Disease Cooperative Study. *N. Engl. J. Med.* **336**, 1216–22.

Saunders, A.M. (2001). Apolipoprotein E as a risk factor for Alzheimer's disease. In *Neurobiology of Alzheimer's disease*, 2nd edn (ed. D. Dawbarn and S.J. Allen), pp. 207–26. Oxford University Press, Oxford.

Saunders, A.M., Strittmatter, W.J., Schmechel, D., *et al.* (1993). Association of apolipoprotein ε4 with late-onset familial and sporadic Alzheimer's disease. *Neurology* **43**, 1462–72.

Schenk, D., Barbour, R., Dunn, W., *et al.* (1999). Immunization with amyloid-β attenuates Alzheimer-disease-like pathology in the PDAPP mouse. *Nature* **400**, 173–7.

Scheuner, D., Eckman, C., Jensen, M., *et al.* (1996). Secreted amyloid β-protein similar to that in the amyloid plaques of Alzheimer's disease is increased in vivo by the presenilin 1 and 2 and APP mutations linked to familial Alzheimer's disease. *Nature Med.* **2**, 864–70.

Sherrington, R., Rogaev, E.I., Liang, Y., *et al.* (1995). Cloning of a gene bearing missense mutations in early-onset familial Alzheimer's disease. *Nature* **375**, 754–60.

Shobab, L.A., Hsiung, G-Y.R., and Feldman, H.H. (2005). Cholesterol in Alzheimer's disease. *Lancet Neurol.* **4**, 841–52.

Shulman, K. and Feinstein, A. (2003). *Quick cognitive screening for clinicians: mini mental, clock drawing and other brief tests.* Martin Dunitz, London.

Shumaker, S.A., Legault, C., Rapp, S.R., *et al.* (2003). Estrogen plus progestin and the incidence of dementia and mild cognitive impairment in postmenopausal women: the Women's Health Initiative Memory Study: a randomized controlled trial. *J. Am. Med. Assoc.* **289**, 2651–62.

Silverman, D., Small, G., Chang, C., *et al.* (2001). Positron emission tomography in evaluation of dementia—regional brain metabolism and long-term outcome. *J. Am. Med. Assoc.* **286**, 2120–7.

Simchowicz, T. (1911). Histologische Studien über die Senile Demenz. In *Histologische und histopathologische Arbeiten über die Grosshirnrinde mit besonderer Beruchsichtigung der pathologischen Anatomie der Geisteskrankheiten* (ed. F. Nissl and A. Alzheimer), Vol. 4, pp. 267–444. Fischer, Jena.

Simons, M., Schwärzler, F., Lütjohann, D., *et al.* (2002). Treatment with simvastatin in normocholesterolemic patients with Alzheimer's disease: a 26-week randomized, placebo-controlled, double-blind trial. *Ann. Neurol.* **52**, 346–50.

Snowdon, D.A., Kemper, S.J., Mortimer, J.A., Greiner, L.H., Wekstein, D.R., and Markesbery, W.R. (1996). Linguistic ability in early life and cognitive function and Alzheimer's disease in late life. *J. Am. Med. Assoc.* **275**, 528–32.

Snowdon, D.A., Greiner, L.H., Mortimer, J.A., *et al.* (1997). Brain infarction and the clinical expression of Alzheimer disease. The Nun Study. *J. Am. Med. Assoc.* **277**, 813–17.

Stern, R.G., Mohs, R.C., Davidson, M., *et al.* (1994). A longitudinal study of Alzheimer's disease: measurement, rate and predictors of cognitive deterioration. *Am. J. Psychiatry* **151**, 390–6.

Stewart, R. (2005). Vascular factors in Alzheimer's disease. In *Dementia*, 3rd edn (ed. A. Burns, J. O'Brien, and D. Ames), pp. 436–43. Hodder Arnold, London.

Tabira, T., Chui, D.H., Nakayama, H., Kuroda, S., and Shibuya, M. (2002). Alzheimer's disease with spastic paresis and cotton wool type plaques. *J. Neurosci. Res.* **70**, 367–72.

Talbot, P.R., Lloyd, J.J., Snowden, J.S., Neary, D., and Testa, H.J. (1998). A clinical role for ^{99m}Tc-HMPAO SPECT in the investigation of dementia? *J. Neurol. Neurosurg. Psychiatry* **64**, 306–13.

Tariot, P.N., Farlow, M.R., Grossberg, G.T., *et al.* (2004). Memantine treatment in patients with moderate to severe Alzheimer disease already receiving donepezil: a randomized controlled trial. *J. Am. Med. Assoc.* **291**, 317–24.

Terry, R.D. (1963). The fine structure of neurofibrillary tangles in Alzheimer's disease. *J. Neuropathol. Exp. Neurol.* **22**, 629–41.

Terry, R.D., Masliah, E., Salmon, D.P., *et al.* (1991). Physical basis of cognitive alterations in Alzheimer's disease: synapse loss is the major correlate of cognitive impairment. *Ann. Neurol.* **30**, 572–80.

Tschampa, H.J., Neumann, M., Zerr, I., *et al.* (2001). Patients with Alzheimer's disease and dementia with Lewy bodies mistaken for Creutzfeldt–Jakob disease. *J. Neurol. Neurosurg. Psychiatry* **71**, 33–9.

Tzourio, C., Anderson, C., Cahpman, N., *et al.* for the PROGRESS Collaborative Group (2003). Effects of blood pressure lowering with perindopril and indapamide therapy on dementia and cognitive decline in patients with cerebrovascular disease. *Arch. Intern. Med.* **163**, 1069–75.

Van Broeckhoven, C., Backhoven, H., Cruts, M., *et al.* (1994). ApoE genotype does not modulate age of onset in families with chromosome 14 encoded Alzheimer's disease. *Neurosci. Lett.* **169**, 179–80.

van Gool, W.A., Aisen, P.S., and Eikelenboom, P. (2003). Anti-inflammatory therapy in Alzheimer's disease: is hope still alive? *J. Neurol.* **250**, 788–92.

Verghese, J., Lipton, R.B., Katz, M.J., *et al.* (2003). Leisure activities and risk of dementia in the elderly. *N. Engl. J. Med.* **348**, 2508–16.

Volicer, L., Harper, D.G., Manning, B.C., Goldstein, R., and Satlin, A. (2001). Sundowning and circadian rhythms in Alzheimer's disease. *Am. J. Psychiatry* **158**, 704–11.

Waegemans, T., Wilsher, C.R., Danniau, A., Ferris, S.H., Kurz, A., and Winblad, B. (2002). Clinical efficacy of piracetam in cognitive impairment: a meta-analysis. *Dementia Geriatr. Cogn. Dis.* **13**, 217–24.

Waldemar, G., Dubois, B., Emre, M., Scheltens, P., Tanska, P., and Rossor, M. (2000). Diagnosis and management of Alzheimer's disease and other disorders associated with dementia. The role of neurologists in Europe. European Federation of Neurological Societies. *Eur. J. Neurol.* **7**, 133–44.

Warren, J.D., Schott, J.M., Fox, N.C., *et al.* (2005). Brain biopsy in dementia. *Brain* **128**, 2016–25.

Whitehouse, P.J., Price, D.L., Struble, R.G., Clark, A.W., Coyle, J.T., and Delon, M.R. (1982). Alzheimer's disease and senile dementia: loss of neurons in the basal forebrain. *Science* **215**, 1237–9.

Wilcock, G.K. (2003). Memantine for the treatment of dementia. *Lancet Neurol.* **2**, 503–5.

Wilcock, G., Birks, J., Whitehead, A., and Evans, J.G. (2002). The effect of selegiline in the treatment of people with Alzheimer's disease; a meta-analysis of published trials. *Int. J. Geriatr. Psychiatry* **17**, 175–83.

Wilcock, G., Howe, I., Coles, H., *et al.* (2003). A long-term comparison of galantamine and donepezil in the treatment of Alzheimer's disease. *Drugs Aging* **20**, 777–89.

Wilson, R.S., Mendes de Leon, C.F., Barnes, L.L., *et al.* (2002). Participation in cognitively stimulating activities and risk of incident Alzheimer disease. *J. Am. Med. Assoc.* **287**, 742–8.

Winblad, B. and Poritis, N. (1999). Memantine in severe dementia: results of the 9M-Best Study. Benefit and efficacy in severely demented patients during treatment with memantine. *Int. J. Geriatr. Psychiatry* **14**, 135–46.

Wischik, C.M., Novak, M., Thogersen, H.C., *et al.* (1988). Isolation of a fragment of tau from the core of the paired helical filament of Alzheimer's disease. *Proc. Natl. Acad. Sci. USA* **85**, 4506–10.

Wisniewski, H.M., Wegiel, J., and Kotula, L. (1996). Some neuropathological aspects of Alzheimer's disease and its relevance to other disciplines. *Neuropathol. Appl. Neurobiol.* **22**, 3–11.

Wolozin, B., Kellman, W., Ruosseau, P., Celesia, G.G., and Siegel, G. (2000). Decreased prevalence of Alzheimer disease associated with 3-hydroxy-3-methylglutaryl coenzyme A reductase inhibitors. *Arch. Neurol.* **57**, 1439–43.

Zandi, P.P., Carlson, M.C., Plassman, B.L., *et al.* (2002). Hormone replacement therapy and incidence of Alzheimer disease in older women: the Cache County Study. *J. Am. Med. Assoc.* **288**, 2123–9.

Zandi, P.P., Anthony, J.C., Khachaturian, A.S., *et al.* (2004). Reduced risk of Alzheimer disease in users of antioxidant vitamin supplements: the Cache County Study. *Arch. Neurol.* **61**, 82–8.

Zandi, P.P., Sparks, D.L., Khachaturian, A.S., *et al.* (2005). Do statins reduce risk of incident dementia and Alzheimer disease? The Cache County Study. *Arch. Gen. Psychiatry* **62**, 217–24.

Chapter 12

Frontotemporal lobar degeneration

Jared Narvid and Maria Luisa Gorno-Tempini

12.1 Definition

- FTLD may present with clinical features of progressive behavioural or linguistic deterioration (or a combination of the two), depending on whether the frontal or temporal lobes are the focus of greatest pathological involvement.
- Linguistic dysfunction may produce either a fluent or nonfluent picture.
- Cases with the fluent variety are often labelled 'semantic dementia' (SD) as the principal deficit seems to be in the brain's ability to represent meaning (or semantics).
- Nonfluent cases exhibit problems with the more peripheral aspects of linguistic processing (e.g. phonology, syntax, articulation, or any combination of these).

Frontotemporal lobar degeneration (FTLD) is a syndrome of focal, often asymmetric neurodegeneration, presenting clinically as a progressive dementia associated with focal atrophy of the frontal and/or temporal lobes. The disease is capable of producing striking changes in personality, behaviour, and language, with a diverse range of clinical presentations.

Two major clinical presentations of FTLD are recognized. In the frontal variant—usually designated frontotemporal dementia (FTD)—the emergence of disinhibition, mental rigidity, stereotyped and perseverative behaviour, hyperorality, and loss of insight give rise to marked changes in personality. An aphasic variant—designated primary progressive aphasia (PPA)—is also recognized. Patients with PPA present with relatively isolated disturbances of language, and can be further categorized on the basis of the fluency of their spontaneous speech. Patients with the fluent variant appear to have difficulty expressing and understanding *meaning*, a syndrome that has been given the name semantic dementia (SD). In contrast, the nonfluent variant—progressive nonfluent aphasia (PNFA)—manifests as a laboured, often agrammatic spoken output, with severe problems in word retrieval but normal comprehension of individual words. Needless to say, these distinctions are not rigid, and many patients present with an amalgamation of behavioural disturbance, progressive aphasia, and semantic deficits. Moreover, because FTLD can be associated with degeneration of cortical and bulbar motor neurons and anterior horn cells of the spinal cord, some patients with FTD, SD, or PNFA also meet clinical criteria for amyotrophic lateral sclerosis (ALS).

FTLD is histopathologically distinct from Alzheimer's disease (AD) but is nonetheless heterogeneous. Recent insights from molecular, biochemical, and genetic investigations of FTLD have raised awareness of this heterogeneity, catalysing debate about the pathological and clinical classification of FTLD, its subvariants, and its related disorders. These factors have made the nosology of FTD controversial and confusing.

Although, as we shall see, the range of pathological processes underpinning FTLD is diverse, the nature of first presenting symptoms probably depends more on the distribution of pathological involvement than on its molecular characteristics.

12.2 **Epidemiology**

- FTLD is as common a cause of dementia as Alzheimer's disease in the under-65 age group.

The lack (until very recently) of complete consensus concerning the criteria for neuropathological diagnosis of FTLD has given rise to widely divergent estimates of its incidence. In a recent study from the UK, record review in the specialty clinic and hospitals in several communities in Cambridge was used to identify dementia cases. In that survey, the prevalence of FTLD in patients aged 45 to 64 from a population of approximately 300 000 individuals in Cambridgeshire, England was estimated to be of the order of 15 per 100 000 (Ratnavalli *et al.* 2002). The figure was identical to the prevalence of early-onset AD in the same population, suggesting that FTLD is a common cause of dementia in patients under 65 years of age. Another study of FTLD prevalence in the Netherlands (Rosso *et al.* 2003) estimated the prevalence of FTD at 3.6 cases per 100 000 between the ages of 50 and 59 years, 9.4 per 100 000 between ages 60 and 69, and 3.8 per 100 000 between ages 70 and 79. The average age of onset was 57.6 years.

12.3 **Aetiological factors**

- As many as 45% of FTLD cases are likely to have a genetic component—mostly with an autosomal dominant pattern.
- Mutations in microtubule-associated protein tau (MAPT) on chromosome 17 have been found to be responsible for up to half of cases with a positive family history, though only in a minority of cases with autopsy proven tau pathology.
- Additional genetic, epigenetic and environmental factors remain to be discovered.

12.3.1 **Genetic (see also Chapter 15)**

A family history of dementia occurs in approximately 29–38% of patients with FTLD, and it has been estimated that having a first-degree relative with FTLD confers a 3.5 times higher risk of developing dementia (Stevens *et al.* 1998). A more recent study suggests that 38–45% of patients with FTLD have a strong hereditary component, with an autosomal dominant inheritance pattern in 80% of cases (Chow *et al.* 1999).

An important subgroup of FTLD has a genetically determined form of the disease that demonstrates linkage to DNA markers on chromosome 17. Individuals in these families often develop parkinsonian features, leading to a designation of FTD with parkinsonism linked to chromosome 17 (FTDP-17; Foster *et al.* 1997). Mutations in the tau gene, MAPT, have been revealed in many of these families (Pickering-Brown *et al.* 2002), leading to the estimate that approximately 10–50% of patients with a positive family history have a mutation in MAPT (Poorkaj *et al.* 2001; Morris and Balota 2001). One of the most common mutations is P301L, which produces a classic clinical phenotype and decreased microtubule binding *in vitro*. Histopathologically, however, P301L can generate changes consistent with corticobasal degeneration (CBD), Pick's disease with or without Pick bodies (PiD), and dementia lacking distinctive histology (DLDH). At this time, routine clinical testing for tau mutations is not available.

Persons with the P301L mutation exhibit a wide range in age of onset (40–75 years of age). Additional genetic and epigenetic factors must play a role in the development to the disease. In fact, mutations in other genes in addition to MAPT are likely to be involved in the development of FTLD. A different locus on chromosome 17q21–22 may lead to familial FTD in one Dutch family (Chan *et al.* 2001*b*). Familial FTLD associated with motor neuron disease has been linked to chromosome 9q21–22 (Hosler *et al.* 2000). A syndrome of hereditary FTLD associated with inclusion body myopathy and Paget's disease of bone has been linked to a locus on chromosome 9 (9p13.3-p12; Kovach *et al.* 2001). A locus in the pericentromeric region of chromosome 3 has also been identified in a Danish FTLD family (Skibinski *et al.* 2005).

12.3.2 Acquired

To date, most cases of FTLD with tau pathology identified at autopsy have been found *not* to harbour a mutation in MAPT, while an analysis of two series of sporadic cases documented this finding in only 5.9–13% of such patients (Rosso and van Swieten 2002). It seems inevitable that further genetic, epigenetic, and environmental factors will be discovered to account for an increasing proportion of the remainder.

12.4 Clinical features

- Behavioural changes in frontal variant FTLD can take a variety of forms. The commonest are:
  - loss of social awareness;
  - disinhibition;
  - impulsivity;
  - apathy;
  - obsessionality (e.g. food faddism and hyperreligiosity).
- Semantic dementia is characterized by profound anomia in the context of fluent well-formed speech, normal day-to-day memory, and non-verbal problem solving, but impoverished knowledge of word and object meaning.
- Progressive nonfluent aphasia presents with distortion of speech output with relatively well preserved comprehension.
- Frontal and language-related features frequently co-occur, particularly at more advanced stages.

12.4.1 History

12.4.1.1 Frontotemporal dementia

Personality change and behavioural abnormalities characterize the patient with FTD. There is a loss of social graces and manners: for example, patients may touch strangers and disregard boundaries of personal space. Disinhibited verbal or physical behaviours often emerge, sometimes coinciding with withdrawal and apathy. Additional behavioural features include changes in dietary habits and eating behaviour, hyperorality, disinhibition, and distractability, stereotyped or perseverative behaviour, and altered speech output. Patients may demonstrate increased food consumption or excessive smoking or alcohol consumption, and initiate a preference for a certain type of food, such as sweets, or may try to eat inedible objects.

Disinhibition and distractability emerge as restlessness, impulsivity, irritiablity, aggressiveness, or excessive sentimentality. Sexual disinhibition can occur, but is usually harmless and easy to deflect. Stereotyped or perseverative behaviours include features such as impulse buying, hoarding, or compulsions. Hyperreligiosity, social withdrawal, and loss of drive have also been reported as common features of FTD (Neary *et al.* 1998).

Most patients deny their problems, or show a lack of concern regarding the condition. Decreased concern may extend to personal grooming and appearance, as well as concern for others. Lack of empathy, self-centredness, emotional coldness, and decreased concern about friends and family are commonly reported (Neary *et al.* 1998; Gregory and Hodges 1996; Rankin *et al.* 2005). Patients may appear self-absorbed and isolated, with a lack of concern for interpersonal relationship. This combination of loss of empathy and abnormal non-verbal communication (e.g. loss of facial expression and prosody) leads to an unnerving affect that makes other people uncomfortable—a phenomenon that stands in stark contrast to AD, where social graces seem to be preserved until late in the disease course.

12.4.1.2 Semantic dementia

Semantic dementia (SD) is a syndrome of progressive degradation of semantic knowledge about people, objects, facts, and words. The syndrome was first described in patients with progressive anomia who were recognized to have lost not only the ability to name objects, but also fundamental information about each item, leading to difficulties with category comprehension and object recognition (Warrington 1975). Following Mesulam's seminal report, more than 100 patients with progressive aphasia have been reported and it is now clear that two different syndromes were described: progressive fluent/semantic dementia (SD) and progressive nonfluent aphasia. Many of the patients with the fluent subtype of primary progressive aphasia described by Mesulam (1982) would now be classified as having SD (Grossman 2002).

The most common presenting complaint in SD involves language, and may be described as a 'loss of memory for words' or difficulties with 'meaning'. The core features of SD have been described as: (1) selective impairment of semantic memory causing severe anomia, impaired spoken and written single-word comprehension, and an impoverished fund of general knowledge about objects, persons, and the meanings of words; (2) relative sparing of other components of language output and comprehension, notably syntax and phonology; (3) normal visuoperceptual and spatial skills, working memory, and non-verbal problem-solving abilities; and (4) relatively preserved autobiographical and day-to-day (episodic) memory (Hodges *et al.* 1992). Although Alzheimer's dementia can also present with progressive difficulty with language, these deficits are virtually always overshadowed by impairments in new learning (episodic memory) (Bayles and Tomoeda 1983; Hodges *et al.* 1990), while the hallmark of SD is the opposite pattern (difficulties with semantic knowledge but relatively preserved episodic memory).

While SD patients are aware of their expressive deficits, they may be unaware of the extent of their comprehension problems. Speech is fluent but there are frequent semantic paraphasias, and use of substitute phrases such as 'thing' or 'stuff'. Errors in speech are almost always of the semantic variety, manifested by the intrusion of semantically related words (e.g. 'horse' for cow, or 'window' for door Poeck and Luzzatti 1988). Again, in contrast to patients with AD, recent memory tends to be preserved early in the course of SD. Instead, there is more difficulty with distant memory, such as autobiographical events, leading to a reversal of the temporally graded memory impairment that is observed in AD (Graham and Hodges 1997).

Repetition, prosody, syntax, and verb generation are generally well preserved. Associative agnosia may lead to difficulty with object recognition, resulting in failure to recognize common household items such as can-openers or pliers. An emergence of artistic talent has been observed in some patients with SD who have significant language impairment (Miller *et al.* 1998).

Most patients diagnosed with SD have prominent involvement of left temporal lobe structures, but a subgroup with more significant right brain involvement may present with progressive prosopagnosia (Evans *et al.* 1995). Unlike the prosopagnosia caused by right occipito-temporal lesions, which is limited to the visual domain, the prosopagnosia of SD extends to other modalities of information (Thompson *et al.* 2003). Similarly, left predominant SD patients have been shown to have greater difficulty with semantic tasks involving words, while right predominant have more trouble with faces (Snowden *et al.* 2004).

Behavioural changes similar to those seen in frontal variant FTD often arise as the disease progresses. Patients with right-sided disease tend to have more severe behavioural abnormalities than those with left-sided disease (Edwards-Lee *et al.* 1997; Thompson *et al.* 2003). The first symptom may be somatic (e.g. weight changes (gain or loss), sleep disturbance, decreased libido) or affective (e.g. irritability or apathy). Patients who present with SD develop behavioural symptoms after a mean of 3 years, while the patients who begin with behavioural symptoms typically develop semantic deficits within a similar time frame. The progression of symptoms most likely represents spread of atrophy to the contralateral temporal pole (Seeley *et al.* 2005).

12.4.1.2 Progressive non-fluent aphasia

This group has been studied less intensively than SD patients but the nature of the deficit represents an important contrast with SD (Hodges and Patterson 1996). Patients present with complaints of speech dysfluency or word finding difficulty. Distortion of speech output with both perturbed articulation and prosody remains the most prominent clinical feature of nonfluent progressive aphasia. Phonologic errors are usually obvious in conversation. Word finding pauses and agrammatic sentence output are also common. In the final stages of disease patients can become mute.

Clinically, PNFA should probably be distinguished from 'logopenic aphasia' in which speech is slow, with frequent word-finding pauses but without motor speech impairments. In addition, logopenic aphasia is characterized by more severely impaired repetition and sentence comprehension and the absence of grammatic errors. Anatomically, atrophy in logopenic aphasia occurs more posteriorly, in parietotemporal regions. This anatomy, along with the high prevalence of ApoE4 carriers in one series, raises suspicion that logopenic aphasia is associated with AD rather than FTLD pathology (Gorno-Tempini *et al.* 2004*a*).

12.4.2 Examination

Neurological examination of patients with FTLD typically reveals frontal release signs or primitive responses such as the grasp or pout reflexes. Extrapyramidal features such as rigidity and gait instability are not uncommon. Some patients may have a masked face, micrographia, and other secondary features of a parkinsonian syndrome, but a resting tremor is rare. Often mild oculomotor abnormalities (such as changes in smooth pursuit or mild ocular apraxia) and subtle reflex asymmetry can be present. At the bedside, tasks such as Luria (fist–hand–palm) and the Frontal Assessment Battery often unveil impairments in these patients. While motor symptoms are rare in SD, PNFA is often accompanied by mild motor slowing and incoordination in the right hand, and buccofacial apraxia (inability to execute or pantomime common actions involving the mouth and tongue) is also common.

Case Study

A 66-year-old, left-handed, retired physician was referred to the clinic due to a multiple-year history of behavioural changes. Approximately 5 years earlier, Dr Z. began to have problems with social function. On one occasion, he abandoned his two young grandchildren suggesting that they return home on their own in the dark. When asked about this incident, Dr Z. seemed unconcerned, and stated that they were familiar with the neighbourhood and should have been able to get home by themselves. Around the same time period, there were several incidents of sexually inappropriate behaviour. At a wedding rehearsal dinner, his sexual advances toward three different women caused considerable embarrassment. Shortly following his retirement in 2002, he began to drink heavily, consuming multiple glasses of wine in rapid succession. Dr Z. was referred for alcohol rehabilitation more than once, but each time left against medical advice after a few days. On several occasions, he entered his neighbour's garage and stole several bottles of expensive liquor. His family stated that his memory was 'excellent'. He did not lose objects such as his wallet or keys. He had no problems with fluency, comprehension, or naming. In the spatial domain, Dr Z. appeared to have no difficulties and gave excellent directions to his daughter on how to get about in central California. He travelled between cities by bus and successfully navigated multiple bus lines and transfers. His past medical history was unremarkable as was his family history. A basic neurological examination was essentially normal.

12.5 **Neuropsychology**

12.5.1 **FTD**

Patients and families typically describe few cognitive perturbations accompanying the behavioural changes. Indeed, some patients require residential care in spite of normal scores on screening cognitive tests such as the Mini-Mental State Exam (Gregory *et al.* 1999). Deficits on frontal/executive tasks are, however, a common finding on neuropsychological testing. These include tests of working memory, attention, set shifting, mental flexibility, verbal fluency, response inhibition, and abstract reasoning (Kramer *et al.* 2003; Rosen *et al.* 2004; Neary *et al.* 2005; Hodges *et al.* 1999). Nonetheless, isolated failure on such tasks is not sufficient to make the diagnosis of FTD, particularly given the considerable overlap with AD. Nonetheless, such findings have engendered the hypothesis that executive tests depend on dorsolateral prefrontal functioning rather than the orbitofrontal and ventromedial frontal areas affected early in FTD (Rosen *et al.* 2005; Liu *et al.* 2004).

On the other hand, poor performance on specific tests of verbal and visual memory is more specific for AD rather than FTD (Kertesz *et al.* 2003; Rosen *et al.* 2004); the same is true for tests of temporal and spatial orientation and praxis (Rascovsky *et al.* 2005). Clinicians must, however, view quantitative scores on visuospatial and memory tasks with a critical eye, due to these patients' poor attention and organization (Varma *et al.* 1999). Qualitative observations of performance on cognitive testing, and especially the presence of rule violations, perseverative errors, and confabulations, may be more helpful than quantitative scores in differentiating FTD from AD (Nedjam *et al.* 2004; Kramer *et al.* 2003).

12.5.2 **SD**

Language testing in SD reveals preserved phonology and syntax. Surface dyslexia is commonly (though not invariably) found, and presents as difficulty in reading words with irregular spellings (e.g. the word 'pint' read as if it rhymed with 'hint' or 'mint'). An analogous disorder of writing, surface dysgraphia, which results in the overgeneralization of sound-to-spelling conventions (e. g. spelling the spoken word *yacht* as 'yot'), is also seen. SD patients have difficulty with generating past tenses from low frequency verbs, which has implications for the role of semantic knowledge in basic linguistic functions (Patterson *et al.* 2001).

Due to their language difficulties, patients with SD may score poorly on bedside screening measures such as the Mini-Mental State Exam. However, more detailed testing reveals a loss of semantic knowledge, with relatively preserved episodic memory for recent events (Graham *et al.* 2000; Garrard and Hodges 2000). Patients are most impaired on tests such as category fluency (i.e. the number of animals or musical instruments generated in one minute), picture naming (Boston Naming Test), and generation of verbal definitions of words and pictures. Hodges and colleagues have shown that errors on these tasks initially reflect a loss of subordinate knowledge, or detailed items within categories, followed by a loss of more superordinate knowledge (the categories themselves). For example, a patient may initially misidentify an orange as a lemon; however with time, both are identified only as citrus, and eventually, only as fruit (Hodges *et al.* 1995).

Non-verbal semantic knowledge may be assessed with tests such as the Pyramids and Palm Trees Test (Howard and Patterson 1992), in which the subject is asked to judge which of two pictures is related to a third (see Fig. 12.1). Patients with SD perform poorly on other tests that do not require language, such as picture sorting, attribute judgement (Garrard and Carroll 2006), and drawing in which distinct category members may display similar generic characteristics (see Fig. 12.2; Bozeat *et al.* 2003). Finally, it should be noted that, in marked contrast to their performance on tests requiring semantic memory, SD patients show normal or near-normal scores performance on testing of auditory–verbal short-term memory (digit span), and visuospatial abilities (Rey–Osterreith complex figure).

12.5.3 **PNFA**

The linguistic profile of patients with PNFA is the mirror image of that found in SD. Nonfluent aphasics are substantially impaired only on tests requiring speech production, while single word

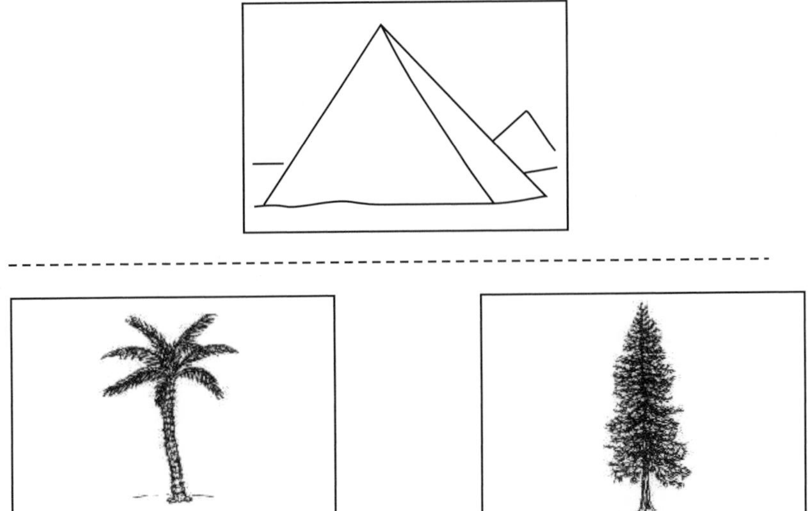

Fig. 12.1 Example of Pyramid and Palm Trees task. SD patients have difficulty due to lack of encyclopaedic knowledge—they cannot associate pyramids with the appropriate desert tree, the palm.

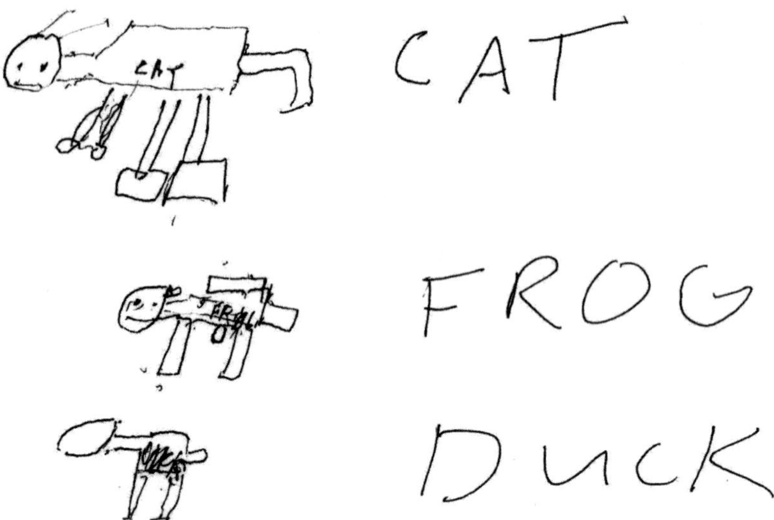

Fig. 12.2 SD patient's drawing of several animals. Notably, the animals are all the same & lack specific, defining characteristics.

comprehension is preserved. Speech may be more fluent when using a picture or other prompt than during spontaneous speech (Vandenberghe *et al.* 2005; Graham *et al.* 2004). Comprehension for syntactically complex constructions may be impaired, such that comprehension of even low frequency nominal terms is superior to performance on tests of syntactic comprehension (Weintraub *et al.* 1990).

Recent research has suggested a differential impairment in processing verbs and nouns (Rhee *et al.* 2001). Subtle speech apraxia can be demonstrated at the bedside by rapid repetition of multisyllabic, consonant-rich words that require moving quickly between articulators (e.g. 'artillery' or 'episcopal'). Impaired speech production in PNFA may, therefore, represent the merging of a language disorder with the failure of sensorimotor integration of speech (speech apraxia). Anatomically, this type of aphasia relates to atrophy of the left frontal operculum (Broca areas 44, 45, and 47), while the apraxia may relate to atrophy of the left anterior insula (Gorno-Tempini *et al.* 2004*a*). Although conversational speech is severely disrupted, the anomia is mild and the errors are phonological (e.g. 'efelant' for elephant). On tests of fluency, semantic category fluency is less profoundly affected than letter fluency. Word–picture matching, synonym tasks, and other semantic tests are usually performed perfectly. Likewise, performance on visuospatial and perceptual function tests is well preserved, as exemplified in Fig. 12.3.

12.6 **Imaging correlates (see Fig. 12.4)**

- Magnetic resonance imaging (MRI), single photon emission computerized tomography (SPECT), and ^{18}F fluorodeoxy-glucose positron emission tomography (FDG-PET) are all useful modalities for distinguishing early FTLD from AD.
- Behavioural and linguistic clinical features have been found to correlate with regional involvement.

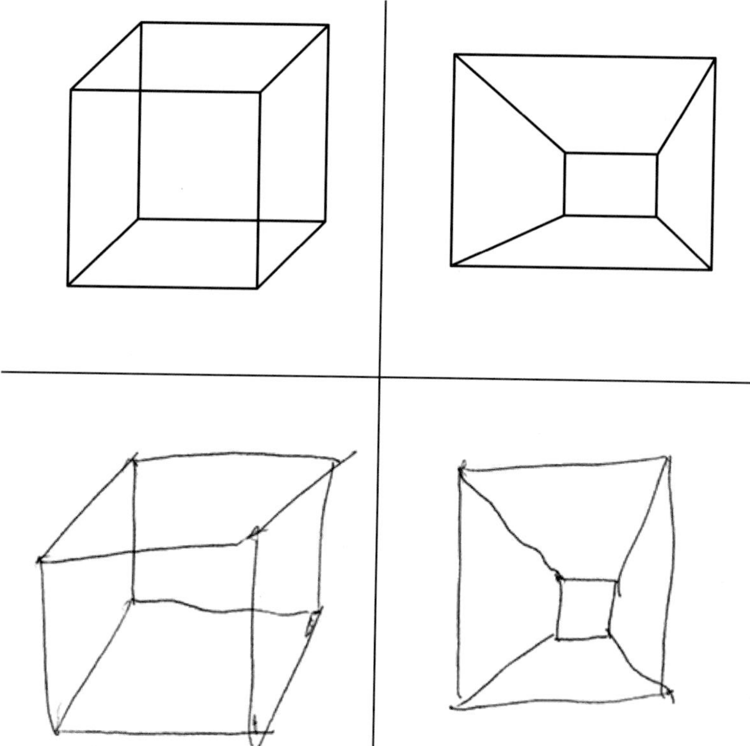

Fig. 12.3 Intact visuospatial processing in an FTD patient.

12.6.1 FTD

Physiological neuroimaging of blood flow abnormalities using Tc99-hexamethylyl-propyleneamine (HMPAO)-SPECT shows bilateral frontal hypoperfusion early in the course of frontal variant FTLD, and reliably differentiates these patients from those with AD (Miller *et al.* 1991). Fluorodeoxy-glucose (FDG)-PET demonstrates frontal hypometabolism in FTD (Hoffman *et al.* 2000). Unbiased analysis of T1-weighted MRI scans from patients with FTD has identified regions of significant atrophy in the ventromedial frontal cortex, the posterior orbital frontal regions bilaterally, the insula bilaterally, the left anterior cingulated cortex, the right dorsolateral frontal cortex, and the left premotor cortex as compared with controls and patients with SD (see Fig. 12.4 (left and centre panels); Rosen *et al.* 2002). Longitudinal measurements of MRI scans of patients with FTD show faster rates of frontal atrophy (4.1–4.5%) and similar rates of parieto-occipital atrophy (2.2–2.4%) as compared to patients with AD (2.4–2.8% per year, globally; Chan *et al.* 2001*b*). The corpus callosum can appear atrophic either anteriorly or more diffusely, differentiating FTD from AD in which the posterior is more prominently affected (Kaufer *et al.* 1997). FTD/ALS patients demonstrate atrophy in motor and premotor cortex, anterior temporal lobes, and middle and inferior frontal gyri (Chang *et al.* 2005).

Recent studies have correlated specific symptoms with patterns of regional atrophy. In this way, behavioural disturbance appears to correlate with degeneration of right hemispheric volumes (Liu *et al.* 2004; Seeley *et al.* 2005). Furthermore, disinhibiton correlates with ventromedial frontal cortex, apathy with anterior cingulate, aberrant motor behaviour with dorsal anterior

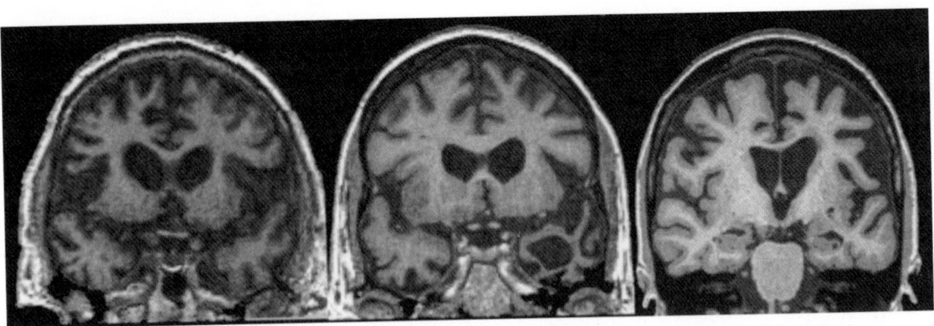

Fig. 12.4 Patterns of brain atrophy in FTD, SD, PNFA (from left to right, respectively). FTD shows marked degeneration of frontal lobes. SD degenerates temporal lobar volumes, often asymmetrically. PNFA is most associated with atrophy in left insula and inferior frontal gyrus.

cingulate and premotor cortex, semantic memory loss with left anterior temporal lobe, and inability to recognize facial emotions with right amygdala (Rosen *et al.* 2005).

New imaging techniques continue to elucidate FTLD pathophyisology. Diffusion tensor imaging—a means of mapping white matter tracts in the brain—has been used to visualize white matter changes, frontal gliosis, and demyelination in FTLD (Larsson *et al.* 2004). Recent PET studies have correlated extrapyramidal signs with decreases in presynaptic dopamine, and have revealed FTD brains' deficits in frontal serotonin (Franceschi *et al.* 2005; Rinne *et al.* 2002).

12.6.2 **Semantic dementia**

As an adjunct to neuropsychological investigations, neuroimaging remains a valuable tool in making the diagnosis. SD patients often have severe, bilateral, but asymmetric atrophy of anterior temporal lobe ('knife edge atrophy') as well as medial temporal lobe structures. Early changes may be visualized as hypoperfusion on HMPAO-SPECT prior to frank atrophy (Garrard and Hodges 2000). Standard MRI sequences can demonstrate anterior temporal lobe atrophy sufficiently dramatic to accurately differentiate SD from AD (Galton *et al.* 2001). More detailed volumetric measurements of temporal lobe structures have demonstrated more severe atrophy of the amygdala, temporal pole, and fusiform and inferolateral temporal gyri with relative sparing of the hippocampal formation (Chan *et al.* 2001*b*; see Fig. 12.4 (centre panel)). Unbiased measurements of T1-weighted MRI scans using the technique of voxel-based morphometry (VBM) suggest that atrophy in SD is much more significant in temporal than extratemporal brain regions (Mummery *et al.* 2000; Gorno-Tempini *et al.* 2004*a*). FDG-PET studies during semantic memory tasks in SD patients show brain activation changes outside the areas of brain atrophy suggesting that neuronal networks involving the temporal lobes are disrupted in SD (Mummery *et al.* 1999).

12.6.3 **Progressive nonfluent aphasia**

VBM has enabled behavioural and anatomical features to be correlated in PNFA as well. One study found significant apraxia of speech and syntactic deficits in a PNFA group correlated with atrophy in the left inferior frontal gyrus, premotor cortex, and anterior insula regions (Gorno-Tempini *et al.* 2004*a*; see Fig. 12.4 (right-hand panel)). These results are consistent with previous findings on the role of these in motor speech and syntax processing. Specifically, the left precentral gyrus of the insula has been associated with apraxia of speech (Dronkers 1996; Harasty *et al.* 2001). Broca's area has been implicated as a source of syntax comprehension, albeit controversially (Alexander *et al.* 1990). Metabolic imaging studies have shown frontal lobe hypometabolism in cases of 'progressive aphemia'. It is likely that PNFA and 'progressive aphemia' represent parts of a clinical spectrum in which damage in the insula/premotor inferior frontal area and/or in more anterior prefrontal regions causes various degrees of speech and/or syntactic impairment.

12.7 **Pathology**

- Many cases of FTLD show tau-related pathology, a feature shared by other sporadic neurodegenerative conditions including Alzheimer's disease, progressive supranuclear palsy (PSP), and corticobasal degeneration (CBD).
- Tau pathology is morphologically different in CBD and PSP (4-repeat tau) from that usually seen in FTLD (3-repeat tau).
- Some FTLD cases are found to have tau-negative pathology. Such cases may show inclusions positive for ubiquitin, or lack any distinctive histological features at all.
- Ubiquitin positive pathology commonly occurs in patients with semantic dementia, and in those with features of both FTLD and motor neuron disease (FTD-MND).
- CBD pathology may present with the syndrome of progressive nonfluent aphasia.
- CBD and PSP clinical phenotypes correlate closely with their respective pathologies.

FTLD and other primary neurodegenerative disorders with prominent tau pathology have been grouped together under the heading of 'tauopathies' to distinguish them from other protein aggregate diseases such as Parkinson's and Lewy body disease, which are characterized by protein aggregates of alpha synuclein (Hardy and Gwinn-Hardy 1998). In addition to FTLD, this pathological criterion brings AD, corticobasal degeneration (CBD), and progressive supranuclear palsy (PSP) into the tauopathy 'family'. The pathological and biochemical classification is based on the morphology and histochemical characterization of neuronal inclusions or their absence, and the type of tau deposits seen. Recent insights into tau protein biology have directly led to a better understanding of the molecular pathogenesis and histopathology of FTLD (Hutton 2001). Tau is a neuronal protein that binds to microtubules, and is thought to be involved in the assembly, and maintenance of stability of these cytoskeletal structural elements. The gene that encodes tau (microtubule-associated protein, or MAPT) is found at chromosome 17q21 and is involved in the regulation of microtubule assembly and disassembly. In the adult human brain, tau protein has six isoforms, all derived from a single gene by alternative splicing. Three isoforms contain three repeats of a sequence which determines binding to microtubules, while the other three contain a fourth repeat region, coded by exon 10, alternative splicing of which therefore controls the number of microtubule binding domains. In the normal adult human brain, there is an approximately 1:1 ratio of 3-repeat to 4-repeat tau. Tauopathies, on the other hand, are classified by the species predominating in the deposits: 3-repeat tau in Pick's disease, and 4-repeat tau in CBD and PSP.

In some patients, the pathology does not include tau deposits. Such patients segregate into two groups: those with the ubiquitin-positive neuronal inclusions typical of amyotrophic lateral sclerosis (ALS) and consequently referred to as FTD-ALS; and those without any inclusions (often referred to as dementia lacking distinctive histology (DLDH)). It has been shown that the FTD-MND type pathology is the most frequent pathological correlate of SD (Davies *et al.* 2005).

A familial form of FTLD has been recognized for many years (Schenk 1959; Groen and Endtz 1982). Most patients with tau gene mutations develop an autosomal dominantly inherited syndrome characterized by early behavioural changes later followed by cognitive disturbances and parkinsonism (Foster *et al.* 1997), giving rise to the designation frontotemporal dementia with parkinsonism linked to chromosome 17 (FTDP-17). These patients usually display predominant frontotemporal atrophy with neuronal loss, gliosis, and cortical spongiform changes. Neuropathologically, they all show the presence of abundant filamentous tau pathology in nerve cells (Spillantini and Goedert 1998). The identification of exonic and intronic tau gene mutations associated with FTDP-17 established that tau dysfunction could cause neurodegeneration.

Analysis of tau mutations found in FTDP-17 has provided insights into the pathogenesis of FTLD. Changes in tau isoform expression are thought to eventually result in the formation of insoluble protein aggregates, which in turn lead to neuronal dysfunction and death. When one or more of the isoforms fails to function, not only does microtubule assembly diminish but microtubule stability also becomes compromised. Thus, excess and unused tau accumulates and is visualized as indigestible residues and inclusions. All analysed cases of FTDP-17 contain abundant filamentous hyperphosphorylated tau protein. However, the morphology, isoform composition, and distribution of tau aggregates appear to vary according to the type of mutation.

A recent consensus statement on clinical and pathological diagnosis of FTLD emphasized the composition of insoluble tau deposits found in brains at autopsy (Hardy and Gwinn-Hardy 1998). Tau protein extracted from PiD brains has revealed that Pick bodies consist of deposits of predominantly 3R tau. Tau deposits in CBD and PSP neurons contain predominantly 4R. On the other hand, neurofibrillary tangles in AD contain an equal mixture of 3R and 4R tau. Other disorders, such as post-encephalitic parkinsonism (Bussiere *et al.* 1999), neurofibrillary tangle dementia (Reed *et al.* 1997), Lytico-Bodig disease (Hof *et al.* 1994), and Niemann–Pick C disease (Love *et al.* 1995), also produce insoluble protein aggregates containing equal ratios of 3R and 4R tau. In this context, Hardy and colleagues suggested, if the insoluble tau aggregates contained predominantly 3R tau, the most likely diagnosis would be PiD or FTDP-17. However, this criteria has been shown to be non-specific (Zhukareva *et al.* 2002). Thus, studies have not only called into question the utility of classifying FTLD pathology by tau isoform expression ratio, but also highlighted the incomplete nature of current understanding regarding the relationship between tau isoform expression and clinical disease.

FTLD brains are often highly atrophic with postmortem weights as low as 750 grams (Dickson 2001). The frontal and anterior temporal lobes are the most substantially affected (see Fig. 12.5,

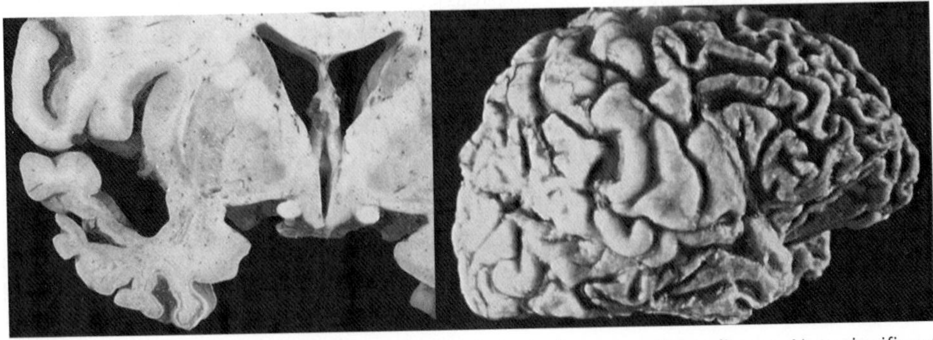

Fig. 12.5 Gross findings at autopsy in a case of pathologically proven Pick's disease. Note significant right frontal and temporal lobar degeneration.

but reduced volumes have been documented in the amygdala and hippocampus, the insula, and variably in subcortical structures such as the caudate, putamen, thalamus, and substantia nigra (Mann *et al.* 1993).

12.7.1 Pick's disease

The microscopic picture of PiD lends detail to the atrophic changes readily apparent on gross examination of the brain. Regions of atrophy confirm a severe loss of large pyramidal neurons with diffuse spongiosis and gliosis. In PiD, superficial cortical layers in affected areas contain small neurons with round inclusion that are intensely argyrophilic on silver stains called Pick bodies. Pick bodies are consistently found in the dentate gyrus, the pyramidal cells of the CA1 sector, and subiculum of the hippocampus, the neocortex, and several subcortical nuclei (Fig. 12.6). In the neocortex they are distributed in layers II and VI, contrasting with the predominance of neurofibrillary tangles in layers III and V in AD. On the other hand, like the neurofibrillary tangles found in AD, the hippocampus and amygdala have the largest numbers of Pick bodies. Anti-paired helical filaments antibodies—used to stain the neurofibrillary tangles (NFTs) observed in AD and PSP—do bind Pick bodies as well. However, the arrangement of

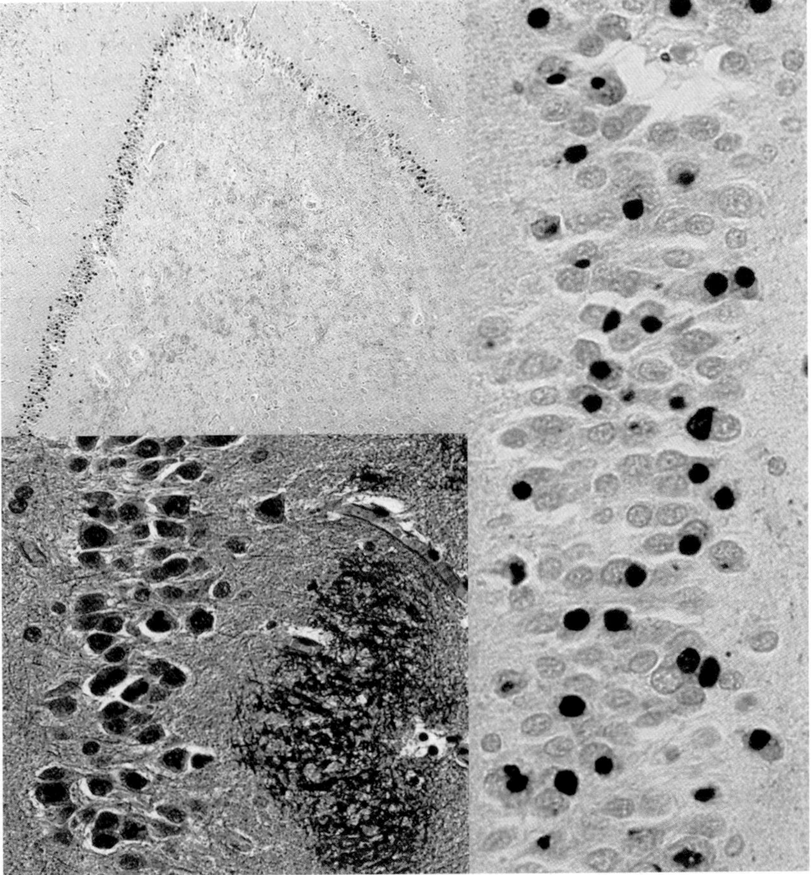

Fig. 12.6 Dentate gyrus. Tau-immunoreactive inclusions (upper left and right). Bielschowsky staining reveals Pick's bodies (lower left). This is a black and white version of Plate 9.

these tau filaments within Pick bodies is random in contrast to those within AD/PSP NFTs (Pollock *et al.* 1986). Accordingly, the most sensitive stain for Pick bodies is the anti-tau antibody (Dickson 2001).

Tau immunoreactivity is sometimes present in ballooned neurons (Dickson 2001). Although the insoluble tau in tissue homogenates has been reported to contain only 3R-isoforms (Delacourte *et al.* 1996), a recent study of PiD has demonstrated much greater biochemical heterogeneity (Zhukareva *et al.* 2002). The composition of hyperphosphorylated tau protein in PiD brains can be used to distinguish PiD from AD. In Western blots of PiD brains there are two abnormal bands that migrate at 55 and 66 kDa, whereas in AD there are three bands: 55, 66, and 69 kDa (Zhukareva *et al.* 2002).

In contrast to AD, PiD is well known to spare the nucleus basalis of Meynert. Thus, patients do not experience the marked decrease in cholinergic signalling that marks AD (Wood *et al.* 1983). Conversely, PiD can affect dopaminergic neurons in the substantia nigra.

12.7.2 **Corticobasal degeneration and progressive supranuclear palsy**

CBD and PSP are the classic 4R-tau tauopathies. CBD, characterized by asymmetric parkinsonism, apraxia, and myoclonus, is also recognized to present with language and personality changes such that distinguishing it from FTLD and AD *in vivo* can be problematic (Boeve *et al.* 2003; Gorno-Tempini *et al.* 2004*b*). It bears pathological similarity to Pick's disease as described below. Progressive supranuclear palsy (PSP), characterized by vertical gaze palsy, rigidity, instability, and dementia, also shows considerable clinical, pathological, biochemical, and genetic overlap with CBD and FTLD. Imaging studies as well as gross examination show atrophy in superior frontal and parasagittal regions in CBD and in midbrain and frontal regions in PSP (Hou *et al.* 2004; Boxer *et al.* 2003).

Histology shows tau deposition in neurons as neurofibrillary tangles and round or oval inclusions. Despite the fact that CBD brains have ballooned neurons similar to those in Pick's, there are no Pick bodies. Ballooned neurons are found throughout the neocortex, and are most abundant in the superior frontal and parietal lobes, unlike Pick's disease, which spares these regions (Bergeron *et al.* 1998). Also, unlike Pick's disease, ballooned cells may be found in primary motor or sensory cortex. Tau-immunoreactive, intracytoplasmic neuronal inclusions of variable morphology and abundant tau-positive glial pathology comprise the tau-related pathology.

12.7.3 **Dementia lacking distinctive histopathology**

DLDH is a common pathological finding in patients with the clinical symptoms of sporadic FTLD (Knopman *et al.* 1990; Bird and Schellenberg 2001). Despite spongiform changes, significant neuronal loss, and gliosis, these brains are devoid of Pick bodies, ballooned neurons, neurofibrillary tangles, or other inclusion bodies. In addition, there is a dramatic reduction of tau protein expression in DLDH brains as compared to that in PiD. Studies have suggested changes at the post-transcriptional level as the cause of this reduced expression (Zhukareva *et al.* 2001).

12.7.4 **Frontotemporal dementia with motor neuron disease**

Frontal lobe degeneration may occur in patients with motor neuron disease (MND; amyotrophic lateral sclerosis). Like DLDH, there are no Pick bodies or ballooned neurons; however, immunohistochemical stains reveal ubiquitin-positive, tau-negative neuronal inclusions in affected areas of cerebral cortex as well as in anterior horn cells (Jackson *et al.* 1996). In a recent series, the most common histological picture of FTD brains revealed these ubiquitinated inclusions (Kertesz *et al.* 2005). Histopathology shows spongiosis, neocortical ubiquitinated neurites, and neuronal inclusions, as well as inclusions in dentate neurons. Degeneration of subcortical nuclei has been described in many cases of MND and in most cases of MND-dementia. Inclusions reported in MND include ubiquitin-immunoreactive filamentous skeins and Lewy-like bodies in brainstem and spinal cord motor neurons. Dense, round or crescentic ubiquitin-immunoreactive inclusions in small neurons of neostriatum have been reported as specific for MND dementia.

Two series of FTLD patients, one with semantic dementia (Rossor *et al.* 2000), the other with frontotemporal dementia (Forno *et al.* 2002), both lacking features of MND, were found to have ubiquitin-positive, tau-negative neuronal inclusions. Three families with autosomal dominant frontotemporal dementia, but without mutations in tau, have also been described with similar pathology (Rosso *et al.* 2001).

A number of large series have investigated correlations between clinical presentation and autopsy-proven FTLD pathology (Kertesz *et al.* 2005; Hodges *et al.* 2004). An important conclusion that has emerged from these studies is that all forms of FTLD pathology can present as any of the FTLD clinical syndromes. For that reason, clinical issues in the diagnosis of disorders in the spectrum of frontotemporal lobar degenerations (FTLD) from the perspective of the underlying pathologies remain challenging. Pathologically, two broad categories emerged, cases with tau pathology (classified as Pick's disease, CBD, PSP, multisystem tauopathy, and frontotemporal dementia and parkinsonism linked to chromosome 17), those without (classified as FTLD with ubiquitin-only inclusions (FTLD-U), or FTLD with motor neuron degeneration (FTLD-MND)), and neurofilament inclusion body disease. Among these non-tauopathy classifications the predominant pathology is that of ubiquitin-only inclusions (UBI). The most secure clinical diagnoses (i.e. supported by pathology at autopsy) are frontotemporal dementia associated clinically with motor neuron disease (FTLD-MND), which was always found to have UBI pathology, and PSP and CBD, which were always found to be tauopathies in one study (Josephs *et al.* 2006). Clinical diagnosis of frontotemporal dementia (FTD) is clearly less predictive of pathology—42% have a tauopathy (usually CBD) but 58% have tau-negative UBI pathology. Likewise, 77% of patients diagnosed with primary non-fluent aphasia (PNFA) had tauopathy and the remainder only UBI pathology. One theme that has emerged from these results maintains that CBD pathology presents clinically both with its classic syndrome but also with an FTD syndrome that is not distinguishable from FTLD-U. In this way, a single pathology (CBD) can present as different clinical syndromes (CBD and FTD) and, accordingly, the same clinical syndrome (FTD) can arise from CBD and FTLD-U (Ince *et al.* 2006).

Prevalence of pathologically diagnosed Pick's disease (not including other tauopathies) is 11–33%, while DLDH is present 13–23% of the time. FTLD-MND is the most prevalent pathology, ranging from 26% to 62% in the various series (Shi *et al.* 2005). FTLD-MND accounts for a large proportion of SD presentations (13/18 cases in one series; Davies *et al.* 2005; Shi *et al.* 2005). Clinically apparent motor neuron disease virtually assures non-tau pathology, and very strongly predicts FTLD-MND (Hodges *et al.* 2004; Kertesz *et al.* 2005). Of the FTLD clinical syndromes, PNFA is more likely to be associated with non-FTLD pathology, such as CBD or AD (Hodges *et al.* 2004; Kertesz *et al.* 2005). Early onset of a movement disorder makes tau-pathology more likely (Kertesz *et al.* 2005), and the clinical syndromes of CBD and PSP often correlate with either CBD or PSP pathology (Kertesz *et al.* 2005; Hodges *et al.* 2004).

12.9 **Clinical course and prognosis**

Cognitive and functional decline are more rapid in FTLD than in AD, and survival relatively shorter (Rascovsky *et al.* 2005; Johnson *et al.* 2005). In this context, median survival from diagnosis and symptom onset is between 3 and 6 years. Of note, FTD-MND is associated with rapid progression and median survival from diagnosis and symptoms onset of between 1 and 2 years, (Hodges *et al.* 2003; Johnson *et al.* 2005).

12.9.1 Management

- At the time of going to press no pharmacological treatments have been proven to be of clinical benefit.

Pharmacological treatments for FTD are limited. Data from neurochemical studies of necropsied brains have revealed abnormalities in serotonin metabolism (Procter *et al.* 1999; Sjogren *et al.* 1998). As well, functional imaging studies have confirmed serotonergic changes in FTLD (Franceschi *et al.* 2005). Serotonin dysfunction is linked with impulsivity, irritability, affective change, and changes in eating behaviour, which are common features of FTD. Some reports describe elevated concentration of serotonin in cases of FTLD (Francis *et al.* 1993). Others have hypothesized that reductions in serotonin receptors on cortical pyramidal neurons may simply result from neuronal cell loss (Neary *et al.* 2005). Thus, it may not seem suprising that trials of serotonin selective reuptake inhibitors have shown equivocal results (Swartz *et al.* 1997; Moretti *et al.* 2003; Lebert *et al.* 2004; Deakin *et al.* 2004). Rivastigmine, an inhibitor of acetylcholinesterase and butyrylcholinesterase used in Alzheimer's disease (Farlow *et al.* 2000), was found to be effective in one open-label study (Moretti *et al.* 2004), but physiological support for this finding is dubious in that there is no cortical cholinergic deficit in FTLD (Hansen *et al.* 1988; Meier-Ruge *et al.* 1984). In light of therapeutic success with anti-glutamatergic therapy in ALS (Bensimon *et al.* 1994), memantine, an NMDA antagonist used in AD, is under investigation (Reisberg *et al.* 2003).

Caring for a demented patient imposes a heavy strain on caregivers. Noncognitive behavioural symptoms commonly prove more burdensome than cognitive impairment and are therefore the commonest reason for nursing home admissions. The most burdensome symptoms of FTD are offensive, egocentric, and quarrelsome behaviours. Of note, FTLD relative to AD strikes at a young age and thus possesses the unfortunate ability to bring dramatic social and economic changes. Caregivers require comprehensive information about the disease to enhance their understanding of the patients and to avoid unnecessary feelings of self-blame and depression (Perry and Miller 2001). The construction of a support network can relieve the burden on families. Psychiatric services for elderly people remain an important avenue in pursuing this support network.

References

Alexander, M.P., Naeser, M.A., *et al.* (1990). Broca's area aphasias: aphasia after lesions including the frontal operculum. *Neurology* **40** (2), 353–62.

Bayles, K.A. and Tomoeda, C.K. (1983). Confrontation naming impairment in dementia. *Brain Lang.* **19**, 98–114.

Bensimon, G., Lacomblez, L., and Meininger, V. (1994). A controlled trial of riluzole in amyotrophic lateral sclerosis. ALS/Riluzole Study Group. *N. Engl. J. Med.* **330**, 585–91.

Bergeron, C., Davis, A., and Lang, A.E. (1998). Corticobasal ganglionic degeneration and progressive supranuclear palsy presenting with cognitive decline. *Brain Pathol.* **8**, 355–65.

Bird, T.D. and Schellenberg, G.D. (2001). The case of the missing tau, or, why didn't the mRNA bark? *Ann. Neurol.* **49**, 144–5.

Boeve, B.F., Lang, A.E., and Litvan, I. (2003). Corticobasal degeneration and its relationship to progressive supranuclear palsy and frontotemporal dementia. *Ann. Neurol.* **54** (Suppl. 5), S15–19.

Boxer, A.L., Rankin, K.P., Miller, B.L., Schuff, N., Weiner, M., Gorno-Tempini, M.L., and Rosen, H.J. (2003). Cinguloparietal atrophy distinguishes Alzheimer disease from semantic dementia. *Arch. Neurol.* **60**, 949–56.

Bozeat, S., Lambon Ralph, M.A., Graham, K., Patterson, K., Wilkin, H., Rowland, J., Rogers, T.T., and Hodges, J. (2003). A duck with four legs: investigating the structure of conceptual knowledge using picture drawing in semantic dementia. *Cogn. Neuropsychol.* **20**, 27–47.

Bussiere, T., Hof, P.R., Mailliot, C., Brown, C.D., Caillet-Boudin, M.L., Perl, D.P., Buee, L., and Delacourte, A. (1999). Phosphorylated serine422 on tau proteins is a pathological epitope found in several diseases with neurofibrillary degeneration. *Acta Neuropathol.* (*Berl.*) **97**, 221–30.

Chan, D., Fox, N.C., Jenkins, R., Scahill, R.I., Crum, W.R., and Rossor, M.N. (2001*a*). Rates of global and regional cerebral atrophy in AD and frontotemporal dementia. *Neurology* **57**, 1756–63.

Chan, D., Fox, N.C., Scahill, R.I., Crum, W.R., Whitwell, J.L., Leschziner, G., Rossor, A.M., Stevens, J.M., Cipolotti, L., and Rossor, M.N. (2001*b*). Patterns of temporal lobe atrophy in semantic dementia and Alzheimer's disease. *Ann. Neurol.* **49**, 433–42.

Chang, J.L., Lomen-Hoerth, C., Murphy, J., Henry, R.G., Kramer, J.H., Miller, B.L., and Gorno-Tempini, M.L. (2005). A voxel-based morphometry study of patterns of brain atrophy in ALS and ALS/FTLD. *Neurology* **65**, 75–80.

Chow, T.W., Miller, B.L., *et al.* (1999). Inheritance of frontotemporal dementia. *Arch. Neurol.* **56** (7), 817–22.

Davies, R.R., Hodges, J.R., Kril, J.J., Patterson, K., Halliday, G.M., and Xuereb, J.H. (2005). The pathological basis of semantic dementia. *Brain* **128**, 1984–95.

Deakin, J.B., Rahman, S., Nestor, P.J., Hodges, J.R., and Sahakian, B.J. (2004). Paroxetine does not improve symptoms and impairs cognition in frontotemporal dementia: a double-blind randomized controlled trial. *Psychopharmacology* (*Berl.*) **172**, 400–8.

Delacourte, A., Robitaille, Y., Sergeant, N., Buee, L., Hof, P.R., Wattez, A., Laroche-Cholette, A., Mathieu, J., Chagnon, P., and Gauvreau, D. (1996). Specific pathological Tau protein variants characterize Pick's disease. *J. Neuropathol. Exp. Neurol.* **55**, 159–68.

Dickson, D.W. (2001). Neuropathology of Pick's disease. *Neurology* **56**, S16–20.

Dronkers, N.F. (1996). A new brain region for coordinating speech articulation. *Nature* **384**, 159–61.

Edwards-Lee, T., Miller, B.L., Benson, D.F., Cummings, J.L., Russell, G.L., Boone, K., and Mena, I. (1997). The temporal variant of frontotemporal dementia. *Brain* **120** (6), 1027–40.

Evans, J.J., Heggs, A.J., Antoun, N., and Hodges, J.R. (1995). Progressive prosopagnosia associated with selective right temporal lobe atrophy. A new syndrome? *Brain* **118** (1), 1–13.

Farlow, M., Anand, R., Messina, J., JR., Hartman, R., and Veach, J. (2000). A 52-week study of the efficacy of rivastigmine in patients with mild to moderately severe Alzheimer's disease. *Eur. Neurol*, **44**, 236–41.

Forno, L.S., Langston, J.W., Herrick, M.K., Wilson, J.D., and Murayama, S. (2002). Ubiquitin-positive neuronal and tau 2-positive glial inclusions in frontotemporal dementia of motor neuron type. *Acta Neuropathol.* (*Berl.*) **103**, 599–606.

Foster, N.L., Wilhelmsen, K., *et al.* (1997). Frontotemporal dementia and parkinsonism linked to chromosome 17: a consensus conference. Conference participants. *Ann. Neurol.* **41** (6), 706–15.

Franceschi, M., Anchisi, D., Pelati, O., Zuffi, M., Matarrese, M., Moresco, R.M., Fazio, F., and Perani, D. (2005). Glucose metabolism and serotonin receptors in the frontotemporal lobe degeneration. *Ann. Neurol.* **57**, 216–25.

Francis, P.T., Holmes, C., *et al.* (1993). Preliminary neurochemical findings in non-Alzheimer dementia due to lobar atrophy. *Dementia* **4** (3–4), 172–7.

Galton, C.J., Patterson, K., Graham, K., Lambon-Ralph, M.A., Williams, G., Antoun, N., Sahakian, B.J., and Hodges, J.R. (2001). Differing patterns of temporal atrophy in Alzheimer's disease and semantic dementia. *Neurology* **57**, 216–25.

Garrard, P. and Carroll, E. (2006). Lost in semantic space: a multi-modal, non-verbal assessment of feature knowledge in semantic dementia. *Brain* **129**, 1152–63.

Garrard, P. and Hodges, J.R. (2000). Semantic dementia: clinical, radiological and pathological perspectives. *J. Neurol.* **247**, 409–22.

Gorno-Tempini, M.L., Dronkers, N.F., Rankin, K.P., Ogar, J.M., Phengrasamy, L., Rosen, H.J., Johnson, J.K., Weiner, M.W., and Miller, B.L. (2004*a*). Cognition and anatomy in three variants of primary progressive aphasia. *Ann. Neurol.* **55**, 335–46.

Gorno-Tempini, M.L., Murray, R.C., Rankin, K.P., Weiner, M.W., and Miller, B.L. (2004*b*). Clinical, cognitive and anatomical evolution from nonfluent progressive aphasia to corticobasal syndrome: a case report. *Neurocase* **10**, 426–36.

Graham, K.S. and Hodges, J.R. (1997). Differentiating the roles of the hippocampal complex and the neocortex in long-term memory storage: evidence from the study of semantic dementia and Alzheimer's disease. *Neuropsychology* **11**, 77–89.

Graham, K.S., Simons, J.S., Pratt, K.H., Patterson, K., and Hodges, J.R. (2000). Insights from semantic dementia on the relationship between episodic and semantic memory. *Neuropsychologia* **38**, 313–24.

Graham, N.L., Patterson, K., and Hodges, J.R. (2004). When more yields less: speaking and writing deficits in nonfluent progressive aphasia. *Neurocase* **10**, 141–55.

Gregory, C.A. and Hodges, J.R. (1996). Clinical features of frontal lobe dementia in comparison to Alzheimer's disease. *J. Neural Transm. Suppl.* **47**, 103–23.

Gregory, C.A., Serra-Mestres, J., *et al.* (1999). Early diagnosis of the frontal variant of frontotemporal dementia: how sensitive are standard neuroimaging and neuropsychologic tests? *Neuropsychiatry Neuropsychol. Behav. Neurol.* **12** (2), 128–35.

Grossman, M. (2002). Progressive aphasic syndromes: clinical and theoretical advances. *Curr. Opin. Neurol.* **15**, 409–13.

Hansen, L.A., Deteresa, R., *et al.* (1988). Neocortical morphometry and cholinergic neurochemistry in Pick's disease. *Am. J. Pathol.* **131** (3), 507–18.

Harasty, J.A., Halliday, G.M., Xuereb, J., Croot, K., Bennett, H., and Hodges, J.R. (2001). Cortical degeneration associated with phonologic and semantic language impairments in AD. *Neurology* **56**, 944–50.

Hardy, J. and Gwinn-Hardy, K. (1998). Genetic classification of primary neurodegenerative disease. *Science* **282**, 1075–9.

Hodges, J.R. and Patterson, K. (1996). Nonfluent progressive aphasia and semantic dementia: a comparative neuropsychological study. *J. Int. Neuropsychol. Soc.* **2** (6), 511–24.

Hodges, J.R., Salmon, D.P., and Butters, N. (1990). Differential impairment of semantic and episodic memory in Alzheimer's and Huntington's diseases: a controlled prospective study. *J. Neurol. Neurosurg. Psychiatry* **53**, 1089–95.

Hodges, J.R., Patterson, K., Oxbury, S., and Funnell, E. (1992). Semantic dementia. Progressive fluent aphasia with temporal lobe atrophy. *Brain* **115** (6), 1783–806.

Hodges, J.R., Graham, N., and Patterson, K. (1995). Charting the progression in semantic dementia: implications for the organisation of semantic memory. *Memory* **3**, 463–95.

Hodges, J.R., Patterson, K., Ward, R., Garrard, P., Bak, T., Perry, R., and Gregory, C. (1999). The differentiation of semantic dementia and frontal lobe dementia (temporal and frontal variants of frontotemporal dementia) from early Alzheimer's disease: a comparative neuropsychological study. *Neuropsychology* **13**, 31–40.

Hodges, J.R., Davies, R., Xuereb, J., Kril, J., and Halliday, G. (2003). Survival in frontotemporal dementia. *Neurology* **61**, 349–54.

Hodges, J.R., Davies, R.R., Xuereb, J.H., Casey, B., Broe, M., Bak, T.H., Kril, J.J., and Halliday, G.M. (2004). Clinicopathological correlates in frontotemporal dementia. *Ann. Neurol.* **56**, 399–406.

Hof, P.R., Perl, D.P., *et al.* (1994). Amyotrophic lateral sclerosis and parkinsonism–dementia from Guam: differences in neurofibrillary tangle distribution and density in the hippocampal formation and neocortex. *Brain Res.* **650** (1), 107–16.

Hoffman, J.M., Welsh-Bohmer, K.A., *et al.* (2000). FDG PET imaging in patients with pathologically verified dementia. *J. Nucl. Med.* **41** (11), 1920–8.

Hosler, B.A., Siddique, T., Sapp, P.C., Sailor, W., Huang, M.C., Hossain, A., Daube, J.R., Nance, M., Fan, C., Kaplan, J., Hung, W.Y., McKenna-Yasek, D., Haines, J.L., Pericak-Vance, M.A., Horvitz, H.R., and Brown, R.H., Jr. (2000). Linkage of familial amyotrophic lateral sclerosis with frontotemporal dementia to chromosome 9q21–q22. *J. Am. Med. Assoc.* **284**, 1664–9.

Hou, C.E., Carlin, D., and Miller, B.L. (2004). Non-Alzheimer's disease dementias: anatomic, clinical, and molecular correlates. *Can. J. Psychiatry* **49**, 164–71.

Howard, D. and Patterson, K. (1992). *Pyramids and Palm Trees: a test of semantic access from pictures and words.* Bury St. Edmunds, Thames Valley Publishing Company.

Hutton, M. (2001). Missense and splice site mutations in tau associated with FTDP-17: multiple pathogenic mechanisms. *Neurology* **56**, S21–5.

Jackson, M., Lennox, G., *et al.* (1996). Motor neurone disease—inclusion dementia. *Neurodegeneration* **5** (4), 339–50.

Johnson, J.K., Diehl, J., Mendez, M.F., Neuhaus, J., Shapira, J.S., Forman, M., Chute, D.J., Roberson, E.D., Pace-Savitsky, C., Neumann, M., Chow, T.W., Rosen, H.J., Forstl, H., Kurz, A., and Miller, B.L. (2005). Frontotemporal lobar degeneration: demographic characteristics of 353 patients. *Arch. Neurol.* **62**, 925–30.

Kaufer, D.I., Miller, B.L., Itti, L., Fairbanks, L.A., Li, J., Fishman, J., Kushi, J., and Cummings, J.L. (1997). Midline cerebral morphometry distinguishes frontotemporal dementia and Alzheimer's disease. *Neurology* **48**, 978–85.

Kertesz, A., Davidson, W., McCabe, P., and Munoz, D. (2003). Behavioral quantitation is more sensitive than cognitive testing in frontotemporal dementia. *Alzheimer Dis. Assoc. Disord.* **17**, 223–9.

Kertesz, A., McMonagle, P., Blair, M., Davidson, W., and Munoz, D.G. (2005). The evolution and pathology of frontotemporal dementia. *Brain* **128**, 1996–2005.

Knopman, D.S., Mastri, A.R., Frey, W.H., 2nd, Sung, J.H., and Rustan, T. (1990). Dementia lacking distinctive histologic features: a common non-Alzheimer degenerative dementia. *Neurology* **40**, 251–6.

Kovach, M.J., Waggoner, B., Leal, S.M., Gelber, D., Khardori, R., Levenstien, M.A., Shanks, C.A., Gregg, G., Al-Lozi, M.T., Miller, T., Rakowicz, W., Lopate, G., Florence, J., Glosser, G., Simmons, Z., Morris, J.C., Whyte, M.P., Pestronk, A., and Kimonis, V.E. (2001). Clinical delineation and localization to chromosome 9p13.3–p12 of a unique dominant disorder in four families: hereditary inclusion body myopathy, Paget disease of bone, and frontotemporal dementia. *Mol. Genet. Metab.* **74**, 458–75.

Kramer, J.H., Jurik, J., Sha, S.J., Rankin, K.P., Rosen, H.J., Johnson, J.K., and Miller, B.L. (2003). Distinctive neuropsychological patterns in frontotemporal dementia, semantic dementia, and Alzheimer disease. *Cogn. Behav. Neurol.* **16**, 211–18.

Larsson, E.M., Englund, E., *et al.* (2004). MRI with diffusion tensor imaging post-mortem at 3.0 T in a patient with frontotemporal dementia. *Dementia Geriatr. Cogn. Disord.* **17**, 316–19.

Lebert, F., Stekke, W., Hasenbroekx, C., and Pasquier, F. (2004). Frontotemporal dementia: a randomised, controlled trial with trazodone. *Dementia Geriatr. Cogn. Disord.* **17**, 355–9.

Liu, W., Miller, B.L., *et al.* (2004). Behavioral disorders in the frontal and temporal variants of frontotemporal dementia. *Neurology* **62** (5), 742–8.

Love, S., Bridges, L.R., *et al.* (1995). Neurofibrillary tangles in Niemann–Pick disease type C. *Brain* **118** (1), 119–29.

Mann, D.M., South, P.W., *et al.* (1993). Dementia of frontal lobe type neuropathology and immunohistochemistry. *J. Neurol. Neurosurg. Psychiatry* **56** (6), 605–14.

Meier-Ruge, W., Iwangoff, P., and Reichlmeier, K. (1984). Neurochemical enzyme changes in Alzheimer's and Pick's disease. *Arch. Gerontol. Geriatr.* **3**, 161–5.

Mesulam, M.M. (1982). Slowly progressive aphasia without generalized dementia. *Ann. Neurol.* **11**, 592–8.

Miller, B.L., Cummings, J.L., *et al.* (1992). Frontal lobe degeneration: clinical, neuropsychological, and SPECT characteristics. *Neurology* **41** (9), 1374–82.

Miller, B.L., Cummings, J., *et al.* (1998). Emergence of artistic talent in frontotemporal dementia. *Neurology* **51** (4), 978–82.

Moretti, R., Torre, P., Antonello, R.M., Cazzato, G., and Bava, A. (2003). Frontotemporal dementia: paroxetine as a possible treatment of behavior symptoms. A randomized, controlled, open 14-month study. *Eur. Neurol.* **49**, 13–19.

Moretti, R., Torre, P., Antonello, R.M., Cattaruzza, T., Cazzato, G., and Bava, A. (2004). Rivastigmine in frontotemporal dementia: an open-label study. *Drugs Aging* **21**, 931–7.

Morris, J.C. and Balota, D.A. (2001). Semantic dementia versus Alzheimer's disease: a matter of semantics? *Neurology* **57**, 173–4.

Mummery, C.J., Patterson, K., Wise, R.J., Vandenbergh, R., Price, C.J., and Hodges, J.R. (1999). Disrupted temporal lobe connections in semantic dementia. *Brain* **122** (1), 61–73.

Mummery, C.J., Patterson, K., Price, C.J., Ashburner, J., Frackowiak, R.S., and Hodges, J.R. (2000). A voxel-based morphometry study of semantic dementia: relationship between temporal lobe atrophy and semantic memory. *Ann. Neurol.* **47**, 36–45.

Neary, D., Snowden, J.S., Gustafson, L., Passant, U., Stuss, D., Black, S., Freedman, M., Kertesz, A., Robert, P.H., Albert, M., Boone, K., Miller, B.L., Cummings, J., and Benson, D.F. (1998). Frontotemporal lobar degeneration: a consensus on clinical diagnostic criteria. *Neurology* **51**, 1546–54.

Neary, D., Snowden, J., and Mann, D. (2005). Frontotemporal dementia. *Lancet Neurol.* **4**, 771–80.

Nedjam, Z., Devouche, E., and Dalla Barba, G. (2004). Confabulation, but not executive dysfunction discriminate AD from frontotemporal dementia. *Eur. J. Neurol.* **11**, 728–33.

Patterson, K., Lambon-Ralph, M.A., *et al.* (2001). Deficits in irregular past-tense verb morphology associated with degraded semantic knowledge. *Neuropsychologia* **39** (7), 709–24.

Perry, R.J. and Miller, B.L. (2001). Behavior and treatment in frontotemporal dementia. *Neurology* **56** (Suppl. 4), S46–51.

Pickering-Brown, S.M., Richardson, A.M., Snowden, J.S., McDonagh, A.M., Burns, A., Braude, W., Baker, M., Liu, W.K., Yen, S.H., Hardy, J., Hutton, M., Davies, Y., Allsop, D., Craufurd, D., Neary, D., and Mann, D.M. (2002). Inherited frontotemporal dementia in nine British families associated with intronic mutations in the tau gene. *Brain* **125**, 732–51.

Poeck, K. and Luzzatti, C. (1988). Slowly progressive aphasia in three patients. The problem of accompanying neuropsychological deficit. *Brain* **111** (1), 151–68.

Pollock, N.J., Mirra, S.S., Binder, L.I., Hansen, L.A., and Wood, J.G. (1986). Filamentous aggregates in Pick's disease, progressive supranuclear palsy, and Alzheimer's disease share antigenic determinants with microtubule-associated protein, tau. *Lancet* **2**, 1211.

Poorkaj, P., Grossman, M., Steinbart, E., Payami, H., Sadovnick, A., Nochlin, D., Tabira, T., Trojanowski, J.Q., Borson, S., Galasko, D., Reich, S., Quinn, B., Schellenberg, G., and Bird, T.D. (2001). Frequency of tau gene mutations in familial and sporadic cases of non-Alzheimer dementia. *Arch. Neurol.* **58**, 383–7.

Procter, A.W., Qume, M., and Francis, P.T. (1999). Neurochemical features of frontotemporal dementia. *Dementia Geriatr. Cogn. Disord.* **10**, 80–4.

Rankin, K.P., Kramer, J.H., and Miller, B.L. (2005). Patterns of cognitive and emotional empathy in frontotemporal lobar degeneration. *Cogn. Behav. Neurol.* **18**, 28–36.

Rascovsky, K., Salmon, D.P., Lipton, A.M., Leverenz, J.B., Decarli, C., Jagust, W.J., Clark, C.M., Mendez, M.F., Tang-Wai, D.F., Graff-Radford, N.R., and Galasko, D. (2005). Rate of progression differs in frontotemporal dementia and Alzheimer disease. *Neurology* **65**, 397–403.

Ratnavalli, E., Brayne, C., Dawson, K., and Hodges, J.R. (2002). The prevalence of frontotemporal dementia. *Neurology* **58**, 1615–21.

Reed, L.A., Grabowski, T.J., Schmidt, M.L., Morris, J.C., Goate, A., Solodkin, A., Van Hoesen, G.W., Schelper, R.L., Talbot, C.J., Wragg, M.A., and Trojanowski, J.Q. (1997). Autosomal dominant dementia with widespread neurofibrillary tangles. *Ann. Neurol.* **42**, 564–72.

Reisberg, B., Doody, R., Stoffler, A., Schmitt, F., Ferris, S., and Mobius, H.J. (2003). Memantine in moderate-to-severe Alzheimer's disease. *N. Engl. J. Med.* **348**, 1333–41.

Rhee, J., Antiquena, P., and Grossman, M. (2001). Verb comprehension in frontotemporal degeneration: the role of grammatical, semantic and executive components. *Neurocase* **7**, 173–84.

Rinne, J.O., Laine, M., Kaasinen, V., Norvasuo-Heila, M.K., Nagren, K., and Helenius, H. (2002). Striatal dopamine transporter and extrapyramidal symptoms in frontotemporal dementia. *Neurology* **58**, 1489–93.

Rosen, H.J., Gorno-Tempini, M.L., Goldman, W.P., Perry, R.J., Schuff, N., Weiner, M., Feiwell, R., Kramer, J.H., and Miller, B.L. (2002). Patterns of brain atrophy in frontotemporal dementia and semantic dementia. *Neurology* **58**, 198–208.

Rosen, H.J., Narvaez, J.M., Hallam, B., Kramer, J.H., Wyss-Coray, C., Gearhart, R., Johnson, J.K., and Miller, B.L. (2004). Neuropsychological and functional measures of severity in Alzheimer disease, frontotemporal dementia, and semantic dementia. *Alzheimer Dis. Assoc. Disord.* **18**, 202–7.

Rosen, H.J., Allison, S.C., Schauer, G.F., Gorno-Tempini, M.L., Weiner, M.W., and Miller, B.L. (2005). Neuroanatomical correlates of behavioural disorders in dementia. *Brain* **128**, 2612–25.

Rosso, S.M. and Van Swieten, J.C. (2002). New developments in frontotemporal dementia and parkinsonism linked to chromosome 17. *Curr. Opin. Neurol.* **15**, 423–8.

Rosso, S.M., Kamphorst, W., De Graaf, B., Willemsen, R., Ravid, R., Niermeijer, M.F., Spillantini, M.G., Heutink, P., and Van Swieten, J.C. (2001). Familial frontotemporal dementia with ubiquitin-positive inclusions is linked to chromosome 17q21–22. *Brain* **124**, 1948–57.

Rosso, S.M., Donker Kaat, L., Baks, T., Joosse, M., De Koning, I., Pijnenburg, Y., De Jong, D., Dooijes, D., Kamphorst, W., Ravid, R., Niermeijer, M.F., Verheij, F., Kremer, H.P., Scheltens, P., Van Duijn, C.M., Heutink, P., and Van Swieten, J.C. (2003). Frontotemporal dementia in The Netherlands: patient characteristics and prevalence estimates from a population-based study. *Brain* **126**, 2016–22.

Rossor, M.N., Revesz, T., Lantos, P.L., and Warrington, E.K. (2000). Semantic dementia with ubiquitin-positive tau-negative inclusion bodies. *Brain* **123** (2), 267–76.

Seeley, W.W., Bauer, A.M., Miller, B.L., Gorno-Tempini, M.L., Kramer, J.H., Weiner, M., and Rosen, H.J. (2005). The natural history of temporal variant frontotemporal dementia. *Neurology* **64**, 1384–90.

Shi, J., Shaw, C.L., Du Plessis, D., Richardson, A.M., Bailey, K.L., Julien, C., Stopford, C., Thompson, J., Varma, A., Craufurd, D., Tian, J., Pickering-Brown, S., Neary, D., Snowden, J.S., and Mann, D.M. (2005). Histopathological changes underlying frontotemporal lobar degeneration with clinicopathological correlation. *Acta Neuropathol. (Berl.)* **110**, 501–12.

Sjogren, M., Minthon, L., Passant, U., Blennow, K., and Wallin, A. (1998). Decreased monoamine metabolites in frontotemporal dementia and Alzheimer's disease. *Neurobiol. Aging* **19**, 379–84.

Skibinski, G., Parkinson, N.J., Brown, J.M., *et al.* (2005). Mutations in the endosomal ESCRTIII-complex subunit CHMP2B in frontotemporal dementia. *Nat. Genet.* **37**, 806–8.

Snowden, J.S., Thompson, J.C., and Neary, D. (2004). Knowledge of famous faces and names in semantic dementia. *Brain* **127**, 860–72.

Spillantini, M.G. and Goedert, M. (1998). Tau protein pathology in neurodegenerative diseases. *Trends Neurosci.* **21** (10), 428–33.

Stevens, M., van Duijin, C.M., *et al.* (1998). Familial aggregation in frontotemporal dementia. *Neurology* **50** (6), 1541–5.

Swartz, J.R., Miller, B.L., Lesser, I.M., and Darby, A.L. (1997). Frontotemporal dementia: treatment response to serotonin selective reuptake inhibitors. *J. Clin. Psychiatry* **58**, 212–16.

Thompson, S.A., Patterson, K., and Hodges, J.R. (2003). Left/right asymmetry of atrophy in semantic dementia: behavioral–cognitive implications. *Neurology* **61**, 1196–203.

Vandenberghe, R.R., Vandenbulcke, M., Weintraub, S., Johnson, N., Porke, K., Thompson, C.K., and Mesulam, M.M. (2005). Paradoxical features of word finding difficulty in primary progressive aphasia. *Ann. Neurol.* **57**, 204–9.

Varma, A.R., Snowden, J.S., Lloyd, J.J., Talbot, P.R., Mann, D.M., and Neary, D. (1999). Evaluation of the NINCDS-ADRDA criteria in the differentiation of Alzheimer's disease and frontotemporal dementia. *J. Neurol. Neurosurg. Psychiatry* **66**, 184–8.

Warrington, E. K. (1975). The selective impairment of semantic memory. *Quart. J. Exp. Psychol.* **27**, 635–57.

Weintraub, S., Rubin, N.P., and Mesulam, M.M. (1990). Primary progressive aphasia. Longitudinal course, neuropsychological profile, and language features. *Arch. Neurol.* **47**, 1329–35.

Wood, P.L., Etienne, P., Lal, S., Nair, N.P., Finlayson, M.H., Gauthier, S., Palo, J., Haltia, M., Paetau, A., and Bird, E.D. (1983). A post-mortem comparison of the cortical cholinergic system in Alzheimer's disease and Pick's disease. *J. Neurol. Sci.* **62**, 211–17.

Zhukareva, V., Vogelsberg-Ragaglia, V., Van Deerlin, V.M., Bruce, J., Shuck, T., Grossman, M., Clark, C.M., Arnold, S.E., Masliah, E., Galasko, D., Trojanowski, J.Q., and Lee, V.M. (2001). Loss of brain tau defines novel sporadic and familial tauopathies with frontotemporal dementia. *Ann. Neurol.* **49**, 165–75.

Zhukareva, V., Mann, D., Pickering-Brown, S., Uryu, K., Shuck, T., Shah, K., Grossman, M., Miller, B.L., Hulette, C.M., Feinstein, S.C., Trojanowski, J.Q., and Lee, V.M. (2002). Sporadic Pick's disease: a tauopathy characterized by a spectrum of pathological tau isoforms in gray and white matter. *Ann. Neurol.* **51**, 730–9.

Chapter 13

Vascular cognitive impairment

John Bowler

13.1 Definition

Vascular cognitive impairment (VCI) is a relatively new term intended to encompass and replace the older concept of vascular dementia (VaD). Put simply, VCI refers to cognitive impairment of any severity arising from cerebrovascular disease of any kind.

As a new concept, the precise definition of VCI and its operational implementation are not yet established. Some understanding of the history of the concept is essential in understanding the current state of VCI and future likely developments.

13.1.1 Historical aspects

Despite the recognition of both Alzheimer's disease (AD) and a form of VaD (Binswanger's disease) at the end of the nineteenth century, for most of the twentieth century dementia was routinely attributed to arteriosclerosis and consequent chronic cerebral ischaemia (Fields 1985). This view changed with the increasing recognition of AD and the demonstration that infarcts and not chronic ischaemia were the basis of what came to be termed multi-infarct dementia (Hachinski *et al.* 1974; Miller Fisher 1968). Cerebral blood flow and metabolism studies later confirmed the absence of chronic cerebral ischaemia. Instead, they showed a modest fall in cerebral blood flow in VaD, which is accompanied by a normal oxygen extraction ratio. Thus, cerebral blood flow is matched to decreased metabolic demands, as is normal (Frackowiak *et al.* 1981). The term 'vascular dementia' subsequently replaced multi-infarct dementia as it was recognized that there were many aetiologies apart from multiple infarcts including single infarcts in eloquent areas, episodes of hypotension, leukoaraiosis, incomplete infarction, and haemorrhage.

However, by the end of the twentieth century, the increasingly recognized AD overshadowed VaD to the extent that some authors reported that multi-infarct dementia was rare (Brust 1988). Because AD was thought to be the major cause of dementia, the criteria for AD (American Psychiatric Association 1994; McKhann *et al.* 1984; World Health Organization 1993) formed the basis for those of all dementia. AD was separated from VaD using clinical features thought to reflect vascular risk factors, vascular events, and the manifestations of systemic and cerebral vascular disease. These elements are typically codified using the ischaemic score (see Table 13.1; Hachinski *et al.* 1975; Moroney *et al.* 1997). This basis for the definition has resulted in the criteria for VaD (Chui *et al.* 1992; Roman *et al.* 1993) emphasizing memory loss and usually the progression and irreversibility of the cognitive decline, none of which are necessarily the case (del Ser *et al.* 1990; Hachinski 1992; Loeb *et al.* 1988).

13.1.2 Old criteria for vascular dementia

Two similar sets of criteria for the identification of VaD have been proposed, the NINDS–AIREN criteria (Roman *et al.* 1993) and the California criteria (Chui *et al.* 1992) but neither has met

Table13.1 The ischaemic scale. Scores over 7 suggest a vascular aetiology for dementia, whereas scores of 4 or less do not support a vascular aetiology

Feature	Value
Abrupt onset	2
Stepwise deterioration	1
Fluctuating course	2
Nocturnal confusion	1
Relative preservation of personality	1
Depression	1
Somatic complaints	1
Emotional incontinence	1
History/presence of hypertension	1
History of strokes	2
Evidence of associated atherosclerosis	1
Focal neurological symptoms	2
Focal neurological signs	2
Total score	

universal acceptance nor been validated. Furthermore, they are difficult to apply consistently and produce very different results, even when applied to the same population (Bowler and Hachinski 2000; Chui *et al.* 2000; Lopez *et al.* 1994; Pohjasvaara *et al.* 1997*b*; Wetterling *et al.* 1996).

Their use in new work is not recommended, but the NINDS–AIREN criteria in particular have been used in much of the published work available to date and an appreciation of these criteria and their deficits is necessary in interpreting the data derived using them.

13.1.2.1 NINDS–AIREN

The NINDS–AIREN (National Institute of Neurological Disorders and Stroke (NINDS) and the Association Internationale pour la Recherche at L'Enseignement en Neurosciences (AIREN)) criteria (Roman *et al.* 1993) define dementia according to the ICD 10, requiring impaired functioning in daily living and a decline in memory and at least two other domains. VaD is excluded in cases with disturbed consciousness, psychosis, severe aphasia, major sensorimotor deficits, or other brain diseases such as AD that could themselves account for the deficit. Mixed dementia is not recognized, but the coexistence of AD is termed AD with cerebrovascular disease (Roman *et al.* 1993).

Probable vascular dementia A diagnosis of probable VaD requires dementia and evidence of cerebrovascular disease on both clinical examination and neuroimaging, and evidence of a relationship between the stroke and cognitive decline, which can be provided by two of the following: (1) onset of dementia within 3 months after a recognized stroke; (2) abrupt deterioration in cognition; and (3) stepwise deterioration. Abnormalities on neuroimaging are only considered to support the diagnosis of VaD if they fulfil criteria regarding site and size, e.g. large vessel strokes in the following sites: bilateral anterior cerebral, posterior cerebral, association areas, or carotid watershed (superior frontal, parietal); small vessel disease in the basal ganglia and frontal white matter; extensive periventricular white matter lesions; or bilateral thalamic lesions.

Haemorrhagic lesions are permitted. The criteria for severity specify that leucoencephalopathy must involve at least 25% of the total white matter. The radiological criteria can be difficult to apply in practice without a combination of experience, operational guidelines, and training (van Straaten *et al.* 2003) and may be invalid, at least for post-stroke dementia (Ballard *et al.* 2004).

Possible vascular dementia A diagnosis of possible VaD is made: (1) if there are no neuroimaging data but there is clinical evidence of cerebrovascular disease; or (2) in the absence of a clear temporal relationship between dementia and stroke; or (3) in those with a subtle onset and variable course.

Definite vascular dementia Definite VaD is diagnosed provided probable dementia exists, it is accompanied by histopathological evidence of cerebrovascular disease, and there is no histopathological evidence of other possible causes of the cognitive loss.

13.1.2.2 California criteria

Details of these criteria are given in Table 13.2. They are not fundamentally different from the NINDS–AIREN criteria, but the details differ sufficiently to produce very different results. Haemorrhagic and anoxic lesions are not included. The number and types of cognitive defects

Table 13.2 Criteria for Alzheimer's disease from the State of California Alzheimer's Disease Diagnostic and Treatment Centers *

Dementia

Dementia is a deterioration from a known or estimated prior level of intellectual function sufficient to interfere broadly with the conduct of the patient's customary affairs of life, which is not isolated to a single narrow category of intellectual performance, and which is independent of level of consciousness. This deterioration should be supported by historical evidence and documented by either bedside mental status testing or ideally by more detailed neuropsychological examination, using tests that are quantifiable, reproducible, and for which normative data are available.

Probable IVD

A The criteria for the clinical diagnosis of **probable** IVD include *all* of the following.

1 Dementia.

2 Evidence of two or more ischaemic strokes by history, neurological signs, and/or neuroimaging studies (CT or T1-weighted MRI) or occurrence of a single stroke with a clearly documented temporal relationship to the onset of dementia.

3 Evidence of at least one infarct outside the cerebellum by CT or T1-weighted MRI.

B The diagnosis of **probable** IVD is supported by the following.

1 Evidence of multiple infarcts in brain regions known to affect cognition.

2 A history of multiple transient ischaemic attacks.

3 History of vascular risk factors (e.g. hypertension, heart disease, diabetes mellitus).

4 Elevated Hachinski ischemic Scale (original or modified version).

C Clinical features that are thought to be associated with IVD, but await further research, include the following.

1 Relatively early appearance of gait disturbance and urinary incontinence.

2 Periventricular and deep white matter changes on T2-weighted MRI that are excessive for age.

3 Focal changes in electrophysiological studies (e.g. EEG, evoked potentials) or physiologic neuroimaging studies (e.g. SPECT, PET, NMR, spectroscopy).

Table 13.2 (continued) Criteria for Alzheimer's disease from the State of California Alzheimer's Disease Diagnostic and Treatment Centers *

D Other clinical features that do not constitute strong evidence either for or against a diagnosis of **probable** IVD include the following.

1 Periods of slowly progressive symptoms.

2 Illusions, psychosis, hallucinations, delusions.

3 Seizures.

E Clinical features that cast doubt on a diagnosis of **probable** IVD include the following.

1 Transcortical sensory aphasia in the absence of corresponding focal lesions on neuroimaging studies.

2 Absence of central neurological symptoms/signs, other than cognitive disturbance.

Possible IVD

A clinical diagnosis of **possible** IVD may be made when there is:

1 Dementia *and* one or more of the following:

2a A history or evidence of a single stroke (but not multiple strokes) without a clearly documented temporal relationship to the onset of dementia *or*

2b Binswanger's syndrome (without multiple strokes) that includes *all* of the following:

i early-onset urinary incontinence not explained by urologic disease, or gait disturbance (e.g. parkinsonian, magnetic, apraxic, or 'senile' gait) not explained by peripheral cause;

ii vascular risk factors;

iii extensive white matter changes on neuroimaging.

Definite IVD

A diagnosis of **definite** IVD requires histopathological examination of the brain, as well as:

1 clinical evidence of dementia.

2 pathological confirmation of multiple infarcts, some outside the cerebellum.

Note. If there is evidence of Alzheimer's disease or some other pathological disorder that is thought to have contributed to the dementia, a diagnosis of **mixed** dementia should be made.

Mixed dementia

A diagnosis of **mixed** dementia should be made in the presence of one or more other systemic or brain disorders that are thought to be causally related to the dementia.

The degree of confidence in the diagnosis of IVD should be specified as possible, probable, or definite, and the other disorder(s) contributing to the dementia should be listed. For example: mixed dementia due to probable IVD and possible Alzheimer's disease or mixed dementia due to definite IVD and hypothyroidism.

Research classification

Classification of IVD for research purposes should specify features of the infarcts that may differentiate subtypes of the disorder, such as:

- Location: cortical, white matter, periventricular, basal ganglia, thalamus
- Size: volume
- Distribution: large, small, or microvessel
- Severity: chronic ischaemia versus infarction
- Aetiology: embolism, atherosclerosis, arteriosclerosis, cerebral amyloid angiopathy, hypoperfusion.

* Modified from Chui *et al*. (1992).

are deliberately not specified but are not confined to a single narrow category and memory loss is not emphasized. The severity should be sufficient to interfere with the conduct of the patient's customary affairs of life and this judgement is to be made on clinical criteria, not by neuropsychological testing. Two or more ischaemic strokes (at least one of which is outside the cerebellum) by history and examination or imaging are required, though rarely one stroke with a clear temporal relationship to the onset of dementia may be allowed. These criteria do not ask for a clear temporal relationship between infarcts and dementia, except where a single infarct is the alleged cause of the dementia. The reason for this is that vascular cases may progress gradually, without a clear-cut association between events and cognitive decline, such that establishing a temporal relationship can be difficult. These points are valid but the criteria risk diagnosing all cases of dementia with two or more infarcts as cases of VaD. Risk factors and some clinical features are included as supportive features, but how these are to be operationalized is not stated (Chui *et al.* 1992).

13.1.3 **Critique of old criteria**

While these criteria are the only operational criteria available, it is important to realize that they are based on supposition and not on fact. The NINDS–AIREN criteria were also developed with a view to epidemiological convenience rather than to clinical accuracy. They are at fault in several fundamental respects, and the reader is encouraged to review them critically and use them cautiously.

13.1.3.1 Pattern of cognitive deficit in vascular dementia

The adoption of criteria from AD, in which the mesial temporal lobes are affected early and prominently, is erroneous as the mesial temporal lobes are not especially involved in cerebrovascular disease. Thus, a diagnostic paradigm based on early memory loss is inappropriate and will fail to identify many cases of VaD. Appropriate criteria will instead emphasize a subcortical, frontal, and executive pattern of dysfunction in most cases.

13.1.3.2 Severity of dementia

Current criteria define dementia on the basis of a clear loss of cognitive function. This will deny early cases the most appropriate opportunity for secondary preventive measures by failing to detect them (Erkinjuntti and Hachinski 1993; Hachinski 1990, 1991, 1992; Hachinski and Bowler 1993).

13.1.3.3 Infarct volume

Early work suggested that an infarct volume over 20 mL and in particular of 50–100 cm^3 distinguished between VaD and 'senile dementia' (Tomlinson *et al.* 1970). However, these data were based on highly selected cases and dementia can exist with much smaller infarct volumes, usually in the range of 1–30 mL in more modern work (del Ser *et al.* 1990; Erkinjuntti *et al.* 1988; Gorelick *et al.* 1992; Liu *et al.* 1992; Loeb *et al.* 1988) and cognitive impairment short of dementia can be seen with very small infarct volumes (Bowler *et al.* 1998*a*; Corbett *et al.* 1994). Correlation between infarct volume and neuropsychological deficit is poor when all aetiologies of VaD are studied together (Bowler 1993; Bowler *et al.* 1994; Liu *et al.* 1992; Neuropathology Group of the Medical Research Council Cognitive Function and Ageing Study (MRC CFAS) 2001). This is not surprising as site is at least as important as size. It is therefore unlikely that there is a precise volume of infarction that can reliably predict VaD other than at meaninglessly large volumes.

The current criteria are not, in any case, concerned with infarct volumes but concentrate on numbers of infarcts. While, in subcortical regions, the number of infarcts correlates more closely with cognitive loss than infarct volume (Corbett *et al.* 1994), infarcts by themselves are found in less than 50% of cases of established VaD (Pohjasvaara *et al.* 2000; Wetterling *et al.* 1996) and the presence of infarcts is therefore not essential for that diagnosis to be made. Microvascular disease is crucial in the development of dementia (Esiri *et al.* 1997) and this further weakens the correlation between infarct volume and cognitive status. Infarct volume should not therefore form part of the criteria for VaD.

13.1.3.4 Infarct site

Infarct location at sites such as the thalamus can be crucial (Katz *et al.* 1987; Ladurner *et al.* 1982). However, the most important locations are disputed, partly because of the application of variable methods to differing populations. Reports have variously favoured the following lesion sites: bilateral (Erkinjuntti *et al.* 1988; Gorelick *et al.* 1992; Ladurner *et al.* 1982); left-sided (Gorelick *et al.* 1992; Liu *et al.* 1992; Tatemichi *et al.* 1993, 1994); anterior cerebral artery territory (Tatemichi *et al.* 1994); and frontal (Fukuda *et al.* 1990). Various patterns important in producing dementia have also been suggested: thalamic plus cortical (Loeb *et al.* 1988); cortical and white matter (Liu *et al.* 1992); dominant hemisphere (Loeb *et al.* 1988). Some work favours a special role for lacunar and other deep lesions over cortical lesions (del Ser *et al.* 1990; Meyer *et al.* 1988, 1989*a*; Parnetti *et al.* 1990; Tatemichi *et al.* 1993), but other work does not (Gorelick *et al.* 1992; Liu *et al.* 1992; Loeb *et al.* 1988; Tatemichi *et al.* 1994). Fisher (1965) felt that dementia in association with lacunae was rare but cognitive impairment in association with small numbers and volumes of subcortical infarcts is readily detectable (Corbett *et al.* 1994; Miyao *et al.* 1992). These contradictory findings will not be resolved until uniform criteria for patient selection and cognitive assessment have been developed. Special emphasis on individual sites is therefore impractical in the formulation of criteria, except perhaps for involvement of the thalamus.

13.1.3.5 Multiple types of vascular dementia

The term 'vascular dementia' describes dementia due to cerebrovascular disease in general (Loeb 1990) and has replaced 'multi-infarct dementia' as multiple infarcts are not the only aetiology. All of the current criteria largely treat VaD as a single condition. This is an important error, since vascular lesions capable of causing cognitive loss arise from many different aetiologies, and differing causes require different treatments. It is more accurate to speak of the vascular dementias. In addition, events falling short of stroke are now known to be important. Episodes of hypotension, leukoaraiosis, and incomplete infarction are all associated with cognitive impairment and all have some vascular basis but do not necessarily cause or consist of infarcts (Almkvist *et al.* 1992; Bowen *et al.* 1990; Breteler *et al.* 1994*a*, *c*; Cummings and Benson 1984; Diaz *et al.* 1991; Goto *et al.* 1989; Kertesz *et al.* 1990; Pujol *et al.* 1991; Skoog *et al.* 1996; Steingart *et al.* 1987*a*; Wahlund *et al.* 1992).

13.1.3.6 Statement of aetiology

The most important aspect of VaD must always be the treatment and prevention of disease. Prevention in particular will depend on aetiology and it is important that this is specified routinely in each case. Current practice does not emphasize this (Erkinjuntti and Hachinski 1993; Hachinski 1990, 1991, 1992; Hachinski and Bowler 1993).

13.1.3.7 Leukoaraiosis

Leukoaraiosis can be associated with neurological signs and psychological deficits, particularly the attention and speed components of executive function (Moser *et al.* 2001). Initial work suggested that only CT-demonstrated leukoaraiosis had clinical correlates, the interpretation being that MR, a more sensitive tool, was detecting numerous asymptomatic lesions (Diaz *et al.* 1991;

Mirsen *et al.* 1991; Steingart *et al.* 1987*a*, *b*). That more than 90% of elderly individuals have some form of leukoaraiosis without necessarily being demented supports this (de Leeuw *et al.* 2001). More recent work using detailed neuropsychological assessment has shown that subtle, predominantly subcortical, deficits are associated with leukoaraiosis in the absence of dementia and in apparently normal aged subjects (Jokinen *et al.* 2006; Kramer *et al.* 2002; Prins *et al.* 2005; Skoog *et al.* 1996; van der Flier *et al.* 2005; Zekry *et al.* 2003). Longitudinal studies have also demonstrated a correlation between increasing leukoaraiosis and declining cognition (Garde *et al.* 2005; Schmidt *et al.* 2005). There is continuing debate over whether there is a difference in the cognitive consequences of periventricular as opposed to deep white matter leukoaraiosis. One MRI-based study has shown that they closely correlate with each other (DeCarli *et al.* 2005) implying a shared aetiology but cognition was not studied. However, data from the Rotterdam scan study suggests a difference in prognosis and pattern of cognitive deficit according to lesion site (Breteler *et al.* 1994*a*; Prins *et al.* 2004).

13.1.3.8 Subcortical vascular cognitive impairment

Subcortical VCI, discussed below in detail, is now recognized to be the single commonest form of VCI but this is not recognized in current criteria.

13.1.3.9 Atrophy

Atrophy is largely ignored in the current criteria but is often assumed to be due to degenerative dementia and its presence is sometimes used as an argument against a patient having VaD (Pohjasvaara *et al.* 1999). However, increasing evidence suggests that atrophy is a common feature in cerebrovascular disease, even where this is limited to leukoaraiosis. The process may begin with risk factors alone, without definite vascular events, which are associated with both a relative increase lateral ventricle volume, suggesting central atrophy (Salerno *et al.* 1992), and cognitive decline (Launer *et al.* 1995, 2000; Wilkie and Eisdorfer 1971). In other words, cognitive impairment may correlate more closely with ventricular enlargement than it does with infarct volume and this trend is continued in more fully established cerebrovascular disease (Barber *et al.* 1999; Bowler *et al.* 1998*a*; Corbett *et al.* 1994; O'Sullivan *et al.* 2004; Pantel *et al.* 1998; Sabri *et al.* 1999; Walters *et al.* 2003). Similar findings have been reported in multiple sclerosis, a condition that can be regarded as closely analogous to subcortical VaD (Zivadinov *et al.* 2001). Atrophy may progress at the same rate in VaD, AD, and Lewy body dementia (O'Brien *et al.* 2001). Atrophy may therefore be associated with both vascular disease and degenerative dementia, rather than just being a hallmark of degenerative dementia as previously supposed.

13.1.3.10 Inclusion of major stroke

Whether major stroke should be included within VaD largely depends on the purpose of the study in question. Major stroke, identified by the production of substantial motor, sensory, visual, or language deficits, is a group of conditions for which the epidemiology, risk factors, primary and secondary preventative therapy, and prognoses are relatively well established. If the purpose of defining VaD is to identify a group of conditions for which there may be special risk factors, perhaps different from stroke in general, for which patients may benefit from appropriate preventative therapy, then the inclusion of patients with major stroke is inappropriate. Alternatively, if, for example, the purpose is to describe the economic burden of cognitive decline due to stroke, a more inclusive approach is necessary. All of the current criteria implicitly or explicitly include major stroke. We would recommend that studies should explicitly state whether or not major stroke is included and present, or make available, their data in such a way that they can be analysed with or without the contribution from major stroke.

13.1.3.11 Inclusion of subarachnoid and intracerebral haemorrhage

The inclusion or exclusion of intracerebral and subarachnoid haemorrhage within VCI is a matter of opinion and, like the inclusion of major stroke, will vary in appropriateness according to the purpose of the study in question. Once again, the solution is to state clearly whether such cases have been included or excluded and to tabulate, or make available to others, the data with and without these cases so that others may interpret the data as necessary.

13.1.3.12 Inclusion of post-stroke dementia

Over one-quarter of patients admitted with stroke become demented (Tatemichi *et al.* 1992, 1993) but much of this is due to coexistent degenerative dementia, either pre-existent or developed subsequently (Barba *et al.* 2000; Desmond *et al.* 2000; Pohjasvaara *et al.* 1997*a*, 1998). Most of these cases therefore fall outside pure VaD and might best be considered as mixed dementia unless there is a high level of confidence that only cerebrovascular disease is present.

13.1.3.13 Mixed dementia

Over the past decade, there has been another major change with the increasing recognition of mixed dementia, where VaD coexists with other causes of dementia, particularly AD. These are now known to be common but are not recognized in current criteria; they are discussed in more detail below.

13.1.4 A solution—vascular cognitive impairment

Given the limitations of the current criteria, progress in this field would best be served by moving away from VaD toward a new concept. Over the past decade there has been a paradigm shift towards such a concept, that of VCI (Hachinski and Bowler 1993), and this is now widely accepted as a more appropriate concept than the old concept of VaD. However, validated criteria for VCI are awaited. Development of these will require alternative rating scales and screening tools that focus on the cognitive domains most affected in vascular disease. The identification of patients with VCI will lead to the identification of risk factors for VCI and in turn will allow the identification of presymptomatic subjects, a stage termed 'brain-at-risk' (Hachinski 1992; Hachinski and Bowler 1993). VCI and 'brain-at-risk' are the most appropriate stages for early secondary and primary preventative therapy, respectively (Fig. 13.1).

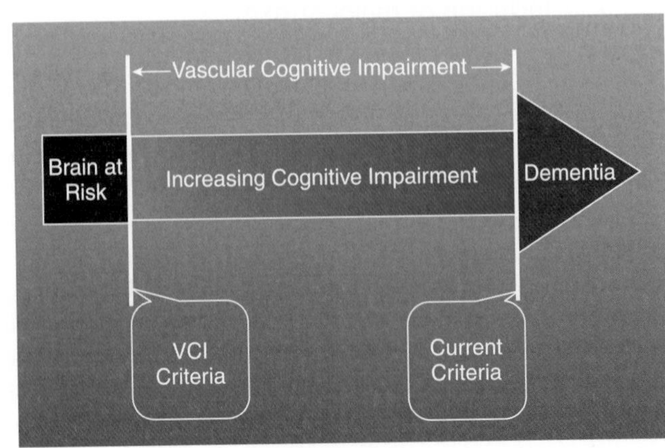

Fig. 13.1 The concept of 'brain-at-risk' and vascular cognitive impairment compared to vascular dementia.

13.1.4.1 Mixed dementia

Eighty per cent of the elderly have evidence of cerebrovascular disease (Neuropathology Group of the Medical Research Council Cognitive Function and Ageing Study (MRC CFAS) 2001) and mixed VaD and AD may account for up to half of all dementia and may be more common than any other single group (Bowler *et al.* 1998*b*; Gold *et al.* 1997; Holmes *et al.* 1999; Lim *et al.* 1999; Neuropathology Group of the Medical Research Council Cognitive Function and Ageing Study (MRC CFAS) 2001; Snowdon *et al.* 1997). In one autopsy-based series based on a dementia clinic, none of 87 patients had pure VaD, while 32 had mixed disease (Nolan *et al.* 1998). Furthermore, the interaction between the vascular component and other components more than doubles the rate of progression when compared to pure AD alone (Heyman *et al.* 1998; Snowdon *et al.* 1997).

Thus mixed dementia is far more important than was realized when the current criteria were prepared and poses a major problem in that no good method yet exists for identifying mixed dementia in life. Criteria that first select AD-like cases and then subselect those with vascular features might form an excellent basis for doing so. Unfortunately, this is precisely what the current criteria for VaD do and it is very likely that much of the reported data about VaD are in fact about mixed disease, albeit not yet recognized as such.

13.1.4.2 Subcortical VCI

Subcortical VCI is now recognized to be the commonest form of VCI, its clinical pattern, risk factors, and imaging features being sufficiently consistent for it to be considered an entity for the purposes of diagnosis, clinical trials, and management. It is recognized as subcortical VaD in the *International classification of diseases*, 10th revision (World Health Organization 1993) but not in the *Diagnostic and statistic manual of mental disorders*, 4th edition (American Psychiatric Association 1994).

Its history dates back to the now outdated concept of Binswanger's disease. By 1987, before the arrival of CT scanning and MRI, only 46 cases had been reported (Babikian and Ropper 1987). Throughout the last two decades of the 20th century, there were numerous reports of 'Binswanger's disease' diagnosed solely by the appearance of extensive white matter changes on neuroimaging without clinical correlates. This is now recognized to be inappropriate as leukoaraiosis without readily apparent clinical correlates is very common in the elderly and the term 'leukoaraiosis' should be used in describing such findings on imaging (Hachinski *et al.* 1987).

Diagnostic criteria for Binswanger's disease have been proposed (Bennett *et al.* 1990) but their use is not recommended. According to these criteria, the following must be present.

1 Dementia.

2 Two of the following:
   (a) a vascular risk factor or evidence of systemic vascular disease;
   (b) evidence of focal cerebrovascular disease (focal neurological signs);
   (c) evidence of what is termed 'subcortical' dysfunction, such as a parkinsonian, magnetic, or senile gait, gegenhalten, or incontinence due to a spastic bladder.

3 Bilateral leukoaraiosis on CT or bilateral multiple or diffuse white matter lesions each measuring more than 2 mm^2 on MR.

4 Absence of multiple or bilateral cortical lesions on CT or MRI.

5 Absence of severe dementia (e.g. MMSE > 10).

These criteria have not been validated and apply only to Binswanger's disease. Knowledge regarding subcortical VaD has increased considerably since these criteria were proposed and they are rarely applicable now. However, new criteria have yet to be developed. New research criteria for subcortical VaD have been proposed, but have not yet been validated (Erkinjuntti *et al.* 2000).

Even when applied to Binswanger's disease, the old Bennett criteria have a number of failings including the following.

1. The use of the term 'dementia' without clarification is not acceptable. The cognitive deficits arising from subcortical white matter disease are predominantly frontal and executive and this needs to be considered in case identification (Corbett *et al.* 1994; Graham *et al.* 2004; Kramer *et al.* 2002; Moser *et al.* 2001; Skoog *et al.* 1996).
2. The use of the MMSE is inappropriate as it is insensitive for deficits in the frontal and executive domains and it should not be used in subcortical VaD. Other tests may be more appropriate and there is some evidence that short batteries of individual neuropsychological tests can separate subcortical VaD from AD (Gainotti *et al.* 2001; O'Sullivan *et al.* 2005; Tierney *et al.* 2001) but this remains to be confirmed. Other tests of executive and frontal function including CLOX, EXIT25, trail making, and digit symbol substitution have also been developed or found particularly sensitive to the changes typically seen in subcortical VCI (Ferris 1999; O'Sullivan *et al.* 2005; Roman and Royall 1999).
3. The radiological guidelines are inappropriate as, on MR, extensive deep white matter lesions sparing the subcortical U-fibres and corpus callosum would be expected and periventricular lesions alone, which may be due in part to ependymal breakdown, are not consistent with Binswanger's disease. The sensitivity of CT to white matter lesions is insufficient for these limitations to be applied to CT. Lesions outside the deep white matter are not part of Binswanger's disease but occur in up to one-third of cases (Babikian and Ropper 1987), presumably as other manifestations of cerebrovascular disease.

A combination of neuropsychological and imaging data provides the most certain way of making a diagnosis although proposals exist at present only for late stage disease (Price *et al.* 2005).

13.2 **Epidemiology**

13.2.1 **Vascular dementia**

The incidence of VaD is about 3.8 per 1000 per annum. The incidence in women rises from between 0.3 and 1.36 in those aged 65 to 69 to 9.3 in those aged 85 or over. For men the corresponding figures are between 1.3 and 2.2 rising to 9.3 and 15.9 in those aged over 90 (Andersen *et al.* 1999; Hebert *et al.* 2000). Dementia from all causes has a prevalence of about 8% of the population over the age of 65. Between 9% and 39% (but typically 13% to 19%) of these cases are vascular (Knopman *et al.* 2003*b*; Ott *et al.* 1995) but VaD may account for half of Japanese cases (Canadian Study of Health and Aging Working Group 1994; Ebly *et al.* 1994; Ikeda *et al.* 2001; Kase *et al.* 1989; Kase 1991; Ueda *et al.* 1992). An additional 11– 43% may be mixed dementia (Kase 1991). The proportion of cases due to VaD falls with increasing age (Ebly *et al.* 1994; Rocca *et al.* 1991) but even so, the prevalence of all dementia rises so rapidly with age that the prevalence of VaD also rises, from 0% to 2% in the 60 to 69 age group to up to 16% for males aged 80 to 89, though more typical figures are between 3% and 6% (Ott *et al.* 1995; Rocca *et al.* 1991). Males are more commonly affected than females in most studies (Gorelick *et al.* 1993; Kase 1991; Meyer *et al.* 1988; Ott *et al.* 1995; Rocca *et al.* 1991).

13.2.2 **Post-stroke dementia**

Dementia after stroke is now increasingly recognized. Initial studies suggested that 30% of all stroke patients were demented 3 months after stroke but that 10% were demented prior to the index stroke. It now appears that these high figures arose because of case selection. In the Framingham study, the 10-year risk of post-stroke dementia was rather lower at 19.3% of cases and dementia developed in 11% of controls suggesting that the risk attributable to an index stroke is lower than had been thought (Ivan *et al.* 2004). However, the study methodology may have produced an underestimate (Bowler 2004). The incidence of cognitive impairment after stroke sufficient to adversely affect outcome but not meeting old criteria for VaD is as high as 35.2% compared to 3.8% with a similar degree of impairment in stroke-free controls (Tatemichi *et al.* 1994).

Even in those without prior dementia, post-stroke dementia correlates with pre-stroke cognitive status suggesting pre-existing pathology in at least some cases. This is supported by the finding that MRI changes more usually associated with degenerative dementia correlate with pre-stroke cognitive decline. Pre-existent disease may also be vascular, cognitive decline after stroke being much more common in those who have small-vessel cerebrovascular disease (Mok *et al.* 2004). Blacks may be at greater risk of post-stroke dementia than Whites. The risk of dementia after stroke increases with age, from 14.8% in those aged 60 to 69 to 52.3% for those over 80, but 36.4% of these had mixed dementia (Barba *et al.* 2000; Pohjasvaara *et al.* 1997*b*, 1999; Tatemichi *et al.* 1992, 1993, 1994). In the Rotterdam study, a history of stroke increased the proportion of subjects aged over 55 with a Mini-Mental State score below 24 from 6.5% to 15.5% and for a score below 26 from 13.5% to 25.6%. Other vascular risk factors had a similar but less powerful action (Breteler *et al.* 1994*b*; Di Carlo *et al.* 2000).

13.2.3 Vascular cognitive impairment

Data are now becoming available concerning the epidemiology of VCI. In patients under 74, VCI may be the commonest cause of cognitive impairment. In those aged 75 to 84, cases of pure VCI, VaD, and those with a vascular component in the context of mixed disease outnumber those with pure AD. Patients with VCI are more likely to die or become institutionalized than those with early AD who are not yet demented (Rockwood *et al.* 2000). VCI is associated with both stroke and death from stroke (Ferrucci *et al.* 1996; Gale *et al.* 1996).

13.3 Aetiological factors

13.3.1 Genetic

The accepted risk factors explain only part of the development of leukoaraiosis (Streifler 2003) and it is a common clinical experience that leukoaraiosis is not directly related in severity to hypertension in all patients, some having more than might be anticipated and others appear remarkably spared. This suggests that genetic factors might affect susceptibility and there is now increasing evidence for this (Atwood *et al.* 2004; Carmelli *et al.* 1998, 2002; Henskens *et al.* 2005; Turner *et al.* 2004). Some of this may be mediated through angiotensin receptor and endothelial nitric oxide synthase gene polymorphisms (Henskens *et al.* 2005), but it seems probable that there are other, as yet unidentified, conditions that are relevant here (Bowler 2003*b*) with evidence of linkage to chromosome 4 (DeStefano *et al.* 2006).

13.3.1.1 Single gene disorders

CADASIL An hereditary multi-infarct dementia consistent with 'cerebral autosomal dominant arteriopathy with subcortical infarcts and leucoencephalopathy' (CADASIL) was first described 30 years ago (Sourander and Walinder 1977) but described in more detail and its cause localized to chromosome 19 in the early 1990s (Tournier Lasserve *et al.* 1991, 1993). It occurs in all racial groups and its prevalence may be of the order of 1:100 000.

It is caused by mutation of the Notch 3 gene, which codes for a large transmembrane receptor. The gene is expressed in vascular smooth muscle cells in a variety of organs and mutated genes cause accumulation of the extracellular portion of the receptor within blood vessel walls. This material was originally noted to be periodic acid–Schiff (PAS)-positive on light microscopy and on electron microscopy is seen as a granular osmiophilic deposit (GOM) within vessel walls adjacent to smooth muscle cells. These changes may be seen in a variety of tissues, but it is in the brain that the pathology gives rise to clinically apparent disease. This seems to be due primarily to mechanical damage to the walls of small arteries (below 400 microns), arterioles, and capillaries. Most of the damage is ischaemic with multiple lacunar infarcts and other areas of leukoaraiosis but haemorrhage has been reported (Fig. 13.2).

The clinical presentation is most characteristically in the fourth decade with recurrent transient ischaemic attacks or strokes but clinical onset as late as the seventh decade has been reported. Migraine, usually with aura, develops in half of cases, usually a few years before the first vascular events. This may be preceded by a decade by psychiatric manifestations, most commonly depression, in a substantial minority. Epilepsy occurs but is uncommon. The disease progresses initially with recurrent vascular events with recovery but, as disability increases, these discrete events gradually merge and the condition becomes gradually progressive. As might be expected with extensive small-vessel disease, the picture is typically pseudobulbar with extrapyramidal features in those where the disease involves the basal ganglia. At this stage subcortical cognitive impairment may be seen and this can proceed to frank dementia but presentation with dementia is unusual. About 10% of cases may present with an acute encephalopathy preceded by migraine and characterized by headache, confusion, pyrexia, and fitting resolving fully over 7 to 14 days (Schon *et al.* 2003).

In the majority of patients, the condition may be suspected with the development of otherwise unexplained small-vessel cerebrovascular disease at a young age and without vascular risk factors, although in those patients with later presentations coincidental vascular risk factors may be present. An accompanying history of migraine with aura and psychiatric illnesses supports the diagnosis as does a family history although new mutations have been reported and the family history may be limited by misdiagnoses in the relatives. Additional evidence for the diagnosis may be apparent on MRI. The bulk of the changes due to CADASIL are identical to those seen in the common forms of small-vessel disease. However, these common forms affect the deep perforating arteries and so tend to spare the external capsule, corpus callosum, and anterior temporal lobe. This pattern is not seen in CADASIL and ischaemic white matter lesions at these sites support the diagnosis. Angiography should be avoided; the vessels affected in CADASIL are smaller than those visible on angiography which is therefore characteristically normal and up to 2/3 of patients may suffer neurological complications that can be permanent (Dichgans and Petersen 1997). See Fig. 13.3.

The diagnosis can be confirmed by genetic analysis in the majority of cases. However, there are over 30 mutations and the Notch 3 gene is large. It is not practical in routine diagnostic work to test the whole gene but the mutations do cluster which facilitates the development of screening protocols. These will generally identify about 2/3 of cases. As the disease affects vessels in many organs, a peripheral biopsy can often be positive. Skin has often been used but may be false negative in almost half of cases. Muscle may be better as the sensitivity of the test is related to the number of smooth muscle cells in arteriolar walls and these are more numerous in muscle (and nerve) than skin. Routine laboratory testing therefore comprises genetic screening and electron microscopy of a suitable biopsy with further genetic analysis where the biopsy confirms GOM.

Other single gene disorders While CADASIL is the best described single-gene condition affecting vessels in this way, it is not the only one. One of the groups studying CADASIL has reported that only a third of skin biopsies are positive for GOM, but that many of the others

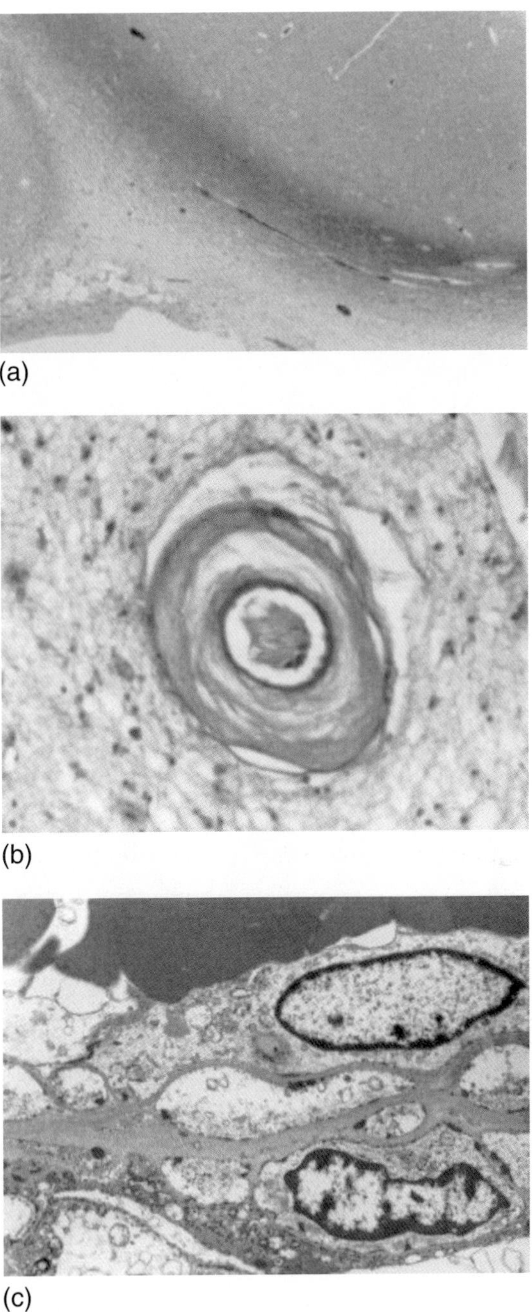

Fig. 13.2 Histopathology in CADASIL. (a) This low power section shows, from top right corner downwards: unremarkable cerebral cortex, spared U fibres (blue), degenerated white matter (grey), and cavitated infarct. Luxol Fast blue and haemoxylin and eosin (H & E). (b) High power view of small artery in the white matter, showing thickened wall almost devoid of cellular elements. Blobs of different colour material are seen apposed to the thick line encircling the lumen H & E. (c) Electron microscopic photograph of a small artery in a skin biopsy. The multiple dark blobs against the basement membrane represent the granular osmophilic deposits. (Courtesy of Dr D.G. Munoz.) This is a black and white version of Plate 10.

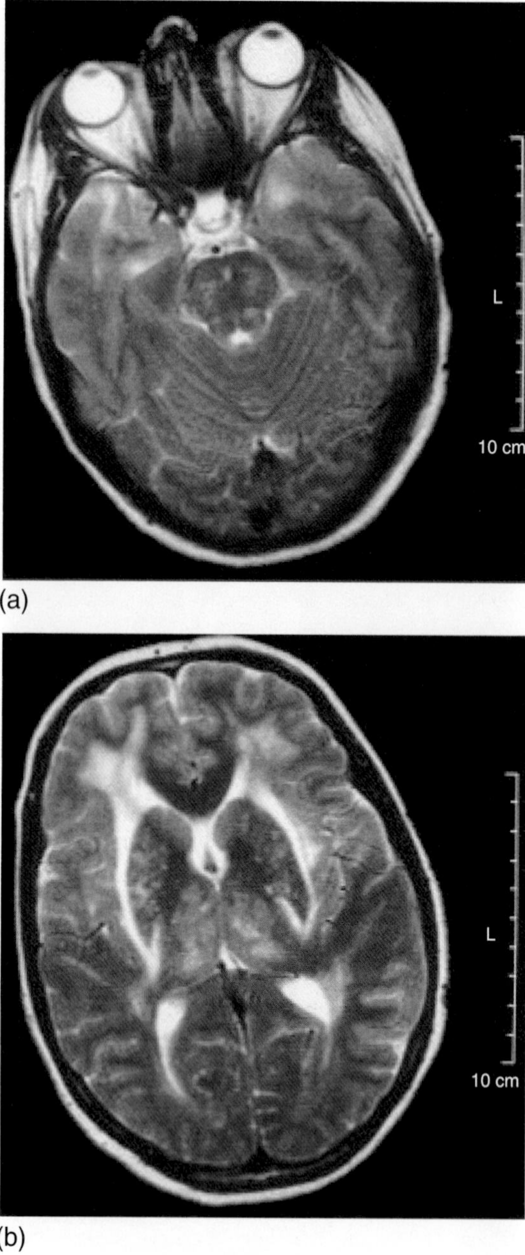

Fig. 13.3 MRI in CADASIL. Image (a) shows confluent high signal in both temporal poles and (b) shows confluent high signal in the external capsule. Neither of these locations are typically involved in small-vessel cerebrovascular disease. (Courtesy Professor H.S. Markus.)

exhibit pathological changes in the vessel walls which they felt could be divided into eight groups, some of which ran in families (Ruchoux *et al.* 2000). The Japanese literature contains a number of reports of a condition with subcortical infarcts and leucoencephalopathy with an autosomal recessive pattern of inheritance (sometimes termed CARASIL), often accompanied by alopecia and degenerative disease in the lumbar spine and knees (Fukutake and Hirayama 1995;

Maeda *et al.* 1976; Yanagawa *et al.* 2002). A family has been reported from Hamburg with a condition resembling CADASIL but without GOM (Hagel *et al.* 2004). There may, therefore, be several as yet poorly characterized inherited diseases of small vessels affecting the cerebral circulation.

13.3.2 Acquired

Many of the commonly recognized vascular risk factors have been identified as risk factors for VaD. These include hypertension, heart disease, atrial fibrillation, diabetes, insulin resistance, hyperlipidaemia, smoking, carotid bruits, age, male sex, education, race, prior stroke, ECG changes, hematocrit, history of myocardial infarction, homocysteine, carotid atherosclerosis, dietary fat, low-density lipoprotein cholesterol, isolated systolic hypertension, and proteinuria (Boston *et al.* 2001; Geroldi *et al.* 2005; Goldstein *et al.* 2005; Gorelick *et al.* 1992, 1993; Gorelick 1997; Hofman *et al.* 1997; Knopman *et al.* 2001; Ladurner *et al.* 1982; Lindsay *et al.* 1997; Loeb *et al.* 1988; Longstreth *et al.* 1996, 2005; Meyer *et al.* 1988; Mielke *et al.* 1998; Moroney *et al.* 1999; Morris *et al.* 2004; O'Connell *et al.* 1998; Ott *et al.* 1995, 1996, 1997, 2004; Slooter *et al.* 1997; Tatemichi *et al.* 1993; Ueda *et al.* 1992; Wright *et al.* 2005; Xu *et al.* 2004; Yaffe *et al.* 2004; Yamamoto *et al.* 2002). Endothelial activation may also have a role in the progression of leukoaraiosis (Markus *et al.* 2005).

Orthostatic hypotension and blood pressure variability may also play a role (Goldstein *et al.* 2005; Watanabe *et al.* 1996, 1997). Nocturnal hypotension superimposed upon limited perfusion reserve and impaired vasoreactivity producing partial ischaemia leading to incomplete infarction has been a proposed mechanism but evidence from Japan suggests that this is not the case and that nocturnal dipping of blood pressure reduces the risk of ischaemic damage (Yamamoto *et al.* 2002, 2005).

Vascular risk factors in middle age may predict both VCI and AD in later life, even when the risk factors themselves have resolved. This has now been shown for hypertension, smoking, diabetes, hypercholesterolaemia, and obesity (Galanis *et al.* 1997; Kivipelto *et al.* 2001*a*, *b*, 2005; Knopman *et al.* 2001; Schnaider Beeri *et al.* 2004; Skoog 1997; Whitmer *et al.* 2005). It has also been shown that blood pressure falls with increasing dementia, leading to a spuriously negative association between dementia and hypertension when measured in cross-sectional studies (Qiu *et al.* 2004; Skoog *et al.* 1998) and not inconceivably to a false association between hypotension and dementia.

Leukoaraiosis is associated with hypertension, a history of stroke, and stroke risk factors in general (Bogousslavsky *et al.* 1987; Inzitari *et al.* 1987; Jeerakathil *et al.* 2004; Kertesz *et al.* 1988; Longstreth *et al.* 1996), suggesting a vascular cause, but is not associated with carotid disease (Streifler *et al.* 1995). Episodic hypotension occurring through transient dysrhythmias, nocturnal hypotension, or carotid sinus hypersensitivity superimposed on a background of diminished vascular reserve (Brown *et al.* 1990; Brun and Englund 1986; De Reuck *et al.* 1999; Kuwabara *et al.* 1996; Rossi *et al.* 1999; Sabri *et al.* 1998; Sulkava and Erkinjuntti 1987) may be one group of aetiological mechanisms for both leukoaraiosis and incomplete infarction but data concerning hypotension as a risk factor for VaD remain contradictory (Lindsay *et al.* 1997; Verghese *et al.* 2003). While most closely associated with hypertension, this is not necessary for the development of leukoaraiosis; measurable changes in the extent of leukoaraiosis can be seen over time with even low-normal systolic pressures (Goldstein *et al.* 2005).

13.4 Clinical features

13.4.1 History

Dementia can be established by the clinical history and examination alone. An assessment for depression should be included in the examination. The description of dysarthria, mild hemiparesis, imbalance, pseudobulbar palsy, small stepping (magnetic) gait, emotional incontinence, some degree of dementia, and incontinence (the 'lacunar state') dates back to the turn of the century and describes a minuscule proportion of all cases of VaD (Fisher 1965, 1982). Neither a clear history of stroke nor of a temporal relationship between strokes and cognitive decline is necessary for VaD to be present (Knopman *et al.* 2003*b*). In 90% of cases where multiple infarcts are responsible there is also a history of stroke or of transient ischemic attacks. However, in cases where subcortical ischemic change is the vascular mechanism, a history of stroke may be absent in up to 40% and focal signs are also less common (Tarvonen-Schröder *et al.* 1996).

13.4.1.1 Subcortical vascular dementia

In cases that have reached the level of severity corresponding to Binswanger's disease and have fulfilled Bennett's criteria (Bennett *et al.* 1990), the clinical picture is that of a patient, slightly more often male than female, in his/her sixth or seventh decade. A history of hypertension is present in 80% or more and is often poorly controlled. A history of stroke at some stage is almost universal, but exceptions occur and rarely focal signs may be absent even late in the disease (Burger *et al.* 1976). Other risk factors for vascular disease, especially diabetes, are often present (Babikian and Ropper 1987; Loizou *et al.* 1981). Dementia is variable and not necessarily the presenting symptom. It evolves over 3 to 10 years and is intermittently progressive but may become gradually progressive without further clear-cut vascular events (Pohjasvaara *et al.* 2003). Aphasia, amnestic intervals, and neglect are seen in some cases. Memory loss is less prominent than in AD, the neuropsychological picture being that of frontal lobe and executive dysfunction (Au *et al.* 2006; Bennett *et al.* 1994; Caplan and Schoene 1978; Cummings 1994; Graham *et al.* 2004). Behavioural changes are early and prominent and may be the presenting feature. Some patients exhibit an early manic phase but, in most, progressively increasing aboulia develops later in the illness (Caplan and Schoene 1978). Depression is common and may be particularly related to frontal deep white matter lesions (Bennett *et al.* 1990; O'Brien *et al.* 2000; Pohjasvaara *et al.* 2003). Fluctuating mood with irritability and outbreaks of rage has also been reported (Delong *et al.* 1974).

Dysarthria, focal motor signs, and a gait disturbance, with features of spasticity, parkinsonism, and ataxia (Thompson and Marsden 1987) evolve during the illness and may be relatively early. Incontinence develops later but may occur while cognition is still, at least grossly, intact (Caplan and Schoene 1978; Delong *et al.* 1974; Pohjasvaara *et al.* 2003; Starr *et al.* 2003). The dysarthria is part of a pseudobulbar palsy and, while both are variable in degree, they are nearly universally present (Caplan and Schoene 1978). Dizziness, faints, and, less commonly, epilepsy also occur (Olszewski 1962).

13.4.2 Examination

13.4.2.1 Subcortical vascular dementia

A detailed description of gait change in Binswanger's has been published (Thompson and Marsden 1987), but some caution is necessary as these cases presented atypically with gait disturbance and were not confirmed by autopsy. The gait is described as having elements of both parkinsonism and ataxia. Difficulty in leg use is out of proportion to other leg movements when lying or seated and also out of proportion to movements of the upper limbs and face, which are relatively preserved. Early cases stand wide-based with the legs, arms, and trunk held straight (contrast parkinsonism). The gait consists of short steps with a tendency to shuffle, especially on turning corners. The arm swing may be slightly reduced. Postural reflexes are preserved. In more severe cases, standing may be difficult but even so, such patients can typically move their legs easily in a bicycling or walking action when seated. These movements are slow and deliberate, but not ataxic. The gait is wide-based and the legs are held stiffly extended. The feet may appear stuck to the ground. Attempts to step forward are accompanied by forward flexing of the trunk and reaching out with the arms for support. When walking the steps are of variable length and accompanied by scraping and shuffling. These patients do not festinate; they would fall before increasing gait speed. Attempted changes of direction precipitate freezing and further loss of balance. In severely affected patients truncal ataxia is prominent and a history of backward falls is often given. These phenomena are explained by disconnection of the leg region of the motor and supplementary motor cortex from the basal ganglia and cerebellum. As a disconnection phenomenon, correlation of the gait abnormality would be expected with leukoaraiosis rather than basal ganglionic ischaemic changes. Supportive evidence comes from the observation that cases of vascular parkinsonism had more frontal white matter changes than cases of Binswanger's disease without gait abnormality, but that there was no difference in ischaemic changes in the basal ganglia (Yamanouchi and Nagura 1997). Gait speed may correlate with cognitive status (Starr *et al.* 2003). Sparing of the face and arms occurs because these fibres are more superficial.

13.5 Neuropsychology

The old criteria for VaD tended to select cases according to the presence of memory and cortical cognitive deficits, historically leading to an inaccurate view of the pattern of cognitive impairment. Data derived using such criteria were even sometimes used to validate them, a tautological process whereby analysis of case series meeting the old criteria for VaD will reveal prominent memory loss in all cases. This has been taken as showing that memory loss is prominent in VaD but this is so only because the cases were selected for memory loss. If the criteria are wrong, so is case identification. A better source of information is to look at the cognitive changes seen in cerebrovascular disease in general. Data derived this way reveal a predominating theme of a primarily subcortical dementia with early impairment of frontal lobe function. Memory impairment is usual but is often not pre-eminent (Babikian *et al.* 1990; Bowler *et al.* 1994, 1997; Gold *et al.* 2005; Graham *et al.* 2004; Hom and Reitan 1990; Loeb *et al.* 1988; Perez *et al.* 1975*a*, *b*, *c*; Sachdev *et al.* 2004; Tatemichi *et al.* 1992, 1994; Wade *et al.* 1986, 1988; Wolfe *et al.* 1990).

The presence of 'patchy' or unequal cognitive deficits is a requirement for a diagnosis of VaD in ICD-10 but this pattern of cognitive loss is only to be expected in true multi-infarct dementia where there are only very few (two or three) cortical infarcts. In VaD in general the extent to which the cognitive deficit is patchy is not different from that in Alzheimer's disease, although the domains affected are different (Boston *et al.* 2001).

That VCI is a subcortical condition means that the screening and simple rating tools used in Alzheimer's disease are not appropriate. This applies particularly to the MMSE. Instruments that include assessment of frontal, executive, and subcortical function are required. Such tests as the EXIT25, CLOX (Roman and Royall 1999; Royall *et al.* 1998), and a modification of the ADAS-Cog termed VaDAS-Cog may all represent appropriate steps in this direction (Ferris 1999; Gauthier and Ferris 2001). Some tests may be able to separate AD and subcortical VaD (Graham *et al.* 2004), but test batteries specifically developed for this purpose are most likely to be useful and some of these are now being reported (O'Sullivan *et al.* 2005; Price *et al.* 2005).

13.6 Imaging correlates

13.6.1 Structural

The term leukoaraiosis encompasses a range of pathologies. The term was originally used in the context of CT white matter changes (Hachinski *et al.* 1987), but it is also used to refer to white matter changes on MRI. However, a wide range of structural changes encompassing increased water content without functional loss through to axon or myelin loss appear similar or identical on MRI. This is one of the reasons for the relatively poor correlation between leukoaraiosis and cognition.

Early reports on the effects of leukoaraiosis on cognition were mixed. In part this was because some studies used insensitive measures of cognition and others used insensitive rating scales to quantify leukoaraiosis. However, there is now clear evidence that leukoaraiosis is associated with both cognitive impairment and focal signs in otherwise normal individuals (Breteler *et al.* 1994*c*; Diaz *et al.* 1991; Steingart *et al.* 1987*a*, *b*). Even in early VCI and in the independent elderly there is an association between leukoaraiosis and cognitive loss (Bowler *et al.* 1998*a*; van der Flier *et al.* 2005). Large population studies also confirm an association between leukoaraiosis and impaired cognition (Longstreth *et al.* 1996) and leukoaraiosis may be the earliest correlate of cognitive symptoms (de Groot *et al.* 2001). Functional imaging (diffusion tensor MRI) shows abnormalities of diffusivity in normal appearing white matter in patients with leukoaraiosis and diffusivity correlates better with cognition than simple lesion load (O'Sullivan *et al.* 2004).

Whether subcortical or periventricular leukoaraiosis is primarily associated with cognitive decline and even whether separating the two is a useful exercise remains uncertain (DeCarli *et al.* 2005; Prins *et al.* 2004; van den Heuvel *et al.* 2006). Lesions in the deep grey matter may have a greater effect than those in deep white matter (Gold *et al.* 2005).

13.6.2 **Functional**

Imaging of cerebral blood flow (CBF) along with cerebral metabolic rate for oxygen ($CMRO_2$) has the potential to help solve two of the principal mysteries surrounding leukoaraiosis. The first of these concerns the pathophysiology. Is leukoaraiosis of ischaemic origin? The second concerns the consequences. If leukoaraiosis causes cognitive decline it probably does so by disconnecting the cortex, producing a subcortical dementia. Disconnected cortex shows lower energy metabolism (diaschisis). This can be imaged directly using positron emission tomography (PET) and measuring the $CMRO_2$ or the cerebral metabolic rate for glucose (CMR_{glu}). Because of flow-metabolism coupling, CBF is diminished in proportion to metabolism and CBF can be imaged both by PET and single photon emission (computerized) tomography (SPECT). However, white matter disease has not been a subject of great importance in functional imaging until recently, partly because of lack of interest and partly because of the difficulty of imaging white matter, which is both located deep to, and generates a lower signal than cortex. The past decade has seen the development of work that begins to answer some of the questions.

13.6.2.1 Functional changes in leukoaraiosis

Functional imaging and the pathogenesis of leukoaraiosis Regions of leukoaraiosis have abnormally low blood flow and low oxygen and glucose metabolism. However, most of this work has been done using subjects in a steady state. Such observations, unless supported by an elevated oxygen extraction ratio (OER), cannot distinguish between the cause and the consequences of ischaemia or other processes leading to the development of leukoaraiosis. Dynamic studies, stressing the blood supply to the lesions and the adjacent regions, will provide more evidence regarding the possible aetiology of the lesions, but this kind of work is relatively uncommon.

Static observations In patients with very extensive white matter disease, the resting CBF and $CMRO_2$ are decreased in the regions of white matter change by about 2/3 such that the OER remains normal (Herholz *et al.* 1990; Meguro *et al.* 1990; Toso 1989; Yao *et al.* 1990). This provides no evidence for an ischaemic aetiology. Some PET studies have demonstrated not only a decrease in CBF and $CMRO_2$, but also an increase in OEF. This was limited to the frontal white matter in the most severely demented patients. In these the $CMRO_2$ in the white matter fell to 50% of that seen in normal elderly control subjects (De Reuck *et al.* 1992).

In a PET study of eight patients, four of whom were demented and two more of whom became so within a year, with leukoaraiosis sufficiently extensive to be confluent in the periventricular regions, the non-demented cases had insignificantly lower CBF and lower $CMRO_2$ than the controls but had a significantly higher OEF. The demented cases with leukoaraiosis had significant falls in both CBF and $CMRO_2$ with an OEF that was, if anything, slightly higher than that of the controls, but not significantly so (Yao *et al.* 1992). While this has the limitations of a cross-sectional study it could be interpreted as suggesting that, in the early stages of leukoaraiosis, ischaemia as indicated by an elevated OEF is present and that, as the condition evolves to completed ischaemic damage, this is replaced by a near-normal OEF in the presence of lowered CBF and $CMRO_2$.

In one study of CBF and leukoaraiosis in VaD, there were falls in CBF in the cortex, the white matter, and in the subcortical grey matter. The extent of the CT leukoaraiosis correlated with CBF in the subcortical grey matter. Leukoaraiosis may therefore either cause the decrease in CBF in grey matter via diaschisis, or more probably shares a common aetiology in VaD as both the deep grey matter and deep white matter are supplied by thin penetrating arterioles (Kawamura *et al.* 1991, 1993).

Dynamic observations In one of the few dynamic studies, Brown *et al.* (1990) used xenon-enhanced CT to measure resting CBF and the dynamic effect of injecting acetazolamide in 12 subjects with known cerebrovascular disease and leukoaraiosis and 10 age-matched controls without leukoaraiosis. Resting white-matter CBF in the patients was only 2/3 that of the controls and reactivity was greatly attenuated in the patients. Conversely, resting grey matter CBF was not different between the patients and the controls but, once again and perhaps unexpectedly, reactivity was lower in the patients, though not to the same degree as in the white matter (Brown *et al.* 1990). These observations support suggestions that the aetiology of leukoaraiosis is ischaemia at the ends of the long penetrating arterioles, occurring perhaps as a result of episodic hypotension on top of impaired reactivity. This could lead to progressive infarction, possibly through an intermediate stage of incomplete infarction (Lassen 1982).

These conclusions are supported by a PET study comparing 17 hypertensive patients with seven normotensive controls and measuring the response to hypercapnia, which produces a similar effect to injection of acetazolamide. At rest no differences in CBF between the groups were found, but once again diminished reactivity was found in the patients, something that increased with increasing severity of leukoaraiosis and dementia (Kuwabara *et al.* 1996).

13.6.2.2 Functional imaging and the cognitive correlates of leukoaraiosis

Having established that in areas of leukoaraiosis there is both diminished CBF and cerebral metabolism and that there is evidence to suggest, by virtue of an elevated OEF and diminished reserve, that this may arise through ischaemia, the next question that functional imaging has been able to shed some light on is that of the functional consequences. One marker for functional effects remote from the site of the causative lesion is remote changes on functional imaging, termed diaschisis.

13.6.2.3 Diaschisis

Diaschisis refers to functional deactivation occurring remotely from the responsible structural lesion (Feeney and Baron 1986) and evidence of this may be seen on functional imaging (Baron *et al.* 1992).

Diaschisis has been extensively reported in association with stroke, most often in the cerebellum contralateral to supratentorial lesions and in the cortex overlying small deep lesions, especially those of the thalamus (Bowler *et al.* 1992). These observations are pertinent to the possible effects of leukoaraiosis and there is a correlation between diaschisis and neuropsychological deficit following small deep lesions (Baron *et al.* 1986, 1992; Perani *et al.* 1987; Vallar *et al.* 1988). Further correlations exist between extensive cortical diaschisis and motor hemineglect (Fiorelli *et al.* 1991) and between performance on the Token test and parietotemporal metabolism (Karbe *et al.* 1989). While these reports show a correlation between diaschisis and deficit, they have been unable to establish whether the association is causal or whether it is simply that appropriately sited lesions produce both the clinical deficit and diaschisis, without the diaschisis adding to the deficit (Baron *et al.* 1986; Bowler *et al.* 1992, 1995).

As would be expected from this, local cortical changes as a result of diaschisis can be identified when large areas of leukoaraiosis lie directly under the cortex. These changes become more diffuse with deeper white matter lesions (Herholz *et al.* 1990; Yao *et al.* 1990).

13.6.2.4 Cognitive changes and diaschisis as a consequence of leukoaraiosis

Having then established that cortical CBF and metabolic changes consistent with diaschisis do occur in association with, and presumably as a consequence of leukoaraiosis, the next question is whether these changes are associated with clinical and, in particular, cognitive changes.

Several studies have shown a correlation between leukoaraiosis, local reductions in cortical CBF and metabolism, often with an emphasis on the frontal lobes, and cognitive status in both symptomatic and asymptomatic individuals (De Carli *et al.* 1995; De Reuck *et al.* 1992; Kobari *et al.* 1990; Shyu *et al.* 1996; Sultzer *et al.* 1995; Yamauchi *et al.* 1996). Callosal atrophy may also occur in association with lacunar infarction and leukoaraiosis and, in a stepwise regression analysis, the severity of white matter changes in the centrum semiovale correlates most closely with callosal atrophy, which also correlates with cognitive loss (Yamauchi *et al.* 1996).

13.7 Pathology

Infarcts contribute to most cases of VaD, but multiple smaller infarcts and small vessel disease are more often a substrate of VaD than single major infarcts (Esiri *et al.* 1997). Leukoaraiosis, haemorrhages, amyloid angiopathy, vasculitides, angioendotheliosis, and incomplete infarction are less common aetiological factors. Incomplete infarction comprises zones of partial neuronal or axonal loss with demyelination, increased perivascular spaces, a reactive astrocytosis, gliosis, and sparse macrophages (Brun and Englund 1986; Chimowitz *et al.* 1989). Silent infarcts also contribute to cognitive decline (Vermeer *et al.* 2003). Ischaemic hippocampal sclerosis may account for a significant proportion of cases (Fig. 13.4; Barker *et al.* 2002; Crystal *et al.* 2000).

13.7.1 Leukoaraiosis

Deep white-matter changes seen on MR correspond to myelin pallor on naked eye examination of slides when the MR changes are over 10 mm. The subcortical U-fibres are spared. Axons, myelinated fibres, and oligodendrocytes are decreased in the affected areas, and spongiosis is seen in the same areas. These changes blend gradually into surrounding tissue (Fig. 13.5; Braffman *et al.* 1988*b*; Munoz *et al.* 1993). Frank infarction is rare in lesions corresponding to leukoaraiosis (Munoz *et al.* 1993) but is otherwise a common part of the pathology of the deep white matter (Braffman *et al.* 1988*a*, *b*; Marshall *et al.* 1988). Small punctate lesions seen on MRI correspond to dilated perivascular (Virchow–Robin) spaces (Braffman *et al.* 1988*a*; Munoz *et al.* 1993). When seen in the periventricular regions, leukoaraiosis is often due to breakdown of the ependyma,

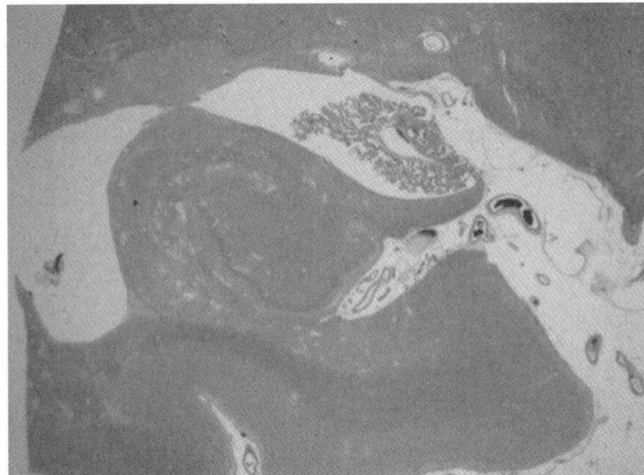

Fig. 13.4 Hippocampal sclerosis. This H & E stained section of the hippocampus shows multiple small infarcts, some of which are cavitated, whereas in others neurons are replaced by glial scars. Dilated perivascular spaces are also seen. (Courtesy of Dr D.G. Munoz.) This is a black and white version of Plate 11.

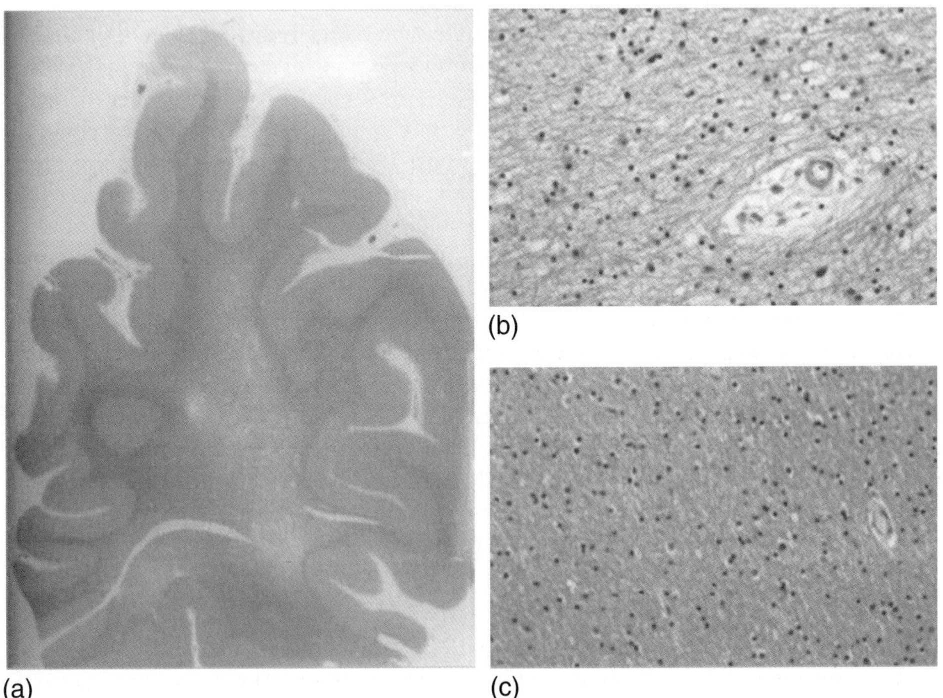

Fig. 13.5 Leukoaraiosis. (a) H & E stained coronal section through a frontal lobe in a patient with prominent leukoaraiosis on magnetic resonance scans. Note extensive, but irregular pallor of white matter in the absence of lacunes. (b) High power view of the pale white matter area, showing rarefaction of the tissue, persistence of oligodendrocytes, and the presence of rare astrocytes. H & E. (c) High power view of the dark white matter area, showing the normal histology. H & E. (Courtesy of Dr D.G. Munoz.) This is a black and white version of Plate 12.

with increased fluid content of the local white matter with some loss of myelin (Sze *et al.* 1985) and dilated perivascular spaces (Awad *et al.* 1986), and is therefore less closely linked to hypertension. There is also evidence of breakdown of the blood–brain barrier in regions of leukoaraiosis and plasma proteins can be found in glial cells in close relation to demonstrable white matter lesions (Akiguchi *et al.* 1998; Pantoni *et al.* 1993; Tomimoto *et al.* 1996; Wallin and Blennow 1991). Whether these changes are causal, or merely consequences of ischaemia remains to be established, though extravasated plasma proteins are known to be neurotoxic.

13.7.2 **Subcortical vascular dementia**

The histopathology in advanced subcortical VaD is characteristic. The only typical gross external abnormality is slight gyral atrophy (Babikian and Ropper 1987). Hydrocephalus ex vacuo is seen on sectioning. Discrete lacunae are seen in 93% of cases, typically in the centrum semiovale, internal capsule, and basal ganglia. Confluent areas of white matter discolouration occur separately from the infarcts and are commonly occipital, periventricular, and sometimes frontal, but the changes are primarily in the centrum semiovale and around the ventricles (Babikian and Ropper 1987). The corpus callosum may be thinned but not ischaemic. In these areas the pathology is variable. The earliest changes are of swollen myelin sheaths and oligodendrocytes. Subsequently incomplete demyelination and loss of oligodendrocytes develop followed by fragmentation of axis cylinders (Fig. 13.6). Axons may be relatively preserved (Pellissier and Poncet 1989). Rarefaction and cavitation with scattered microcystic areas of infarction follow. Gliosis is invariable. Subcortical association fibres are characteristically spared from direct lesions (Olszewski 1962; Tomonaga *et al.* 1982), but axons in the white matter remote from the lesions are reduced in number (Yamanouchi *et al.* 1989), presumably by Wallerian degeneration. Atheromatous changes at the base of the brain occur in up to 93%, but are not severe enough to cause haemodynamic change (Babikian and Ropper 1987). Carotid disease may also coexist (Pellissier and Poncet 1989). Cortical infarcts occur in up to one third (Babikian and Ropper 1987) but are not universally found (Janota 1981) and simply represent other manifestations of vascular disease. Enlargement of the lateral ventricles is typical (Pellissier and Poncet 1989). The arterioles supplying the deep white matter exhibit lipohyalinosis with perivascular lymphocytes, thickened walls and basal lamina, increased deposition of normal collagen, some of which is type I, which is not seen normally, deposition of type IV collagen in the adventitia which is also not seen normally, disruption of the media, narrowed lumina, splitting of the internal elastic lamina, and some occluded vessels but often an intact endothelium although the endothelial cells may be swollen (Fig. 13.7). Some vessels show hypertrophy of smooth muscle cells and others, where fibrosis has, occurred, show a decrease (Akiguchi *et al.* 1997; Lin *et al.* 2000; Zhang and Olsson 1997).

13.8 **Clinical course and prognosis**

13.8.1 **Complications**

Depression is common in VaD, occurring in up to 20% of cases, and is disproportionately prominent in those cases with small amounts of infarction. It may be particularly related to frontal deep white matter lesions (Ballard *et al.* 2000*a*, *b*; Newman 1999; O'Brien *et al.* 2000; Pohjasvaara *et al.* 2000).

13.8.2 **Prognosis**

The prognosis of VaD varies considerably according to the criteria used to make the diagnosis and hence to the severity of the population being studied. Mortality in the most severe populations

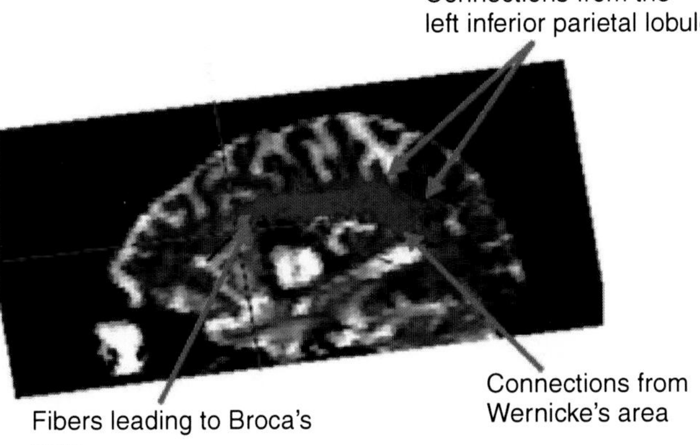

Plate 1 Diffusion tensor imaging (DTI) and the reconstruction of the left arcuate fasciculus in a patient with a left basal ganglia haemorrhage. (See also Fig. 4.2, p. 59.)

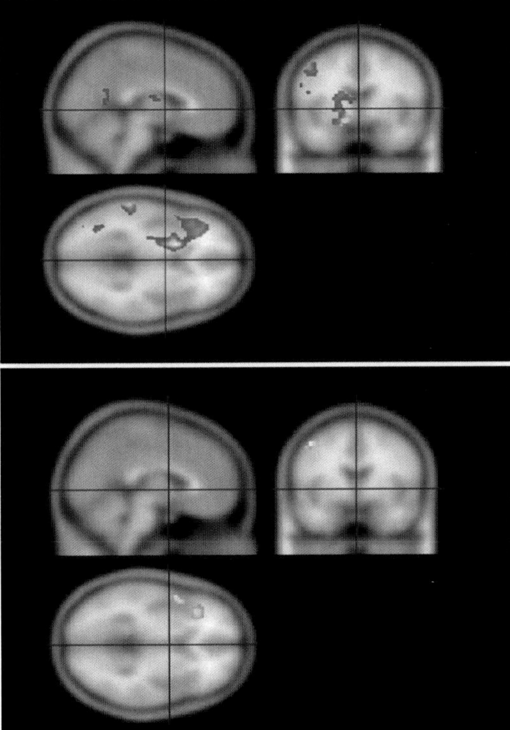

Plate 2 Brain plasticity as observed during different stages of literacy acquisition. (See also Fig. 4.3, p. 60.)

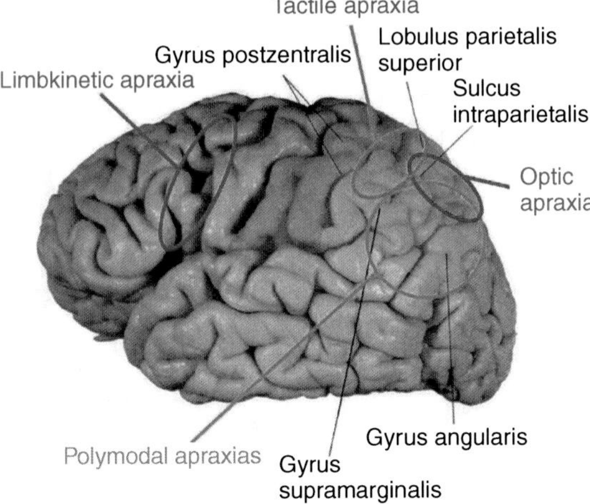

Plate 3 Schematic drawing demonstrating the predominant localizations of lesions in the individual forms of apraxia. (See also Fig. 5.1, p. 68.)

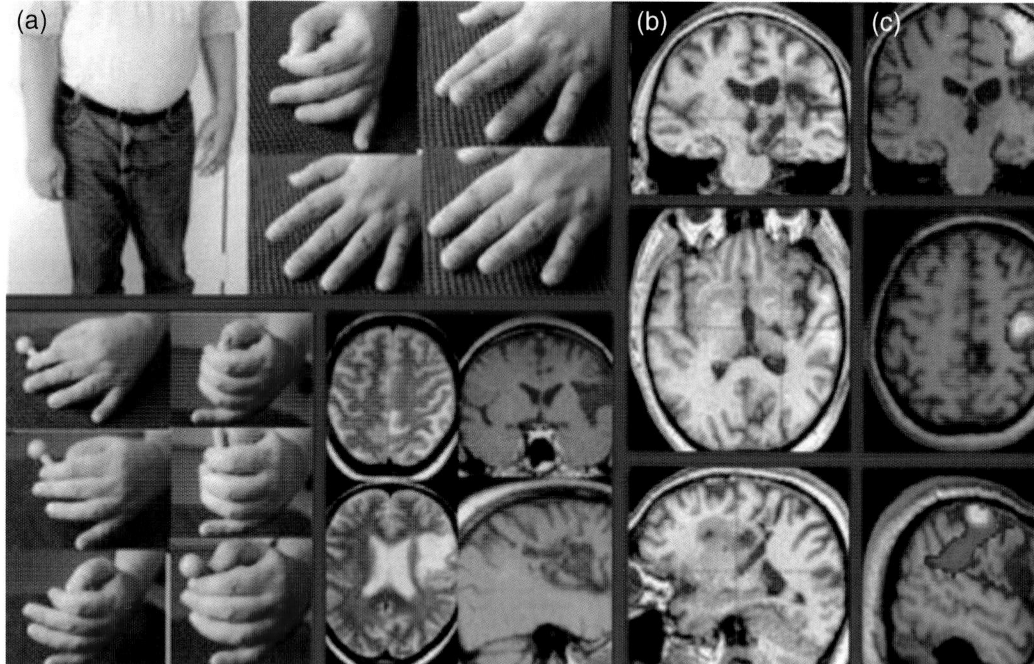

Plate 4 Limb-kinetic apraxia. (See also Fig. 5.2, p. 70.)

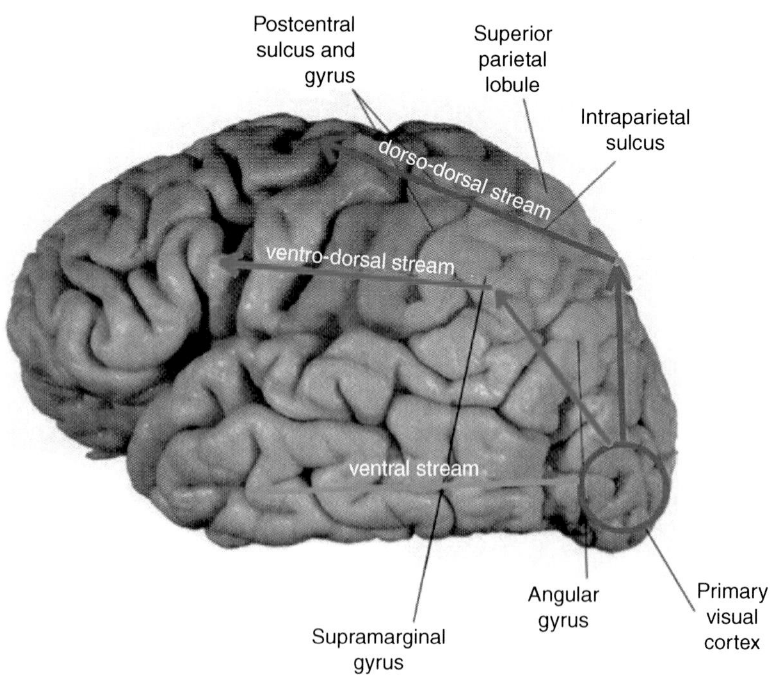

Plate 5 Schematic representation of the dorsal ('where') and the ventral ('what') streams. The dorsal stream can be subdivided into the dorso-dorsal (red) and the ventro-dorsal (green) stream. The dorso-dorsal stream is responsible for the fast 'online' control of visually guided movements. The ventro-dorsal stream is responsible for the complex spatio-temporal planning of movements. The ventral stream (blue) is responsible for the visual object recognition (Rizzolatti and Matelli 2003). (See also Fig. 5.6, p. 75.)

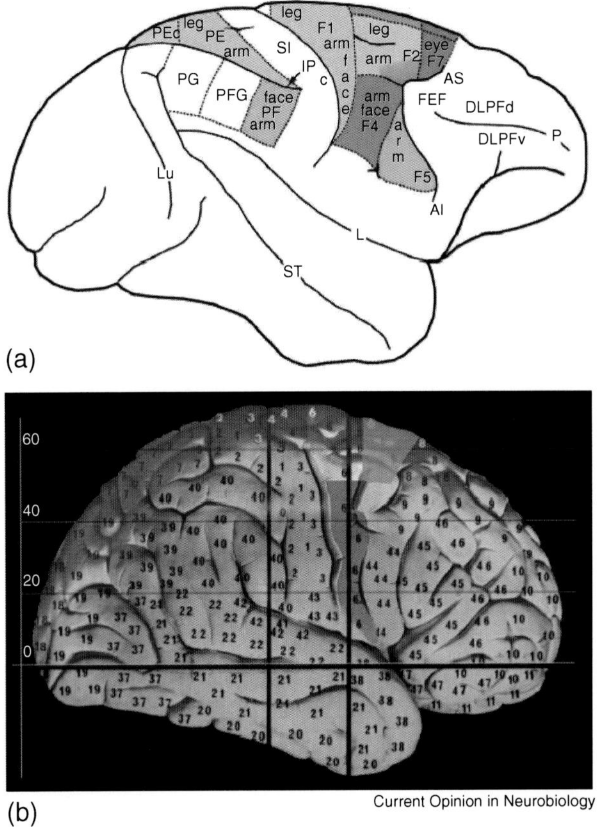

Plate 6 The cortical motor system in monkey and man. (Taken with permission from Rizzolatti et al. 2002.) (See also Fig. 9.1, p. 163.)

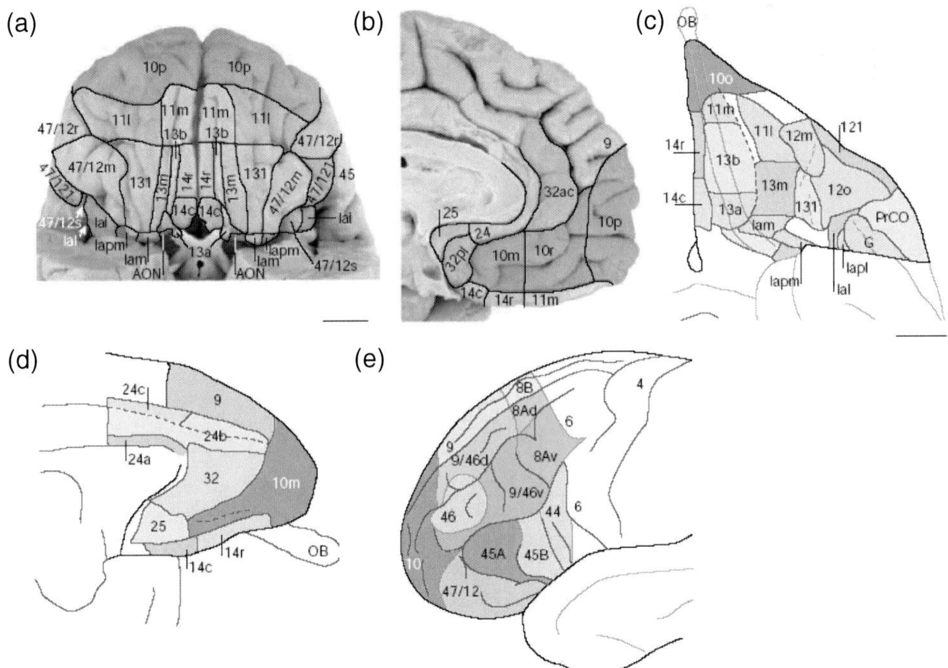

Plate 7 The orbitofrontal cortex in: (a), (b) man and (c), (d) monkey, (e) human lateral prefrontal cortex. (Taken with permission from Petrides and Pandya 1994.) (See also Fig. 9.5, p. 171).

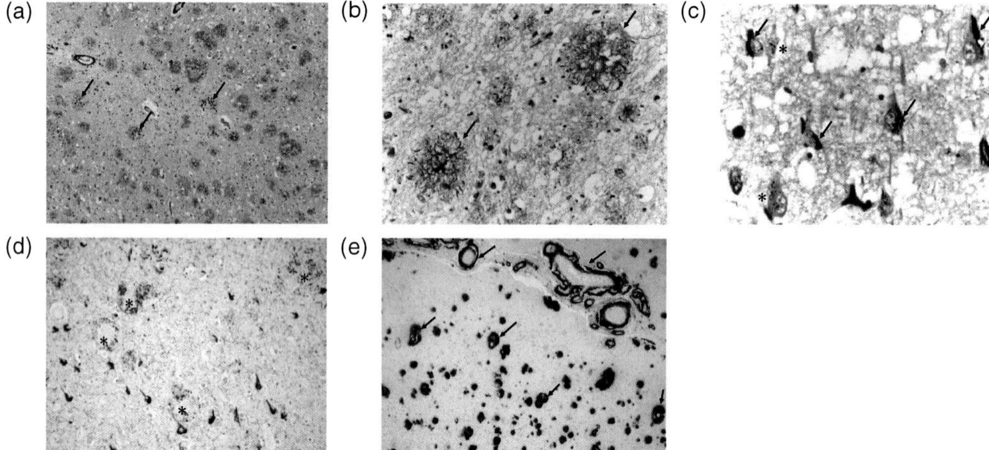

Plate 8 (a) Neocortex showing a high density of silver staining amyloid plaques. Diffuse, primitive and mature/neuritic plaques (arrows) are evident. (b) Neocortex containing diffuse, primitive and mature/neuritic amyloid plaques (arrows). The neuritic plaques consist of an amyloid core surrounded by a corona of silver staining thickened, distorted dystrophic neurites. (c) Hippocampal pyramidal neurons containing silver staining neurofibrillary tangles (arrows). The neurons also show granulovacuolar degeneration (*). (d) Neocortex containing a high density of tau-immunopositive neurofibrillary tangles, neuropil threads, and neuritic plaques (*), the latter delineated by immunopositive dystrophic neurites. (e) Cortex showing prominent leptomeningeal and intracortical amyloid angiopathy (arrows), the latter often extending into the surrounding parenchyma. Numerous dense cortical amyloid plaques, some vessel-derived. (Courtesy of Dr D.G. DuPlessis, Greater Manchester Neurosciences Centre, Salford.) (See also Fig. 11.2, p. 211.)

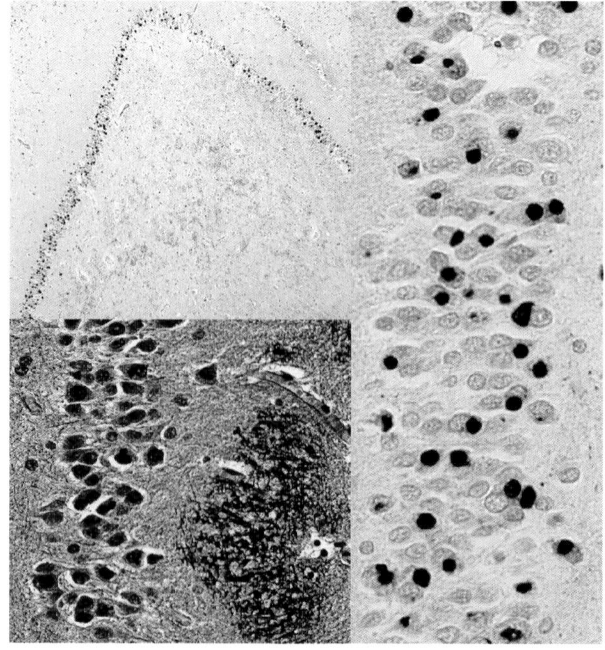

Plate 9 Dentate gyrus. Tau-immunoreactive inclusions (upper left and right). Bielschowsky staining reveals Pick's bodies (lower left). (See also Fig. 12.6, p. 241.)

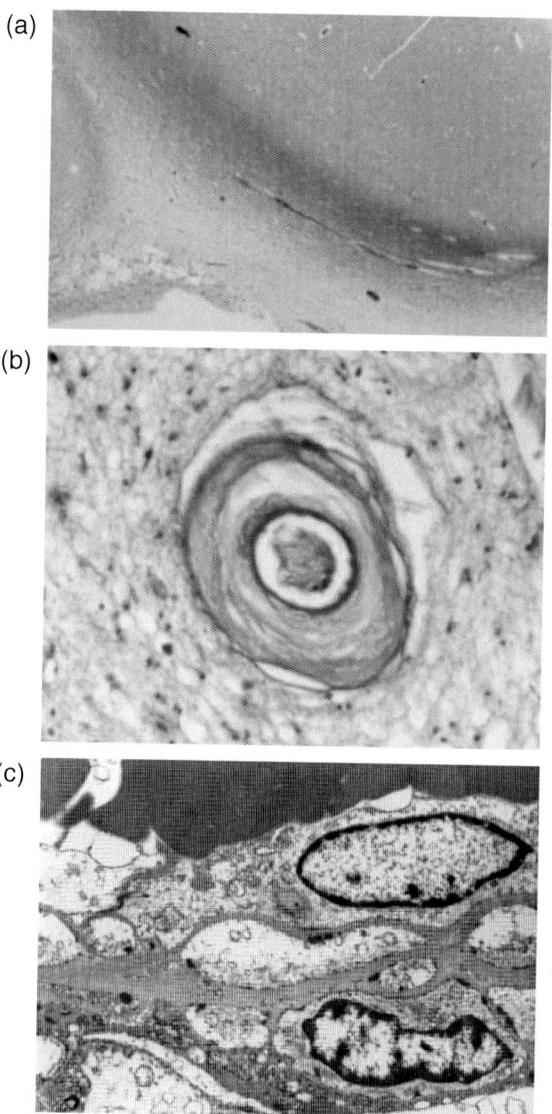

Plate 10 Histopathology in CADASIL. (Courtesy of Dr D.G. Munoz.) (See also Fig. 13.2, p. 263.)

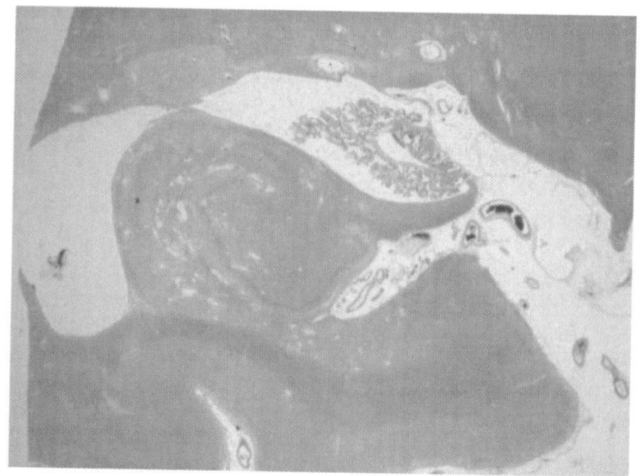

Plate 11 Hippocampal sclerosis. (Courtesy of Dr D.G. Munoz.) (See also Fig. 13.4, p. 271.)

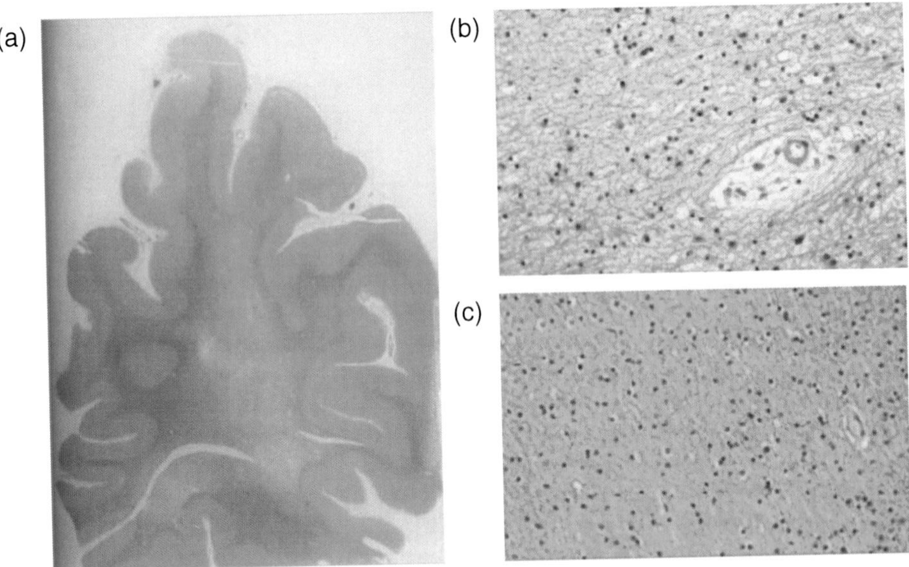

Plate 12 Leukoaraiosis. (Courtesy of Dr D.G. Munoz.) (See also Fig. 13.5, p. 271.)

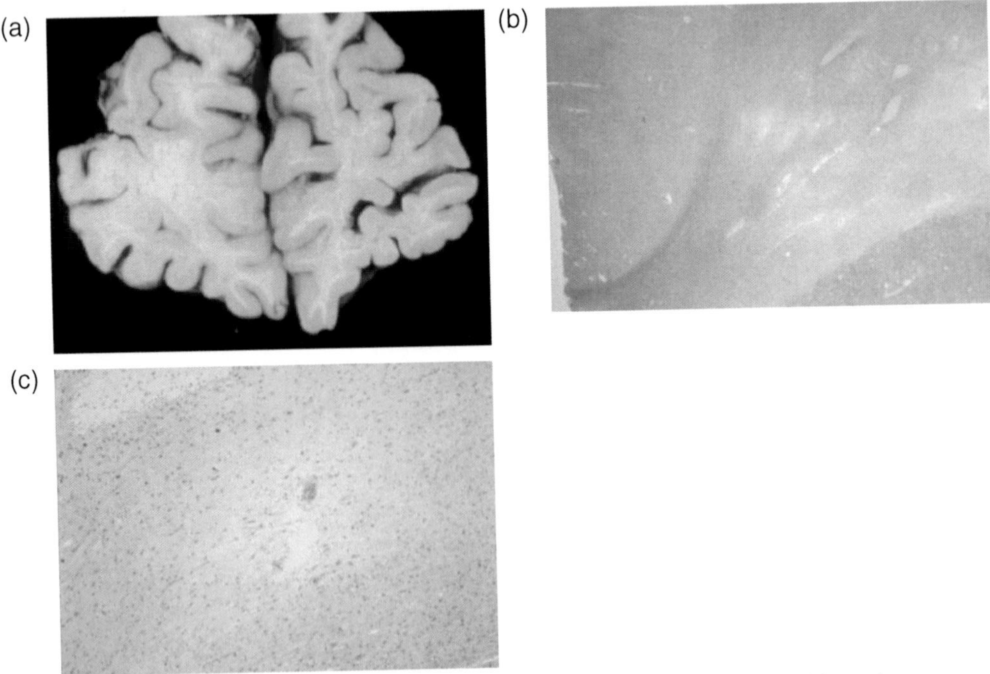

Plate 13 Advanced subcortical vascular cognitive impairment. (Courtesy of Dr D.G. Munoz.) (See also Fig. 13.6, p. 273.)

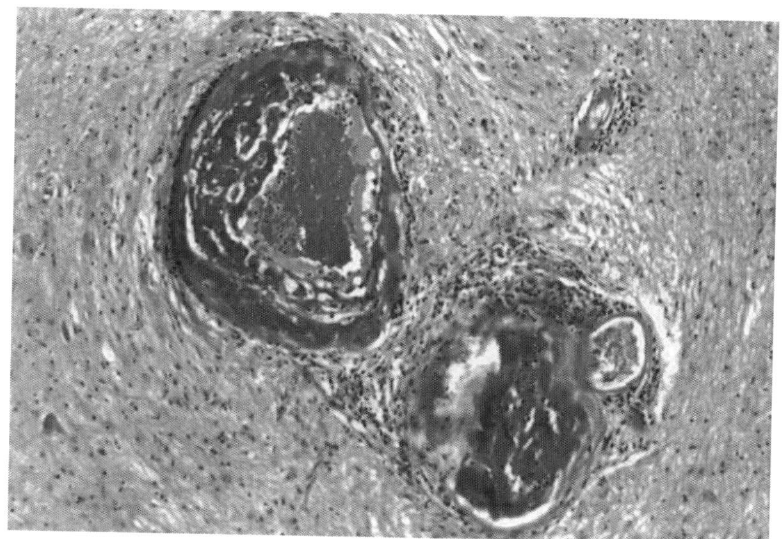

Plate 14 Lipohyalinosis. (Courtesy of Dr D.G. Munoz.) (See also Fig. 13.7, p. 274.)

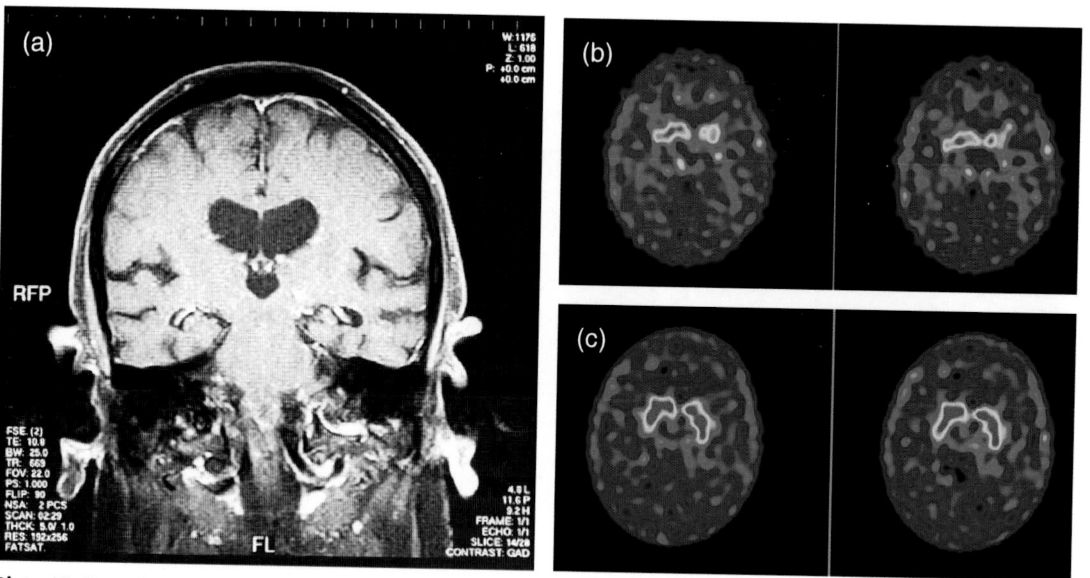

Plate 15 Neuroimaging in cortical Lewy body diseases. (SPECT images courtesy of Dr Andrew Newberg, University of Pennsylvania.) (See also Fig. 14.2, p. 304.)

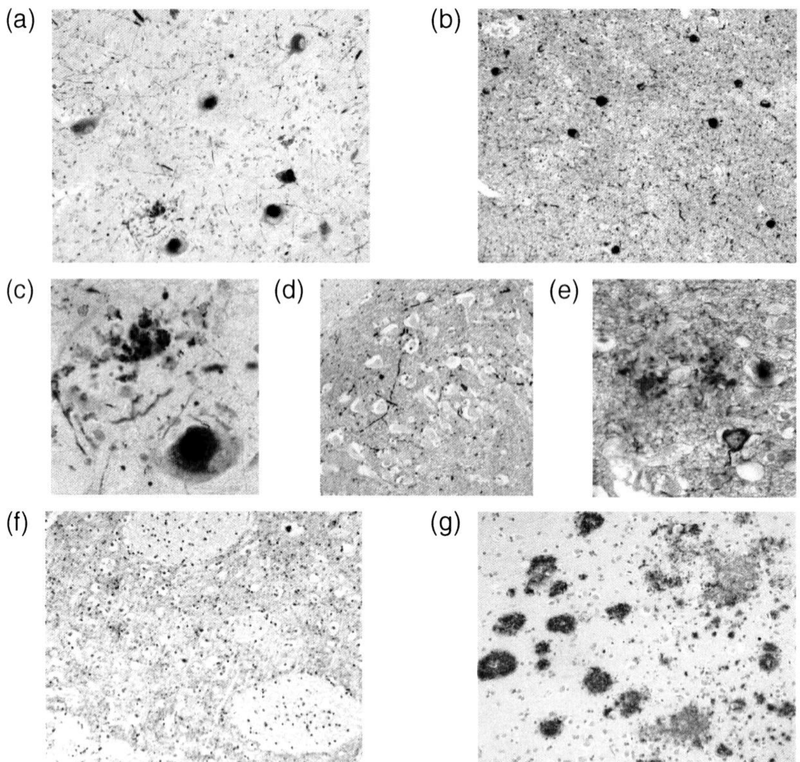

Plate 16 Neuropathology of cortical Lewy body diseases. (See also Fig. 14.3, p. 306.)

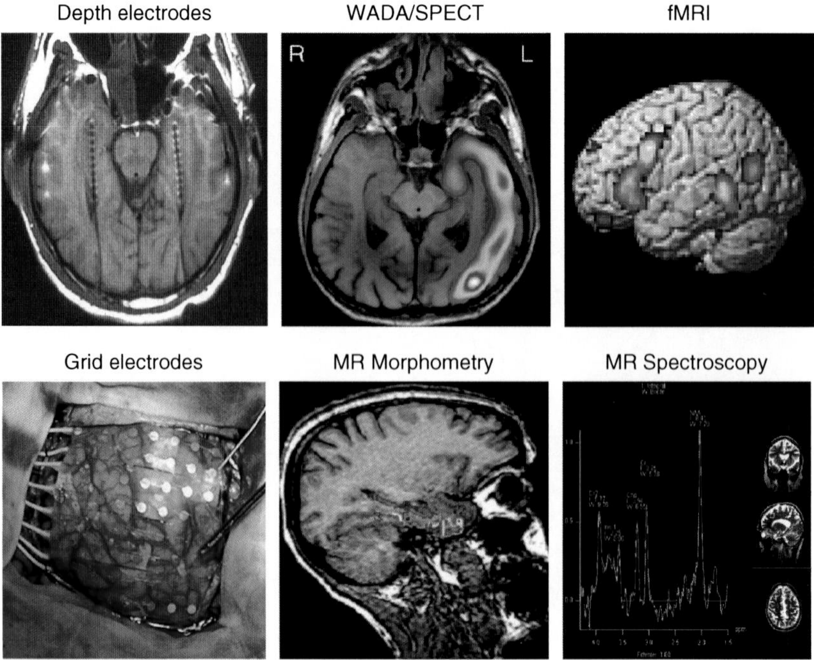

Plate 17 Selection of diagnostic approaches to the brain and its function in presurgical evaluation of patients with pharmacoresistant epilepsy. Information from these tools can serve for correlation/validation of behavioural neuropsychological data. (See also Fig. 18.7, p. 400.)

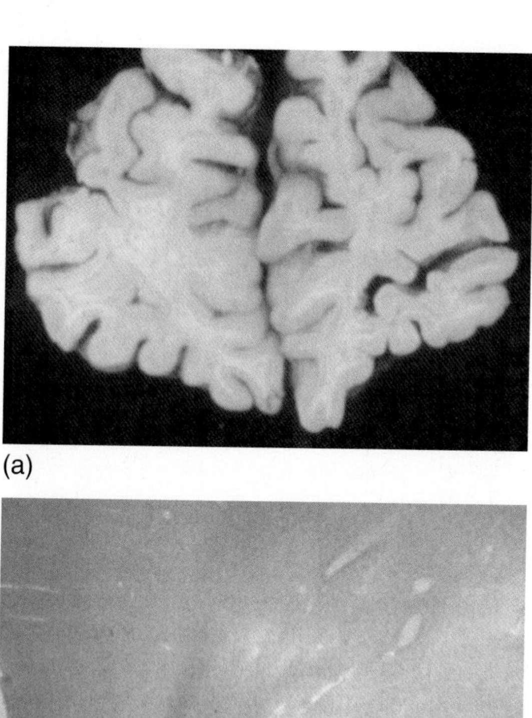

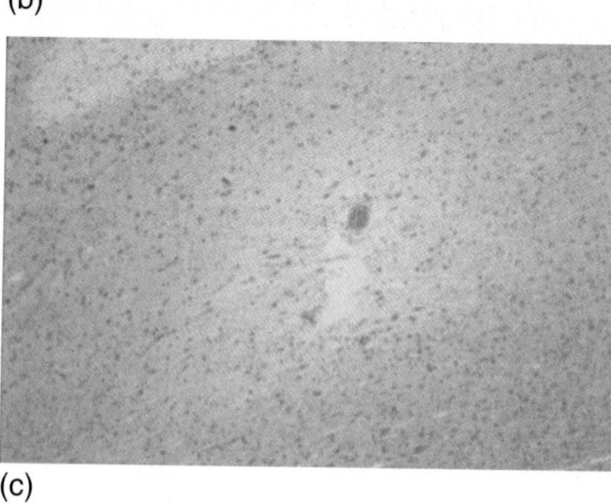

Fig. 13.6 Advanced subcortical vascular cognitive impairment. (a) Coronal section through the frontal lobes, demonstrating the inhomogeneous loss of myelin and sparing of the cortex. (b) Section of cortex (left) and underlying white matter, stained with luxol fast blue–H & E, showing the sparing of subcortical U fibres. (c) Medium power view of the white matter stained with H & E. A small cavitated infarct is located in the region around the '(c)'. The area surrounding the central vessels shows accentuation of the oligodendroglial loss present throughout the field. (Courtesy of Dr D.G. Munoz.) This is a black and white version of Plate 13.

reported is almost twice that of the mildest (Knopman *et al.* 2003*a*). Multi-infarct dementia shortens life expectancy to about 50% of normal at 4 years from initial evaluation, but females, those with higher education, and those who perform well on some neuropsychological tests do better (Barclay *et al.* 1985; Hier *et al.* 1989; Martin *et al.* 1987). In the very elderly, 3-year mortality may reach two thirds, almost three times that of controls (Skoog *et al.* 1993). In one study, the 6-year survival was only 11.9%, about a quarter of that expected (Molsa *et al.* 1986), though

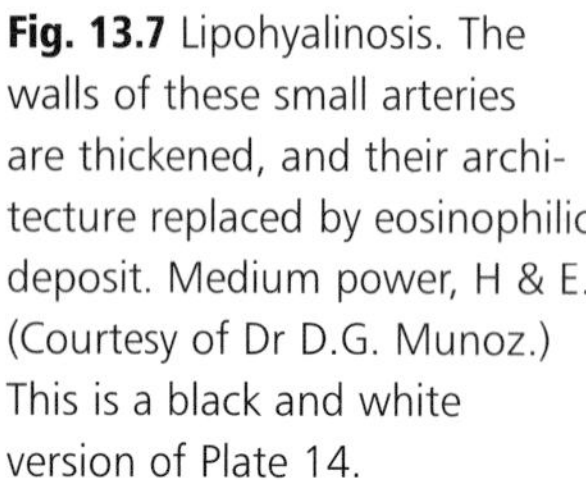
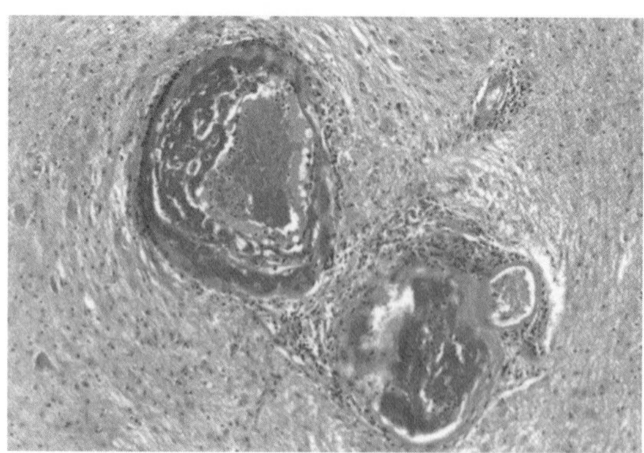

Fig. 13.7 Lipohyalinosis. The walls of these small arteries are thickened, and their architecture replaced by eosinophilic deposit. Medium power, H & E. (Courtesy of Dr D.G. Munoz.) This is a black and white version of Plate 14.

many of these patients were elderly and severely demented at entry. About a third die from complications of the dementia itself, one-third from cerebrovascular disease, 8% from other cardiovascular disease, and the rest from miscellaneous causes, including malignancy (Molsa *et al.* 1986). Overall, the effect of VaD on mortality is similar to, or mildly worse than that of AD (Aevarsson *et al.* 1998; Aguero-Torres *et al.* 1998; Knopman *et al.* 2003*a*).

Cognitive impairment short of dementia (VCI) increased the likelihood of subsequent dementia from 8% to 42% after 9 years of follow-up in Japan (Yamamoto *et al.* 2002) and, in the Canadian Study of Health and Aging, approximately half were dead and half institutionalized after 5 years. However, in 16% there was no cognitive decline, or even improvement, reflecting the diversity of potential outcomes in this condition (Wentzel *et al.* 2001).

13.8.2.1 Subcortical VCI

In those aged over 65 studied in the Cardiovascular Health Study, white matter disease increased in 28% of subjects over 5 years, the increase usually being modest but nonetheless correlated with cognitive decline (Longstreth, Jr. *et al.* 2005). Progression of established Binswanger's disease seems to be more rapid, typically over 3 to 10 years (Bennett *et al.* 1990; Delong *et al.* 1974) suggesting that more advanced disease progresses more rapidly. There are insufficient data to comment on spontaneous or therapeutic remission.

13.9 Management strategies

13.9.1 Prevention and arrest of progression

The management of VaD is primarily that of the underlying cause although care must be taken to identify and treat depression. Data regarding cognitive outcomes from drug trials directed at vascular risk factors are relatively sparse.

Hypertension is the best investigated. The Syst-Eur study showed that a reduction of 7 mmHg in systolic and 3.2 mmHg in diastolic blood pressure over 3.9 years halved incident dementia (Forette *et al.* 1998, 2002) although the absolute figures are a little less impressive at 3 cases per 100 patient years. The PROGRESS study (Tzourio *et al.* 2003) demonstrated a reduction, over 3.9 years of follow-up, in risk of dementia from 7.1% to 6.3% (non-significant) and in cognitive decline from 11% to 9.1%, this benefit being attributable to the prevention of recurrent stroke. In the SCOPE study (Lithell *et al.* 2003) of candesartan therapy in 5000 individuals aged 70 to 89, the blood pressure difference between cases and controls was 3.2/1.6 mmHg and no effect on cognition was demonstrable over a mean of 3.7 years. Importantly, both groups enjoyed a fall in blood pressure of approximately 20/10 due to permitted add-on therapy and both maintained a stable MMSE. It is likely that both groups were, in effect, treatment groups. Primary prevention by control of blood pressure seems to make little difference (Prince *et al.* 1996) but, importantly, the Honolulu–Asia ageing study has reported that treatment of midlife hypertension can reduce the risk of subsequent dementia (Forette *et al.* 1998; Launer *et al.* 2000).

Chronically hypertensive patients have an autoregulatory range for cerebral blood flow shifted to accommodate higher perfusion pressures. Even with treatment this will not fully return to normal (Barry 1989; Paulson *et al.* 1990; Strandgaard 1976). They are thus readily susceptible to hypotension, even at pressures that would otherwise be considered normal. This may be important, as periodic hypotension is a suggested mechanism for the white matter changes seen in these patients (Sulkava and Erkinjuntti 1987). Pravastatin may improve cerebral vasomotor reactivity in subcortical small-vessel disease (Sterzer *et al.* 2001), but whether this has cognitive benefits is as yet unknown.

Evidence that the statins protect against cognitive loss is relatively weak. The PROSPER study of 6000 individuals aged 70 to 82 was unable to demonstrate any benefit on stroke, cognition, or activities of daily living but did show a benefit on myocardial infarction and TIA (Shepherd *et al.* 2002). In a 4-year observational study of 1000 post-menopausal women, statin users had a trivially (1%) higher score on a modified MMSE (Yaffe *et al.* 2002). The Cardiovascular Health study also showed no benefit (Rea *et al.* 2005). Given the established benefits of the statins in preventing adverse vascular events, the discrepancy between these and antihypertensive therapy requires some explanation. This may lie in the fact that subcortical VaD is the commonest form of VaD and that hypertension is, by a very considerable margin, the most powerful treatable risk factor. Cholesterol has little association with small-vessel disease and the plaque-stabilizing, antioxidant, and other properties attributed to the statins may not be relevant to lipohyalinosis and so to small-vessel disease. Taking these observations together, it is readily possible to see why different treatments may have differing effects.

Aspirin may be helpful (Meyer *et al.* 1989*b*). Other non-steroidal analgesics do not protect against VaD (in't Veld *et al.* 2001). The consumption of antioxidant vitamins in mid-life may also protect against VaD (Masaki *et al.* 2000).

13.9.1.2 Subcortical VCI

There are few data on this subject separate from VCI as a whole. Particular emphasis might be given to hypertension, which reduces the rate of development of leukoaraiosis (de Leeuw *et al.* 2002). Carotenoids are also associated with less extensive leukoaraiosis (den Heijer *et al.* 2001). Nimodipine may slow progression in subcortical VaD (Pantoni *et al.* 1996, 2000*b*, 2005) but is of limited help in other types of VaD (Lopez-Arrieta and Birks 2002; Pantoni *et al.* 2000*a*). It may reduce the risk of other cardiovascular events (Pantoni *et al.* 2005).

13.9.2 **Symptomatic relief**

Memantine may help in dementia in general (including mixed disease), may reduce the burden on caregivers (Winblad and Poritis 1999), and offers some benefit in VaD alone without major side-effects (Areosa and Sherriff 2003; Mobius and Stoffler 2002; Orgogozo *et al.* 2002; Wilcock *et al.* 2002). Propentofylline may improve cognitive function on formal testing but does not seem to affect activities of daily living (Kittner 1999; Mielke *et al.* 1996, 1998; Rother *et al.* 1998). Some evidence exists for vincamine (Fischhof *et al.* 1996), vinpocetine (Szatmari and Whitehouse 2003), pentoxifylline (European Pentoxifylline Multi-Infarct Dementia Study Group 1996; Sha and Callahan 2003), and posatirelin (Parnetti *et al.* 1996) but as yet there is no convincing evidence for any single drug and none of these can be recommended. The acetylcholinesterase inhibitors may be more helpful with modest benefits for galantamine, rivastigmine, and donepezil over placebo in both cognition and activities of daily living (Black *et al.* 2003; Erkinjuntti *et al.* 2002; Moretti *et al.* 2002; Wilkinson *et al.* 2003), although there remains a question as to how much of these benefits are due to the drugs' effect on coexistent AD (Bowler 2003*a*).

The typical apraxic gait is not amenable to therapy but, where the burden of vascular disease lies in the basal ganglia or substantia nigra and the gait disturbance is that of vascular parkinsonism, this may be amenable to treatment with L-dopa (Zijlmans *et al.* 2004).

References

Aevarsson, O., Svanborg, A., and Skoog, I. (1998). Seven-year survival rate after age 85 years: relation to Alzheimer disease and vascular dementia. *Arch. Neurol.* **55** (9), 1226–32.

Aguero-Torres, H., Fratiglioni, L., Guo, Z., Viitanen, M., and Winblad, B. (1998). Prognostic factors in very old demented adults: a seven-year follow-up from a population-based survey in Stockholm. *J. Am. Geriatr. Soc.* **46** (4), 444–52.

Akiguchi, I., Tomimoto, H., Suenaga, T., Wakita, H., and Budka, H. (1997). Alterations in glia and axons in the brains of Binswanger's disease patients. *Stroke* **28** (7), 1423–9.

Akiguchi, I., Tomimoto, H., Suenaga, T., Wakita, H., and Budka, H. (1998). Blood–brain barrier dysfunction in Binswanger's disease: an immunohistochemical study. *Acta Neuropathol. (Berl.)* **95** (1), 78–84.

Almkvist, O., Wahlund, L., Andersson-Lundman, G., Bäsun, H., and Bäckman, L. (1992). White-matter hyperintensity and neuropsychological functions in dementia and healthy aging. *Arch. Neurol.* **49**, 626–32.

American Psychiatric Association (1994). *Diagnostic and statistical manual of mental disorders*, 4th edn. American Psychiatric Association, Washington, DC.

Andersen, K., Launer, L.J., Dewey, M.E., Letenneur, L., Ott, A., Copeland, J.R., Dartigues, J.F., Kragh-Sørensen P., Baldereschi, M., Brayne, C., Lobo, A., Martinez-Lage, J.M., Stijnen, T., and Hofman, A. (1999). Gender differences in the incidence of AD and vascular dementia: The EURODEM Studies. EURODEM Incidence Research Group. *Neurology* **53** (9), 1992–7.

Areosa, S.A. and Sherriff, F. (2003). Memantine for dementia. *Cochrane Database Syst. Rev.* no. 1, CD003154.

Atwood, L.D., Wolf, P.A., Heard-Costa, N.L., Massaro, J.M., Beiser, A., D'Agostino, R.B., and DeCarli, C. (2004). Genetic variation in white matter hyperintensity volume in the Framingham study. *Stroke* **35** (7), 1609–13.

Au, R., Massaro, J.M., Wolf, P.A., Young, M.E., Beiser, A., Seshadri, S., D'Agostino, R.B., and DeCarli, C. (2006). Association of white matter hyperintensity volume with decreased cognitive functioning: the Framingham Heart Study. *Arch. Neurol.* **63** (2), 246–50.

Awad, I.A., Johnson, P.C., Spetzler, R.F., and Hodak, J.A. (1986). Incidental subcortical lesions identified on magnetic resonance imaging in the elderly. II. Postmortem pathological correlations. *Stroke* **17**, 1090–7.

Babikian, V. and Ropper, A.H. (1987). Binswanger's disease: a review. *Stroke* **18**, 2–12.

Babikian, V.L., Wolfe, N., Linn, R., Knoefel, J.E., and Albert, M.L. (1990). Cognitive changes in patients with multiple cerebral infarcts. *Stroke* **21**, 1013–18.

Ballard, C., McKeith, I., O'Brien, J., Kalaria, R., Jaros, E., Ince, P., and Perry, R. (2000*a*). Neuropathological substrates of dementia and depression in vascular dementia, with a particular focus on cases with small infarct volumes. *Dement. Geriatr. Cogn. Disord.* **11** (2), 59–65.

Ballard, C., Neill, D., O'Brien, J., McKeith, I.G., Ince, P., and Perry, R. (2000*b*). Anxiety, depression and psychosis in vascular dementia: prevalence and associations. *J. Affect. Disord.* **59** (2), 97–106.

Ballard, C.G., Burton, E.J., Barber, R., Stephens, S., Kenny, R.A., Kalaria, R.N., and O'Brien, J.T. (2004). NINDS AIREN neuroimaging criteria do not distinguish stroke patients with and without dementia. *Neurology* **63** (6), 983–8.

Barba, R., Martínez-Espinosa, S., Rodríguez-Garcia, E., Pondal, M., Vivancos, J., and del Ser, T. (2000). Poststroke dementia: clinical features and risk factors. *Stroke* **31** (7), 1494–501.

Barber, R., Gholkar, A., Scheltens, P., Ballard, C., McKeith, I.G., and O'Brien, J.T. (1999). Medial temporal lobe atrophy on MRI in dementia with Lewy bodies. *Neurology* **52** (6), 1153–8.

Barclay, L.L., Zemcov, A., Blass, J.P., and Sansone, J. (1985). Survival in Alzheimer's disease and vascular dementias. *Neurology* **35**, 834–40.

Barker, W.W., Luis, C.A., Kashuba, A., Luis, M., Harwood, D.G., Loewenstein, D., Waters, C., Jimison, P., Shepherd, E., Sevush, S., Graff-Radford, N., Newland, D., Todd, M., Miller, B., Gold, M., Heilman, K., Doty, L., Goodman, I., Robinson, B., Pearl, G., Dickson, D., and Duara, R. (2002). Relative frequencies of Alzheimer disease, Lewy body, vascular and frontotemporal dementia, and hippocampal sclerosis in the state of Florida brain bank. *Alzheimer Dis. Assoc. Disord.* **16** (4), 203–12.

Baron, J.C., D'Antona, R., Pantano, P., Serdaru, M., Samson, Y., and Bousser, M.G. (1986). Effects of thalamic stroke on energy metabolism of the cerebral cortex. A positron tomography study in man. *Brain* **109**, 1243–59.

Baron, J.C., Levasseur, M., Mazoyer, B., Legault Demare, F., Mauguiere, F., Pappata, S., Jedynak, P., Derome, P., Cambier, J., Tran Dinh, S., and Cambon, H. (1992). Thalamocortical diaschisis: positron emission tomography in humans. *J. Neurol. Neurosurg. Psychiatry* **55**, 935–42.

Barry, D.I. (1989). Cerebrovascular aspects of antihypertensive treatment. *Am. J. Cardiol.* **63**, 14C–18C.

Bennett, D.A., Wilson, R.S., Gilley, D.W., and Fox, J.H. (1990). Clinical diagnosis of Binswanger's disease. *J. Neurol. Neurosurg. Psychiatry* **53**, 961–5.

Bennett, D.A., Gilley, D.W., Lee, S., and Cochran, E.J. (1994). White matter changes: neurobehavioral manifestations of Binswanger's disease and clinical correlates in Alzheimer's disease. *Dementia* **5** (3–4), 148–52.

Black, S., Roman, G.C., Geldmacher, D.S., Salloway, S., Hecker, J., Burns, A., Perdomo, C., Kumar, D., and Pratt, R. (2003). Efficacy and tolerability of donepezil in vascular dementia. Positive results of a 24-week, multicenter, international, randomized, placebo-controlled clinical trial. *Stroke* **34**, 2323–30.

Bogousslavsky, J., Regli, F., and Uske, A. (1987). Leukoencephalopathy in patients with ischemic stroke. *Stroke* **18**, 896–9.

Boston, P.F., Dennis, M.S., Jagger, C., Jarman, M., and Lamers, C. (2001). Unequal distribution of cognitive deficits in vascular dementia—is this a valid criterion in the ICD-10? *Int. J. Geriatr. Psychiatry* **16** (4), 422–6.

Bowen, B.C., Barker, W.W., Loewenstein, D.A., Sheldon, J., and Duara, R. (1990). MR signal abnormalities in memory disorder and dementia. *Am. J. Neuroradiol.* **11**, 283–90.

Bowler, J.V. (1993). Cerebral infarction and $^{99}Tc^{m}$ HMPAO SPECT. MD Thesis, University of London.

Bowler, J.V. (2003*a*). Acetylcholinesterase inhibitors for vascular dementia and Alzheimer's disease combined with cerebrovascular disease. *Stroke* **34** (2), 584–6.

Bowler, J.V. (2003*b*). The progression of leukoaraiosis. *Stroke* **34** (8), 1916–17.

Bowler, J.V. (2004). Dementia after stroke—the Framingham study. *Stroke* **35** (6), 1268–9.

Bowler, J.V. and Hachinski, V. (2000). Criteria for vascular dementia: replacing dogma with data. *Arch. Neurol.* **57** (2), 170–1.

Bowler, J.V., Costa, D.C., Jones, B.E., Steiner, T.J., and Wade, J.P.H. (1992). High resolution SPECT, small deep infarcts and diaschisis. *J. R. Soc. Med.* **85**, 142–6.

Bowler, J.V., Hadar, U., and Wade, J.P.H. (1994). Cognition in stroke. *Acta Neurol. Scand.* **90**, 424–9.

Bowler, J.V., Wade, J. P.H., Jones, B.E., Nijran, K., Jewkes, R.F., Cummins, R., and Steiner, T.J. (1995). The contribution of diaschisis to the clinical deficit in human cerebral infarction. *Stroke* **26**, 1000–6.

Bowler, J.V., Eliasziw, M., Steenhuis, R., Munoz, D.G., Fry, R., Merskey, H., and Hachinski, V.C. (1997). Comparative evolution of Alzheimer disease, vascular dementia and mixed dementia. *Arch. Neurol.* **54**, 697–703.

Bowler, J.V., Hachinski, V., Steenhuis, R., and Lee, D. (1998*a*). Vascular cognitive impairment; clinical, neuropsychological and imaging findings in early vascular dementia. *Lancet* **352** (Suppl. 4), 63.

Bowler, J.V., Munoz, D.G., Merskey, H., and Hachinski, V.C. (1998*b*). Fallacies in the pathological confirmation of the diagnosis of Alzheimer's disease. *J. Neurol. Neurosurg. Psychiatry* **64** (1), 18–24.

Braffman, B.H., Zimmerman, R.A., Trojanowski, J.Q., Gonatas, N.K., Hickey, W.F., and Schlaepfer, W.W. (1988*a*). Brain MR: pathologic correlation with gross and histopathology. 1. Lacunar infarction and Virchow–Robin spaces. *Am. J. Roentgenol.* **151**, 551–8.

Braffman, B.H., Zimmerman, R.A., Trojanowski, J.Q., Gonatas, N.K., Hickey, W.F., and Schlaepfer, W.W. (1988*b*). Brain MR: pathologic correlation with gross and histopathology. 2. Hyperintense white-matter foci in the elderly. *Am. J. Roentgenol.* **151**, 559–66.

Breteler, M.M., van Amerongen, N.M., van Swieten, J.C., Claus, J.J., Grobbee, D.E., van Gijn, J., Hofman, A., and van Harskamp, F. (1994*a*). Cognitive correlates of ventricular enlargement and cerebral white matter lesions on magnetic resonance imaging. The Rotterdam Study. *Stroke* **25**, 1109–15.

Breteler, M.M.B., Claus, J.J., Grobbee, D.E., and Hofman, A. (1994*b*). Cardiovascular disease and distribution of cognitive function in elderly people: the Rotterdam study. *Br. Med. J.* **308**, 1604–8.

Breteler, M.M.B., van Swieten, J.C., Bots, M.L., Grobbee, D.E., Claus, J.J., van den Hout, J.H.W., von Harskamp, F., Tanghe, H.L.J., de Jong, P.T.V.M., van Gijn, J., and Hofman, A. (1994*c*). Cerebral white matter lesions, vascular risk factors, and cognitive function in a population-based study: the Rotterdam Study. *Neurology* **44**, 1246–52.

Brown, M.M., Pelz, D.M., and Hachinski, V. (1990). Xenon-enhanced CT measurement of cerebral blood flow in cerebrovascular disease. *J. Neurol. Neurosurg. Psychiatry* **53**, 815.

Brun, A. and Englund, E. (1986). A white matter disorder in dementia of the Alzheimer type: a pathoanatomical study. *Ann. Neurol.* **19**, 253–62.

Brust, J.C. (1988). Vascular dementia is overdiagnosed. *Arch. Neurol.* **45**, 799–801.

Burger, P.C., Burch, J.G., and Kunze, U. (1976). Subcortical arteriosclerotic encephalopathy (Binswanger's disease). A vascular etiology of dementia. *Stroke* **7**, 626–31.

Canadian Study of Health and Aging Working Group (1994). The Canadian study of health and aging: study methods and prevalence of dementia. *Can. Med. Assoc. J.* **150** (6), 899–913.

Caplan, L.R. and Schoene, W.C. (1978). Clinical features of subcortical arteriosclerotic encephalopathy (Binswanger disease). *Neurology* **28**, 1206–15.

Carmelli, D., DeCarli, C., Swan, G.E., Jack, L.M., Reed, T., Wolf, P.A., and Miller, B.L. (1998). Evidence for genetic variance in white matter hyperintensity volume in normal elderly male twins. *Stroke* **29**, 1177–81.

Carmelli, D., Reed, T., and DeCarli, C. (2002). A bivariate genetic analysis of cerebral white matter hyperintensities and cognitive performance in elderly male twins. *Neurobiol. Aging* **23** (3), 413–20.

Chimowitz, M.I., Awad, I.A., and Furlan, A.J. (1989). Periventricular lesions on MRI. Facts and theories. *Stroke* **20**, 963–7.

Chui, H.C., Victoroff, J.I., Margolin, D., Jagust, W., Shankle, R., and Katzman, R. (1992). Criteria for the diagnosis of ischemic vascular dementia proposed by the State of California Alzheimer's Disease Diagnostic and Treatment Centers. *Neurology* **42**, 473–80.

Chui, H.C., Mack, W., Jackson, J.E., Mungas, D., Reed, B.R., Tinklenberg, J., Chang, F.L., Skinner, K., Tasaki, C., and Jagust, W.J. (2000). Clinical criteria for the diagnosis of vascular dementia: a multi-center study of comparability and inter-rater reliability. *Arch. Neurol.* **57** (2), 191–6.

Corbett, A., Bennett, H., and Kos, S. (1994). Cognitive dysfunction following subcortical infarction. *Arch. Neurol.* **51**, 999–1007.

Crystal, H.A., Dickson, D., Davies, P., Masur, D., Grober, E., and Lipton, R.B. (2000). The relative frequency of 'dementia of unknown etiology' increases with age and is nearly 50% in nonagenarians. *Arch. Neurol.* **57** (5), 713–19.

Cummings, J.L. (1994). 'Vascular subcortical dementias: clinical aspects. *Dementia* **5** (3–4), 177–80.

Cummings, J.L. and Benson, D.F. (1984). Subcortical dementia. Review of an emerging concept. *Arch. Neurol.* **41**, 874–9.

De Carli, C., Murphy, D.G., Tranh, M., Grady, C.L., Haxby, J.V., Gillette, J.A., Salerno, J.A., Gonzales, A., Horwitz, B., Rapoport, S.I., *et al.* (1995). The effect of white matter hyperintensity volume on brain structure, cognitive performance, and cerebral metabolism of glucose in 51 healthy adults. *Neurology* **45** (11), 2077–84.

DeCarli, C., Fletcher, E., Ramey, V., Harvey, D., and Jagust, W.J. (2005). Anatomical mapping of white matter hyperintensities (WMH): exploring the relationships between periventricular WMH, deep WMH, and total WMH burden. *Stroke* **36** (1), 50–5.

de Groot, J.C., de Leeuw, F.E., Oudkerk, M., Hofman, A., Jolles, J., and Breteler, M.M. (2001). Cerebral white matter lesions and subjective cognitive dysfunction: the Rotterdam Scan Study. *Neurology* **56** (11), 1539–45.

de Leeuw, F.E., de Groot, J.C., Achten, E., Oudkerk, M., Ramos, L.M., Heijboer, R., Hofman, A., Jolles, J., van Gijn, J., and Breteler, M.M. (2001). Prevalence of cerebral white matter lesions in elderly people: a population based magnetic resonance imaging study. The Rotterdam Scan Study. *J. Neurol. Neurosurg. Psychiatry* **70** (1), 9–14.

de Leeuw, F.E., de Groot, J.C., Oudkerk, M., Witteman, J.-C.M., Hofman, A., van Gijn, J., and Breteler, M.-M.B. (2002). Hypertension and cerebral white matter lesions in a prospective cohort study. *Brain* **125** (4), 765–72.

Delong, G.R., Kemper, T.L., Pogacar, S., and Lee, H.Y. (1974). Clinical neuropathological conference. *Dis. Nerv. Syst.* **35**, 286–91.

del Ser, T., Bermejo, F., Portera, A., Arredondo, J.M., Bouras, C., and Constantinidis, J. (1990). Vascular dementia. A clinicopathological study. *J. Neurol. Sci.* **96**, 1–17.

den Heijer, T., Launer, L.J., de Groot, J.C., de Leeuw, F.E., Oudkerk, M., van Gijn, J., Hofman, A., and Breteler, M.M. (2001). Serum carotenoids and cerebral white matter lesions: the Rotterdam scan study. *J. Am. Geriatr. Soc.* **49** (5), 642–6.

De Reuck, J., Decoo, D., Strijckmans, K., and Lemahieu, I. (1992). Does the severity of leukoaraiosis contribute to senile dementia? A comparative computerized and positron emission tomographic study. *Eur. Neurol.* **32**, 199–205.

De Reuck, J., Decoo, D., Hasenbroekx, M.C., Lamont, B., Santens, P., Goethals, P., Strijckmans, K., and Lemahieu, I. (1999). Acetazolamide vasoreactivity in vascular dementia: a positron emission tomographic study. *Eur. Neurol.* **41** (1), 31–6.

Desmond, D.W., Moroney, J.T., Paik, M.C., Sano, M., Mohr, J.P., Aboumatar, S., Tseng, C.L., Chan, S., Williams, J.B., Remien, R.H., Hauser, W.A., and Stern, Y. (2000). Frequency and clinical determinants of dementia after ischemic stroke. *Neurology* **54** (5), 1124–31.

DeStefano, A.L., Atwood, L.D., Massaro, J.M., Heard-Costa, N., Beiser, A., Au, R., Wolf, P.A., and DeCarli, C. (2006). Genome-wide scan for white matter hyperintensity: the Framingham Heart Study. *Stroke* **37** (1), 77–81.

Diaz, J.F., Merskey, H., Hachinski, V.C., Lee, D.H., Boniferro, M., Wong, C.J., Mirsen, T.R., and Fox, H. (1991). Improved recognition of leukoaraiosis and cognitive impairment in Alzheimer's disease. *Arch. Neurol.* **48**, 1022–5.

Di Carlo, A., Baldereschi, M., Amaducci, L., Maggi, S., Grigoletto, F., Scarlato, G., and Inzitari, D. (2000). Cognitive impairment without dementia in older people: prevalence, vascular risk factors, impact on disability. The Italian Longitudinal Study on Aging. *J. Am. Geriatr. Soc.* **48** (7), 775–82.

Dichgans, M. and Petersen, D. (1997). Angiographic complications in CADASIL. *Lancet* **349**, 776–77.

Ebly, E.M., Parhad, I.M., Hogan, D.B., and Fung, T.S. (1994). Prevalence and types of dementia in the very old: results from the Canadian Study of Health and Aging. *Neurology* **44** (9), 1593–600.

Erkinjuntti, T. and Hachinski, V.C. (1993). Rethinking vascular dementia. *Cerebrovasc. Dis.* **3**, 3–23.

Erkinjuntti, T., Haltia, M., Palo, J., Sulkava, R., and Paetau, A. (1988). Accuracy of the clinical diagnosis of vascular dementia: a prospective clinical and post-mortem neuropathological study. *J. Neurol. Neurosurg. Psychiatry* **51**, 1037–44.

Erkinjuntti, T., Inzitari, D., Pantoni, L., Wallin, A., Scheltens, P., Rockwood, K., Roman, G.C., Chui, H., and Desmond, D. W. (2000). Research criteria for subcortical vascular dementia in clinical trials. *J. Neural Trans. (Suppl.)* **59**, 23–30.

Erkinjuntti, T., Kurz, A., Gauthier, S., Bullock, R., Lilienfeld, S., and Damaraju, C.V. (2002). Efficacy of galantamine in probable vascular dementia and Alzheimer's disease combined with cerebrovascular disease: a randomised trial. *Lancet* **359** (9314), 1283–90.

Esiri, M.M., Wilcock, G.K., and Morris, J.H. (1997). Neuropathological assessment of the lesions of significance in vascular dementia. *J. Neurol. Neurosurg. Psychiatry* **63** (12), 749–53.

European Pentoxifylline Multi-Infarct Dementia Study Group (1996). European Pentoxifylline Multi-Infarct Dementia Study. *Eur. Neurol.* **36** (5), 315–21.

Feeney, D.M. and Baron, J.C. (1986). Diaschisis. *Stroke* **17**, 817–30.

Ferris, S.H. (1999). Cognitive outcome measures. *Alzheimer Dis. Assoc. Disord.* **13** (Suppl. 3), S140–S142.

Ferrucci, L., Guralnik, J.M., Salive, M.E., Pahor, M., Corti, M.C., Baroni, A., and Havlik, R.J. (1996). Cognitive impairment and risk of stroke in the older population. *J. Am. Geriatr. Soc.* **44**, 237–41.

Fields, W. S. (1985). 'Vascular disease and dementia. In *Interdisciplinary topics in gerontology* (ed. H.P. von Hahn), pp. 12–17. S. Karger, Basel.

Fiorelli, M., Blin, J., Bakchine, S., Laplane, D., and Baron, J.C. (1991). PET studies of cortical diaschisis in patients with motor hemi-neglect. *J. Neurol. Sci.* **104**, 135–42.

Fischhof, P.K., Moslinger, G.R., Herrmann, W.M., Friedmann, A., and Russmann, D.L. (1996). Therapeutic efficacy of vincamine in dementia. *Neuropsychobiology* **34** (1), 29–35.

Fisher, C.M. (1965). Lacunes: small, deep cerebral infarcts. *Neurology* **15**, 774–84.

Fisher, C.M. (1982). Lacunar strokes and infarcts: a review. *Neurology* **32**, 871–6.

Forette, F., Seux, M.-L., Staessen, J.A., Thijs, L., Birkenhager, W.H., Babarskiene, Babeanu, S., Bossini, A., Gil-Extremera, B., Girerd, X., Laks, T., Lilov, E., Moisseyev, V., Tuomilehto, J., Vanhanen, H., Webster, J., Yodfat, Y., and Fagard, R. (1998). Prevention of dementia in randomised double-blind placebo-controlled systolic hypertension in Europe (Syst-Eur) trial. *Lancet* **352** (9137), 1347–51.

Forette, F., Seux, M.L., Staessen, J.A., Thijs, L., Babarskiene, M.R., Babeanu, S., Bossini, A., Fagard, R., Gil-Extremera, B., Laks, T., Kobalava, Z., Sarti, C., Tuomilehto, J., Vanhanen, H., Webster, J., Yodfat, Y., and Birkenhager, W.H. (2002). The prevention of dementia with antihypertensive treatment: new evidence from the systolic hypertension in Europe (Syst-Eur) study. *Arch. Intern. Med.* **162** (18), 2046–52.

Frackowiak, R.S., Pozzilli, C., Legg, N.J., Du Boulay, G.H., Marshall, J., Lenzi, G.L., and Jones, T. (1981). Regional cerebral oxygen supply and utilisation in dementia. *Brain* **104**, 753–78.

Fukuda, H., Kobayashi, S., Okada, K., and Tsunematsu, T. (1990). Frontal white matter lesions and dementia in lacunar infarction. *Stroke* **21**, 1143–9.

Fukutake, T. and Hirayama, K. (1995). Familial young-adult-onset arteriosclerotic leukoencephalopathy with alopecia and lumbago without arterial hypertension. *Eur. Neurol.* **35** (2), 69–79.

Gainotti, G., Marra, C., and Villa, G. (2001). A double dissociation between accuracy and time of execution on attentional tasks in Alzheimer's disease and multi-infarct dementia. *Brain* **124** (4), 731–8.

Galanis, D.J., Petrovitch, H., Launer, L.J., Harris, T.B., Foley, D.J., and White, L.R. (1997). Smoking history in middle age and subsequent cognitive performance in elderly Japanese-American men. The Honolulu-Asia Aging Study. *Am. J. Epidemiol.* **145** (6), 507–15.

Gale, C.R., Martyn, C.N., and Cooper, C. (1996). Cognitive impairment and mortality in a cohort of elderly people. *Br. Med. J.* **312**, 608–11.

Garde, E., Lykke Mortensen, E., Rostrup, E., and Paulson, O.B. (2005). Decline in intelligence is associated with progression in white matter hyperintensity volume. *J. Neurol. Neurosurg. Psychiatry* **76** (9), 1289–91.

Gauthier, S. and Ferris, S. (2001). Outcome measures for probable vascular dementia and Alzheimer's disease with cerebrovascular disease. *Int. J. Clin. Pract. Suppl.* **120**, 29–39.

Geroldi, C., Frisoni, G.B., Paolisso, G., Bandinelli, S., Lamponi, M., Abbatecola, A.M., Zanetti, O., Guralnik, J.M., and Ferrucci, L. (2005). Insulin resistance in cognitive impairment: the InCHIANTI Study. *Arch. Neurol.* **62** (7), 1067–72.

Gold, G., Giannakopoulos, P., Montes-Paixao, J.C., Herrmann, F.R., Mulligan, R., Michel, J.P., and Bouras, C. (1997). Sensitivity and specificity of newly proposed clinical criteria for possible vascular dementia. *Neurology* **49** (3), 690–4.

Gold, G., Kovari, E., Herrmann, F.R., Canuto, A., Hof, P.R., Michel, J.P., Bouras, C., and Giannakopoulos, P. (2005). Cognitive consequences of thalamic, basal ganglia, and deep white matter lacunes in brain aging and dementia. *Stroke* **36** (6), 1184–8.

Goldstein, I.B., Bartzokis, G., Guthrie, D., and Shapiro, D. (2005). Ambulatory blood pressure and the brain: a 5-year follow-up. *Neurology* **64** (11), 1846–52.

Gorelick, P. B. (1997). Status of risk factors for dementia associated with stroke. *Stroke* **28** (2), 459–63.

Gorelick, P.B., Chatterjee, A., Patel, D., Flowerdew, G., Dollear, W., Taber, J., and Harris, Y. (1992). Cranial computed tomographic observations in multi-infarct dementia. A controlled study. *Stroke* **23**, 804–11.

Gorelick, P.B., Brody, J., Cohen, D., Freels, S., Levy, P., Dollear, W., Forman, H., and Harris, Y. (1993). Risk factors for dementia associated with multiple cerebral infarcts. A case-control analysis in predominantly African-American hospital-based patients. *Arch. Neurol.* **50**, 714–20.

Goto, K., Ishii, N., and Fukasawa, H. (1989). Diffuse white matter disease in the geriatric population. A clinical, neuropathological and CT study. *Radiology* **141**, 687–95.

Graham, N.L., Emery, T., and Hodges, J.R. (2004). Distinctive cognitive profiles in Alzheimer's disease and subcortical vascular dementia. *J. Neurol. Neurosurg. Psychiatry* **75** (1), 61–71.

Hachinski, V.C. (1990). The decline and resurgence of vascular dementia. *Can. Med. Assoc. J.* **142**, 107–11.

Hachinski, V.C. (1991). Multi-infarct dementia: a reappraisal. *Alzheimer Dis. Assoc. Disord.* **5**, 64–8.

Hachinski, V.C. (1992). Preventable senility: a call for action against the vascular dementias. *Lancet* **340**, 645–7.

Hachinski, V.C. and Bowler, J.V. (1993). Vascular dementia. *Neurology* **43**, 2159–60.

Hachinski, V.C., Lassen, N.A., and Marshall, J. (1974). Multi-infarct dementia: a cause of mental deterioration in the elderly. *Lancet* **ii**, 207–9.

Hachinski, V.C., Iliff, L.D., Zilkha, E., Du Boulay, G.H., McAllister, V.L., Marshall, J., Ross Russell, R.W., and Symon, L. (1975). Cerebral blood flow in dementia. *Arch. Neurol.* **32**, 632–7.

Hachinski, V.C., Potter, P., and Merskey, H. (1987). Leuko-araiosis. *Arch. Neurol.* **44**, 21–3.

Hagel, C., Groden, C., Niemeyer, R., Stavrou, D., and Colmant, H.J. (2004). Subcortical angiopathic encephalopathy in a German kindred suggests an autosomal dominant disorder distinct from CADASIL. *Acta Neuropathol. (Berl.)* **108** (3), 231–40.

Hebert, R., Lindsay, J., Verreault, R., Rockwood, K., Hill, G., and Dubois, M.F. (2000). Vascular dementia: incidence and risk factors in the Canadian study of health and aging. *Stroke* **31** (7), 1487–93.

Henskens, L.H.G., Kroon, A.A., van Boxtel, M.P.J., Hofman, P.A.M., and de Leeuw, P.W. (2005). Associations of the angiotensin II type 1 receptor A1166C and the endothelial NO synthase G894T gene polymorphisms with silent subcortical white matter lesions in essential hypertension. *Stroke* **36** (9), 1869–73.

Herholz, K., Heindel, W., Rackl, A., Neubauer, I., Steinbrich, W., Pietrzyk, U., Erasmi-Korber, H., and Heiss, W.D. (1990). Regional cerebral blood flow in patients with leuko-araiosis and atherosclerotic carotid artery disease. *Arch. Neurol.* **47**, 392–6.

Heyman, A., Fillenbaum, G.G., Welsh-Bohmer KA, Gearing, M., Mirra, S.S., Mohs, R.C., Peterson, B.L., and Pieper, C.F. (1998). Cerebral infarcts in patients with autopsy-proven Alzheimer's disease: CERAD, part XVIII. Consortium to Establish a Registry for Alzheimer's Disease. *Neurology* **51** (1), 159–62.

Hier, D.B., Warach, J.D., Gorelick, P.B., and Thomas, J. (1989). Predictors of survival in clinically diagnosed Alzheimer's disease and multi-infarct dementia. *Arch. Neurol.* **46**, 1213–16.

Hofman, A., Ott, A., Breteler, M.M.B., Bots, M.L., Slooter, A.J.C., van Harskamp, F., van Duijn, C.N., Van Broeckhoven, C., and Grobbee, D.E. (1997). Atherosclerosis, apolipoprotein E, and prevalence of dementia and Alzheimer's disease in the Rotterdam Study. *Lancet* **349** (9046), 151–4.

Holmes, C., Cairns, N., Lantos, P., and Mann, A. (1999). Validity of current clinical criteria for Alzheimer's disease, vascular dementia and dementia with Lewy bodies. *Br. J. Psychiatry* **174**, 45–50.

Hom, J. and Reitan, R.M. (1990). Generalized cognitive function after stroke. *J. Clin. Exp. Neuropsychol.* **12**, 644–54.

Ikeda, M., Hokoishi, K., Maki, N., Nebu, A., Tachibana, N., Komori, K., Shigenobu, K., Fukuhara, R., and Tanabe, H. (2001). Increased prevalence of vascular dementia in Japan: a community-based epidemiological study. *Neurology* **57** (5), 839–44.

in't Veld, B.A., Ruitenberg, A., Hofman, A., Launer, L.J., van Duijn, C.M., Stijnen, T., Breteler, M.M.B., and Stricker, B.H.C. (2001). Nonsteroidal antiinflammatory drugs and the risk of Alzheimer's disease. *N. Engl. J. Med.* **345** (21), 1515–21.

Inzitari, D., Diaz, F., Fox, A., Hachinski, V.C., Steingart, A., Lau, C., Donald, A., Wade, J. P.H., Mulic, H., and Merskey, H. (1987). Vascular risk factors and leuko-araiosis. *Arch. Neurol.* **44**, 42–7.

Ivan, C.S., Seshadri, S., Beiser, A., Au, R., Kase, C.S., Kelly-Hayes, M., and Wolf, P. A. (2004). Dementia after stroke: the Framingham Study. *Stroke* **35** (6), 1264–8.

Janota, I. (1981). Dementia, deep white matter damage and hypertension: 'Binswanger's disease'. *Psychol. Med.* **11**, 39–48.

Jeerakathil, T., Wolf, P.A., Beiser, A., Massaro, J., Seshadri, S., D'Agostino, R.B., and DeCarli, C. (2004). Stroke risk profile predicts white matter hyperintensity volume: the Framingham Study. *Stroke* **35** (8), 1857–61.

Jokinen, H., Kalska, H., Mantyla, R., Pohjasvaara, T., Ylikoski, R., Hietanen, M., Salonen, O., Kaste, M., and Erkinjuntti, T. (2006). Cognitive profile of subcortical ischaemic vascular disease. *J. Neurol. Neurosurg. Psychiatry* **77** (1), 28–33.

Karbe, H., Herholz, K., Szelies, B., Pawlik, G., Wienhard, K., and Heiss, W.D. (1989). Regional metabolic correlates of Token test results in cortical and subcortical left hemispheric infarction. *Neurology* **39**, 1083–8.

Kase, C.S. (1991). Epidemiology of multi-infarct dementia. *Alzheimer Dis. Assoc. Disord.* **5**, 71–6.

Kase, C.S., Wolf, P.A., Bachman, D.L., Linn, R.T., and Cupples, L.A. (1989). Dementia and stroke: The Framingham study. In *Cerebrovascular diseases. Sixteenth research (Princeton) conference* (ed. M.D. Ginsberg and W.D. Dietrich), pp. 193–7. Raven Press, New York.

Katz, D.I., Alexander, M.P., and Mandell, A.M. (1987). Dementia following strokes in the mesencephalon and diencephalon. *Arch. Neurol.* **44**, 1127–33.

Kawamura, J., Meyer, J.S., Terayama, Y., and Weathers, S. (1991). Leukoaraiosis correlates with cerebral hypoperfusion in vascular dementia. *Stroke* **22**, 609–14.

Kawamura, J., Meyer, J.S., Ichijo, M., Kobari, M., Terayama, Y., and Weathers, S. (1993). Correlations of leuko-araiosis with cerebral atrophy and perfusion in elderly normal subjects and demented patients. *J. Neurol. Neurosurg. Psychiatry* **56**, 182–7.

Kertesz, A., Black, S.E., Tokar, G., Benke, T., Carr, T., and Nicholson, L. (1988). Periventricular and subcortical hyperintensities on magnetic resonance imaging. 'Rims, caps, and unidentified bright objects'. *Arch. Neurol.* **45**, 404–8.

Kertesz, A., Polk, M., and Carr, T. (1990). Cognition and white matter changes on magnetic resonance imaging in dementia. *Arch. Neurol.* **47**, 387–91.

Kittner, B. (1999). Clinical trials of propentofylline in vascular dementia. European/Canadian Propentofylline Study Group. *Alzheimer Dis. Assoc. Disord.* **13** (Suppl. 3), S166–S171.

Kivipelto, M., Helkala, E.L., Hanninen, T., Laakso, M.P., Hallikainen, M., Alhainen, K., Soininen, H., Tuomilehto, J., and Nissinen, A. (2001*a*). Midlife vascular risk factors and late-life mild cognitive impairment: a population-based study. *Neurology* **56** (12), 1683–9.

Kivipelto, M., Helkala, E.L., Laakso, M.P., Hanninen, T., Hallikainen, M., Alhainen, K., Soininen, H., Tuomilehto, J., and Nissinen, A. (2001*b*). Midlife vascular risk factors and Alzheimer's disease in later life: longitudinal, population based study. *Br. Med. J.* **322** (7300), 1447–51.

Kivipelto, M., Ngandu, T., Fratiglioni, L., Viitanen, M., Kareholt, I., Winblad, B., Helkala, E.L., Tuomilehto, J., Soininen, H., and Nissinen, A. (2005). Obesity and vascular risk factors at midlife and the risk of dementia and Alzheimer disease. *Arch. Neurol.* **62** (10), 1556–60.

Knopman, D., Boland, L.L., Mosley, T., Howard, G., Liao, D., Szklo, M., McGovern, P., and Folsom, A.R. (2001). Cardiovascular risk factors and cognitive decline in middle-aged adults. *Neurology* **56** (1), 42–8.

Knopman, D.S., Rocca, W.A., Cha, R.H., Edland, S.D., and Kokmen, E. (2003*a*). Survival study of vascular dementia in Rochester, Minnesota. *Arch. Neurol.* **60** (1), 85–90.

Knopman, D.S., Parisi, J.E., Boeve, B.F., Cha, R.H., Apaydin, H., Salviati, A., Edland, S.D., and Rocca, W.A. (2003*b*). Vascular dementia in a population-based autopsy study. *Arch. Neurol.* **60** (4), 569–75.

Kobari, M., Meyer, J.S., Ichijo, M., and Oravez, W.T. (1990). Leukoaraiosis: correlation of MR and CT findings with blood flow, atrophy, and cognition. *Am. J. Neuroradiol.* **11**, 273–81.

Kramer, J.H., Reed, B.R., Mungas, D., Weiner, M.W., and Chui, H.C. (2002). Executive dysfunction in subcortical ischaemic vascular disease. *J. Neurol. Neurosurg. Psychiatry* **72** (2), 217–20.

Kuwabara, Y., Ichiya, Y., Sasaki, M., Yoshida, T., Fukumura, T., Masuda, K., Ibayashi, S., and Fujishima, M. (1996). Cerebral blood flow and vascular response to hypercapnia in hypertensive patients with leukoaraiosis. *Ann. Nuclear Med.* **10** (3), 293–8.

Ladurner, G., Iliff, L.D., and Lechner, H. (1982). Clinical factors associated with dementia in ischaemic stroke. *J. Neurol. Neurosurg. Psychiatry* **45**, 97–101.

Lassen, N. A. (1982). Incomplete cerebral infarction—focal incomplete ischaemic tissue necrosis not leading to emollision. *Stroke* **13**, 522–3.

Launer, L.J., Masaki, K., Petrovitch, H., Foley, D., and Havlik, R.J. (1995). The association between midlife blood pressure levels and late-life cognitive function. The Honolulu–Asia Aging Study. *J. Am. Med. Assoc.* **274** (23), 1846–51.

Launer, L.J., Ross, G.W., Petrovitch, H., Masaki, K., Foley, D., White, L.R., and Havlik, R.J. (2000). Midlife blood pressure and dementia: the Honolulu–Asia aging study. *Neurobiol. Aging* **21** (1), 49–55.

Lim, A., Tsuang, D., Kukull, W., Nochlin, D., Leverenz, J., McCormick, W., Bowen, J., Teri, L., Thompson, J., Peskind, E.R., Raskind, M., and Larson, E.B. (1999). Clinico-neuropathological correlation of Alzheimer's disease in a community-based case series. *J. Am. Geriatr. Soc.* **47** (5), 564–9.

Lin, J.X., Tomimoto, H., Akiguchi, I., Matsuo, A., Wakita, H., Shibasaki, H., and Budka, H. (2000). Vascular cell components of the medullary arteries in Binswanger's disease brains: a morphometric and immunoelectron microscopic study. *Stroke* **31** (8), 1838–42.

Lindsay, J., Hebert, R., and Rockwood, K. (1997). The Canadian Study of Health and Aging: risk factors for vascular dementia. *Stroke* **28** (3), 526–30.

Lithell, H., Hansson, L., Skoog, I., Elmfeldt, D., Hofman, A., Olofsson, B., Trenkwalder, P., and Zanchetti, A. (2003). The Study on Cognition and Prognosis in the Elderly (SCOPE): principal results of a randomized double-blind intervention trial. *J. Hypertens.* **21** (5), 875–86.

Liu, C.K., Miller, B.L., Cummings, J.L., Mehringer, C.M., Goldberg, M.A., Howng, S.L., and Benson, D.F. (1992). A quantitative MRI study of vascular dementia. *Neurology* **42**, 138–43.

Loeb, C. (1990). Vascular dementia. *Dementia* **1**, 175–84.

Loeb, C., Gandolfo, C., and Bino, G. (1988). Intellectual impairment and cerebral lesions in multiple cerebral infarcts. A clinical-computed tomography study. *Stroke* **19**, 560–5.

Loizou, L.A., Kendall, B.E., and Marshall, J. (1981). Subcortical arteriosclerotic encephalopathy: a clinical and radiological investigation. *J. Neurol. Neurosurg. Psychiatry* **44**, 294–304.

Longstreth, W.T., Manolio, T.A., Arnold, A., Burke, G.L., Bryan, N., Jungreis, C.A., Enright, P.L., O'Leary, D., and Fried, L. (1996). Clinical correlates of white matter findings on cranial magnetic resonance imaging of 3301 elderly people. The Cardiovascular Health Study. *Stroke* **27** (8), 1274–82.

Longstreth, W.T., Jr., Arnold, A.M., Beauchamp, N.J., Jr., Manolio, T.A., Lefkowitz, D., Jungreis, C., Hirsch, C.H., O'Leary, D.H., and Furberg, C.D. (2005). Incidence, manifestations, and predictors of worsening white matter on serial cranial magnetic resonance imaging in the elderly: the Cardiovascular Health Study. *Stroke* **36** (1), 56–61.

Lopez, O.L., Larumbe, M.R., Becker, J.T., Rezek, D., Rosen, J., Klunk, W., and Dekosky, S.T. (1994). Reliability of NINDS-AIREN clinical criteria for the diagnosis of vascular dementia. *Neurology* **44**, 1240–5.

Lopez-Arrieta, J.M. and Birks, J. (2002). Nimodipine for primary degenerative, mixed and vascular dementia. *Cochrane Database Syst. Rev.* **3**, CD000147.

Maeda, S., Nakayama, H., Isaka, K., Aihara, Y., and Nemoto, S. (1976). Familial unusual encephalopathy of Binswanger's type without hypertension. *Folia Psychiatr. Neurol. Jpn* **30**, 165–77.

Markus, H.S., Hunt, B., Palmer, K., Enzinger, C., Schmidt, H., and Schmidt, R. (2005). Markers of endothelial and hemostatic activation and progression of cerebral white matter hyperintensities: longitudinal results of the Austrian Stroke Prevention Study. *Stroke* **36** (7), 1410–14.

Marshall, V.G., Bradley, W.G., Jr., Marshall, C.E., Bhoopat, T., and Rhodes, R.H. (1988). Deep white matter infarction: correlation of MR imaging and histopathologic findings. *Radiology* **167**, 517–22.

Martin, D.C., Miller, J.K., Kapoor, W., Arena, V.C., and Boller, F. (1987). A controlled study of survival with dementia. *Arch. Neurol.* **44**, 1122–6.

Masaki, K.H., Losonczy, K.G., Izmirlian, G., Foley, D.J., Ross, G.W., Petrovitch, H., Havlik, R., and White, L.R. (2000). Association of vitamin E and C supplement use with cognitive function and dementia in elderly men. *Neurology* **54** (6), 1265–72.

McKhann, G., Drachman, D., Folstein, M., Katzman, R., Price, D., and Stadlan, E.M. (1984). Clinical diagnosis of Alzheimer's disease: report of the NINCDS-ADRDA Work Group under the auspices of Department of Health and Human Services Task Force on Alzheimer's Disease. *Neurology* **34**, 939–44.

Meguro, K., Hatazawa, J., Yamaguchi, T., Itoh, M., Matsuzawa, T., Ono, S., Miyazawa, H., Hishinuma, T., Yanai, K., Sekita, Y., and Yamada, K. (1990). Cerebral circulation and oxygen metabolism associated with subclinical periventricular hyperintensity as shown by magnetic resonance imaging. *Ann. Neurol.* **28**, 378–83.

Meyer, J.S., McClintic, K.L., Rogers, R.L., Sims, P., and Mortel, K.F. (1988). Aetiological considerations and risk factors for multi-infarct dementia. *J. Neurol. Neurosurg. Psychiatry* **51**, 1489–97.

Meyer, J.S., Rogers, R.L., and Mortel, K.F. (1989*a*). Multi-infarct dementia: demography, risk factors and therapy. In *Cerebrovascular diseases. Sixteenth research (Princeton) conference* (ed. M.D. Ginsberg and W.D. Dietrich), pp. 199–206. Raven Press, New York,.

Meyer, J.S., Rogers, R.L., McClintic, K., Mortel, K.F., and Lotfi, J. (1989*b*). Randomized clinical trial of daily aspirin therapy in multi- infarct dementia. A pilot study. *J. Am. Geriatr. Soc.* **37**, 549–55.

Mielke, R., Kittner, B., Ghaemi, M., Kessler, J., Szelies, B., Herholz, K., and Heiss, W.D. (1996). Propentofylline improves regional cerebral glucose metabolism and neuropsychologic performance in vascular dementia. *J. Neurol. Sci.* **141** (1–2), 59–64.

Mielke, R., Moller, H.J., Erkinjuntti, T., Rosenkranz, B., Rother, M., and Kittner, B. (1998). Propentofylline in the treatment of vascular dementia and Alzheimer-type dementia: overview of phase I and phase II clinical trials. *Alzheimer Dis. Assoc. Disord.* **12** (Suppl. 2), S29–S35.

Miller Fisher, C. (1968). Dementia in cerebrovascular disease. In *Cerebral vascular diseases. Sixth Conference* (ed. J.F. Toole, R.G. Siekert, and J.P. Whisnant), pp. 232–6. Grune and Stratton, New York.

Mirsen, T.R., Lee, D.H., Wong, C.J., Diaz, J.F., Fox, A.J., Hachinski, V.C., and Merskey, H. (1991). Clinical correlates of white-matter changes on magnetic resonance imaging scans of the brain. *Arch. Neurol.* **48**, 1015–1021.

Miyao, S., Takano, A., Teramoto, J., and Takahashi, A. (1992). Leukoaraiosis in relation to prognosis for patients with lacunar infarction. *Stroke* **23**, 1434–8.

Mobius, H.J. and Stoffler, A. (2002). New approaches to clinical trials in vascular dementia: memantine in small vessel disease. *Cerebrovasc. Dis.* **13** (Suppl. 2), 61–6.

Mok, V.C.T., Wong, A., Lam, W. W.M., Fan, Y.H., Tang, W.K., Kwok, T., Hui, A.C.F., and Wong, K.S. (2004). Cognitive impairment and functional outcome after stroke associated with small vessel disease. *J. Neurol. Neurosurg. Psychiatry* **75** (4), 560–6.

Molsa, P.K., Marttila, R.J., and Rinne, U.K. (1986). Survival and cause of death in Alzheimer's disease and multi- infarct dementia. *Acta Neurol. Scand.* **74**, 103–7.

Moretti, R., Torre, P., Antonello, R.M., Cazzato, G., and Bava, A. (2002). Rivastigmine in subcortical vascular dementia: an open 22-month study. *J. Neurol. Sci.* **203–204**, 141–6.

Moroney, J.T., Bagiella, E., Desmond, D.W., Hachinski, V.C., Molsa, P.K., Gustafson, L., Brun, A., Fischer, P., Erkinjuntti, T., Rosen, W., Paik, M.C., and Tatemichi, T.K. (1997). Meta-analysis of the Hachinski Ischemic Score in pathologically verified dementias. *Neurology* **49**, 1096–105.

Moroney, J.T., Tang, M.X., Berglund, L., Small, S., Merchant, C., Bell, K., Stern, Y., and Mayeux, R. (1999). Low-density lipoprotein cholesterol and the risk of dementia with stroke. *J. Am. Med. Assoc.* **282** (3), 254–60.

Morris, M.C., Evans, D.A., Bienias, J.L., Tangney, C.C., and Wilson, R.S. (2004). Dietary fat intake and 6-year cognitive change in an older biracial community population. *Neurology* **62** (9), 1573–9.

Moser, D.J., Cohen, R.A., Paul, R.H., Paulsen, J.S., Ott, B.R., Gordon, N.M., Bell, S., and Stone, W.M. (2001). Executive function and magnetic resonance imaging subcortical hyperintensities in vascular dementia. *Neuropsychiatry Neuropsychol. Behav. Neurol.* **14** (2), 89–92.

Munoz, D.G., Hastak, S.M., Harper, B., Lee, D., and Hachinski, V.C. (1993). Pathologic correlates of increased signals of the centrum ovale on magnetic resonance imaging. *Arch. Neurol.* **50**, 492–7.

Neuropathology Group of the Medical Research Council Cognitive Function and Ageing Study (MRC CFAS) (2001). Pathological correlates of late-onset dementia in a multicentre, community-based population in England and Wales. *Lancet* **357** (9251), 169–75.

Newman, S.C. (1999). The prevalence of depression in Alzheimer's disease and vascular dementia in a population sample. *J. Affect. Disord.* **52** (1–3), 169–76.

Nolan, K.A., Lino, M.M., Seligmann, A.W., and Blass, J.P. (1998). Absence of vascular dementia in an autopsy series from a dementia clinic. *J. Am. Geriatr. Soc.* **46** (5), 597–604.

O'Brien, J., Perry, R., Barber, R., Gholkar, A., and Thomas, A. (2000). The association between white matter lesions on magnetic resonance imaging and noncognitive symptoms. *Ann. NY Acad. Sci.* **903**, 482–9.

O'Brien, J.T., Paling, S., Barber, R., Williams, E.D., Ballard, C., McKeith, I.G., Gholkar, A., Crum, W.R., Rossor, M.N., and Fox, N.C. (2001). Progressive brain atrophy on serial MRI in dementia with Lewy bodies, AD, and vascular dementia. *Neurology* **56** (10), 1386–8.

O'Connell, J.E., Gray, C.S., French, J.M., and Robertson, I.H. (1998). Atrial fibrillation and cognitive function: case-control study. *J. Neurol. Neurosurg. Psychiatry* **65** (3), 386–9.

Olszewski, J. (1962). Subcortical arteriosclerotic encephalopathy: review of the literature on the so-called Binswanger's disease and presentation of two cases. *World Neurol.* **3**, 359–75.

Orgogozo, J.M., Rigaud, A.S., Stoffler, A., Mobius, H.J., and Forette, F. (2002). Efficacy and safety of memantine in patients with mild to moderate vascular dementia: a randomized, placebo-controlled trial (MMM 300). *Stroke* **33** (7), 1834–9.

O'Sullivan, M., Morris, R.G., Huckstep, B., Jones, D.K., Williams, S. C.R., and Markus, H.S. (2004). Diffusion tensor MRI correlates with executive dysfunction in patients with ischaemic leukoaraiosis. *J. Neurol. Neurosurg. Psychiatry* **75** (3), 441–7.

O'Sullivan, M., Morris, R.G., and Markus, H.S. (2005). Brief cognitive assessment for patients with cerebral small vessel disease. *J. Neurol. Neurosurg. Psychiatry* **76** (8), 1140–5.

Ott, A., Breteler, M.M., van Harskamp, F., Claus, J.J., van der Cammen, T.J., Grobbee, D.E., and Hofman, A. (1995). Prevalence of Alzheimer's disease and vascular dementia: association with education. The Rotterdam study. *Br. Med. J.* **310** (6985), 970–3.

Ott, A., Stolk, R.P., Hofman, A., van Harskamp, F., Grobbee, D.E., and Breteler, M.M. (1996). Association of diabetes mellitus and dementia: the Rotterdam Study. *Diabetologia* **39** (11), 1392–7.

Ott, A., Breteler, M.M., de Bruyne, M.C., van Harskamp, F., Grobbee, D.E., and Hofman, A. (1997). Atrial fibrillation and dementia in a population-based study. The Rotterdam Study. *Stroke* **28** (2), 316–21.

Ott, A., Andersen, K., Dewey, M.E., Letenneur, L., Brayne, C., Copeland, J. R.M., Dartigues, J.F., Kragh-Sorensen, P., Lobo, A., Martinez-Lage, J.M., Stijnen, T., Hofman, A., and Launer, L.J. (2004). Effect of smoking on global cognitive function in nondemented elderly. *Neurology* **62** (6), 920–4.

Pantel, J., Schroder, J., Essig, M., Jauss, M., Schneider, G., Eysenbach, K., von, K.R., Baudendistel, K., Schad, L.R., and Knopp, M.V. (1998). In vivo quantification of brain volumes in subcortical vascular dementia and Alzheimer's disease. An MRI-based study. *Dement. Geriatr. Cogn. Disord.* **9** (6), 309–16.

Pantoni, L., Inzitari, D., Pracucci, G., Lolli, F., Giordano, G., Bracco, L., and Amaducci, L. (1993). Cerebrospinal fluid proteins in patients with leucoaraiosis: possible abnormalities in blood-brain barrier function. *J. Neurol. Sci.* **115**, 125–131.

Pantoni, L., Carosi, M., Amigoni, S., Mascalchi, M., and Inzitari, D. (1996). A preliminary open trial with nimodipine in patients with cognitive impairment and leukoaraiosis. *Clin. Neuropharmacol.* **19** (6), 497–506.

Pantoni, L., Bianchi, C., Beneke, M., Inzitari, D., Wallin, A., and Erkinjuntti, T. (2000*a*). The Scandinavian Multi-Infarct Dementia Trial: a double-blind, placebo-controlled trial on nimodipine in multi-infarct dementia. *J. Neurol. Sci.* **175** (2), 116–23.

Pantoni, L., Rossi, R., Inzitari, D., Bianchi, C., Beneke, M., Erkinjuntti, T., and Wallin, A. (2000*b*). Efficacy and safety of nimodipine in subcortical vascular dementia: a subgroup analysis of the Scandinavian Multi-Infarct Dementia Trial. *J. Neurol. Sci.* **175** (2), 124–34.

Pantoni, L., Del Ser, T., Soglian, A.G., Amigoni, S., Spadari, G., Binelli, D., and Inzitari, D. (2005). Efficacy and safety of nimodipine in subcortical vascular dementia: a randomized placebo-controlled trial. *Stroke* **36** (3), 619–24.

Parnetti, L., Mecocci, P., Santucci, C., Gaiti, A., Petrini, A., Longo, A., Cadini, D., Caputo, N., Signorini, E., and Senin, U. (1990). Is multi-infarct dementia representative of vascular dementias? A retrospective study. *Acta Neurol. Scand.* **81**, 484–7.

Parnetti, L., Ambrosoli, L., Agliati, G., Caratozzolo, P., Fossati, L., Frattola, L., Martucci, N., Murri, L., Nappi, G., Puca, F.M., Poli, A., Girardello, R., and Senin, U. (1996). Posatirelin in the treatment of vascular dementia: a double-blind multicentre study vs placebo. *Acta Neurol. Scand.* **93** (6), 456–63.

Paulson, O.B., Strandgaard, S., and Edvinsson, L. (1990). Cerebral autoregulation. *Cerebrovasc. Brain Metab. Rev.* **2**, 161–92.

Pellissier, J.-F. and Poncet, M. (1989). Binswanger's encephalopathy. In *Handbook of clinical neurology. Vascular diseases Part II*, Vol. 54 (ed. P.J. Vinken *et al.*), pp. 221–33. Elsevier Science Publishers, Amsterdam.

Perani, D., Vallar, G., Cappa, S., Messa, C., and Fazio, F. (1987). Aphasia and neglect after subcortical stroke. A clinical/cerebral perfusion correlation study. *Brain* **110**, 1211–29.

Perez, F.I., Gay, J.R., Taylor, R.L., and Rivera, V.M. (1975*a*). Patterns of memory performance in the neurologically impaired aged. *Can. J. Neurol. Sci.* **2**, 347–55.

Perez, F.I., Rivera, V.M., Meyer, J.S., Gay, J.R., Taylor, R.L., and Mathew, N.T. (1975*b*). Analysis of intellectual and cognitive performance in patients with multi-infarct dementia, vertebrobasilar insufficiency with dementia, and Alzheimer's disease. *J. Neurol. Neurosurg. Psychiatry* **38**, 533–40.

Perez, F.I., Gay, J.R., and Taylor, R.L. (1975*c*). WAIS performance of neurologically impaired aged. *Psychol. Rep.* **37**, 1043–7.

Pohjasvaara, T., Erkinjuntti, T., Vataja, R., and Kaste, M. (1997*a*). Comparison of stroke features and disability in daily life in patients with ischemic stroke aged 55 to 70 and 71 to 85 years. *Stroke* **28** (4), 729–35.

Pohjasvaara, T., Erkinjuntti, T., Vataja, R., and Kaste, M. (1997*b*). Dementia three months after stroke. Baseline frequency and effect of different definitions of dementia in the Helsinki Stroke Aging Memory Study (SAM) cohort. *Stroke* **28** (4), 785–92.

Pohjasvaara, T., Erkinjuntti, T., Ylikoski, R., Hietanen, M., Vataja, R., and Kaste, M. (1998). Clinical determinants of poststroke dementia. *Stroke* **29** (1), 75–81.

Pohjasvaara, T., Mantyla, R., Aronen, H.J., Leskela, M., Salonen, O., Kaste, M., and Erkinjuntti, T. (1999). Clinical and radiological determinants of prestroke cognitive decline in a stroke cohort. *J. Neurol. Neurosurg. Psychiatry* **67** (6), 742–8.

Pohjasvaara, T., Mantyla, R., Ylikoski, R., Kaste, M., and Erkinjuntti, T. (2000). Comparison of different clinical criteria (DSM-III, ADDTC, ICD-10, NINDS-AIREN, DSM-IV) for the diagnosis of vascular dementia. National Institute of Neurological Disorders and Stroke-Association Internationale pour la Recherche et l'Enseignement en Neurosciences. *Stroke* **31** (12), 2952–7.

Pohjasvaara, T., Mantyla, R., Ylikoski, R., Kaste, M., and Erkinjuntti, T. (2003). Clinical features of MRI-defined subcortical vascular disease. *Alzheimer Dis. Assoc. Disord.* **17** (4), 236–42.

Price, C.C., Jefferson, A.L., Merino, J.G., Heilman, K.M., and Libon, D.J. (2005). Subcortical vascular dementia: integrating neuropsychological and neuroradiologic data. *Neurology* **65** (3), 376–82.

Prince, M., Bird, A.S., Blizard, R.A., and Mann, A.H. (1996). Is the cognitive function of older patients affected by antihypertensive treatment? Results from 54 months of the Medical Research Council's treatment trial of hypertension in older adults. *Br. Med. J.* **312**, 801–5.

Prins, N.D., van Dijk, E.J., den Heijer, T., Vermeer, S.E., Koudstaal, P.J., Oudkerk, M., Hofman, A., and Breteler, M.M.B. (2004). Cerebral white matter lesions and the risk of dementia. *Arch. Neurol.* **61** (10), 1531–4.

Prins, N.D., van Dijk, E.J., den Heijer, T., Vermeer, S.E., Jolles, J., Koudstaal, P.J., Hofman, A., and Breteler, M.M.B. (2005). Cerebral small-vessel disease and decline in information processing speed, executive function and memory. *Brain* **128** (9), 2034–41.

Pujol, J., Junque, C., Vendrell, P., Capdevila, A., and Marti-Vilalta, J.L. (1991). Cognitive correlates of ventricular enlargement in vascular patients with leukoaraiosis. *Acta Neurol. Scand.* **84**, 237–42.

Qiu, C., von Strauss, E., Winblad, B., and Fratiglioni, L. (2004). Decline in blood pressure over time and risk of dementia: a longitudinal study From the Kungsholmen Project. *Stroke* **35** (8), 1810–15.

Rea, T.D., Breitner, J.C., Psaty, B.M., Fitzpatrick, A.L., Lopez, O.L., Newman, A.B., Hazzard, W.R., Zandi, P.P., Burke, G.L., Lyketsos, C.G., Bernick, C., and Kuller, L.H. (2005). Statin use and the risk of incident dementia: the Cardiovascular Health Study. *Arch. Neurol.* **62** (7), 1047–51.

Rocca, W.A., Hofman, A., Brayne, C., Breteler, M.M., Clarke, M., Copeland, J.R., Dartigues, J.F., Engedal, K., Hagnell, O., Heeren, T.J., Jonker, C., Lindesay, J., Lobo, A., Mann, A.H., Molsa, P.K., Morgan, K., O'Connor, D.W., da Silva Droux, A., Sulkava, R., Kay, D.W.K., and Amaducci, L. (1991). The prevalence of vascular dementia in Europe: facts and fragments from 1980–1990 studies. EURODEM-Prevalence Research Group. *Ann. Neurol.* **30**, 817–24.

Rockwood, K., Wentzel, C., Hachinski, V., Hogan, D.B., MacKnight, C., McDowell, I., and Vascular Cognitive Impairment Investigators of the Canadian Study of Health and Aging (2000). Prevalence and outcomes of vascular cognitive impairment. *Neurology* **54** (2), 447–51.

Roman, G.C. and Royall, D.R. (1999). Executive control function: a rational basis for the diagnosis of vascular dementia. *Alzheimer Dis. Assoc. Disord.* **13** (Suppl. 3), S69–80.

Roman, G.C., Tatemichi, T.K., Erkinjuntti, T., Cummings, J.L., Masdeu, J.C., Garcia, J.H., Amaducci, L., Orgogozo, J.M., Brun, A., Hofman, A., Moody, D.M., O'Brien, M.D., Yamaguchi, T., Grafman, J., Drayer, B.P., Bennett, D.A., Fisher, M., Ogata, J., Kokmen, E., Bermejo, F., Wolf, P.A., Gorelick, P.B., Bick, K.L., Pajeau, A.K., Bell, M.A., DeCarli, C., Culebras, A., Korczyn, A.D., Bogousslavsky, J., Hartmann, A., and Scheinberg, P. (1993). Vascular dementia: diagnostic criteria for research studies. Report of the NINDS-AIREN international workshop. *Neurology* **43**, 250–60.

Rossi, R., Inzitari, D., Pantoni, L., del Ser, T., Erkinjuntti, T., Wallin, A., Bianchi, C., Badenas, J.M., and Beneke, M. (1999). Nimodipine in subcortical vascular dementia trial. *Alzheimer Dis. Assoc. Disord.* **13** (Suppl. 3), S159–65.

Rother, M., Erkinjuntti, T., Roessner, M., Kittner, B., Marcusson, J., and Karlsson, I. (1998). Propentofylline in the treatment of Alzheimer's disease and vascular dementia: a review of phase III trials. *Dement. Geriatr. Cogn. Disord.* **9** (Suppl. 1), 36–43.

Royall, D.R., Cordes, J.A., and Polk, M. (1998). CLOX: an executive clock drawing task. *J. Neurol. Neurosurg. Psychiatry* **64** (5), 588–594.

Ruchoux, M.M., Brulin, P., Leteurtre, E., and Maurage, C.A. (2000). Skin biopsy value and leukoaraiosis. *Ann. NY Acad. Sci.* **903**, 285–92.

Sabri, O., Hellwig, D., Schreckenberger, M., Cremerius, U., Schneider, R., Kaiser, H.J., Doherty, C., Mull, M., Ringelstein, E.B., and Buell, U. (1998). Correlation of neuropsychological, morphological and functional (regional cerebral blood flow and glucose utilization) findings in cerebral microangiopathy. *J. Nucl. Med.* **39** (1), 147–54.

Sabri, O., Ringelstein, E.B., Hellwig, D., Schneider, R., Schreckenberger, M., Kaiser, H.J., Mull, M., and Buell, U. (1999). Neuropsychological impairment correlates with hypoperfusion and hypometabolism but not with severity of white matter lesions on MRI in patients with cerebral microangiopathy. *Stroke* **30** (3), 556–66.

Sachdev, P.S., Brodaty, H., Valenzuela, M.J., Lorentz, L., Looi, J. C.L., Wen, W., and Zagami, A. S. (2004). The neuropsychological profile of vascular cognitive impairment in stroke and TIA patients. *Neurology* **62** (6), 912–19.

Salerno, J.A., Murphy, D. G.M., Horwitz, B., DeCarli, C., Haxby, J.V., Rapoport, S.I., and Schapiro, M.B. (1992). Brain atrophy in hypertension. A volumetric magnetic resonance imaging study. *Hypertension* **20**, 340–8.

Schmidt, R., Ropele, S., Enzinger, C., Petrovic, K., Smith, S., Schmidt, H., Matthews, P.M., and Fazekas, F. (2005). White matter lesion progression, brain atrophy, and cognitive decline: the Austrian stroke prevention study. *Ann. Neurol.* **58** (4), 610–16.

Schnaider Beeri, M., Goldbourt, U., Silverman, J.M., Noy, S., Schmeidler, J., Ravona-Springer, R., Sverdlick, A., and Davidson, M. (2004). Diabetes mellitus in midlife and the risk of dementia three decades later. *Neurology* **63** (10), 1902–7.

Schon, F., Martin, R.J., Prevett, M., Clough, C., Enevoldson, T.P., and Markus, H.S. (2003). 'CADASIL coma': an underdiagnosed acute encephalopathy. *J. Neurol. Neurosurg. Psychiatry* **74** (2), 249–52.

Sha, M.C. and Callahan, C.M. (2003). The efficacy of pentoxifylline in the treatment of vascular dementia: a systematic review. *Alzheimer Dis. Assoc. Disord.* **17** (1), 46–54.

Shepherd, J., Blauw, G.J., Murphy, M.B., Bollen, E.L., Buckley, B.M., Cobbe, S.M., Ford, I., Gaw, A., Hyland, M., Jukema, J.W., Kamper, A.M., Macfarlane, P.W., Meinders, A.E., Norrie, J., Packard, C.J., Perry, I.J., Stott, D.J., Sweeney, B.J., Twomey, C., and Westendorp, R.G. (2002). Pravastatin in elderly individuals at risk of vascular disease (PROSPER): a randomised controlled trial. *Lancet* **360** (9346), 1623–30.

Shyu, W.C., Lin, J.C., Shen, C.C., Hsu, Y.D., Lee, C.C., Shiah, I.S., and Tsao, W.L. (1996). Vascular dementia of Binswanger's type: clinical, neuroradiological and 99mTc-HMPAO SPECT study. *Eur. J. Nuclear Med.* **23** (10), 1338–44.

Skoog, I. (1997). The relationship between blood pressure and dementia: a review. *Biomed. Pharmacother.* **51**, 367–75.

Skoog, I., Nilsson, L., Palmertz, B., Andreasson, L.-A., and Svanborg, A. (1993). A population-based study of dementia in 85-year-olds. *N. Engl. J. Med.* **328**, 153–8.

Skoog, I., Berg, S., Johansson, B., Palmertz, B., and Andreasson, L.A. (1996). The influence of white matter lesions on neuropsychological functioning in demented and non-demented 85-year-olds. *Acta Neurol. Scand.* **93** (2–3), 142–8.

Skoog, I., Andreasson, L.-A., Landahl, S., and Lernfelt, B. (1998). A population-based study on blood pressure and brain atrophy in 85-year-olds. *Hypertension* **32**, 404–9.

Slooter, A.J., Tang, M.X., van Duijn, C.M., Stern, Y., Ott, A., Bell, K., Breteler, M.M., Van Broeckhoven, C., Tatemichi, T.K., Tycko, B., Hofman, A., and Mayeux, R. (1997). Apolipoprotein E ε4 and the risk of dementia with stroke. A population-based investigation. *J. Am. Med. Assoc.* **227** (10), 818–21.

Snowdon, D.A., Greiner, L.H., Mortimer, J.A., Riley, K.P., Greiner, P.A., and Markesbery, W.R. (1997). Brain infarction and the clinical expression of Alzheimer disease. The nun study. *J. Am. Med. Assoc.* **227**, 813–17.

Sourander, P. and Walinder, J. (1977). Hereditary multi-infarct dementia. Morphological and clinical studies of a new disease. *Acta Neuropathol. (Berl.)* **39**, 247–54.

Starr, J.M., Leaper, S.A., Murray, A.D., Lemmon, H.A., Staff, R.T., Deary, I.J., and Whalley, L.J. (2003). Brain white matter lesions detected by magnetic resonance imaging are associated with balance and gait speed. *J. Neurol. Neurosurg. Psychiatry* **74** (1), 94–8.

Steingart, A., Hachinski, V.C., Lau, C., Fox, A.J., Diaz, F., Cape, R., Lee, D., Inzitari, D., and Merskey, H. (1987*a*). Cognitive and neurologic findings in subjects with diffuse white matter lucencies on computed tomographic scan (leukoaraiosis). *Arch. Neurol.* **44**, 32–5.

Steingart, A., Hachinski, V.C., Lau, C., Fox, A.J., Fox, H., Lee, D., Inzitari, D., and Merskey, H. (1987*b*). Cognitive and neurologic findings in demented patients with diffuse white matter lucencies on computed tomographic scan (leukoaraiosis). *Arch. Neurol.* **44**, 36–9.

Sterzer, P., Meintzschel, F., Rosler, A., Lanfermann, H., Steinmetz, H., and Sitzer, M. (2001). Pravastatin improves cerebral vasomotor reactivity in patients with subcortical small-vessel disease. *Stroke* **32** (12), 2817–20.

Strandgaard, S. (1976). Autoregulation of cerebral blood flow in hypertensive patients. The modifying influence of prolonged antihypertensive treatment on the tolerance to acute drug-induced hypotension. *Circulation* **53**, 720–7.

Streifler, J.Y., Eliasziw, M., Benavente, O.R., Hachinski, V.C., Fox, A.J., and Barnett, H.J.M. (1995). Lack of relationship between leukoaraiosis and carotid artery disease. *Arch. Neurol.* **52**, 21–4.

Streifler, J.Y., Eliasziw, M., Benavente, O.R.; North American Symptomatic Carotid Endarterectomy Trial Group (2003). Development and progression of leukoaraiosis in patients with brain ischemia and carotid artery disease. *Stroke* **34** (8), 1913–16.

Sulkava, R. and Erkinjuntti, T. (1987). Vascular dementia due to cardiac arrhythmias and systemic hypotension. *Acta Neurol. Scand.* **76**, 123–8.

Sultzer, D.L., Mahler, M.E., Cummings, J.L., Van Gorp, W.G., Hinkin, C.H., and Brown, C. (1995). Cortical abnormalities associated with subcortical lesions in vascular dementia: clinical and positron emission tomographic findings. *Arch. Neurol.* **52**, 773–80.

Szatmari, S.Z. and Whitehouse, P.J. (2003). Vinpocetine for cognitive impairment and dementia. *Cochrane Database Syst. Rev.* **1**, CD003119.

Sze, G., De Armond, S., Brant-Zawadzki, M., Davis, R., De Groot, J., Norman, D., and Newton, T. H. (1985). 'Abnormal' MRI foci anterior to the frontal horns: pathologic correlates of an ubiquitous finding. *Am. J. Neuroradiol.* **6**, 467–8.

Tarvonen-Schröder, S., Röyttä, M., Räihä, I., Kurki, T., Rajala, T., and Sourander, L. (1996). Clinical features of leuko-araiosis. *J. Neurol. Neurosurg. Psychiatry* **60** (4), 431–6.

Tatemichi, T.K., Desmond, D.W., Mayeux, R., Paik, M., Stern, Y., Sano, M., Remien, R.H., Williams, J.B., Mohr, J.P., Hauser, W.A., and Figueroa, M. (1992). Dementia after stroke: baseline frequency, risks, and clinical features in a hospitalized cohort. *Neurology* **42**, 1185–93.

Tatemichi, T.K., Desmond, D.W., Paik, M., Figueroa, M., Gropen, T.I., Stern, Y., Sano, M., Remien, R., Williams, J. B.W., Mohr, J.P., and Mayeux, R. (1993). Clinical determinants of dementia related to stroke. *Ann. Neurol.* **33**, 568–75.

Tatemichi, T.K., Desmond, D.W., Stern, Y., Paik, M., Sano, M., and Bagiella, E. (1994). Cognitive impairment after stroke: frequency, patterns, and relationship to functional abilities. *J. Neurol. Neurosurg. Psychiatry* **57**, 202–7.

Thompson, P.D. and Marsden, C.D. (1987). Gait disorder of subcortical arteriosclerotic encephalopathy: Binswanger's disease. *Movem. Disord.* **2**, 1–8.

Tierney, M.C., Black, S.E., Szalai, J.P., Snow, W.G., Fisher, R.H., Nadon, G., and Chui, H.C. (2001). Recognition memory and verbal fluency differentiate probable Alzheimer disease from subcortical ischemic vascular dementia. *Arch. Neurol.* **58** (10), 1654–9.

Tomimoto, H., Akiguchi, I., Suenaga, T., Nishimura, M., Wakita, H., Nakamura, S., and Kimura, J. (1996). Alterations of the blood–brain barrier and glial cells in white-matter lesions in cerebrovascular and Alzheimer's disease patients. *Stroke* **27** (11), 2069–74.

Tomlinson, B.E., Blessed, G., and Roth, M. (1970). Observations on the brains of demented old people. *J. Neurol. Sci.* **11**, 205–42.

Tomonaga, M., Yamanouchi, H., Tohgi, H., and Kameyama, M. (1982). Clinicopathologic study of progressive subcortical vascular encephalopathy (Binswanger type) in the elderly. *J. Am. Geriatr. Soc.* **30**, 524–9.

Toso, V. (1989). Single photon emission tomography findings in lacunar lesions. *Eur. Neurol.* **29** (Suppl. 2), 36–8.

Tournier Lasserve, E., Iba Zizen, M.T., Romero, N., and Bousser, M.G. (1991). Autosomal dominant syndrome with strokelike episodes and leukoencephalopathy. *Stroke* **22**, 1297–302.

Tournier Lasserve, E., Joutel, A., Melki, J., Weissenbach, J., Lathrop, G.M., Chabriat, H., Mas, J.-L., Cabanis, E.-A., Baudrimont, M., Maciazek, J., Bach, M.-A., and Bousser, M.G. (1993). Cerebral autosomal dominant arteriopathy with subcortical infarcts and leukoencephalopathy maps to chromosome 19q12. *Nature Genet.* **3**, 256–9.

Turner, S.T., Jack, C.R., Fornage, M., Mosley, T.H., Boerwinkle, E., and de Andrade, M. (2004). Heritability of leukoaraiosis in hypertensive sibships. *Hypertension* **43** (2), 483–7.

Tzourio, C., Anderson, C., The PROGRESS Collaborative Group, Chapman, N., Woodward, M., Neal, B., MacMahon, S., and Chalmers, J. (2003). Effects of blood pressure lowering with perindopril and indapamide therapy on dementia and cognitive decline in patients with cerebrovascular disease. *Arch. Intern. Med.* **163** (9), 1069–75.

Ueda, K., Kawano, H., Hasuo, Y., and Fujishima, M. (1992). Prevalence and etiology of dementia in a Japanese community. *Stroke* **23**, 798–803.

Vallar, G., Perani, D., Cappa, S.F., Messa, C., Lenzi, G.L., and Fazio, F. (1988). Recovery from aphasia and neglect after subcortical stroke: neuropsychological and cerebral perfusion study. *J. Neurol. Neurosurg. Psychiatry* **51**, 1269–76.

van den Heuvel, D.M.J., ten Dam, V.H., de Craen, A.J.M., Admiraal-Behloul, F., Olofsen, H., Bollen, E.L.E.M., Jolles, J., Murray, H.M., Blauw, G.J., Westendorp, R.G.J., and van Buchem, M.A. (2006). Increase in periventricular white matter hyperintensities parallels decline in mental processing speed in a non-demented elderly population. *J. Neurol. Neurosurg. Psychiatry* **77** (2), 149–53.

van der Flier, W.M., van Straaten, E. C.W., Barkhof, F., Verdelho, A., Madureira, S., Pantoni, L., Inzitari, D., Erkinjuntti, T., Crisby, M., Waldemar, G., Schmidt, R., Fazekas, F., Scheltens, P., and on behalf of the LADIS Study Group (2005). Small vessel disease and general cognitive function in nondisabled elderly: the LADIS Study. *Stroke* **36** (10), 2116–20.

van Straaten, E. C.W., Scheltens, P., Knol, D.L., van Buchem, M.A., van Dijk, E.J., Hofman, P. A.M., Karas, G., Kjartansson, O., de Leeuw, F.E., Prins, N.D., Schmidt, R., Visser, M.C., Weinstein, H.C., and Barkhof, F. (2003). Operational definitions for the NINDS-AIREN criteria for vascular dementia: an interobserver study. *Stroke* **34** (8), 1907–12.

Verghese, J., Lipton, R.B., Hall, C.B., Kuslansky, G., and Katz, M.J. (2003). Low blood pressure and the risk of dementia in very old individuals. *Neurology* **61** (12), 1667–72.

Vermeer, S.E., Prins, N.D., den Heijer, T., Hofman, A., Koudstaal, P.J., and Breteler, M.M. (2003). Silent brain infarcts and the risk of dementia and cognitive decline. *N. Engl. J. Med.* **348** (13), 1215–22.

Wade, D.T., Parker, V., and Langton Hewer, R. (1986). Memory disturbance after stroke: frequency and associated losses. *Int. Rehabil. Med.* **8**, 60–4.

Wade, D.T., Wood, V.A., and Hewer, R.L. (1988). Recovery of cognitive function soon after stroke: a study of visual neglect, attention span and verbal recall. *J. Neurol. Neurosurg. Psychiatry* **51**, 10–13.

Wahlund, L.O., Andersson-Lundman, G., Julin, P., Nordstrom, M., Viitanen, M., and Saaf, J. (1992). Quantitative estimation of brain white matter abnormalities in elderly subjects using magnetic resonance imaging. *Magn. Reson. Imaging* **10**, 859–65.

Wallin, A. and Blennow, K. (1991). Pathogenetic basis of vascular dementia. *Alzheimer Dis. Assoc. Disord.* **5**, 91–102.

Walters, R. J.L., Fox, N.C., Schott, J.M., Crum, W.R., Stevens, J.M., Rossor, M.N., and Thomas, D.J. (2003). Transient ischaemic attacks are associated with increased rates of global cerebral atrophy. *J. Neurol. Neurosurg. Psychiatry* **74** (2), 213–16.

Watanabe, M., Miura, T., Ito, H., Mano, K., and Watanabe, H. (1996). Change of blood pressure in head-up tilting test in patients with Binswanger-type infarction. *Clin. Neurol.* **36** (11), 1221–4.

Watanabe, M., Nishimura, R., Ito, H., Mano, K., and Watanabe, H. (1997). Clinical significance of orthostatic blood pressure decline in patients with Binswanger-type infarction. *Clin. Neurol.* **37** (10), 868–72.

Wentzel, C., Rockwood, K., MacKnight, C., Hachinski, V., Hogan, D.B., Feldman, H., Ostbye, T., Wolfson, C., Gauthier, S., Verreault, R., and McDowell, I. (2001). Progression of impairment in patients with vascular cognitive impairment without dementia. *Neurology* **57** (4), 714–16.

Wetterling, T., Kanitz, R.D., and Borgis, K. J. (1996). Comparison of different diagnostic criteria for vascular dementia (ADDTC, DSM-IV, ICD-10, NINDS–AIREN). *Stroke* **27**, 30–6.

Whitmer, R.A., Sidney, S., Selby, J., Johnston, S.C., and Yaffe, K. (2005). Midlife cardiovascular risk factors and risk of dementia in late life. *Neurology* **64** (2), 277–81.

Wilcock, G., Mobius, H.J., and Stoffler, A. (2002). A double-blind, placebo-controlled multicentre study of memantine in mild to moderate vascular dementia (MMM500). *Int. Clin. Psychopharmacol.* **17** (6), 297–305.

Wilkie, F. and Eisdorfer, C. (1971). Intelligence and blood pressure in the aged. *Science* **172**, 959–62.

Wilkinson, D., Doody, R., Helme, R., Taubman, K., Mintzer, J., Kertesz, A., and Pratt, R.D. (2003). Donepezil in vascular dementia: a randomized, placebo-controlled study. *Neurology* **61** (4), 479–86.

Winblad, B. and Poritis, N. (1999). Memantine in severe dementia: results of the 9M-Best Study (benefit and efficacy in severely demented patients during treatment with memantine). *Int. J. Geriatr. Psychiatry* **14** (2), 135–46.

Wolfe, N., Linn, R., Babikian, V.L., Knoefel, J.E., and Albert, M.L. (1990). Frontal systems impairment following multiple lacunar infarcts. *Arch. Neurol.* **47**, 129–32.

World Health Organization (1993). *The ICD-10 classification of mental and behavioural disorders. Diagnostic criteria for research.* World Health Organization, Geneva.

Wright, C.B., Paik, M.C., Brown, T.R., Stabler, S.P., Allen, R.H., Sacco, R.L., and DeCarli, C. (2005). Total homocysteine is associated with white matter hyperintensity volume: the Northern Manhattan Study. *Stroke* **36** (6), 1207–11.

Xu, W.L., Qiu, C.X., Wahlin, A., Winblad, B., and Fratiglioni, L. (2004). Diabetes mellitus and risk of dementia in the Kungsholmen project: a 6-year follow-up study. *Neurology* **63** (7), 1181–6.

Yaffe, K., Barrett-Connor, E., Lin, F., and Grady, D. (2002). Serum lipoprotein levels, statin use, and cognitive function in older women. *Arch. Neurol.* **59** (3), 378–84.

Yaffe, K., Kanaya, A., Lindquist, K., Simonsick, E.M., Harris, T., Shorr, R.I., Tylavsky, F.A., and Newman, A.B. (2004). The metabolic syndrome, inflammation, and risk of cognitive decline. *J. Am. Med. Assoc.* **292** (18), 2237–42.

Yamamoto, Y., Akiguchi, I., Oiwa, K., Hayashi, M., Kasai, T., and Ozasa, K. (2002). Twenty-four-hour blood pressure and MRI as predictive factors for different outcomes in patients with lacunar infarct. *Stroke* **33** (1), 297–305.

Yamamoto, Y., Akiguchi, I., Oiwa, K., Hayashi, M., Ohara, T., and Ozasa, K. (2005). The relationship between 24-hour blood pressure readings, subcortical ischemic lesions and vascular dementia. *Cerebrovasc. Dis.* **19** (5), 302–8.

Yamanouchi, H. and Nagura, H. (1997). Neurological signs and frontal white matter lesions in vascular parkinsonism. A clinicopathologic study. *Stroke* **28** (5), 965–9.

Yamanouchi, H., Sugiura, S., and Tomonaga, M. (1989). Decrease in nerve fibres in cerebral white matter in progressive subcortical vascular encephalopathy of Binswanger type. An electron microscopic study. *J. Neurol.* **236**, 382–7.

Yamauchi, H., Fukuyama, H., Nagahama, Y., Katsumi, Y., Dong, Y., Konishi, J., and Kimura, J. (1996). Atrophy of the corpus callosum associated with cognitive impairment and widespread cortical hypometabolism in carotid artery occlusive disease. *Arch. Neurol.* **53** (11), 1103–9.

Yanagawa, S., Ito, N., Arima, K., and Ikeda-Si, S.I. (2002). Cerebral autosomal recessive arteriopathy with subcortical infarcts and leukoencephalopathy. *Neurology* **58** (5), 817–20.

Yao, H., Sadoshima, S., Kuwabara, Y., Ichiya, Y., and Fujishima, M. (1990). Cerebral blood flow and oxygen metabolism in patients with vascular dementia of the Binswanger type. *Stroke* **21**, 1694–9.

Yao, H., Sadoshima, S., Ibayashi, S., Kuwabara, Y., Ichiya, Y., and Fujishima, M. (1992). Leukoaraiosis and dementia in hypertensive patients. *Stroke* **23**, 1673–7.

Zekry, D., Duyckaerts, C., Belmin, J., Geoffre, C., Herrmann, F., Moulias, R., and Hauw, J.J. (2003). The vascular lesions in vascular and mixed dementia: the weight of functional neuroanatomy. *Neurobiol. Aging* **24** (2), 213–19.

Zhang, W.W. and Olsson, Y. (1997). The angiopathy of subcortical arteriosclerotic encephalopathy (Binswanger's disease): immunohistochemical studies using markers for components of extracellular matrix, smooth muscle actin and endothelial cells. *Acta Neuropathol. (Berl.)* **93** (3), 219–24.

Zijlmans, J. C.M., Katzenschlager, R., Daniel, S.E., and Lees, A.J.L. (2004). The L-dopa response in vascular parkinsonism. *J. Neurol. Neurosurg. Psychiatry* **75** (4), 545–7.

Zivadinov, R., Sepcic, J., Nasuelli, D., De Masi, R., Bragadin, L.M., Tommasi, M.A., Zambito-Marsala, S., Moretti, R., Bratina, A., Ukmar, M., Grop, A., Cazzato, G., and Zorzon, M. (2001). A longitudinal study of brain atrophy and cognitive disturbances in the early phase of relapsing–remitting multiple sclerosis. *J. Neurol. Neurosurg. Psychiatry* **70** (6), 773–80.

Chapter 14

Cortical Lewy body disease: dementia with Lewy bodies and Parkinson's disease with dementia

John E. Duda and Ian G. McKeith

14.1 Definition

One of the most hotly debated topics in the field of neurodegenerative disease is the relationship between what has recently been described as dementia with Lewy bodies (DLB) and the condition of patients with Parkinson's disease (PD) who subsequently develop dementia (PDD). Recent advances in our understanding of the pathophysiology of DLB and PDD support the proposition that both of these entities represent points on a spectrum of cortical Lewy body disease (LBD), characterized by accumulation of Lewy pathology—which includes Lewy bodies (LBs) and Lewy neurites (LNs)—within susceptible populations of both cortical and subcortical neurons.

There are two widely accepted diagnostic schemes for PD (Gelb *et al.* 1999; Hughes *et al.* 1992), stipulating progressive parkinsonism of undetermined cause without features suggestive of an alternative diagnosis and responding to dopaminergic therapy (Tolosa *et al.* 2006). There are as yet no formal criteria for the diagnosis of PDD and the generally accepted convention has been to apply DSM III or IV criteria for dementia to patients who have PD. The DSM IV text revision (America Psychiatric Association 2000) has for the first time included a diagnosis of *Dementia Due to Parkinson's Disease* (294.1) but, instead of PD-specific diagnostic criteria, the *Diagnostic Criteria for Dementia Due to Other General Medical Conditions* are to be utilized. These criteria, applied to PD, include:

A The development of multiple cognitive deficits manifested by both (i) memory impairment and (ii) one (or more) of the following cognitive disturbances: aphasia; apraxia; agnosia; or disturbance in executive function.

B The cognitive deficits each cause significant impairment in social or occupational functioning and represent a significant decline from a previous level of functioning.

C There is evidence from the history, physical examination, or laboratory findings that the disturbance is the direct physiological consequence of PD.

D The deficits do not occur exclusively during the course of a delirium.

In addition, the diagnosis is further clarified based on whether it is 'with behavioural disturbance' (294.10) or 'without behavioural disturbance' (294.11).

Limitations of the current diagnostic criteria include mandatory impairment of memory, which may be preserved in many cases of PDD particularly early in the course, and the difficulty in determining if the cognitive deficits cause significant impairment in social or occupational function independently of motor impairments of PD. Originally delineated in 1996 (McKeith *et al.* 1996), consensus criteria for DLB have continued to evolve and are currently defined by the third report of the DLB Consortium (McKeith *et al.* 2005). These revised criteria include a central feature of dementia, three core features including fluctuating cognition, recurrent visual hallucinations, and spontaneous parkinsonism, three suggestive features, and 10 supportive features (Table 14.1). Core features are common symptoms that can be used alone with the central feature to diagnose possible DLB (one core feature) or probable DLB (two core features). In an attempt to increase the sensitivity of the diagnostic criteria, suggestive features were added and can be used in the absence of core features to make a diagnosis of possible DLB, but cannot be used in isolation to make a diagnosis of probable DLB. Supportive features occur commonly in DLB, but are not disease-specific. These diagnostic criteria also continue to define research criteria for PDD as dementia occurring in the context of patients who have had parkinsonism for at least 1 year before the onset of dementia.

Table 14.1 Diagnostic criteria for dementia with Lewy bodies

1 Central feature (essential for a diagnosis of possible or probable DLB)

Dementia defined as progressive cognitive decline of sufficient magnitude to interfere with normal social or occupational function

2 Core features (two core features are sufficient for a diagnosis of probable DLB; one for possible DLB)

a Fluctuating cognition with pronounced variations in attention and alertness

b Recurrent visual hallucinations that are typically well formed and detailed

c Spontaneous features of parkinsonism

3 Suggestive features (If one or more of these is present in the presence of one or more core features, a diagnosis of probable DLB can be made. In the absence of any core features, one or more suggestive features is sufficient for possible DLB. Probable DLB should not be diagnosed on the basis of suggestive features alone.)

a REM sleep behaviour disorder

b Severe neuroleptic sensitivity

c Low dopamine transported uptake in basal ganglia demonstrated by SPECT or PET imaging

4 Supportive features (commonly present but not proven to have diagnostic specificity)

a Repeated falls and syncope

b Transient, unexplained loss of consciousness

c Severe autonomic dysfunction, e.g. orthostatic hypotension, urinary incontinence

d Hallucinations in other modalities

e Systematized delusions

f Depression

g Relative preservation of medial temporal lobe structures on CT/MRI scan

h Generalized low uptake on SPECT/PET perfusion scan with reduced occipital activity

i Abnormal (low uptake) MIBG myocardial scintigraphy

j Prominent slow wave activity on EEG with temporal lobe transient sharp waves

5 A diagnosis of DLB is less likely

a In the presence of cerebrovascular disease evident as focal neurologic signs or on brain imaging

Table 14.1 (Continued) Diagnostic criteria for dementia with Lewy bodies

b In the presence of any other physical illness or brain disorder sufficient to account in part or in total for the clinical picture
c If the parkinsonism only appears for the first time at a stage of severe dementia
6 Temporal sequence of symptoms
DLB should be diagnosed when dementia occurs before or concurrently with parkinsonism (if it is present). The term Parkinson's disease dementia (PDD) should be used to describe dementia that occurs in the context of well-established Parkinson's disease. In a practice setting the term that is most appropriate to the clinical situation should be used and generic terms such as LB disease are often helpful. In research studies in which distinction needs to be made between DLB and PDD, the existing 1-year rule between the onset of dementia and parkinsonism continues to be recommended

14.2 **Epidemiology**

Systematic reviews of the epidemiology of PDD (Aarsland *et al.* 2005*b*) and DLB (Zaccai *et al.* 2005) report the mean proportion of PD subjects with dementia as 24.5% with a range of 17.4% to 31.5%. The estimated prevalence of PDD in the general population was 30.0 per 100 000 persons (range 19.0–41.1) rising to 500 per 100 000 in persons aged 65 years or older. Considering studies of all persons with dementia, the prevalence of PDD was considered to be 3.6% (range 3.1–4.1%) and 0.2% in subjects 65 years or older. Regarding the incidence of dementia in PD, yearly estimates range from 2.6% to 9.5% (Apaydin *et al.* 2002), while two other studies suggested the cumulative risk of developing dementia in PD was 78% at 8 years (Aarsland *et al.* 2003*a*) and more than 65% by the age of 85 (Mayeux *et al.* 1990).

In DLB, there are fewer studies and wider variation due to the use of multiple definitions of DLB. Prevalence estimates range from 0 to 5% within the general population, representing 0 to 30.5% of all dementia cases (Zaccai *et al.* 2005). In one population-based study of subjects aged 75 or older using the original consensus criteria, probable DLB occurred in 3.3% and possible DLB in 1.7% (Rahkonen *et al.* 2003). DLB incidence is estimated to be 0.1% a year for the general population and 3.2% a year for all new dementia cases (Zaccai *et al.* 2005).

14.3 **Aetiological factors**

14.3.1 **Genetic**

While neither PDD nor DLB commonly occur in Mendelian inheritance patterns, several kindreds that include subjects with these phenotypes have been described. The first autopsy confirmed kindred with an identified pathogenic mutation was the Contursi kindred (Polymeropoulos *et al.* 1997), which now includes at least 13 families of mostly Greek and Italian heritage (Golbe *et al.* 1993; Langston *et al.* 1998) with a PDD phenotype and harbouring an A53T mutation in the alpha-synuclein (a-syn), gene. The most recently described pathogenic point mutation in a-syn, the E46K mutation, also presents as PDD in nearly all subjects (Zarranz *et al.* 2004). An interesting observation regarding the clinical relationship between mutations of a-syn and clinical phenotypes is the observation that triplications of the a-syn gene have a higher propensity to cause PDD than duplications, suggesting a gene dosage effect between PD with and without dementia (Chartier-Harlin *et al.* 2004; Farrer *et al.* 2004; Ibanez *et al.* 2004; Singleton and Gwinn-Hardy 2004; Singleton *et al.* 2003). Mutations in the gene for the leucine-rich repeat kinase 2 (LRRK2) are possibly the most common cause of autosomal dominant PD and may produce a PDD phenotype (Paisan-Ruiz *et al.* 2004; Zimprich *et al.* 2004).

Several studies have examined the relationship between the apolipoprotein E (ApoE) gene gene and DLB or PDD, some reporting that the ApoE4 allele, which is an independent risk factor in AD, is overrepresented in DLB (Dickson *et al.* 1996; Hansen *et al.* 1994; Harrington *et al.* 1995; Lippa *et al.* 1995; Singleton *et al.* 2002) but not in PDD.

Recently, several kindreds of familial DLB have been described (Brett *et al.* 2002; Galvin *et al.* 2002; Ohara *et al.* 1999; Tsuang *et al.* 2002, 2004), and one analysis suggested that cortical LB disease, defined as encompassing DLB and PDD, was more likely than PD to occur in a pattern consistent with an autosomal dominant inheritance (Harding *et al.* 2004). LB pathology has also been demonstrated in several kindreds with amyloid precursor protein or presenilin mutations proteins (Houlden *et al.* 2001; Lippa *et al.* 1998, 2001; Revesz *et al.* 1997), as well as in patients with Down's syndrome (Lippa *et al.* 1999*b*). Many of these cases involved LB pathology limited to the amygdala, but the significance of this finding remains uncertain. Novel mutations in the presenilin 1 gene have been shown to be associated with widespread LB pathology in familial AD kindreds (Ishikawa *et al.* 2005; Snider *et al.* 2005), and several familial AD kindreds with LB pathology have been linked to chromosome 12 (Trembath *et al.* 2003). One kindred with a clinical phenotype of frontotemporal dementia and LB pathology has been described (Bonner *et al.* 2003).

14.3.2 **Acquired**

In both DLB and PDD, age stands out as an important risk factor. In a population-based study the presence of LBs and LNs at autopsy was found to increase with age (Wakisaka *et al.* 2003) and to occur in 25.2% of non-demented and 41.4% of demented individuals. Older age and older age of onset are associated with an increased risk of becoming demented in PD (Aarsland *et al.* 2001; Hughes *et al.* 2000; Stern *et al.* 1993). Subtle frontal-executive dysfunction, which will be discussed in greater detail below, has also been shown to precede the onset of dementia in PD (Jacobs *et al.* 1995; Woods and Troster 2003). Severity of motor symptoms has also been found to be a risk factor for PDD (Aarsland *et al.* 2001; Hughes *et al.* 2000; Marder *et al.* 1995; Stern *et al.* 1993) and some studies have found that the more akinetic/rigid phenotypes are more susceptible (Aarsland *et al.* 2003*a*; Burn *et al.* 2002). Depression has also been associated with risk of developing dementia in some studies (Marder *et al.* 1995; Starkstein *et al.* 1992; Stern *et al.* 1993), though others have failed to replicate this finding (Aarsland *et al.* 2001; Hughes *et al.* 2000). Not surprisingly, given the association of psychosis and dementia in DLB, patients with PD and psychosis are also at greater risk of becoming demented (Factor *et al.* 2003; Goetz *et al.* 1998; Stern *et al.* 1993).

14.4 **Clinical features**

14.4.1 **History**

While the progression of symptoms begins at different points in DLB and PDD, both conditions eventually proceed along similar courses from a phase of cognitive impairment insufficient to be diagnosed as dementia, to a stage of impairment sufficient to warrant a diagnosis of dementia. Ultimately, both converge on a similar end-stage characterized by severe impairment and immobility.

Current consensus diagnostic criteria dictate that a diagnosis of DLB be reserved for patients who develop dementia 'before or concurrently with parkinsonism' (if it is present), while PDD should be used for the patients who develop dementia 'that occurs in the context of well-established Parkinson disease' (McKeith *et al.* 2005). Therefore, by definition, the early stages of DLB and PDD will differ in that PDD will begin with typical non-demented PD (see the two case vignettes). Although there have been no large, prospective analyses of autopsy-confirmed DLB utilizing the current diagnostic criteria that have addressed the question of early symptoms, most patients present with either a dementia syndrome, neurobehavioural symptoms, or rapid eye movement (REM) sleep behaviour disorder (RBD). Differentiating the dementia syndrome from other causes of dementia begins by examining the pattern of cognitive dysfunction: DLB patients tend to have relatively preserved short-term memory and recognition memory and worse performance on measures of attention, verbal memory, and visuospatial abilities than patients with AD (Calderon *et al.* 2001; Collerton *et al.* 2003; Noe *et al.* 2004). Simple global cognitive assessment tools such as the Mini-Mental State Examination (MMSE) or the Clock Draw test may help to distinguish between DLB and AD (Ala *et al.* 2004; Gnanalingham *et al.* 1997), but most authors find these simple tests lack the sensitivity and specificity required

Case vignette: Parkinson's disease dementia

At age 53 a left-handed male public works manager developed a right upper extremity resting tremor that was worse when he was working 'on a deadline'. He had previously had intermittent depression and anxiety for which he was treated adequately and was otherwise healthy. On examination he was also noted to have masked facies, decreased arm swing on the right while walking, mild rigidity in the right arm, and intact cognitive abilities for someone of his education and age. He was diagnosed with possible Parkinson's disease and was started on the anticholinergic trihexyphenidyl with some benefit and then a year later a dopamine agonist monotherapy was added with better response to the combined therapy. Over the next 8 years, he continued to respond well to therapy but experienced symptom progression including resting tremor, rigidity, and bradykinesia of both upper extremities and shuffling gait requiring adjunctive therapy with levodopa. He also began to develop motor fluctuations in the form of wearing off symptoms and was started on entacapone with good results.

At age 56, he admitted to occasionally forgetting names and appointments and had a brief neuropsychological examination including a Folstein MMSE score of 28 with points deducted for delayed recall and pentagon copying. Results of testing revealed a mildly reduced learning curve on the Hopkins Verbal Learning Test-Revised (HVLT-R), with little improvement over the course of trials. After a 20 minute delay, he was able to recall most of what he originally encoded, showing good retention. His recall was aided by use of a recognition format, falling in the average range. Cognitive flexibility and inhibition skills were generally in the low average range of functioning. He also scored in the average range on both forms of the Trails Making Test. At this time, his anticholinergic therapy was discontinued without worsening of his parkinsonism but with some subjective improvement in his cognition. Several times over these years he experienced exacerbation of his depression and anxiety symptoms requiring adjustment of his antidepressant therapy. He also developed apathy concerning the activities that had previously given him great pleasure including golf and gardening.

Case vignette: Parkinson's disease dementia *(continued)*

At age 59, his wife reported that he was more forgetful and at age 60 he underwent formal neuropsychological assessment at a time when he felt his depressive symptoms were well controlled. Speech was fluent and goal-directed. Comprehension of simple and complex instructions was intact. Affect appeared mildly flat. His performance on the HVLT-R was in the mildly to moderately impaired range over the course of three learning trials. There was evidence of increased intrusive responding in free recall. Recall after a 25 minute delay was also in the mildly to moderately impaired range with mildly to moderately impaired retention of material already encoded. Recognition memory was poor with false-positive responding evident. Mental status examination revealed a borderline Folstein MMSE score of 23 with points deducted for orientation to time, delayed recall, attention, and pentagon copying. His performance on both forms of the Trail Making Test was severely impaired, indicating very impaired cognitive flexibility and psychomotor speed. Phonemic fluency was borderline, while semantic fluency was low average. Luria sequential hand movements were impaired bilaterally. In sum, he demonstrated moderate impairments in verbal memory, characterized by deficits in both encoding and free recall. Retention of material already encoded was mildly to moderately impaired, while recognition memory was very poor. Basic attentional skills were good, but there was evidence of severe frontal system dysfunction characterized by poor cognitive flexibility, perceptual speed, and disrupted sequential movements. At this time, all laboratory studies for treatable causes of dementia were unremarkable and an MRI of his brain revealed only age-appropriate atrophy and no evidence of hydrocephalus, significant vascular disease, or space-occupying lesions. Acetylcholinesterase therapy was initiated without definite benefit or detriment and a second agent was tried with similar results. Increased structure and supervision of his day-to-day activities was recommended. The patient tolerated weaning of his dopamine agonist but preferred to stay on low-dose therapy rather than to discontinue it completely.

Over the next several years, he demonstrated an accelerated pattern of symptom progression with worsening of motor fluctuations. Off time was marked by severe panic attacks that would resolve following a dose of clonazepam and levodopa. At age 62, he experienced an acute psychotic episode with severe aggression and paranoid delusions. Dopamine agonist therapy was discontinued and quetiapine was started with resolution of psychosis at 25 mg nightly. From this point on, the treatment focus shifted to the management of psychiatric and cognitive complications while trying to stabilize motor symptoms and minimize panic attacks.

In his last few years, he developed several non-motor symptoms with onset of dysphagia, urinary incontinence, and occasional orthostatic symptoms. Anxiety and panic attacks persisted as well as motor fluctuations. At age 66, he experienced rather rapid cognitive deterioration while on levodopa monotherapy. His last Folstein MMSE score was 7/30. By age 67 he was wheelchair bound and dependent in all ADLs. He experienced intermittent periods of lucidity but was disoriented and lethargic most of the day. By age 68, he was bed bound and began choking on his saliva. He began refusing his medications and his appetite diminished with significant weight loss. Eventually, he was nearly mute and unable to follow simple directions. He expired of presumed aspiration pneumonia while in hospice care.

Case vignette: dementia with Lewy bodies

A right-handed male accountant initially presented at age 63 with a complaint of inability to complete his accounting activities as fast as previously with trouble at his job because of report discrepancies. On history-taking, he admitted that he had been 'slowing down' for the past couple of years, that he had been experiencing some word-finding difficulty, and had a past history of REM sleep behaviour disorder symptoms that had subsided in the last couple of years. On examination, he was found to have very mild bradykinesia in his upper extremities, slightly masked facies, and a slightly stooped posture with decreased arm swing bilaterally on walking, but no observable tremor or rigidity. On neuropsychological examination, speech was fluent, but mild word-finding problems were evident. Comprehension of simple and complex instructions was intact. Affect was euthymic. Results of testing revealed a moderately impaired learning curve on the Hopkins Verbal Learning Test-Revised (HVLT-R), with overall recall falling in the moderately impaired range. Recall after a 20 minute delay was also poor, and he was able to recall only 43% of what he previously encoded, his score falling in the impaired range. Recognition memory performance was better than free recall, falling in the mildly impaired range. His score on the Trail Making Test part A was in the low average range, suggesting generally intact visual–perceptual attentional skills. In contrast, his performance on part B was impaired, indicating poor cognitive flexibility and set-shifting skills. His performance on both forms of the Trail Making Test revealed impaired visuoperceptual speed and cognitive flexibility. His performance on the Stroop Colour–Word Test also revealed poor speed and freedom from interference. His Folstein MMSE was 22/30 with points deducted for orientation to time, delayed recall, attention, 3 part command, and pentagon copying. Overall, these data supported a moderate level of cognitive dysfunction characterized by significant frontal system dysfunction and poor memory.

At this time, he was started on acetylcholinesterase therapy with some subjective benefit and a slight improvement on follow-up Folstein MMSE scores, but was still experiencing difficulty with his accounting responsibilities and retired at the age of 64. At that time, he admitted to occasionally seeing small animals that he knew were not real and did not bother him. His wife admitted that he had periods when 'it was like talking to a wall'. At age 65, he had a short period of unresponsiveness, without clear loss of consciousness, and was admitted to his local hospital for comprehensive cardiac and neurological evaluation that was unrevealing.

Over the next several years, his parkinsonism became progressively worse with symmetric rigidity and bradykinesia of all four extremities and gait difficulty that led to rare falls with more frequent near-falls. A course of outpatient physical therapy was completed with some benefit in the frequency of his falls. Levodopa was initiated with some subjective benefit at moderate doses, but his visual hallucinations became more prominent and he complained of excessive daytime sleepiness so that therapy was reduced to low doses with some resolution of side-effects.

Eventually, he developed worsening of hallucinations and confusion. Because of this, his Sinemet was weaned off and he noticed improvement in his cognition and ambulation without dramatic worsening of his parkinsonism. His memory continued to deteriorate to the point that he allowed his wife to take care of the important business affairs and to dispense his medications. He was frequently losing his train of thought. Hallucinations persisted when he was off dopaminergic medications and quetiapine was added but was not tolerated due to a reaction that his nurse daughter described as a 'catatonic state'. He continued to have frequent

Case vignette: Parkinson's disease dementia *(continued)*

hallucinations of people in his house without retained insight and delusions that they were trying to hurt his wife. He flagged down truckers to try to help him rid his house of these 'intruders'. His psychosis progressed to include olfactory hallucinations and paranoid delusions of marital infidelity. Seroquel was restarted, without evidence of neuroleptic sensitivity reaction and with some control of his psychosis at relatively higher dose. He was also noticed to have significant cognitive fluctuations with some lucid periods lasting up to a day. Over the course of the year, he had a rapid decline in cognitive function with an MMSE score of 15. Follow-up neuropsychological examination revealed that his thoughts were generally clear and goal-directed, but very slow and somewhat concrete. Comprehension of simple and complex instructions was variable. Affect was euthymic. His performance on the HVLT-R was severely impaired in initial encoding of verbal information, with poor overall level of recall over the course of three learning trials. His free recall was notable for increased perseverative responding as well as intrusion errors. Recall after a 25 minute delay was also severely impaired with only 25% retention of material previously encoded. He did benefit somewhat from the provision of recognition prompts. His performance on both forms of the Trail Making Test revealed impaired visuoperceptual speed and cognitive flexibility. His performance on the Stroop Colour–Word Test also revealed poor speed and freedom from interference. Phonemic and semantic fluency was also severely impaired, with a marked reduction in his ability to efficiently generate language. For example, he was only able to generate six animal names in the course of 1 minute. Phonemic fluency was notably worse than this performance. Notably, he showed great difficulty in keeping the concept of the task in memory and had to be frequently prompted with the parameters of the task.

At age 68, he had a rapid decline in ability to perform ADLs and started living in the nursing home of the life care community. He continued to have delusions, hallucinations, sundowning, and cognitive fluctuations, which led to numerous titrations of Seroquel and a trial of a second acetylcholinesterase inhibitor. He had more problems with his swallowing and drooling as well as constipation. He also had significant problems with excessive daytime sleepiness and ambulation requiring assistive devices and assistance to walk. He continued to live in the nursing home over the next 2 years, with multiple exacerbations of psychosis and parkinsonism as well as several bouts of pneumonia. By age 69, he was no longer able to make the 60 minute drive to our clinic.

At age 70, he became essentially mute and unable to follow commands, completely dependent for ADLs, but was still able to assist somewhat with transfers. He eventually became unable to swallow and after a short period expired of unknown cause.

and recommend more thorough neuropsychological assessments (McKeith *et al.* 2005; Walker *et al.* 1997).

In addition to variations in the neuropsychological profile, DLB may be differentiated from other dementing illnesses by the early appearance of neuropsychiatric symptoms, particularly visual hallucinations. (Ballard *et al.* 1999; Noe *et al.* 2004). Cognitive fluctuations may also be particularly useful in distinguishing DLB and AD (Ballard *et al.* 2001; Bradshaw *et al.* 2004; Ferman *et al.* 2004) and recently developed tools for their assessment (Ferman *et al.* 2004; M.P. Walker *et al.* 2000) should facilitate this. RBD, if present, is also very helpful in differentiating early DLB and PDD from other disorders, and may present years before other symptoms

(Boeve *et al.* 2001, 2004; Ferman *et al.* 2002), but it will often go undiagnosed unless the clinical history includes questions specific to RBD symptoms.

14.4.2 Examination

Examination of the patient with suspected DLB or PDD should begin with enquiry about the symptoms encompassed in the core, suggestive, and supportive categories of the diagnostic criteria. This should include specific questions regarding fluctuations in cognition, alertness, and awareness, and may be supplemented by recently developed assessment tools mentioned above.

Mental status examination should include a global assessment scale of cognitive function such as in the Mini-Mental State Examination, with the recognition that these tools cannot absolutely differentiate DLB or PDD from AD, and that patients with these conditions often score in the low normal range of performance on these measures. A recently published practice parameter suggests that the MMSE and the CAMCog are suitable for screening PD patients for dementia. They are both equally sensitive: the MMSE is quicker but the CAMCog is more specific (Miyasaki *et al.* 2006).

More detailed bedside testing will often be required using scales specifically designed to assess frontal executive function such as the Exit-25 (Royall *et al.* 1992), more detailed examination of visuospatial and constructional abilities using the Clock Draw test, or additional tests of verbal fluency and attention. Formal neuropsychological examination is often necessary and should include assessments of frontal executive function including attention, visuospatial abilities, language, and memory. Tests useful for the assessment of frontal executive function in DLB/PDD include the Tower of London–Drexel (Culbertson *et al.* 2004), the Trail making Test Part B, the Stroop Colour–Word Test, the Wisconsin Card Sorting Test, or the Exit 25. In the research setting, attention may also be assessed with computerized assessments such as the CDR computerized cognitive assessment system (Wesnes *et al.* 2005), and cognitive performance may be assessed with an instrument recently developed as a short, reliable, and valid assessment of cognitive deficits specific to PD (Marinus *et al.* 2003).

In addition to a screening neurological examination, the physical examination should include a complete assessment of parkinsonian motor signs, similar to part 3 of the Unified Parkinson's Disease Rating Scale (Fahn *et al.* 1987), which includes assessments of facial movement, speech, resting, postural and action tremor, brady- and hypokinesia, postural stability, and gait. Assessment of autonomic function should include orthostatic blood pressure and pulse measurements.

In addition to brain imaging modalites, which will be discussed separately, there are several ancillary tests that have proved useful in the evaluation of particular symptoms in PDD and DLB. In the patient with a clinical history suggestive of REM sleep behaviour disorder, polysomnography is useful for confirmation and differentiation from other parasomnias. Electroencephalography is useful in differentiating cognitive fluctuations from epileptiform activity, and can show abnormalities in some patients with DLB or PDD (P.A. Barber *et al.* 2000; Briel *et al.* 1999), but is not routinely utilized in the diagnostic evaluation of these disorders. As demonstrated by its inclusion as a supportive feature in the current consensus criteria for DLB, meta-iodobenzylguanidine (MIBG) myocardial scintigraphy has proven efficacious in the differentiation of DLB from AD (Oide *et al.* 2003; Watanabe *et al.* 2001; Yoshita *et al.* 2001) but is still primarily used in the research setting. Currently, there are no laboratory markers useful in the diagnostic evaluation of DLB or PDD, other than to rule out other treatable causes of dementia (Knopman *et al.* 2001; McKeith *et al.* 2004).

14.5 **Neuropsychology**

As discussed above, the cardinal clinical difference between DLB and PDD is the symptomatology at disease onset, with PDD presenting with parkinsonism and DLB presenting either with dementia or a combination of the two. Therefore, the early diagnosis of DLB includes differentiation from other dementing illnesses, especially AD, which is often the first diagnosis for patients with DLB (Merdes *et al.* 2003). In contrast, in PDD patients, while the initial diagnosis involves differentiation between alternative causes of parkinsonism, when dementia develops there is also a need to distinguish whether the patient has developed concomitant AD, or whether the cause of the dementia is more likely to be due to diffuse LB, as is often the case (Apaydin *et al.* 2002). It is not surprising that such distinctions can be difficult given that many DLB patients also meet pathological criteria for AD. However, in addition to the core and suggestive features of the DLB consensus criteria, there are neuropsychological features that can be useful in differentiating DLB from AD—though not usually from PDD.

In an early examination comparing autopsy-proven DLB and AD, DLB patients (who all had sufficient plaque and tangle pathology to make a diagnosis of concomitant AD) were shown to perform significantly worse in tests of attention, verbal fluency, visuospatial ability, and constructional ability (Hansen *et al.* 1990). Since then, many studies have shown patterns of dysfunction that have led to what has been termed a 'double discrimination' (McKeith *et al.* 2005) in neuropsychological function between DLB and AD patients, the former displaying greater deficits on tests of verbal fluency, visual perception, and performance tasks, with relative sparing of confrontation naming, short- and medium-term recall as well as recognition (Connor *et al.* 1998; Walker *et al.* 1997). In a recent retrospective examination of the first clinical visit for patients with autopsy-confirmed DLB ($n = 23$) and AD ($n = 94$), it was determined that a

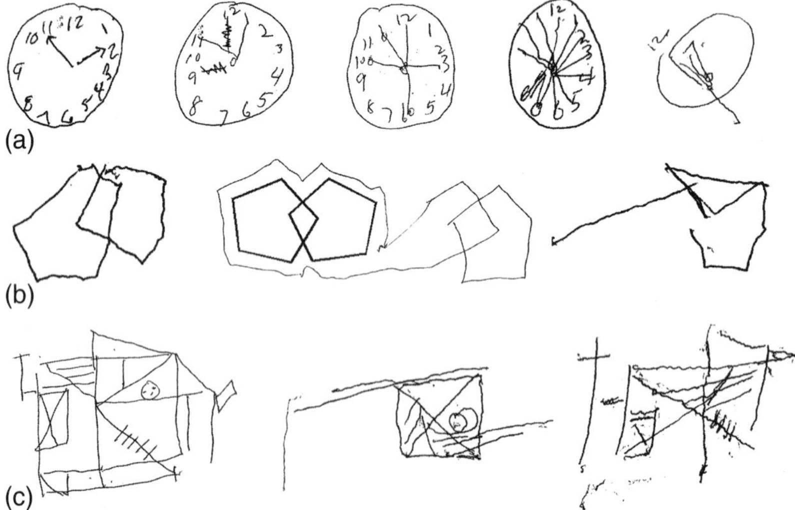

Fig. 14.1 Visuospatial dysfunction in cortical Lewy body diseases. Typical progressive deterioration of visuospatial and constructive abilities is demonstrated in these sequential attempts on: (a) the Clock Draw Test; (b) copying interlocking pentagons; and (c) copying the Rey–Osterrieth complex figure. Note the progressive deterioration in performance on sequential attempts at each task over time. The Rey–Osterrieth complex figures depicted were produced with the sample figure visible, as a copying task, rather than as a memory task.

combination of history of recurrent visual hallucinations and performance on tasks of visuospatial ability, such as the intersecting pentagons of the MMSE, are the best discriminators with a positive predictive value of 83% and negative predictive value of 90% (Tiraboschi *et al.* 2006). For examples of visuospatial dysfunction in PDD and DLB patients see Fig. 14.1.

Similar to the pattern seen in DLB, the neuropsychological profile of patients with PDD includes deficits in executive function, visuospatial and constructional abilities, and attention (Dubois and Pillon 1997; Emre 2003). In fact, many PD patients exhibit deficits in these areas in the absence of frank dementia (Foltynie *et al.* 2004; Green *et al.* 2002; Janvin *et al.* 2003). Moreover, early executive and visuospatial dysfunction has been associated with later onset of dementia in PD patients (Caparros-Lefebvre *et al.* 1995; Janvin *et al.* 2005; Levy *et al.* 2002; Mahieux *et al.* 1998). In comparison studies, most investigations have found very similar neuropsychological performance in PDD and DLB (Ballard *et al.* 2002; Cormack *et al.* 2004; Horimoto *et al.* 2003; Noe *et al.* 2004). However, one possible distinction is that, in well-characterized cohorts of PDD and DLB that are matched for mild to moderate dementia severity, DLB patients tend to have more profound executive dysfunction (Aarsland *et al.* 2003*b*; Downes *et al.* 1998). In a comparison of 35 PDD, 60 DLB, and 29 AD patients tested with the Mattis Dementia Rating Scale and matched by total score, the only difference between PDD and DLB was observed in mild to moderate patients, with the PDD patients performing slightly better on the conceptualization subscale, while performance on the other four subscales was indistinguishable (Aarsland *et al.* 2003*b*).

Furthermore, within PDD and DLB there appears to be variability in the pattern of executive impairment and memory dysfunction between patients that may reflect variable burdens of AD pathology (Janvin *et al.* 2006; Weintraub *et al.* 2004, 2005). In a pooled assessment of 50 PDD, 62 DLB, and 39 AD patients given the Mattis Dementia Rating Scale and the MMSE, four patterns of cognitive dysfunction were observed based on the severity of dementia and the pattern of dysfunction. The four patterns included mild and moderate subcortical profiles, a moderate cortical profile, and a global cognitive impairment profile that included patients with severe dementia and reduced performance on all tests. Interestingly, while the majority of PDD and DLB patients exhibited the subcortical or global profiles and the majority of the AD patients exhibited either the cortical or global profiles, there were exceptions with 30% and 26% of PDD and DLB patients, respectively, exhibiting the cortical profile. Further studies will be needed to determine if these patients have greater burdens of AD pathology than their counterparts.

14.6 **Imaging correlates**

While there are no imaging modalities with sufficient sensitivity and specificity to serve as an independent biomarker of DLB or PDD, several have proved useful as supportive features in the diagnostic evaluation of these disorders.

14.6.1 **Structural**

In addition to being useful in eliminating alternative causes of dementia including normal pressure hydrocephalus, cerebrovascular disease, and subdural haematomas, structural neuroimaging has some utility in the diagnosis but not the differentiation of DLB and PDD. Probably the most relevant structural observation in the diagnosis of DLB and PDD is a relative preservation of the medial temporal lobes (see Fig. 14.2). This finding may be helpful in distinguishing DLB from AD (R. Barber *et al.* 1999, 2000) but not necessarily PDD from AD with one study showing more atrophy in PDD than AD (Laakso *et al.* 1996) and another reporting the reverse

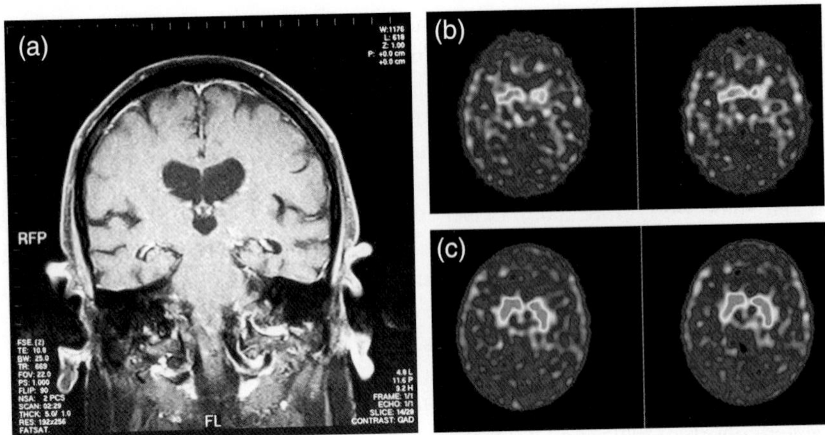

Fig. 14.2 Neuroimaging in cortical Lewy body diseases. (a) Structural imaging of a typical patient with PDD or DLB is presented in this coronal T1-weighted image of a patient with PDD. Note the minimal cortical atrophy and preservation of the medial temporal lobe including the hippocampal formation. (b), (c) Functional imaging of the dopaminergic system, in this case $[^{99m}\text{Tc}]$TRODAT SPECT imaging, can be helpful in differentiating (b) patients with PDD and DLB who can display diminished uptake of dopaminergic ligands in the striatum, compared with (c) normal controls and Alzheimer's disease patients who frequently have normal uptake. (SPECT images courtesy of Dr Andrew Newberg, University of Pennsylvania.) This is a black and white version of Plate 15.

(Camicioli *et al.* 2003). Differential atrophy between DLB and AD has been observed in the putamen (Cousins *et al.* 2003), but not in the caudate nucleus (R. Barber *et al.* 2002). A recent investigation into generalized cortical atrophy in DLB brains showed relative preservation of grey matter in the medial temporal lobe, hippocampus, and amygdala compared to AD patients in the context of atrophy of the temporal, frontal, and insular cortices compared to control subjects (Burton *et al.* 2002). In the only imaging study to date comparing rigorously defined PD, PDD, and DLB, it was found that cortical atrophy was limited to the frontal lobe in PD while involving temporal, parietal, and occipital lobes in PDD, but that PDD could not be distinguished from DLB (Burton *et al.* 2004). Other investigators have also examined the volume of the substantia innominata, including the cholinergic nucleus basalis of Meynert (NBM), and found that PDD could be distinguished from normal controls, but not from other causes of dementia that also exhibited atrophy in this region (Hanyu *et al.* 2002). Cholinergic input from the NBM is required for cognitive functions, including memory, and degeneration of the NBM in DLB and PDD is believed to contribute to cognitive decline in these disorders.

A recently developed method for examining intracranial structures, transcranial sonography (TCS), has also been used to examine structural abnormalities in PDD and DLB (Walter *et al.* 2006). TCS involves an ultrasound assessment of brain echogenicity through the periauricular acoustic bone window and in PD has focused on echogenicity of the substantia nigra, with PD patients exhibiting hyperechogenicity relative to most controls and atypical forms of parkinsonism (Walter *et al.* 2002, 2003). In a study of 14 patients with consensus-criteria-defined possible or probable DLB, 31 with PDD, and 73 patients with non-demented PD, Walter and colleagues were able to distinguish DLB from PDD with a sensitivity of 96%, a specificity of 80%, and a positive predictive value of 93% using a combination of the size and symmetry of substantia nigra hyperechogenicity and age at disease onset. Interestingly, DLB patients had more profound and symmetric hyperechogenicity than PDD and non-demented PD patients, even though less neuronal loss is typically seen in the substantia nigra in DLB (Tsuboi *et al.* 2005). To account for this discrepancy, the authors hypothesize that hyperechogenicity is not a marker of neuronal loss or LB accumulation, but rather a marker of accumulated abnormally bound iron that occurs early in life, increasing susceptibility to PD and DLB, and does not progress during the disease course.

14.6.2 **Functional**

Functional imaging modalities are gaining ground in the clinical setting for most neurodegenerative diseases, including dementia and parkinsonism. In general, techniques can be divided by modality, into functional (functional magnetic resonance imaging (fMRI), positron emission tomography (PET), single photon emission computerized tomography (SPECT)) and physiological (perfusion and ligand-specific imaging). To date, there have been no fMRI studies of PDD or DLB. Cerebral blood flow studies utilizing either glucose metabolism with PET imaging or non-specific blood flow markers and SPECT have revealed biparietal hypoperfusion with or without concomitant change in the frontal and temporal lobes in DLB (Donnemiller *et al.* 1997; Ishii *et al.* 1999, 2004; Lobotesis *et al.* 2001; Minoshima *et al.* 2001). Comparing DLB and AD, several studies have shown profound hypoperfusion of the occipital lobes with relative sparing of the temporal lobes in DLB (Colloby *et al.* 2002; Donnemiller *et al.* 1997; Ishii *et al.* 1999; Lobotesis *et al.* 2001). Indeed, some authors have suggested that occipital hypoperfusion is sufficient to serve as a biomarker, differentiating DLB from AD with a specificity of 86–90% and a sensitivity of 68–80% (Lobotesis *et al.* 2001; Minoshima *et al.* 2001). Ligand-specific functional imaging investigations have mainly utilized markers of dopaminergic function (in particular the dopamine transporter) to differentiate DLB or PDD from AD. In general, either PET or SPECT imaging of transporter ligands has revealed decreased uptake in the striatum when compared to AD (see Fig. 14.2; Donnemiller *et al.* 1997; O'Brien *et al.* 2004; Walker *et al.* 2002). In an examination of cortical acetylcholinesterase function, Bohnen and colleagues made the somewhat unexpected observation that non-demented patients with PD as well as those with PDD had lower activity levels than AD patients of the same relative dementia severity (Bohnen *et al.* 2003; Donnemiller *et al.* 1997; Walker *et al.* 2002).

14.7 **Pathology**

Lewy bodies (LB) in the substantia nigra have been associated with Parkinson's disease (PD) for almost a century, but the relevance of LB to dementia has only been fully ascertained in the past two decades (Kosaka *et al.* 1984; McKeith *et al.* 1996; Perry *et al.* 1990), and has put a spotlight on the significance of non-nigral pathology. Similarly, although LNs were first described with ubiquitin immunochemistry (Dickson *et al.* 1991; Gai *et al.* 1995), the arrival of a-synuclein immunochemistry has engendered a recognition of LN burden that was previously underappreciated (Braak *et al.* 1999; Gomez-Tortosa *et al.* 2000; Irizarry *et al.* 1998). Since then, many reports have highlighted the abundance of LNs in the LB disorders, including the report that novel antibodies raised against oxidized a-synuclein provide an even more sensitive method for recognizing LNs, including a burden of neuritic dystrophy within the striatum in LB disorders (Duda *et al.* 2002) that may contribute to the parkinsonism in these disorders (see Fig. 14.3). Together with the recognition that LNs appear to accumulate prior to LBs (Braak *et al.* 2003; Marui *et al.* 2002) and the suggestion of axonal degeneration in an alpha-synuclein transgenic mouse model (Giasson *et al.* 2002), such studies have led to a hypothesis that neuritic dystrophy is an early and important component in the Lewy neurodegeneration cascade (Duda 2004).

The presence of Lewy pathology (LP)—a term that recognizes the similarity between LBs and LNs—is considered the pathological hallmark of DLB, PDD, and PD, just as senile (amyloid)

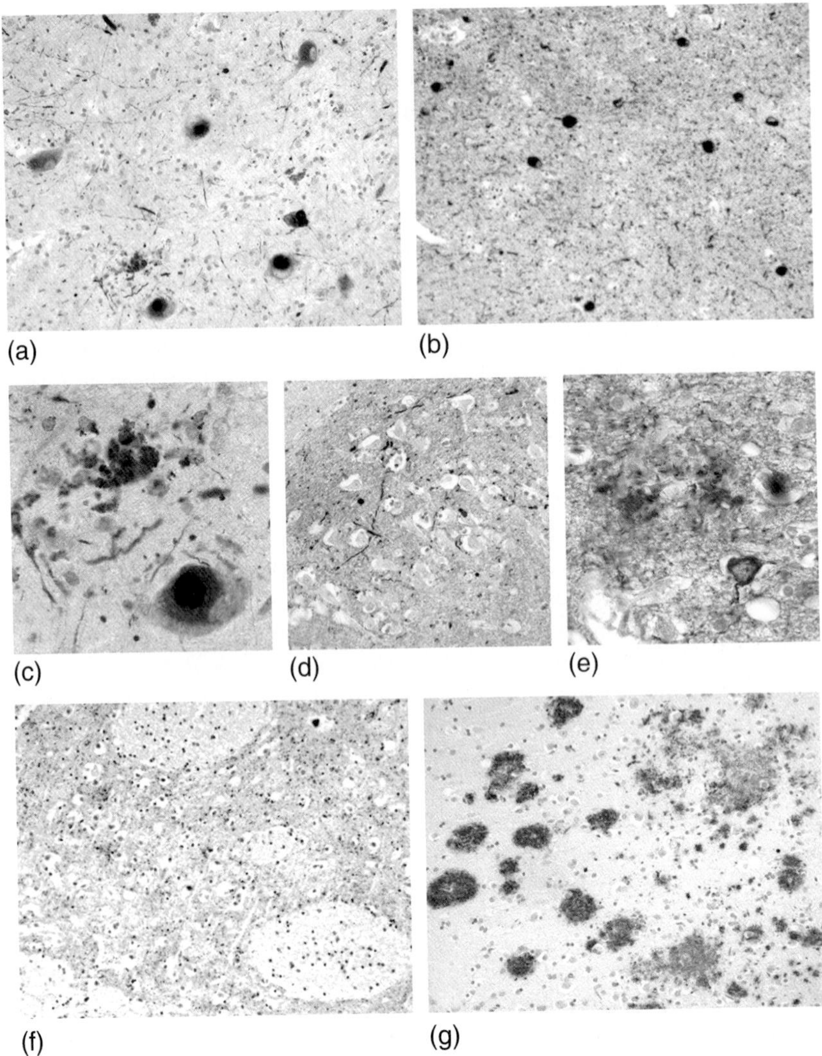

Fig. 14.3 Neuropathology of cortical Lewy body diseases. Lewy pathology (LP) is the predominant neuropathological hallmark of PDD and DLB including deposition in many areas of the brain and brainstem including: (a), (c) the substantia nigra; (b), (d) cerebral cortex; and (f) striatum. (a), (c) Note that in the substantia nigra most remaining pigmented neurons have Lewy aggregates. (c) Occasional 'ghost' neurons, which are the remnants of pigmented neurons with extracellular neuromelanin, can be observed. Cortical LP may take on several patterns with a combination of: (b) LBs, LNs, and granular inclusions in limbic cortices; (d) predominantly LNs in the CA2/3 region of Ammon's horn; and (f) predominantly granular inclusions in the striatum. (e) In addition to LP, tau aggregates are also present in many cases of PDD and DLB, including neurofibrillary tangles (lower right) and neuritic plaques (middle), as well as (g) cortical senile plaques composed of β-amyloid protein, which are found in most cases of PDD and DLB. Slides stained by immunohistochemistry with antibodies directed against: (a)–(d), (f) α-synuclein; (e) tau; and (g) β-amyloid. Slides are counterstained with haematoxylin. Original magnification: (a), (b), (d), (f), (g) 200X; (c), (e) 600X. This is a black and white version of Plate 16.

plaques (SP) and neurofibrillary tangles (NFT) are the hallmarks of AD. However, two or more identifying morphological features frequently coexist in patients with dementia and, in some cases, make it difficult to discern the pathological source of the dementia (Galasko *et al.* 1994; Merdes *et al.* 2003; Samuel *et al.* 1997*b*; Szpak *et al.* 2001). Although there is no direct evidence for an aetiological link between DLB or PDD and AD, the frequency of concurrent pathology in these diseases suggests that there may be a common underlying aetiology (Pompeu and Growdon 2002). In addition, it has been recognized that the burden of concomitant AD pathology alters the phenotype of DLB (Del Ser *et al.* 2001; Lopez *et al.* 2002; Merdes *et al.* 2003), making it more difficult to diagnose and contributing to the low sensitivity of diagnostic criteria. The most recent modifications to the consensus criteria for the clinicopathological diagnosis of DLB attempt to address this complex interaction by assigning probability statements of the likelihood that a specific combination of LP and AD pathology is likely to manifest the DLB phenotype (McKeith *et al.* 2005).

Degeneration of the cholinergic nucleus basalis of Meynert (NBM) in the basal forebrain is universal in DLB and PDD with extensive LP and more profound neuronal loss found in DLB compared to AD (Lippa *et al.* 1999*a*). As discussed above, a number of studies have proposed that it is degeneration in the NBM that leads to the development of dementia in PD (Gaspar and Gray 1984; Whitehouse *et al.* 1983), which may be independent of AD pathology (Tagliavini *et al.* 1984).

Recently, several studies have been conducted to further investigate the role of LP in the generation of dementia in DLB and PDD and the majority have demonstrated a correlation between LP and dementia in DLB (Haroutunian *et al.* 2000; Lennox *et al.* 1989; Samuel *et al.* 1996, 1997*b*) and PD (Apaydin *et al.* 2002; Hurtig *et al.* 2000; Kovari *et al.* 2003; Mattila *et al.* 1998, 2000). There may also be a synergistic effect between LP and AD pathology: Samuel and colleagues found that patients with dual pathology are much more severely demented than DLB patients with the same cortical LB count (Samuel *et al.* 1997*a*), while Serby and colleagues found that dementia is more severe and LBs are more frequent when AD and Lewy pathology coexist. In general, AD pathology present in DLB and PDD is primarily the diffuse type of senile plaques and a relative paucity of NFTs (Hansen *et al.* 1993; Mann *et al.* 1998; Samuel *et al.* 1997*a*).

In an effort to understand the role of LP in neurodegenerative disease, a staging system was developed that suggests that LP may progress in a systematic fashion through the brain. The first efforts to stage LP began when Kosaka and colleagues proposed a three-tiered system that was later adapted as the brainstem, limbic, and neocortical stages of disease of the consensus guidelines for DLB (Kosaka *et al.* 1984; McKeith *et al.* 1996). In a more comprehensive analysis of LP distribution, Braak and colleagues have examined the brains of 41 patients clinically diagnosed with PD and a second group of 69 brains from patients who were not known to have symptoms of PD, PDD, or DLB, but did have LP at autopsy (Braak *et al.* 2003). Many of the brains in the second group can be thought of as having preclinical or incidental LP that may have progressed to become PD or DLB. Interestingly, the authors observed that, in the 20 most mildly affected cases, the LP is found almost exclusively in the medulla and the anterior olfactory nucleus, areas that were not previously recognized as early sites of LP aggregation. The authors developed a staging system of LP with six stages that characterize a progression from the medulla, through the pontine tegmentum, into the midbrain, into the basal prosencephalon and mesocortex, and finally through the neocortex. Further investigations are needed to confirm the progression of LP through the brain, as well as to determine whether the clinical diagnosis of dementia, either in DLB or PDD, or the presence of concomitant AD pathology alters this progression.

14.8 **Clinical course and prognosis**

14.8.1 **Complications**

Many of the symptomatic complications of DLB and PDD have been incorporated as core, suggestive, or supportive features in the DLB consensus criteria (Section 14.1 and Table 14.1). These include psychosis, cognitive fluctuations, RBD, autonomic dysfunction, and depression. One further suggestive feature, severe neuroleptic sensitivity, deserves special attention due to its iatrogenic nature and potentially devastating consequences. Severe neuroleptic sensitivity reactions typically include acute worsening of parkinsonism in association with sudden impairments of consciousness ranging from sedation to coma that often lead to shortened survival with death occasionally occurring in weeks to months (McKeith *et al.* 1992). Although originally described in 1992, severe neuroleptic sensitivity is still underrecognized, especially in the setting of PD and PDD. However, a recent prospective study of neuroleptic exposure in 15 DLB, 26 PD, 39 PDD, and 17 AD patients, found a significant risk in all disease categories except AD (Aarsland *et al.* 2005*a*). As expected, severe neuroleptic sensitivity reactions occurred in over half of the DLB subjects (53%) but, interestingly, large numbers with not only PDD (39%) but also PD (27%) also experienced severe reactions. These reactions have been described not only with 'typical' neuroleptics (such as haloperidol and chlorpromazine) but also with 'atypical' neuroleptics including olanzapine, risperidone, and clozapine. Caution is therefore warranted when prescribing any neuroleptic medications to patients in any of these diagnostic groups.

14.8.2 **Prognosis**

Studies of survival in PD suggest that concomitant dementia is an independent risk factor for nursing home placement and death, with survival significantly shorter than in non-demented patients (Louis *et al.* 1997; Marder *et al.* 1991; Mindham *et al.* 1982). In DLB, most survival comparisons have been made with AD and, while early studies reported reduced survival in DLB, subsequent surveys have found no survival difference between the two conditions (Ala *et al.* 1997; Klatka *et al.* 1996; Z. Walker *et al.* 2000). As in AD, patients with DLB and PDD eventually progress to an end-stage illness characterized by immobility and limited communication, indistinguishable from the advanced stages of most other neurodegenerative conditions.

14.9 **Management strategies**

For most practical purposes, the management strategies for PDD and DLB are very similar, with therapeutic decisions based on each particular patient's combination of symptoms. Just as patients with DLB have varying degrees of psychosis, parkinsonism, and cognitive dysfunction, some PDD patients will have severe parkinsonism with mild psychosis and dementia, while in others dementia and psychosis become the predominant symptoms (even if these features were not prominent at onset). In each case, management will vary with therapeutics directed at the most troublesome and disabling symptoms, bearing in mind that treatment of some symptoms may exacerbate others (Barber *et al.* 2001).

The therapeutic option with the strongest evidence for efficacy in these disorders is the use of acetylcholinesterase inhibitors (AChEIs). While initially developed for AD (see Chapter 11), these agents—which now include donepezil, rivastigmine, galantamine, and tacrine (rarely used due to a risk of severe hepatotoxicity)—have proved beneficial for many symptom domains in PDD and DLB. Indeed, efficacy in these conditions has been shown to be better than in AD (Samuel *et al.* 2000). Responsive symptoms have included dementia, cognitive fluctuations, hallucinations, apathy, and disturbed sleep. Placebo-controlled, double-blinded trials have been conducted in PDD and DLB for both donepezil (Aarsland *et al.* 2002*b*; Ravina *et al.* 2005) and rivastigmine

(Aarsland *et al.* 2002*a*; Emre *et al.* 2004; McKeith *et al.* 2000; Ravina *et al.* 2005). In all of these trials, benefit has been demonstrated with mimimal exacerbation of parkinsonism. The side-effect profile is similar to that seen in AD, with the addition of hypersalivation, urinary problems, and orthostatic hypotension (Thomas *et al.* 2005). A recent evidence-based review concluded that donepezil should be considered for the treatment of dementia in PD and that rivastigmine should be considered for the treatment of dementia in PD or DLB (Miyasaki *et al.* 2006). While no double-blinded placebo-controlled trials of memantine have been conducted in DLB or PDD, there is anecdotal evidence of symptom worsening in these patients (Menendez-Gonzalez *et al.* 2005; Ridha *et al.* 2005; Sabbagh *et al.* 2005).

One of the more idiosyncratic differences in the practical management of PDD and DLB is the approach to the treatment of psychosis in these two conditions. In general, most movement disorder specialists use atypical neuroleptics, particularly quetiapine and clozapine, as first-line agents while many dementia specialists will use AChEIs instead. Limited controlled data is available for the atypical neuroleptics, and the risk of severe sensitivity reactions in both DLB and PDD (Aarsland *et al.* 2005*a*) argues for careful consideration and patient education when choosing one of these agents. A recent evidence-based review concluded that, for patients with PD and psychosis, lozapine should be considered (Miyasaki *et al.* 2006), though this drug is associated with potentially fatal agranulocytosis, so the absolute neutrophil count must be monitored. Quetiapine is preferable to olanzapine in these patients, as two studies have suggested that the latter worsens motor function without improving the psychotic symptoms (Miyasaki *et al.* 2006). Double-blind, placebo-controlled studies have provided evidence for the value of rivastigmine and donepezil in the management of psychosis in these disorders, though rapid cessation of the latter in successfully treated PDD patients may provoke a dramatic recrudescence of neuropsychiatric symptoms (Minett *et al.* 2003).

Although there is little controlled data, parkinsonism in these disorders is normally managed with an emphasis on carbidopa/levodopa monotherapy. By contrast, anticholinergics, dopamine agonists, amantadine, and selegiline tend to be avoided because of a perceived propensity for worsening cognition and psychosis. Carbidopa/levodopa may also worsen psychosis, excessive daytime sleepiness, and orthostatic symptoms, and may be less efficacious in DLB than PDD (Molloy *et al.* 2005). Since motor symptoms increase the overall functional disability of DLB and PDD patients compared with AD with cognitive impairment of the same global severity (McKeith *et al.* 2006), a carefully monitored trial of carbidopa/levodopa should be offered whenever significant parkinsonism is detected.

References

Aarsland, D., Andersen, K., Larsen, J.P., Lolk, A., Nielsen, H., and Kragh-Sorensen, P. (2001). Risk of dementia in Parkinson's disease: a community-based, prospective study. *Neurology* **56** (6), 730–6.

Aarsland, D., Laake, K., Larsen, J.P., and Janvin, C. (2002*a*). Donepezil for cognitive impairment in Parkinson's disease: a randomised controlled study. *J. Neurol. Neurosurg. Psychiatry* **72** (6), 708–12.

Aarsland, D., Laake, K., Larsen, J.P., and Janvin, C. (2002*b*). Donepezil for cognitive impairment in Parkinson's disease: a randomised controlled study. *J. Neurol. Neurosurg. Psychiatry* **72** (6), 708–12.

Aarsland, D., Andersen, K., Larsen, J. P., Lolk, A., and Kragh-Sorensen, P. (2003*a*). Prevalence and characteristics of dementia in Parkinson disease: an 8-year prospective study. *Arch. Neurol.* **60** (3), 387–92.

Aarsland, D., Litvan, I., Salmon, D., Galasko, D., Wentzel-Larsen, T., and Larsen, J.P. (2003*b*). Performance on the dementia rating scale in Parkinson's disease with dementia and dementia with Lewy bodies: comparison with progressive supranuclear palsy and Alzheimer's disease. *J. Neurol. Neurosurg. Psychiatry* **74** (9), 1215–20.

Aarsland, D., Perry, R., Larsen, J.P., McKeith, I.G., O'Brien, J.T., Perry, E.K., Burn, D., and Ballard, C.G. (2005*a*). Neuroleptic sensitivity in Parkinson's disease and parkinsonian dementias. *J. Clin. Psychiatry* **66** (5), 633–7.

Aarsland, D., Zaccai, J., and Brayne, C. (2005*b*). A systematic review of prevalence studies of dementia in Parkinson's disease. *Mov. Disord.* **20** (10), 1255–63.

Ala, T.A., Yang, K.H., Sung, J.H., and Frey, W.H. (1997). Hallucinations and signs of parkinsonism help distinguish patients with dementia and cortical Lewy bodies from patients with Alzheimer's disease at presentation: a clinicopathological study. *J. Neurol. Neurosurg. Psychiatry* **62** (1), 16–21.

Ala, T., Hughes, L.F., Kyrouac, G.A., Ghobrial, M.W., and Elble, R.J. (2004). Use of MMSE to differentiate Alzheimer's disease from dementia with Lewy bodies—response to Larner. *Int. J. Geriatr. Psychiatry* **19** (12), 1209–10.

America Psychiatric Association (2000). *Diagnostic and statistical manual of mental disorders*, 4th edn, Text Revision. American Psychiatric Association, Washington, DC.

Apaydin, H., Ahlskog, J.E., Parisi, J.E., Boeve, B.F., and Dickson, D.W. (2002). Parkinson disease neuropathology: later-developing dementia and loss of the levodopa response. *Arch. Neurol.* **59** (1), 102–12.

Ballard, C., Holmes, C., McKeith, I., Neill, D., O'Brien, J., Cairns, N., Lantos, P., Perry, E., Ince, P., and Perry, R. (1999). Psychiatric morbidity in dementia with Lewy bodies: a prospective clinical and neuropathological comparative study with Alzheimer's disease. *Am. J. Psychiatry* **156** (7), 1039–45.

Ballard, C., O'Brien, J., Gray, A., Cormack, F., Ayre, G., Rowan, E., Thompson, P., Bucks, R., McKeith, I., Walker, M., and Tovee, M. (2001). Attention and fluctuating attention in patients with dementia with Lewy bodies and Alzheimer disease. *Arch. Neurol.* **58** (6), 977–82.

Ballard, C.G., Aarsland, D., McKeith, I., O'Brien, J., Gray, A., Cormack, F., Burn, D., Cassidy, T., Starfeldt, R., Larsen, J.P., Brown, R., and Tovee, M. (2002). Fluctuations in attention: PD dementia vs DLB with parkinsonism. *Neurology* **59** (11), 1714–20.

Barber, P.A., Varma, A.R., Lloyd, J.J., Haworth, B., Snowden, J.S., and Neary, D. (2000). The electroencephalogram in dementia with Lewy bodies. *Acta Neurol. Scand.* **101** (1), 53–6.

Barber, R., Gholkar, A., Scheltens, P., Ballard, C., McKeith, I.G., and O'Brien, J.T. (1999). Medial temporal lobe atrophy on MRI in dementia with Lewy bodies. *Neurology* **52** (6), 1153–8.

Barber, R., Ballard, C., McKeith, I.G., Gholkar, A., and O'Brien, J.T. (2000). MRI volumetric study of dementia with Lewy bodies: a comparison with AD and vascular dementia. *Neurology* **54** (6), 1304–9.

Barber, R., Panikkar, A., and McKeith, I.G. (2001). Dementia with Lewy bodies: diagnosis and management. *Int. J. Geriatr. Psychiatry* **16** (Suppl. 1), S12–S18.

Barber, R., McKeith, I., Ballard, C., and O'Brien, J. (2002). Volumetric MRI study of the caudate nucleus in patients with dementia with Lewy bodies, Alzheimer's disease, and vascular dementia. *J. Neurol. Neurosurg. Psychiatry* **72** (3), 406–7.

Boeve, B.F., Silber, M.H., Ferman, T.J., Lucas, J.A., and Parisi, J.E. (2001). Association of REM sleep behavior disorder and neurodegenerative disease may reflect an underlying synucleinopathy. *Mov Disord.* **16** (4), 622–30.

Boeve, B.F., Silber, M.H., and Ferman, T.J. (2004). REM sleep behavior disorder in Parkinson's disease and dementia with Lewy bodies. *J. Geriatr. Psychiatry Neurol.* **17** (3), 146–57.

Bohnen, N.I., Kaufer, D.I., Ivanco, L.S., Lopresti, B., Koeppe, R.A., Davis, J.G., Mathis, C.A., Moore, R.Y., and DeKosky, S.T. (2003). Cortical cholinergic function is more severely affected in parkinsonian dementia than in Alzheimer disease: an in vivo positron emission tomographic study. *Arch. Neurol.* **60** (12), 1745–8.

Bonner, L.T., Tsuang, D.W., Cherrier, M.M., Eugenio, C.J., Du, J.Q., Steinbart, E.J., Limprasert, P., La Spada, A.R., Seltzer, B., Bird, T.D., and Leverenz, J.B. (2003). Familial dementia with Lewy bodies with an atypical clinical presentation. *J. Geriatr. Psychiatry Neurol.* **16** (1), 59–64.

Braak, H., Sandmann-Keil, D., Gai, W., and Braak, E. (1999). Extensive axonal Lewy neurites in Parkinson's disease: a novel pathological feature revealed by alpha-synuclein immunocytochemistry. *Neurosci. Lett.* **265** (1), 67–9.

Braak, H., Del Tredici, K., Rub, U., de Vos, R.A., Jansen Steur, E.N., and Braak, E. (2003). Staging of brain pathology related to sporadic Parkinson's disease. *Neurobiol. Aging* **24** (2), 197–211.

Bradshaw, J., Saling, M., Hopwood, M., Anderson, V., and Brodtmann, A. (2004). Fluctuating cognition in dementia with Lewy bodies and Alzheimer's disease is qualitatively distinct. *J. Neurol. Neurosurg. Psychiatry* **75** (3), 382–7.

Brett, F.M., Henson, C., and Staunton, H. (2002). Familial diffuse Lewy body disease, eye movement abnormalities, and distribution of pathology. *Arch. Neurol.* **59** (3), 464–7.

Briel, R.C., McKeith, I.G., Barker, W.A., Hewitt, Y., Perry, R.H., Ince, P.G., and Fairbairn, A.F. (1999). EEG findings in dementia with Lewy bodies and Alzheimer's disease. *J. Neurol. Neurosurg. Psychiatry* **66** (3), 401–3.

Burn, D.J., Rowan, E.N., McKeith, I.G., O'Brien, J.T., Minett, T., and Myint, P. (2002). Is parkinsonism phenotype predictive of dementia: a cross-sectional study. *Mov. Disord.* **17** (Suppl. 5), S22.

Burton, E.J., Karas, G., Paling, S.M., Barber, R., Williams, E.D., Ballard, C.G., McKeith, I.G., Scheltens, P., Barkhof, F., and O'Brien, J.T. (2002). Patterns of cerebral atrophy in dementia with Lewy bodies using voxel-based morphometry. *Neuroimage.* **17** (2), 618–30.

Burton, E.J., McKeith, I.G., Burn, D.J., Williams, E.D., and O'Brien, J.T. (2004). Cerebral atrophy in Parkinson's disease with and without dementia: a comparison with Alzheimer's disease, dementia with Lewy bodies and controls. *Brain* **127** (4), 791–800.

Calderon, J., Perry, R.J., Erzinclioglu, S.W., Berrios, G.E., Dening, T.R., and Hodges, J.R. (2001). Perception, attention, and working memory are disproportionately impaired in dementia with Lewy bodies compared with Alzheimer's disease. *J. Neurol. Neurosurg. Psychiatry* **70** (2), 157–64.

Camicioli, R., Moore, M.M., Kinney, A., Corbridge, E., Glassberg, K., and Kaye, J.A. (2003). Parkinson's disease is associated with hippocampal atrophy. *Mov Disord.* **18** (7), 784–90.

Caparros-Lefebvre, D., Pecheux, N., Petit, V., Duhamel, A., and Petit, H. (1995). Which factors predict cognitive decline in Parkinson's disease?. *J. Neurol. Neurosurg. Psychiatry* **58** (1), 51–5.

Chartier-Harlin, M.C., Kachergus, J., Roumier, C., Mouroux, V., Douay, X., Lincoln, S., Levecque, C., Larvor, L., Andrieux, J., Hulihan, M., Waucquier, N., Defebvre, L., Amouyel, P., Farrer, M., and Destee, A. (2004). Alpha-synuclein locus duplication as a cause of familial Parkinson's disease. *Lancet* **364** (9440), 1167–9.

Collerton, D., Burn, D., McKeith, I., and O'Brien, J. (2003). Systematic review and meta-analysis show that dementia with Lewy bodies is a visual-perceptual and attentional-executive dementia. *Dement. Geriatr. Cogn Disord.* **16** (4), 229–37.

Colloby, S.J., Fenwick, J.D., Williams, E.D., Paling, S.M., Lobotesis, K., Ballard, C., McKeith, I., and O'Brien, J.T. (2002). A comparison of (99m)Tc-HMPAO SPET changes in dementia with Lewy bodies and Alzheimer's disease using statistical parametric mapping. *Eur. J. Nucl. Med. Mol. Imaging* **29** (5), 615–22.

Connor, D.J., Salmon, D.P., Sandy, T.J., Galasko, D., Hansen, L.A., and Thal, L.J. (1998). Cognitive profiles of autopsy-confirmed Lewy body variant vs pure Alzheimer disease. *Arch. Neurol.* **55** (7), 994–1000.

Cormack, F., Aarsland, D., Ballard, C., and Tovee, M.J. (2004). Pentagon drawing and neuropsychological performance in dementia with Lewy bodies, Alzheimer's disease, Parkinson's disease and Parkinson's disease with dementia. *Int. J. Geriatr. Psychiatry* **19** (4), 371–7.

Cousins, D.A., Burton, E.J., Burn, D., Gholkar, A., McKeith, I.G., and O'Brien, J.T. (2003). Atrophy of the putamen in dementia with Lewy bodies but not Alzheimer's disease: an MRI study. *Neurology* **61** (9), 1191–5.

Culbertson, W.C., Moberg, P.J., Duda, J.E., Stern, M.B., and Weintraub, D. (2004). Assessing the executive function deficits of patients with Parkinson's disease: utility of the Tower of London–Drexel. *Assessment* **11** (1), 27–39.

Del Ser, T., Hachinski, V., Merskey, H., and Munoz, D.G. (2001). Clinical and pathologic features of two groups of patients with dementia with Lewy bodies: effect of coexisting Alzheimer-type lesion load. *Alzheimer Dis. Assoc. Disord.* **15** (1), 31–44.

Dickson, D.W., Ruan, D., Crystal, H., Mark, M.H., Davies, P., Kress, Y., and Yen, S.H. (1991). Hippocampal degeneration differentiates diffuse Lewy body disease (DLBD) from Alzheimer's disease: light and electron microscopic immunocytochemistry of CA2–3 neurites specific to DLBD. *Neurology* **41** (9), 1402–9.

Dickson, D.W., Crystal, H.A., Davies, P., and Hardy, J. (1996). Cytoskeletal and Alzheimer-type pathology in Lewy body disease. In *Dementia with Lewy bodies* (ed. R. Perry, I. McKeith, and E. Perry), pp. 224–37. Cambridge University Press, Cambridge.

Donnemiller, E., Heilmann, J., Wenning, G.K., Berger, W., Decristoforo, C., Moncayo, R., Poewe, W., and Ransmayr, G. (1997). Brain perfusion scintigraphy with 99mTc-HMPAO or 99mTc-ECD and 123I-beta-CIT single-photon emission tomography in dementia of the Alzheimer-type and diffuse Lewy body disease. *Eur. J. Nucl. Med.* **24** (3), 320–5.

Downes, J.J., Priestley, N.M., Doran, M., Ferran, J., Ghadiali, E., and Cooper, P. (1998). Intellectual, mnemonic, and frontal functions in dementia with Lewy bodies: a comparison with early and advanced Parkinson's disease. *Behav. Neurol.* **11** (3), 173–83.

Dubois, B. and Pillon, B. (1997). Cognitive deficits in Parkinson's disease. *J. Neurol.* **244** (1), 2–8.

Duda, J. E. (2004). Pathology and neurotransmitter abnormalities of dementia with Lewy bodies. *Dement. Geriatr. Cogn Disord.* **17** (Suppl. 1), 3–14.

Duda, J.E., Giasson, B.I., Mabon, M.E., Lee, V.M., and Trojanowski, J.Q. (2002). Novel antibodies to synuclein show abundant striatal pathology in Lewy body diseases. *Ann. Neurol.* **52** (2), 205–10.

Emre, M. (2003). Dementia associated with Parkinson's disease. *Lancet Neurol.* **2** (4), 229–37.

Emre, M., Aarsland, D., Albanese, A., Byrne, E.J., Deuschl, G., De Deyn, P.P., Durif, F., Kulisevsky, J., van Laar, T., Lees, A., Poewe, W., Robillard, A., Rosa, M.M., Wolters, E., Quarg, P., Tekin, S., and Lane, R. (2004). Rivastigmine for dementia associated with Parkinson's disease. *N. Engl. J. Med.* **351** (24), 2509–18.

Factor, S.A., Feustel, P.J., Friedman, J.H., Comella, C.L., Goetz, C.G., Kurlan, R., Parsa, M., and Pfeiffer, R. (2003). Longitudinal outcome of Parkinson's disease patients with psychosis. *Neurology* **60** (11), 1756–61.

Fahn, S., Elton, R., and UPDRS Program Members (1987). Unified Parkinson's disease rating scale. In *Recent developments in Parkinson's disease*, Vol. 2 (ed. S. Fahn *et al.*), pp. 153–63. Macmillan Healthcare Information, Florham Park, New Jersey.

Farrer, M., Kachergus, J., Forno, L., Lincoln, S., Wang, D.S., Hulihan, M., Maraganore, D., Gwinn-Hardy, K., Wszolek, Z., Dickson, D., and Langston, J.W. (2004). Comparison of kindreds with parkinsonism and alpha-synuclein genomic multiplications. *Ann. Neurol.* **55** (2), 174–9.

Ferman, T.J., Boeve, B.F., Smith, G.E., Silber, M.H., Lucas, J.A., Graff-Radford, N.R., Dickson, D.W., Parisi, J.E., Petersen, R.C., and Ivnik, R.J. (2002). Dementia with Lewy bodies may present as dementia and REM sleep behavior disorder without parkinsonism or hallucinations. *J. Int. Neuropsychol. Soc.* **8** (7), 907–14.

Ferman, T.J., Smith, G.E., Boeve, B.F., Ivnik, R.J., Petersen, R.C., Knopman, D., Graff-Radford, N., Parisi, J., and Dickson, D. W. (2004). DLB fluctuations: specific features that reliably differentiate DLB from AD and normal aging. *Neurology* **62** (2), 181–7.

Foltynie, T., Brayne, C.E., Robbins, T.W., and Barker, R.A. (2004). The cognitive ability of an incident cohort of Parkinson's patients in the UK. The CamPaIGN study. *Brain* **127** (3), 550–60.

Gai, W.P., Blessing, W.W., and Blumbergs, P.C. (1995). Ubiquitin-positive degenerating neurites in the brainstem in Parkinson's disease. *Brain* **118** (6)), 1447–59.

Galasko, D., Hansen, L.A., Katzman, R., Wiederholt, W., Masliah, E., Terry, R., Hill, L.R., Lessin, P., and Thal, L.J. (1994). Clinical–neuropathological correlations in Alzheimer's disease and related dementias. *Arch. Neurol.* **51** (9), 888–95.

Galvin, J.E., Lee, S.L., Perry, A., Havlioglu, N., McKeel, D.W., Jr., and Morris, J.C. (2002). Familial dementia with Lewy bodies: clinicopathologic analysis of two kindreds. *Neurology* **59** (7), 1079–82.

Gaspar, P. and Gray, F. (1984). Dementia in idiopathic Parkinson's disease. A neuropathological study of 32 cases. *Acta Neuropathol. (Berl.)* **64** (1), 43–52.

Gelb, D.J., Oliver, E., and Gilman, S. (1999). Diagnostic criteria for Parkinson disease. *Arch. Neurol.* **56** (1), 33–9.

Giasson, B.I., Duda, J.E., Quinn, S.M., Zhang, B., Trojanowski, J.Q., and Lee, V. M. (2002). Neuronal alpha-synucleinopathy with severe movement disorder in mice expressing A53T human alpha-synuclein. *Neuron* **34** (4), 521–33.

Gnanalingham, K.K., Byrne, E.J., Thornton, A., Sambrook, M.A., and Bannister, P. (1997). Motor and cognitive function in Lewy body dementia: comparison with Alzheimer's and Parkinson's diseases. *J. Neurol. Neurosurg. Psychiatry* **62** (3), 243–52.

Goetz, C.G., Vogel, C., Tanner, C.M., and Stebbins, G.T. (1998). Early dopaminergic drug-induced hallucinations in parkinsonian patients. *Neurology* **51** (3), 811–14.

Golbe, L.I., Lazzarini, A.M., Schwarz, K.O., Mark, M.H., Dickson, D.W., and Duvoisin, R.C. (1993). Autosomal dominant parkinsonism with benign course and typical Lewy-body pathology. *Neurology* **43** (11), 2222–7.

Gomez-Tortosa, E., Newell, K., Irizarry, M.C., Sanders, J.L., and Hyman, B. T. (2000). Alpha-Synuclein immunoreactivity in dementia with Lewy bodies: morphological staging and comparison with ubiquitin immunostaining. *Acta Neuropathol. (Berl.)* **99** (4), 352–7.

Green, J., McDonald, W.M., Vitek, J.L., Evatt, M., Freeman, A., Haber, M., Bakay, R.A., Triche, S., Sirockman, B., and DeLong, M.R. (2002). Cognitive impairments in advanced PD without dementia. *Neurology* **59** (9), 1320–4.

Hansen, L., Salmon, D., Galasko, D., Masliah, E., Katzman, R., DeTeresa, R., Thal, L., Pay, M.M., Hofstetter, R., Klauber, M., *et al.* (1990). The Lewy body variant of Alzheimer's disease: a clinical and pathologic entity. *Neurology* **40** (1), 1–8.

Hansen, L.A., Masliah, E., Galasko, D., and Terry, R. D. (1993). Plaque-only Alzheimer disease is usually the lewy body variant, and vice versa. *J. Neuropathol. Exp. Neurol.* **52** (6), 648–54.

Hansen, L.A., Galasko, D., Samuel, W., Xia, Y., Chen, X., and Saitoh, T. (1994). Apolipoprotein-E epsilon-4 is associated with increased neurofibrillary pathology in the Lewy body variant of Alzheimer's disease. *Neurosci. Lett.* **182** (1), 63–5.

Hanyu, H., Asano, T., Sakurai, H., Tanaka, Y., Takasaki, M., and Abe, K. (2002). MR analysis of the substantia innominata in normal aging, Alzheimer disease, and other types of dementia. *Am. J. Neuroradiol.* **23** (1), 27–32.

Harding, A.J., Das, A., Kril, J.J., Brooks, W.S., Duffy, D., and Halliday, G.M. (2004). Identification of families with cortical Lewy body disease. *Am. J. Med. Genet. B Neuropsychiatr. Genet.* **128** (1), 118–22.

Haroutunian, V., Serby, M., Purohit, D.P., Perl, D.P., Marin, D., Lantz, M., Mohs, R.C., and Davis, K.L. (2000). Contribution of Lewy body inclusions to dementia in patients with and without Alzheimer disease neuropathological conditions. *Arch. Neurol.* **57** (8), 1145–50.

Harrington, C.R., Roth, M., Xuereb, J.H., McKenna, P.J., and Wischik, C.M. (1995). Apolipoprotein E type epsilon 4 allele frequency is increased in patients with schizophrenia. *Neurosci. Lett.* **202** (1–2), 101–4.

Horimoto, Y., Matsumoto, M., Nakazawa, H., Yuasa, H., Morishita, M., Akatsu, H., Ikari, H., Yamamoto, T., and Kosaka, K. (2003). Cognitive conditions of pathologically confirmed dementia with Lewy bodies and Parkinson's disease with dementia. *J. Neurol. Sci.* **216** (1), 105–8.

Houlden, H., Crook, R., Dolan, R.J., McLaughlin, J., Revesz, T., and Hardy, J. (2001). A novel presenilin mutation (M233V) causing very early onset Alzheimer's disease with Lewy bodies. *Neurosci. Lett.* **313** (1–2), 93–5.

Hughes, A.J., Daniel, S.E., Kilford, L., and Lees, A.J. (1992). Accuracy of clinical diagnosis of idiopathic Parkinson's disease: a clinico-pathological study of 100 cases. *J. Neurol. Neurosurg. Psychiatry* **55** (3), 181–4.

Hughes, T.A., Ross, H.F., Musa, S., Bhattacherjee, S., Nathan, R.N., Mindham, R.H., and Spokes, E.G. (2000). A 10-year study of the incidence of and factors predicting dementia in Parkinson's disease. *Neurology* **54** (8), 1596–602.

Hurtig, H.I., Trojanowski, J.Q., Galvin, J., Ewbank, D., Schmidt, M.L., Lee, V.M., Clark, C.M., Glosser, G., Stern, M.B., Gollomp, S.M., and Arnold, S.E. (2000). Alpha-synuclein cortical Lewy bodies correlate with dementia in Parkinson's disease. *Neurology* **54** (10), 1916–21.

Ibanez, P., Bonnet, A.M., Debarges, B., Lohmann, E., Tison, F., Pollak, P., Agid, Y., Durr, A., and Brice, A. (2004). Causal relation between alpha-synuclein gene duplication and familial Parkinson's disease. *Lancet* **364** (9440), 1169–71.

Irizarry, M.C., Growdon, W., Gomez-Isla, T., Newell, K., George, J.M., Clayton, D.F., and Hyman, B.T. (1998). Nigral and cortical Lewy bodies and dystrophic nigral neurites in Parkinson's disease and cortical Lewy body disease contain alpha-synuclein immunoreactivity. *J. Neuropathol. Exp. Neurol.* **57** (4), 334–7.

Ishii, K., Yamaji, S., Kitagaki, H., Imamura, T., Hirono, N., and Mori, E. (1999). Regional cerebral blood flow difference between dementia with Lewy bodies and AD. *Neurology* **53** (2), 413–16.

Ishii, K., Hosaka, K., Mori, T., and Mori, E. (2004). Comparison of FDG-PET and IMP-SPECT in patients with dementia with Lewy bodies. *Ann. Nucl. Med.* **18** (5), 447–51.

Ishikawa, A., Piao, Y.S., Miyashita, A., Kuwano, R., Onodera, O., Ohtake, H., Suzuki, M., Nishizawa, M., and Takahashi, H. (2005). A mutant PSEN1 causes dementia with Lewy bodies and variant Alzheimer's disease. *Ann. Neurol.* **57** (3), 429–34.

Jacobs, D.M., Marder, K., Cote, L.J., Sano, M., Stern, Y., and Mayeux, R. (1995). Neuropsychological characteristics of preclinical dementia in Parkinson's disease. *Neurology* **45** (9), 1691–6.

Janvin, C., Aarsland, D., Larsen, J.P., and Hugdahl, K. (2003). Neuropsychological profile of patients with Parkinson's disease without dementia. *Dement. Geriatr. Cogn Disord.* **15** (3), 126–31.

Janvin, C.C., Aarsland, D., and Larsen, J.P. (2005). Cognitive predictors of dementia in Parkinson's disease: a community-based, 4-year longitudinal study. *J. Geriatr. Psychiatry Neurol.* **18** (3), 149–54.

Janvin, C.C., Larsen, J.P., Salmon, D.P., Galasko, D., Hugdahl, K., and Aarsland, D. (2006). Cognitive profiles of individual patients with Parkinson's disease and dementia: comparison with dementia with lewy bodies and Alzheimer's disease. *Mov Disord.* **21** (3), 337–42.

Klatka, L.A., Louis, E.D., and Schiffer, R.B. (1996). Psychiatric features in diffuse Lewy body disease: a clinicopathologic study using Alzheimer's disease and Parkinson's disease comparison groups. *Neurology* **47** (5), 1148–52.

Knopman, D.S., DeKosky, S.T., Cummings, J.L., Chui, H., Corey-Bloom, J., Relkin, N., Small, G.W., Miller, B., and Stevens, J.C. (2001). Practice parameter: diagnosis of dementia (an evidence-based review). Report of the Quality Standards Subcommittee of the American Academy of Neurology. *Neurology* **56** (9), 1143–53.

Kosaka, K., Yoshimura, M., Ikeda, K., and Budka, H. (1984). Diffuse type of Lewy body disease: progressive dementia with abundant cortical Lewy bodies and senile changes of varying degree–a new disease?. *Clin. Neuropathol.* **3** (5), 185–92.

Kovari, E., Gold, G., Herrmann, F.R., Canuto, A., Hof, P.R., Bouras, C., and Giannakopoulos, P. (2003). Lewy body densities in the entorhinal and anterior cingulate cortex predict cognitive deficits in Parkinson's disease. *Acta Neuropathol. (Berl.)* **106** (1), 83–8.

Laakso, M.P., Partanen, K., Riekkinen, P., Lehtovirta, M., Helkala, E.L., Hallikainen, M., Hanninen, T., Vainio, P., and Soininen, H. (1996). Hippocampal volumes in Alzheimer's disease, Parkinson's disease with and without dementia, and in vascular dementia: an MRI study. *Neurology* **46** (3), 678–81.

Langston, J.W., Sastry, S., Chan, P., Forno, L.S., Bolin, L.M., and Di Monte, D.A. (1998). Novel alpha-synuclein-immunoreactive proteins in brain samples from the Contursi kindred, Parkinson's, and Alzheimer's disease. *Exp. Neurol.* **154** (2), 684–90.

Lennox, G., Lowe, J., Morrell, K., Landon, M., and Mayer, R. J. (1989). Anti-ubiquitin immunocytochemistry is more sensitive than conventional techniques in the detection of diffuse Lewy body disease. *J. Neurol. Neurosurg. Psychiatry* **52** (1), 67–71.

Levy, G., Jacobs, D.M., Tang, M.X., Cote, L.J., Louis, E.D., Alfaro, B., Mejia, H., Stern, Y., and Marder, K. (2002). Memory and executive function impairment predict dementia in Parkinson's disease. *Mov Disord.* **17** (6), 1221–6.

Lippa, C.F., Smith, T.W., Saunders, A.M., Crook, R., Pulaski-Salo, D., Davies, P., Hardy, J., Roses, A.D., and Dickson, D. (1995). Apolipoprotein E genotype and Lewy body disease. *Neurology* **45** (1), 97–103.

Lippa, C.F., Fujiwara, H., Mann, D.M., Giasson, B., Baba, M., Schmidt, M.L., Nee, L.E., O'Connell, B., Pollen, D.A., George-Hyslop, P., Ghetti, B., Nochlin, D., Bird, T.D., Cairns, N.J., Lee, V.M., Iwatsubo, T., and Trojanowski, J.Q. (1998). Lewy bodies contain altered alpha-synuclein in brains of many familial Alzheimer's disease patients with mutations in presenilin and amyloid precursor protein genes. *Am. J. Pathol.* **153** (5), 1365–70.

Lippa, C.F., Ozawa, K., Mann, D.M., Ishii, K., Smith, T.W., Arawaka, S., and Mori, H. (1999*a*). Deposition of beta-amyloid subtypes 40 and 42 differentiates dementia with Lewy bodies from Alzheimer disease. *Arch. Neurol.* **56** (9), 1111–18.

Lippa, C.F., Schmidt, M.L., Lee, V.M., and Trojanowski, J.Q. (1999*b*). Antibodies to alpha-synuclein detect Lewy bodies in many Down's syndrome brains with Alzheimer's disease. *Ann. Neurol.* **45** (3), 353–7.

Lippa, C.F., Schmidt, M.L., Lee, V.M., and Trojanowski, J.Q. (2001). Alpha-synuclein in familial Alzheimer disease: epitope mapping parallels dementia with Lewy bodies and Parkinson disease. *Arch. Neurol.* **58** (11), 1817–20.

Lobotesis, K., Fenwick, J.D., Phipps, A., Ryman, A., Swann, A., Ballard, C., McKeith, I.G., and O'Brien, J.T. (2001). Occipital hypoperfusion on SPECT in dementia with Lewy bodies but not AD. *Neurology* **56** (5), 643–9.

Lopez, O.L., Becker, J.T., Kaufer, D.I., Hamilton, R.L., Sweet, R.A., Klunk, W., and DeKosky, S.T. (2002). Research evaluation and prospective diagnosis of dementia with Lewy bodies. *Arch. Neurol.* **59** (1), 43–6.

Louis, E.D., Marder, K., Cote, L., Tang, M., and Mayeux, R. (1997). Mortality from Parkinson disease. *Arch. Neurol.* **54** (3), 260–4.

Mahieux, F., Fenelon, G., Flahault, A., Manifacier, M.J., Michelet, D., and Boller, F. (1998). Neuropsychological prediction of dementia in Parkinson's disease. *J. Neurol. Neurosurg. Psychiatry* **64** (2), 178–83.

Mann, D.M., Brown, S.M., Owen, F., Baba, M., and Iwatsubo, T. (1998). Amyloid beta protein (A beta) deposition in dementia with Lewy bodies: predominance of A beta 42(43) and paucity of A beta 40 compared with sporadic Alzheimer's disease. *Neuropathol. Appl. Neurobiol.* **24** (3), 187–94.

Marder, K., Leung, D., Tang, M., Bell, K., Dooneief, G., Cote, L., Stern, Y., and Mayeux, R. (1991). Are demented patients with Parkinson's disease accurately reflected in prevalence surveys? A survival analysis. *Neurology* **41** (8), 1240–3.

Marder, K., Tang, M.X., Cote, L., Stern, Y., and Mayeux, R. (1995). The frequency and associated risk factors for dementia in patients with Parkinson's disease. *Arch. Neurol.* **52** (7), 695–701.

Marinus, J., Visser, M., Verwey, N.A., Verhey, F.R., Middelkoop, H.A., Stiggelbout, A.M., and van Hilten, J.J. (2003). Assessment of cognition in Parkinson's disease. *Neurology* **61** (9), 1222–8.

Marui, W., Iseki, E., Nakai, T., Miura, S., Kato, M., Ueda, K., and Kosaka, K. (2002). Progression and staging of Lewy pathology in brains from patients with dementia with Lewy bodies. *J. Neurol. Sci.* **195** (2), 153–9.

Mattila, P.M., Roytta, M., Torikka, H., Dickson, D.W., and Rinne, J.O. (1998). Cortical Lewy bodies and Alzheimer-type changes in patients with Parkinson's disease. *Acta Neuropathol. (Berl.)* **95** (6), 576–82.

Mattila, P.M., Rinne, J.O., Helenius, H., Dickson, D.W., and Roytta, M. (2000). Alpha-synuclein-immunoreactive cortical Lewy bodies are associated with cognitive impairment in Parkinson's disease. *Acta Neuropathol. (Berl.)* **100** (3), 285–90.

Mayeux, R., Chen, J., Mirabello, E., Marder, K., Bell, K., Dooneief, G., Cote, L., and Stern, Y. (1990). An estimate of the incidence of dementia in idiopathic Parkinson's disease. *Neurology* **40** (10), 1513–17.

McKeith, I., Fairbairn, A., Perry, R., Thompson, P., and Perry, E. (1992). Neuroleptic sensitivity in patients with senile dementia of Lewy body type. *Br. Med. J.* **305** (6855), 673–8.

McKeith, I.G., Galasko, D., Kosaka, K., Perry, E.K., Dickson, D.W., Hansen, L.A., Salmon, D.P., Lowe, J., Mirra, S.S., Byrne, E.J., Lennox, G., Quinn, N.P., Edwardson, J.A., Ince, P.G., Bergeron, C., Burns, A., Miller, B.L., Lovestone, S., Collerton, D., Jansen, E.N., Ballard, C., de Vos, R.A., Wilcock, G.K., Jellinger, K.A., and Perry, R.H. (1996). Consensus guidelines for the clinical and pathologic diagnosis of dementia with Lewy bodies (DLB): report of the consortium on DLB international workshop. *Neurology* **47** (5), 1113–24.

McKeith, I., Del Ser, T., Spano, P., Emre, M., Wesnes, K., Anand, R., Cicin-Sain, A., Ferrara, R., and Spiegel, R. (2000). Efficacy of rivastigmine in dementia with Lewy bodies: a randomised, double-blind, placebo-controlled international study. *Lancet* **356** (9247), 2031–6.

McKeith, I., Mintzer, J., Aarsland, D., Burn, D., Chiu, H., Cohen-Mansfield, J., Dickson, D., Dubois, B., Duda, J.E., Feldman, H., Gauthier, S., Halliday, G., Lawlor, B., Lippa, C., Lopez, O.L., Carlos, M.J., O'Brien, J., Playfer, J., and Reid, W. (2004). Dementia with Lewy bodies. *Lancet Neurol.* **3** (1), 19–28.

McKeith, I.G., Dickson, D.W., Lowe, J., Emre, M., O'Brien, J.T., Feldman, H., Cummings, J., Duda, J.E., Lippa, C., Perry, E.K., Aarsland, D., Arai, H., Ballard, C.G., Boeve, B., Burn, D.J., Costa, D., Del Ser, T., Dubois, B., Galasko, D., Gauthier, S., Goetz, C.G., Gomez-Tortosa, E., Halliday, G., Hansen, L.A., Hardy, J., Iwatsubo, T., Kalaria, R.N., Kaufer, D., Kenny, R.A., Korczyn, A., Kosaka, K., Lee, V.M., Lees, A., Litvan, I., Londos, E., Lopez, O.L., Minoshima, S., Mizuno, Y., Molina, J.A., Mukaetova-Ladinska, E.B., Pasquier, F., Perry, R.H., Schulz, J.B., Trojanowski, J.Q., and Yamada, M. (2005). Diagnosis and management of dementia with Lewy bodies: third report of the DLB Consortium. *Neurology* **65** (12), 1863–72.

McKeith, I.G., Rowan, E., askew, K., Naidu, A., Allan, L., Barnett, N., *et al.* (2006). More severe functional impairment in dementia with Lewy bodies than Alzheimer disease is related to extrapyramidal motor dysfunction. *J. Am. Geriatr. Soc.* **14**, 582–8.

Menendez-Gonzalez, M., Calatayud, M.T., and Blazquez-Menes, B. (2005). Exacerbation of Lewy bodies dementia due to memantine. *J. Alzheimers. Dis.* **8** (3), 289–91.

Merdes, A.R., Hansen, L.A., Jeste, D.V., Galasko, D., Hofstetter, C.R., Ho, G.J., Thal, L.J., and Corey-Bloom, J. (2003). Influence of Alzheimer pathology on clinical diagnostic accuracy in dementia with Lewy bodies. *Neurology* **60** (10), 1586–90.

Mindham, R.H., Ahmed, S.W., and Clough, C.G. (1982). A controlled study of dementia in Parkinson's disease. *J. Neurol. Neurosurg. Psychiatry* **45** (11), 969–74.

Minett, T.S., Thomas, A., Wilkinson, L.M., Daniel, S.L., Sanders, J., Richardson, J., Littlewood, E., Myint, P., Newby, J., and McKeith, I.G. (2003). What happens when donepezil is suddenly withdrawn? An open label trial in dementia with Lewy bodies and Parkinson's disease with dementia. *Int. J. Geriatr. Psychiatry* **18** (11), 988–93.

Minoshima, S., Foster, N.L., Sima, A.A., Frey, K.A., Albin, R.L., and Kuhl, D.E. (2001). Alzheimer's disease versus dementia with Lewy bodies: cerebral metabolic distinction with autopsy confirmation. *Ann. Neurol.* **50** (3), 358–65.

Miyasaki, J.M., Shannon, K., Voon, V., Ravina, B., Kleiner-Fisman, G., Anderson, K., Shulman, L.M., Gronseth, G., and Weiner, W.J. (2006). Practice parameter: evaluation and treatment of depression, psychosis, and dementia in Parkinson disease (an evidence-based review): report of the Quality Standards Subcommittee of the American Academy of Neurology. *Neurology* **66** (7), 996–1002.

Molloy, S., McKeith, I.G., O'Brien, J.T., and Burn, D.J. (2005). The role of levodopa in the management of dementia with Lewy bodies. *J. Neurol. Neurosurg. Psychiatry* **76** (9), 1200–3.

Noe, E., Marder, K., Bell, K.L., Jacobs, D.M., Manly, J.J., and Stern, Y. (2004). Comparison of dementia with Lewy bodies to Alzheimer's disease and Parkinson's disease with dementia. *Mov Disord.* **19** (1), 60–7.

O'Brien, J.T., Colloby, S., Fenwick, J., Williams, E.D., Firbank, M., Burn, D., Aarsland, D., and McKeith, I.G. (2004). Dopamine transporter loss visualized with FP-CIT SPECT in the differential diagnosis of dementia with Lewy bodies. *Arch. Neurol.* **61** (6), 919–25.

Ohara, K., Takauchi, S., Kokai, M., Morimura, Y., Nakajima, T., and Morita, Y. (1999). Familial dementia with Lewy bodies (DLB). *Clin. Neuropathol.* **18** (5), 232–9.

Oide, T., Tokuda, T., Momose, M., Oguchi, K., Nakamura, A., Ohara, S., and Ikeda, S. (2003). Usefulness of [123I]metaiodobenzylguanidine ([123I]MIBG) myocardial scintigraphy in differentiating between Alzheimer's disease and dementia with Lewy bodies. *Intern. Med.* **42** (8), 686–90.

Paisan-Ruiz, C., Jain, S., Evans, E.W., Gilks, W.P., Simon, J., van der, B.M., Lopez, d.M., Aparicio, S., Gil, A.M., Khan, N., Johnson, J., Martinez, J.R., Nicholl, D., Carrera, I.M., Pena, A.S., de Silva, R., Lees, A., Marti-Masso, J.F., Perez-Tur, J., Wood, N.W., and Singleton, A.B. (2004). Cloning of the gene containing mutations that cause PARK8-linked Parkinson's disease. *Neuron* **44** (4), 595–600.

Perry, R.H., Irving, D., Blessed, G., Fairbairn, A., and Perry, E.K. (1990). Senile dementia of Lewy body type. A clinically and neuropathologically distinct form of Lewy body dementia in the elderly. *J. Neurol. Sci.* **95** (2), 119–39.

Polymeropoulos, M.H., Lavedan, C., Leroy, E., Ide, S.E., Dehejia, A., Dutra, A., Pike, B., Root, H., Rubenstein, J., Boyer, R., Stenroos, E.S., Chandrasekharappa, S., Athanassiadou, A., Papapetropoulos, T., Johnson, W.G., Lazzarini, A.M., Duvoisin, R.C., Di Iorio, G., Golbe, L.I., and Nussbaum, R.L. (1997). Mutation in the alpha-synuclein gene identified in families with Parkinson's disease. *Science* **276** (5321), 2045–7.

Pompeu, F. and Growdon, J.H. (2002). Diagnosing dementia with Lewy bodies. *Arch. Neurol.* **59** (1), 29–30.

Rahkonen, T., Eloniemi-Sulkava, U., Rissanen, S., Vatanen, A., Viramo, P., and Sulkava, R. (2003). Dementia with Lewy bodies according to the consensus criteria in a general population aged 75 years or older. *J. Neurol. Neurosurg. Psychiatry* **74** (6), 720–4.

Ravina, B., Putt, M., Siderowf, A., Farrar, J.T., Gillespie, M., Crawley, A., Fernandez, H.H., Trieschmann, M.M., Reichwein, S., and Simuni, T. (2005). Donepezil for dementia in Parkinson's disease: a randomised, double blind, placebo controlled, crossover study. *J. Neurol. Neurosurg. Psychiatry* **76** (7), 934–9.

Revesz, T., McLaughlin, J.L., Rossor, M.N., and Lantos, P.L. (1997). Pathology of familial Alzheimer's disease with Lewy bodies. *J. Neural Transm. Suppl.* **51**, 121–35.

Ridha, B.H., Josephs, K.A., and Rossor, M. N. (2005). Delusions and hallucinations in dementia with Lewy bodies: worsening with memantine. *Neurology* **65** (3), 481–482.

Royall, D.R., Mahurin, R.K., and Gray, K.F. (1992). Bedside assessment of executive cognitive impairment: the executive interview. *J. Am. Geriatr. Soc.* **40** (12), 1221–6.

Sabbagh, M.N., Hake, A.M., Ahmed, S., and Farlow, M.R. (2005). The use of memantine in dementia with Lewy bodies. *J. Alzheimers Dis.* **7** (4), 285–9.

Samuel, W., Galasko, D., Masliah, E., and Hansen, L.A. (1996). Neocortical lewy body counts correlate with dementia in the Lewy body variant of Alzheimer's disease. *J. Neuropathol. Exp. Neurol.* **55** (1), 44–52.

Samuel, W., Alford, M., Hofstetter, C.R., and Hansen, L. (1997*a*). Dementia with Lewy bodies versus pure Alzheimer disease: differences in cognition, neuropathology, cholinergic dysfunction, and synapse density. *J. Neuropathol. Exp. Neurol.* **56** (5), 499–508.

Samuel, W., Crowder, R., Hofstetter, C.R., and Hansen, L. (1997*b*). Neuritic plaques in the Lewy body variant of Alzheimer disease lack paired helical filaments. *Neurosci. Lett.* **223** (2), 73–6.

Samuel, W., Caligiuri, M., Galasko, D., Lacro, J., Marini, M., McClure, F.S., Warren, K., and Jeste, D. V. (2000). Better cognitive and psychopathologic response to donepezil in patients prospectively diagnosed as dementia with Lewy bodies: a preliminary study. *Int. J. Geriatr. Psychiatry* **15** (9), 794–802.

Singleton, A. and Gwinn-Hardy, K. (2004). Parkinson's disease and dementia with Lewy bodies: a difference in dose? *Lancet* **364** (9440), 1105–7.

Singleton, A.B., Wharton, A., O'Brien, K.K., Walker, M.P., McKeith, I.G., Ballard, C.G., O'Brien, J., Perry, R.H., Ince, P.G., Edwardson, J.A., and Morris, C.M. (2002). Clinical and neuropathological correlates of apolipoprotein E genotype in dementia with Lewy bodies. *Dement. Geriatr. Cogn Disord.* **14** (4), 167–75.

Singleton, A.B., Farrer, M., Johnson, J., Singleton, A., Hague, S., Kachergus, J., Hulihan, M., Peuralinna, T., Dutra, A., Nussbaum, R., Lincoln, S., Crawley, A., Hanson, M., Maraganore, D., Adler, C., Cookson, M.R., Muenter, M., Baptista, M., Miller, D., Blancato, J., Hardy, J., and Gwinn-Hardy, K. (2003). Alpha-synuclein locus triplication causes Parkinson's disease. *Science* **302** (5646), 841.

Snider, B.J., Norton, J., Coats, M.A., Chakraverty, S., Hou, C.E., Jervis, R., Lendon, C.L., Goate, A.M., McKeel, D.W., Jr., and Morris, J.C. (2005). Novel presenilin 1 mutation (S170F) causing Alzheimer disease with Lewy bodies in the third decade of life. *Arch. Neurol.* **62** (12), 1821–30.

Starkstein, S.E., Mayberg, H.S., Leiguarda, R., Preziosi, T.J., and Robinson, R.G. (1992). A prospective longitudinal study of depression, cognitive decline, and physical impairments in patients with Parkinson's disease. *J. Neurol. Neurosurg. Psychiatry* **55** (5), 377–82.

Stern, Y., Marder, K., Tang, M.X., and Mayeux, R. (1993). Antecedent clinical features associated with dementia in Parkinson's disease. *Neurology* **43** (9), 1690–2.

Szpak, G.M., Lewandowska, E., Lechowicz, W., Bertrand, E., Wierzba-Bobrowicz, T., Gwiazda, E., Pasennik, E., Kosno-Kruszewska, E., Lipczynska-Lojkowska, W., Bochynska, A., and Fiszer, U. (2001). Lewy body variant of Alzheimer's disease and Alzheimer's disease: a comparative immunohistochemical study. *Folia Neuropathol.* **39** (2), 63–71.

Tagliavini, F., Pilleri, G., Bouras, C., and Constantinidis, J. (1984). The basal nucleus of Meynert in idiopathic Parkinson's disease. *Acta Neurol. Scand.* **70** (1), 20–8.

Thomas, A.J., Burn, D.J., Rowan, E.N., Littlewood, E., Newby, J., Cousins, D., Pakrasi, S., Richardson, J., Sanders, J., and McKeith, I.G. (2005). A comparison of the efficacy of donepezil in Parkinson's disease with dementia and dementia with Lewy bodies. *Int. J. Geriatr. Psychiatry* **20** (10), 938–44.

Tiraboschi, P., Salmon, D.P., Hansen, L.A., Hofstetter, R.C., Thal, L.J., and Corey-Bloom, J. (2006). What best differentiates Lewy body from Alzheimer's disease in early-stage dementia? *Brain* **129**, 729–35.

Tolosa, E., Wenning, G., and Poewe, W. (2006). The diagnosis of Parkinson's disease. *Lancet Neurol.* **5** (1), 75–86.

Trembath, Y., Rosenberg, C., Ervin, J.F., Schmechel, D.E., Gaskell, P., Pericak-Vance, M., Vance, J., and Hulette, C.M. (2003). Lewy body pathology is a frequent co-pathology in familial Alzheimer's disease. *Acta Neuropathol. (Berl.)* **105** (5), 484–8.

Tsuang, D.W., Dalan, A.M., Eugenio, C.J., Poorkaj, P., Limprasert, P., La Spada, A.R., Steinbart, E.J., Bird, T.D., and Leverenz, J.B. (2002). Familial dementia with Lewy bodies: a clinical and neuropathological study of 2 families. *Arch. Neurol.* **59** (10), 1622–30.

Tsuang, D.W., DiGiacomo, L., and Bird, T.D. (2004). Familial occurrence of dementia with Lewy bodies. *Am. J. Geriatr. Psychiatry* **12** (2), 179–88.

Tsuboi, Y. and Dickson, D.W. (2005). Dementia with Lewy bodies and Parkinson's disease with dementia: are they different? *Parkinsonism Relat Disord.* **11** (Suppl. 1), S47–S51.

Wakisaka, Y., Furuta, A., Tanizaki, Y., Kiyohara, Y., Iida, M., and Iwaki, T. (2003). Age-associated prevalence and risk factors of Lewy body pathology in a general population: the Hisayama study. *Acta Neuropathol. (Berl.)* **106** (4), 374–82.

Walker, M.P., Ayre, G.A., Cummings, J.L., Wesnes, K., McKeith, I.G., O'Brien, J.T., and Ballard, C.G. (2000). The clinician assessment of fluctuation and the one day fluctuation Assessment scale. Two methods to assess fluctuating confusion in dementia. *Br. J. Psychiatry* **177**, 252–6.

Walker, Z., Allen, R.L., Shergill, S., and Katona, C.L. (1997). Neuropsychological performance in Lewy body dementia and Alzheimer's disease. *Br. J. Psychiatry* **170**, 156–8.

Walker, Z., Allen, R.L., Shergill, S., Mullan, E., and Katona, C.L. (2000). Three years survival in patients with a clinical diagnosis of dementia with Lewy bodies. *Int. J. Geriatr. Psychiatry* **15** (3), 267–73.

Walker, Z., Costa, D.C., Walker, R.W., Shaw, K., Gacinovic, S., Stevens, T., Livingston, G., Ince, P., McKeith, I.G., and Katona, C.L. (2002). Differentiation of dementia with Lewy bodies from Alzheimer's disease using a dopaminergic presynaptic ligand. *J. Neurol. Neurosurg. Psychiatry* **73** (2), 134–40.

Walter, U., Wittstock, M., Benecke, R., and Dressler, D. (2002). Substantia nigra echogenicity is normal in non-extrapyramidal cerebral disorders but increased in Parkinson's disease. *J. Neural Transm.* **109** (2), 191–6.

Walter, U., Niehaus, L., Probst, T., Benecke, R., Meyer, B.U., and Dressler, D. (2003). Brain parenchyma sonography discriminates Parkinson's disease and atypical parkinsonian syndromes. *Neurology* **60** (1), 74–7.

Walter, U., Dressler, D., Wolters, A., Wittstock, M., Greim, B., and Benecke, R. (2006). Sonographic discrimination of dementia with Lewy bodies and Parkinson's disease with dementia. *J. Neurol.* **253** (4), 448–54.

Watanabe, H., Ieda, T., Katayama, T., Takeda, A., Aiba, I., Doyu, M., Hirayama, M., and Sobue, G. (2001). Cardiac (123)I-meta-iodobenzylguanidine (MIBG) uptake in dementia with Lewy bodies: comparison with Alzheimer's disease. *J. Neurol. Neurosurg. Psychiatry* **70** (6), 781–3.

Weintraub, D., Moberg, P.J., Culbertson, W.C., Duda, J.E., and Stern, M.B. (2004). Evidence for impaired encoding and retrieval memory profiles in Parkinson disease. *Cogn Behav. Neurol.* **17** (4), 195–200.

Weintraub, D., Moberg, P.J., Culbertson, W.C., Duda, J.E., Katz, I.R., and Stern, M.B. (2005). Dimensions of executive function in Parkinson's disease. *Dement. Geriatr. Cogn Disord.* **20** (2–3), 140–4.

Wesnes, K.A., McKeith, I., Edgar, C., Emre, M., and Lane, R. (2005). Benefits of rivastigmine on attention in dementia associated with Parkinson disease. *Neurology* **65** (10), 1654–6.

Whitehouse, P.J., Hedreen, J.C., White, C.L., III, and Price, D.L. (1983). Basal forebrain neurons in the dementia of Parkinson disease. *Ann. Neurol.* **13** (3), 243–8.

Woods, S. P. and Troster, A. I. (2003). Prodromal frontal/executive dysfunction predicts incident dementia in Parkinson's disease. *J. Int. Neuropsychol. Soc.* **9** (1), 17–24.

Yoshita, M., Taki, J., and Yamada, M. (2001). A clinical role for [(123)I]MIBG myocardial scintigraphy in the distinction between dementia of the Alzheimer's-type and dementia with Lewy bodies. *J. Neurol. Neurosurg. Psychiatry* **71** (5), 583–8.

Zaccai, J., McCracken, C., and Brayne, C. (2005). A systematic review of prevalence and incidence studies of dementia with Lewy bodies. *Age Ageing* **34** (6), 561–566.

Zarranz, J.J., Alegre, J., Gomez-Esteban, J.C., Lezcano, E., Ros, R., Ampuero, I., Vidal, L., Hoenicka, J., Rodriguez, O., Atares, B., Llorens, V., Gomez, T.E., Del Ser, T., Munoz, D.G., and de Yebenes, J.G. (2004). The new mutation, E46K, of alpha-synuclein causes Parkinson and Lewy body dementia. *Ann. Neurol.* **55** (2), 164–73.

Zimprich, A., Biskup, S., Leitner, P., Lichtner, P., Farrer, M., Lincoln, S., Kachergus, J., Hulihan, M., Uitti, R.J., Calne, D.B., Stoessl, A.J., Pfeiffer, R.F., Patenge, N., Carbajal, I.C., Vieregge, P., Asmus, F., Muller-Myhsok, B., Dickson, D.W., Meitinger, T., Strom, T.M., Wszolek, Z.K., and Gasser, T. (2004). Mutations in LRRK2 cause autosomal-dominant parkinsonism with pleomorphic pathology. *Neuron* **44** (4), 601–7.

Chapter 15

Genetics of dementia

William S. Brooks, Clement T. Loy, John B. J. Kwok, and Peter R. Schofield

15.1 Introduction

- Most cases of dementia are sporadic and occur with increasing age.
- Dementia with a genetic cause tends to present in younger patients.
- Alzheimer's disease, frontotemporal lobar degeneration, prion disease, and Huntington's disease are the most frequently encountered genetically determined forms.

The clinical syndrome of dementia can occur in a range of conditions. Some dementia-causing diseases are clearly genetic in origin, such as Huntington's disease (HD) or familial Alzheimer's disease (AD). However, most people with dementia have no obvious cause for their condition. The clearest risk factor for dementia is increasing age, with prevalence approximately doubling with each increase of 5.1 years (Jorm *et al.* 1987). Many patients with dementia have one or more affected first-degree relatives, which most people believe points to a genetic influence rather than a shared environmental one. Rarely, the family history reveals multiple affected members over several generations in a pattern consistent with Mendelian dominant inheritance. Such families are of great importance as they have the potential to increase our understanding of the dementia-causing diseases in general. Although most studies have found that familial dementia is more likely to have a young onset age, it is not uncommon for quite convincing family histories to be encountered in families with onset ages above 70 years. The discovery of disease-causing mutations in recent years has provided explanations for many families with AD and some with familial frontotemporal dementia (FTD), and it is true that the majority of people in such families have a young onset age. The search for genetic influences in later-onset dementia has been less rewarding, though the ε4 allele of the apolipoprotein E gene (APOE) on chromosome 19 is accepted as a risk factor in most population groups studied.

In this chapter we provide an overview of familial AD and its causative genes, familial frontotemporal dementias, and related conditions with non-Alzheimer pathology: these are the most common conditions likely to be seen in memory clinics. We then mention rarer dementia-causing diseases, including HD and familial prion diseases, and conclude by considering some practical questions that occur in clinical settings.

15.2 Familial Alzheimer's disease

- Mutations in three genes have been identified in kindreds with familial AD:
  - amyloid precursor protein (APP) on chromosome 21;
  - presenilin-1 (PS-1) on chromosome 14;
  - presenilin-2 (PS-2) on chromosome 1.
- The mechanisms connecting mutation to disease are complex and incompletely understood. Although many appear to be linked to an increase in amyloid deposition, some PS-1 mutations may be associated with non-amyloid based or even non-Alzheimer processes.

Families with two or more affected members have been reported since the 1930s. The inheritance pattern is usually autosomal dominant. Alzheimer's second case, Johann F., was later found to be the index case of a family with 17 probably affected members in six generations (Klunemann *et al.* 2002), though the absence of neurofibrillary tangles (NFTs) meant that the neuropathology was atypical. A number of large kindreds were studied in the search for a genetic marker: the discovery of the amyloid precursor protein in 1985 and the location of the gene responsible on chromosome 21 led to hopes that this gene would account for all familial AD and provide major insights into the biology of non-familial cases. The association between AD and Down syndrome (DS) made this particularly attractive.

Mutations in three genes have now been identified in kindreds with dominantly inherited familial AD. Two websites maintain an online directory of published mutations in the familial AD genes and the tau gene, which has been implicated in familial frontotemporal dementia. They are the Alzheimer Disease and Frontotemporal Dementia Mutation Database, curated by Marc Cruts and Roos Rademakers (*http://www.molgen.ua.ac.be/ADMutations/default.cfm*) and the Alzheimer Research Forum (*http://www.alzforum.org*) curated by John Hardy and Jennifer Kwon.

15.2.1 Amyloid precursor protein (APP) gene

The Aβ peptide is the major constituent of senile, neuritic, and diffuse plaques in AD. It is produced in two main isoforms, 40 and 42 amino acids long, and is a breakdown product of the much longer amyloid precursor protein (APP), which has a putative structure suggesting that it is a cell membrane receptor. The gene for this protein is on the long arm of chromosome 21. People with DS develop the pathological changes of AD in their thirties, though not all develop typical Alzheimer dementia. They develop AD pathology because of a gene dosage effect—the extra copy of chromosome 21 causes increased expression of APP and increased production (secretion) of the Aβ peptide. It was hoped that this gene would prove to be the sole gene responsible for AD and, indeed, some families with hereditary AD showed linkage to a locus on chromosome 21, though others did not. Eventually, a mutation at position 717 of the APP gene (V717I) was found in two families with hereditary AD (Goate *et al.* 1991). Screening for this mutation in other families showed that it was found in only a few, with many remaining unexplained. Nonetheless, 29 families from various ethnic backgrounds have now been reported with this mutation (for details, see AD and FTD Mutation Database as above), and three other mutations have been found at the same site (V717L, 3 families, V717F, 3 families and V717G, 1 family).

Three enzymes are involved in the cleavage of APP. α-secretase cleaves the gene product between codons 687 and 688, which is well within the Aβ-coding region so no intact Aβ is released. Processing by β-secretase and γ-secretase produces the two main isoforms of Aβ peptide of differing length, with the shorter, 40 amino acid form, Aβ40, being more abundant. The longer 42 amino acid form, Aβ42, is more likely to aggregate and hence become deposited in the brain. Most AD-associated APP mutations are located near the secretase cleavage sites and presumably make the precursor protein either less amenable to α-secretase activity or more amenable to β-secretase and γ-secretase, thus promoting the release of intact Aβ peptide.

The mutations at position 717 are located just beyond the *C*-terminal end of the Aβ-coding region, near the putative γ-secretase site. Mutations have also been found at positions 716, 715, 714, and 713, though mutations at position 713 have been found in unaffected individuals and their causative status remains to be confirmed. A single Australian family has been reported with a mutation at position 723 (L723P; Kwok *et al.* 2000), the most *C*-terminal so far described.

Only one familial AD (FAD)-associated mutation has been found at the *N*-terminal end of the Aβ coding segment. This is a double mutation at positions 670 and 671 (K670N/M671L; Mullan *et al.* 1992*a*) and was found in two large Swedish families that were probably related. The β-secretase cleavage site is between codons 671 and 672.

Other mutations reported in this region have not been shown to segregate with AD or have been found in individuals with other conditions such as schizophrenia.

Mutations within the Aβ coding region are associated with amyloid deposits in the cerebral vessel walls, known as cerebral amyloid angiopathy (CAA), either alone or in combination with AD neuropathology. The first to be described was E693Q, 6 codons *C*-terminal of the α-secretase site, in a Dutch kindred with hereditary cerebral haemorrhage as the main clinical manifestation; progressive dementia occurred in some cases (Haan *et al.* 1990; Levy *et al.* 1990). The neuropathology of affected members of this kindred showed angiopathy with amyloid deposition. Diffuse plaques were present but only minimal tangles. The amyloid was found to be identical to that deposited in the plaques in AD and in the blood vessels of patients with AD and CAA, but three residues shorter (39 instead of 42; Natte *et al.* 2001; Prelli *et al.* 1988). The condition is known as hereditary cerebral haemorrhage with amyloidosis—Dutch type (HCHWA-D). A different mutation at the same site, E693G, was reported in a patient with autopsy-confirmed AD with onset at 56 years (Kamino *et al.* 1992). An affected sibling did not have the mutation, however. This mutation, known as the 'Arctic mutation', was later found in six affected members of a Swedish family with a mean age of onset of 57 years (range, 54–61 years; Nilsberth *et al.* 2001). The adjacent Flemish mutation, A692G, was found in a kindred in which the clinical features included recurrent cerebral haemorrhage and, in some cases, progressive dementia (Hendriks *et al.* 1992). The neuropathology, in contrast to that associated with the neighbouring E693Q mutation, included plaques and tangles as well as CAA and cerebral haemorrhage. A second family reported with this mutation is of British origin, with affected members having progressive dementia and only one of six so far having haemorrhage in addition (Brooks *et al.* 2004). Studies are underway to see whether the two families are related. Other mutations in this region, E693K, found in an Italian family (Miravalle *et al.* 2000), and D694N, found in families from Iowa (USA) and Spain, also have prominent haemorrhage and CAA (Grabowski *et al.* 2001; Greenberg *et al.* 2003). Other mutations within the Aβ coding region, more remote from the α-secretase site, include D678N, found in two affected members of a Japanese family with clinically diagnosed AD (Wakutani *et al.* 2004), and L705V, with CAA and haemorrhage but without AD neuropathology (Obici *et al.* 2005).

Finally, a recent report of five French families with a duplication of the APP locus in association with AD, CAA, and cerebral haemorrhage provides further support for the crucial role of amyloid in the pathogenesis of AD (Rovelet-Lecrux *et al.* 2006). In these families, mutation screening had not revealed mutations in APP, PS-1, or PS-2, but further studies indicated that a short segment of chromosome 21 including the APP gene and a variable number of other genes had been duplicated, presumably leading to increased production of APP and hence Aβ isoforms, as occurs in DS. The duplication was presumably inherited, as in each family a parent of the proband had died with either stroke, presenile dementia, or both. Clearly, though, the duplication did not include the full DS-related segment of chromosome 21.

APOE genotype influences onset age in AD families with APP mutations, with the APOEε4 allele being associated in general with an earlier onset age and the APOEε2 allele with a later one, though these conclusions are based on small numbers of cases (Alzheimer's Disease Collaborative Group 1993; Nacmias *et al.* 1995; Sorbi *et al.* 1995). An individual with an APP V717I mutation was found to be unaffected at an age two standard deviations higher than the mean for affected members of the family. This was thought possibly attributable to an APOEε2 allele (St George-Hyslop *et al.* 1994). This possible gene–gene interaction may provide an explanation for the apparent non-penetrance of the APP mutation. The Italian family FLO33 also included an asymptomatic mutation carrier aged 60, six years older than the latest recorded onset age in the family, and also having an APOE ε2/ε3 genotype (Sorbi *et al.* 1995). In counselling individuals who seek predictive testing, clinicians need to take into account cases like these. Although they are the only recorded instances of possible non-penetrance of an APP mutation, the absolute number of individuals studied worldwide remains low: it is not known whether this represents an incidence of the order of 1%, or much lower, or indeed whether these individuals have since developed symptoms.

APOE genotype has not been found to influence onset age in families with the Dutch (E693Q) and Flemish (A692G) APP mutations (Haan *et al.* 1994).

15.2.2 **Presenilin-1 gene**

Many families remained unexplained by sequencing for mutations in APP. Linkage to chromosome 14 was established in 1992 by several groups (Schellenberg *et al.* 1992; Mullan *et al.* 1992*b*; St George-Hyslop *et al.* 1992; Van Broeckhoven *et al.* 1992), but it was 3 years before mutations were reported in a new AD gene, subsequently called presenilin-1 (PS-1). In an international collaborative effort, five different mutations were found in eight pedigrees with dominantly inherited familial AD (Sherrington *et al.* 1995). The families were of diverse ethnic background, with two Ashkenazi Jewish families, two southern Italian, and one each of Anglo-Saxon-Celt, American Caucasian, French-Canadian, and German origin. Each of the mutations changed a residue in a highly conserved domain of the putative protein, suggesting that the mutations were pathogenic. Soon after this, the Alzheimer's Disease Collaborative Group (1995) described the structure of the gene, and reported six novel mutations, two of which (M146V and H163Y) were at the same sites as mutations reported previously.

In contrast to APP, the PS-1 gene product initially had no apparent connection with AD pathogenesis. It was homologous to a sperm transport protein found in the worm, *Caenorhabditis elegans*. PS-1 consists of 13 exons, of which 10 (exons 4 to 13) are translated (Rogaev *et al.* 1997); mutations have been found in nine of them (exons 4 to 12). With mutations being spread throughout the gene, screening of PS-1 is more difficult than screening APP where the mutations are concentrated in two exons. In addition, several kindreds have been described in which the causative mutation is a complete genomic deletion of exon 9, from flanking intron to intron (Prihar *et al.* 1999; Smith *et al.* 2001). DNA sequencing of exons therefore does not reveal the genetic abnormality.

PS-1 is the most common gene to be implicated in familial AD, with more than 100 mutations having been reported. In general, the onset age tends to be younger than in families with

APP mutations, being mostly in the fourth and fifth decades, though some individuals in these families do not develop symptoms until age 60 or older.

15.2.2.1 Phenotypic variability

Some PS-1 mutations are associated with a phenotypic variant in that some affected members develop spastic paraparesis, either as a presenting feature or as an additional feature accompanying dementia. Typically in such families there is considerable variability, with some members having typical presenile dementia while others have prominent spasticity as their main cause of disability, with little noticeable cognitive impairment until very late in the course of their illness. Sometimes the spastic paraparesis phenotype is associated with a later age at onset of symptoms, so at-risk individuals in such families cannot be reassured that they have passed through the period of risk simply on the basis of age. In the Australian Aus-1/EOFAD1 pedigree, the mean onset age of 10 individuals with dementia was 44.4 years, compared with 49.5 years in the four individuals with spastic paraparesis (Karlstrom *et al.* 2005). The association between spasticity and later onset age is far from universal, however, as spasticity has been reported to occur in younger patients as well, including some in their thirties or even late twenties (Ataka *et al.* 2004; Beck *et al.* 2004; Kwok *et al.* 1997).

The Finnish kindred that was the first to be described with spastic paraparesis, AD, and a deletion of PS-1 exon 9 had another unusual feature in that the neuropathological appearance was atypical, with prominent large non-neuritic plaques having the appearance of cotton wool balls (Crook *et al.* 1998). Such 'cotton wool' plaques have since been reported in other families, not always in association with spastic paraparesis (Kwok *et al.* 2003); their significance is not yet completely understood.

Other neuropathological features reported in some AD patients with PS-1 mutations include Lewy bodies (Lippa *et al.* 1995) and Pick bodies (Halliday *et al.* 2005). Patients with these additional neuropathological features do not seem to have clinical features that reliably distinguish them from other AD patients. In contrast to this is the recent report of a PS-1 mutation (G183V) in a family with clinical and pathologically confirmed Pick disease with no amyloid deposition (Dermaut *et al.* 2004). Another PS-1 mutation (insArg352) was found in a familial case with the clinical features of frontotemporal dementia (Tang-Wai *et al.* 2002), though the proband has since come to autopsy and was found to have, in addition, a mutation in the progranulin gene in association with non-AD, ubiquitin-positive neuropathology (S. Pickering-Brown and B. Boeve, personal communication).

APOE genotype has in general not been found to influence onset age in families with PS-1 mutations. The exception is the very large Colombian kindred, where possession of the APOE ε4 allele was associated with an earlier onset age in a study of 109 affected family members with the E280A mutation (Pastor *et al.* 2003).

15.2.2.2 Incomplete penetrance

There is one report of apparent non-penetrance. Rossor *et al.* (1996) described a novel mutation (I143F) in a family with autosomal dominant FAD. The median onset age was 55 years. Two affected members with onset ages 53 and 57 were shown to carry the mutation; it was also found in an asymptomatic relative aged 68 years. Three further mutations have been reported at this site (I143T, I143N, I143M). The mutation was not found in 100 controls.

15.2.2.3 E318G polymorphism

E318G was first reported as a mutation but is now thought to be a polymorphism. This change was first reported in an individual with symptoms beginning at 47 years but no known family history of dementia (Sandbrink *et al.* 1996). It was subsequently found in two affected siblings with familial AD, onset 60 and 68 years, respectively, whose mother (age at death 69) and brother (onset age 60) had also been affected by dementia (Forsell *et al.* 1997). An unaffected sibling did not carry the mutation.

A further patient with symptom onset at 57 years was found to have this change (Cruts *et al.* 1998). His mother had been affected and had died at 47 years but, despite the convincing family history, only the proband was available for DNA studies. The authors noted that E318G was located in exon 9, a functionally less important region, and that the region was less conserved in PS-2 and in presenilins of other species. In view of this and the wide variation in onset age in reported cases, Cruts and Van Broeckhoven (1998) surmised that E318G was a rare polymorphism and not a disease-causing mutation. Further evidence for this was provided when Mattila *et al.* (1998) found E318G in four of 59 control subjects without clinical evidence of neurological or psychiatric disease who had come to autopsy. These subjects were aged 74, 76, 79, and 87 years; the oldest had neither senile plaques nor NFTs and, in the others, plaques and tangles were said to be within the normal range (Mattila *et al.* 1998). Dermaut *et al.* (1999) found E318G in 1.6% of 676 individuals from the Rotterdam study, including 4.1% of randomly selected age-matched controls without dementia. Functional studies in cell cultures showed no difference in Aβ42 levels between cells transfected with E318G and those transfected with wild-type PS-1, in contrast to studies in cells transfected with disease-causing PS-1 mutations. E318G was shown not to affect beta-catenin trafficking (Nishimura *et al.* 1999), unlike other disease-causing presenilin mutations.

15.2.3 **Presenilin-2 gene**

In 1988 Bird *et al.* from Seattle described five large families with hereditary AD who were American descendants of an ethnic group known as the Volga Germans. In the 1760s immigrants from Germany, at the invitation of Catherine the Great of Russia, settled along the Volga, where they remained a distinct community for more than a century. During the nineteenth and early twentieth centuries, many migrated to the USA, and the ancestors of the families described by Bird were known to have lived in two adjacent villages in Russia. This, and the presence of several shared surnames among the families, suggested a genetic founder effect. It was hoped that the study of these kindreds would reveal a single gene for familial AD. When the APP and PS-1 genes were discovered, however, no mutations were found in the Volga German families. Linkage studies were eventually fruitful in 1995 and the Seattle group identified a locus on chromosome 1, with affected members from five of seven Volga German families sharing a haplotype at this locus (Levy-Lahad *et al.* 1995*a*, *b*). In Boston, researchers were seeking homologous gene sequences to the recently discovered PS-1 (then called S182). The gene coding for the appropriate sequence was found to map to the same locus on chromosome 1, and a missense mutation (N141I) was found in seven of nine Volga German families (Levy-Lahad *et al.* 1995). Similar work by the Toronto group confirmed the N141I mutation in three of four Volga German kindreds and identified another mutation in the same gene, M239V, in all four affected members of the Italian kindred FLO10 (Rogaev *et al.* 1995).

In contrast to families with APP or PS-1 mutations, Volga German families with the N141I PS-2 mutation range widely in onset age (44–75 years in the original report). Some later-onset individuals in these families were phenocopies, however, and did not carry the mutation. There is one example of apparent non-penetrance: an individual who died at 89 without dementia and who was inferred to have the mutation as he had affected children (in whom the mutation was confirmed) and an affected father, sibling, and nephews (Bird *et al.* 1996). Onset age in Volga German families appears to be influenced to some extent by APOE genotype (Wijsman *et al.* 2005). No other mutations in APP, presenilin-1, or presenilin-2 have been reported in Volga German families.

Although the N141I mutation has been found only in Volga German families, several other mutations in PS-2 have been reported. The most convincing are at codons 239 (M239V and M239I) and 122 (T122P and T122R). The M239V mutation was found in the Italian family FLO10, in which AD was present in 18 members across four generations, confirmed by autopsy in two cases. The mutation was found in all eight affected members studied and none of the 14 unaffected members, with onset age among mutation carriers ranging from 45 to 83 years. There were no at-risk mutation carriers older than 51 years (Marcon *et al.* 2004). A second mutation at the same site (M239I) was found in another Italian kindred with four affected members over two generations (Finckh *et al.* 2000). The onset age ranged from 44 to 58, with autopsy confirmation in one case; an asymptomatic mutation carrier aged 68 may represent incomplete penetrance, or variability in onset age as has been seen with other PS-2 mutations.

Two mutations at position 122 (T122P and T122R) have been reported in families from Germany (not Volga German in origin; Finckh *et al.* 2000, 2005) and Italy (Binetti *et al.* 2003). Although few individuals have had DNA studies and post mortem confirmation has not been reported, there is a convincing family history of dominantly inherited presenile dementia in these families. Other mutations reported in PS-2 have not yet been shown to segregate consistently with AD: the status of these may become clearer with time.

The oldest reported affected individual with a confirmed PS-2 mutation (M239V) developed symptoms at 83 years (Rogaev *et al.* 1995). Another member of the FLO10 kindred developed symptoms at 88 years, but no DNA was available, so the possibility that this was a phenocopy cannot be excluded. In summary, despite the report by Bird *et al.* of an 89-year-old apparent N141I escapee, it cannot be assumed that an older individual with a PS-2 mutation will never develop symptoms. Conversely, members of PS-2 families who have reached even their ninth decade without symptoms cannot be reassured that they (and by implication their offspring) have not inherited the family mutation, unless this is confirmed by DNA studies.

Two PS-2 mutations have been included in functional studies involving transfected cell lines. The Volga German mutation, N141I (Citron *et al.* 1997) was found to be associated with a major increase in total Aβ42 levels (six- to eightfold more than the PS-1 mutations). Similar results were found for the Italian M239 mutation (Xia *et al.* 1997).

15.2.4 **Evidence for causation**

How do mutations act to cause or promote the pathogenic processes leading to neurodegeneration and clinical dementia? Although many aspects of this complex process are still poorly understood, a considerable body of experimental evidence fits well with our current concepts of the pathogenesis of AD and FTD. Most functional studies of AD mutations are concerned with their effect on APP processing and amyloid aggregation and deposition: how these mutations are involved in the development of NFTs remains to be explained.

One line of evidence for the pathogenicity of mutations comes from measuring Aβ40 and Aβ42(43) levels in plasma from AD mutation-carriers and controls, or from cultured lymphocytes or fibroblasts from individuals with and without mutations. Differences between cases and controls in such studies, however, could be related to some cause other than the mutation itself. More convincing evidence comes from studies where specific mutations are introduced into cell cultures or transgenic mice. In such studies the differences between groups are presumably attributable to the effects of the mutation.

Not all mutations have been subjected to such functional studies. Those that have been studied, however, have generally shown an increase in the levels of the more amyloidogenic A42(43) isoform, or an increase in the ratio of Aβ42(43) to Aβ40. The Swedish double mutation APP K670N, M671L, which is located just at the amino terminal end of the Aβ peptide sequence, adjacent to the β-secretase site, is associated with increases in both Aβ40 and Aβ42 levels (Citron *et al.* 1994). An exception is the PS-1 E318G mutation, discussed above, which is now considered to be a rare polymorphism with no functional consequences. Table 15.1 summarizes published functional studies of AD-associated mutations.

A recent finding of a PS-1 mutation (G183V) found in association with pathologically confirmed Pick disease with no amyloid deposition (Dermaut *et al.* 2004) and another (insArg352) in a family with the clinical features of frontotemporal dementia (Tang-Wai *et al.* 2002) have led to functional studies suggesting loss of function of PS-1, rather than toxic gain of function, as a mechanism in this presumably non-amyloid-based neurodegenerative process (reviewed in Dermaut *et al.* 2005), though the finding of a progranulin mutation in the second of these families makes this less likely.

Table 15.1 Functional studies of familial AD-associated APP and presenilin mutations

Author	Mutations	Type of study*	Outcome measure and results
Martins *et al.* 1995	PS1: A246E	Aβ levels in cultured skin fibroblast media	Detectable Aβ in one cell line only
Scheuner *et al.* 1996	APP: V717I, APP K670N/M671L (Swedish) PS1: E120D, M146V, H163R, G209V PS2: N141I (Volga German)	Plasma Aβ levels	Increased plasma Aβ1-42(43) in all mutation carriers; increased plasma Aβ1-40 with Swedish mutation only
Scheuner *et al.* 1996	PS1: A246E, L286V, G209V, M146V PS2: N141I (Volga German)	Fibroblast cultures from mutation carriers	Increased Aβ1-42(43)
Citron *et al.* 1997	PS1: H163R, L286V, L392V PS2: N1411 (Volga German)	Transfected HEK cell lines	Increased Aβ1-42; increased ratio of Aβ1-42 to total Aβ
Citron *et al.* 1997	PS1: M146L, L286V	Transgenic mice	Increased Aβ levels in brain
Xia *et al.* 1997	PS1: M146L, C410Y PS2: M239V	Transfected CHO cell lines	Increased Aβ1-42
Mehta *et al.* 1998	PS1: M146V, M146L, Δ9, A246E, L250S, L286V	Transfected HEK cell lines	Increased Aβ42(43) levels
Kwok *et al.* 2000	APP: L723P	Transfected CHO cell lines	Increased Aβ42(43) levels

* HEK, Human embryonic kidney; CHO, Chinese hamster ovary.

15.3 Late-onset Alzheimer disease

- There is almost certainly a genetic contribution to sporadic AD; to date the only factor to have been identified is apolipoprotein E (ApoE) genotype.
- An ApoE E4/E4 genotype is associated with an eightfold increased risk of developing AD compared to the E3/E3 genotype. Individuals with ApoE E2/E2 appear to be at a slightly lower risk.
- First-degree relatives of people with AD are about 2.5 times more likely to develop AD compared to the general population, and this appears to be independent of apolipoprotein E (ApoE) status (Green *et al.* 2002).

Although there have been many encouraging preliminary studies (Kamboh 2004), the only consistently validated genetic risk factor for late onset AD remains ApoE genotype (Tanzi and Bertram 2005). ApoE is a cholesterol transporter coded by a gene on chromosome 19. The at-risk allele (E4) is present in about 15% of the general population, and roughly twice that in the AD population (Tanzi and Bertram 2005). The association between ApoE and AD has been confirmed in over 300 studies. Compared to people with the common ApoE E3/E3 genotype, people with the ApoE E2/E2, E3/E4, and E4/E4 genotypes are 0.5-, 3-, and 8-fold more likely to develop AD, respectively (Pericak-Vance and Haines 2002).

Despite its robust epidemiological association, ApoE lacks the necessary characteristics required for, and cannot be used as, a clinical diagnostic test. Up to 50% of people with AD do not carry the at-risk E4 allele, and up to 75% of people carrying one copy of the E4 allele remain free of AD (ACMG/ASHG 1995). Use of ApoE as a predictive genetic test is therefore not recommended.

15.4 Frontotemporal dementia

- Mutations in the microtubule associated protein Tau (MAPT) gene on chromosome 17 are present in around a quarter of patients with a family history suggesting dominantly inherited FTD, and around 4% of those without.
- 40 mutations have been described in 113 families.
- Mutations either cause structural or splicing anomalies in Tau protein. Both types of defect impair the function of cytoskeletal microtubules.
- Families with the commonly found tau-negative, ubiquitin-positive pathology have been found to carry mutations in the neighbouring progranulin gene.
- Mutations on chromosomes 3 and 9 have also been found in kindreds with FTD.

Frontotemporal dementia (FTD) is a heterogeneous group of disorders characterized by behavioural and specific language deficits due to lobar degeneration of the frontal and/or temporal lobes (Neary *et al.* 1998). Clinical presentation varies according to the pattern of lobar atrophy—with the frontal, left perisylvian temporal, and left anterior temporal lobes being most affected in the behavioural, primary non-fluent progressive aphasia, and semantic dementia variants, respectively (Whitwell *et al.* 2004). Frontotemporal dementia can also be caused by a diversity of underlying pathological processes, including Pick-bodies Pick disease, tau-based pathology, ubiquitin-based pathology, and dementia lacking distinctive histology (DLDH). Clinical features provide some indication of the underlying pathology (Hodges *et al.* 2004). For example, patients with primary non-fluent progressive aphasia are more likely to have a tau-based pathology, whilst patients with semantic dementia are more likely to have a ubiquitin-based pathology (Hodges *et al.* 2004). Patients with FTD and features of motor-neuron disease (MND) often have ubiquitin-based pathology – although, this again, is not without exceptions (Zarranz *et al.* 2005).

Patients with FTD frequently have a positive family history. One study found that a family history of organic dementia in first-degree relatives was 10 times more common in FTD compared to the general population (Grasbeck *et al.* 2005). Another found such a history in 43% of people with FTD (Rosso *et al.* 2003). Precise estimates vary between research groups but, in our experience, mutations in the microtubule-associated protein tau gene can be found in about 25% of the cases with a family history of dominantly inherited frontotemporal dementia and 4% of the cases without (Stanford *et al.* 2004).

15.4.1 Microtubule-associated protein tau

Tau is a microtubule binding protein involved in cellular trafficking. In 1998, mutations in the tau gene on chromosome 17 were found to be associated with FTD in a number of families via a positional cloning approach (Hutton *et al.* 1998). Mutant tau has since been demonstrated to be associated with cognitive function in a transgenic mouse model, independent of the accumulation of neurofibrillary tangles (Santacruz *et al.* 2005).

The original families described with tau mutations presented with FTD associated with parkinsonism (Hutton *et al.* 1998). This phenotype has since been expanded to include a progressive supranuclear palsy-like picture (Stanford *et al.* 2000), a semantic dementia-like picture (Garrard and Carroll 2005), and even FTD associated with motor neuron disease (Zarranz *et al.* 2005). Indeed, the parkinsonian features in tau-mutation related FTD appear to be mediated via the H1 tau haplotype (Baba *et al.* 2005).

To date, 40 mutations in the tau gene have been described in 113 families—see *http://www.molgen.ua.ac.be/FTDmutations* for an annotated database. Tau mutations generally cause disease with an autosomal dominant mode of inheritance. However, there is one report of possible autosomal recessive inheritance in a consanguineous family (Nicholl *et al.* 2003). Non-penetrance has been observed in an 82-year-old woman with the L315R mutation (Van Herpen *et al.* 2003), but from the information available so far the penetrance is high.

Mutations in the tau gene can cause disease either by directly disrupting tau protein structure or by altering the proportion of different tau protein isoforms available (Brandt *et al.* 2005; Neary *et al.* 2005). Mutations in the coding region tend to disrupt tau protein structure, thus impairing microtubule assembly or axonal transport. Some of these mutations may also promote pathological tau filament aggregation. Mutations in exon 10 or intron 9, however, affect tau protein splicing and impair microtubule function by altering the proportion of tau protein isoforms available. Mutations in intron 10 are named after nucleotide location in the splice donor site. For example, a mutation affecting the 16th nucleotide in the splice donor site is designated '+16'.

Regardless of the mechanism of disease causation, neuropathology for tau mutations is characterized macroscopically by atrophy predominantly in the frontal and temporal lobes, and microscopically by neuron loss, spongiform changes, gliosis, and filamentous tau deposition. Genotype–phenotype correlation has been attempted in the past, but phenotype can vary even within single families and there appear to be more exceptions than rules (Rademakers *et al.* 2004).

Finally, the tau haplotype, formed by a number of polymorphisms extending the full length of the tau gene, has also been associated with progressive supranuclear palsy (Baker *et al.* 1999) and corticobasal degeneration (Houlden *et al.* 2001) in replicated studies. This reflects the role of tau in genetically complex disease, and has no clinical role in predictive testing.

15.4.2 Other genes

Frontotemporal dementia has also been found to be associated with mutations in a number of other genes.

There are a number of dominant FTD families linked to 17q21–22 near the tau gene, where no tau mutations have been found on sequencing (Mackenzie *et al.* 2006; Rademakers *et al.* 2002; Rosso *et al.* 2001). Interestingly, instead of tau-based pathology, these families were found to have tau-negative, ubiquitin-positive inclusion bodies. These families have since been found to carry mutations in the progranulin gene (Baker *et al.* 2006; Cruts *et al.* 2006). Further clinical and prevalence data for progranulin mutations are yet to be published, but these mutations are probably at least as common as tau mutations within FTD families. Wilhelmsen *et al.* (2004) also reported a dominant family with FTD and motor neuron disease (MND) linked to 17q, distal to the tau gene. However, the region of linkage is different, and the pathology in this family includes tau and alpha-synuclein inclusions.

Mutations in the chromosome 3 gene CHMP-2B had been found in a large autosomal-dominant Danish pedigree and one other sporadic case to date (Skibinski *et al.* 2005). CHMP-2B is involved in vesicular transport and this family has typical FTD phenotype and ubiquitin-positive pathology. Mutations in the chromosome 9 valosin-containing protein gene also cause an autosomal-dominant FTD phenotype (Watts *et al.* 2004). The phenotype of this is more distinctive, since it is accompanied by inclusion-body myositis and Paget disease of the bone.

Mutations in two other genes may also present as FTD in an atypical fashion. Mutation in the chromosome 2 dynactin-1 gene, typically associated with MND, has been associated with a clinical picture of FTD without MND (Munch *et al.* 2005). Pathological confirmation is not yet available for this family. Mutation in the chromosome 14 presenilin-1 gene has also been reported to be associated with pathologically proven FTD (Dermaut *et al.* 2004; Halliday *et al.* 2005). This, however, may reflect the role of presenilin-1 as a gene-modifier.

15.4.3 Other genetic loci under investigation

Two other dominant families with FTD and MND have been linked to loci on chromosome 9p, with substantial overlap in their regions of genetic linkage (Morita *et al.* 2006; Vance *et al.* 2006). Tau-negative, ubiquitin-positive inclusions were found in these families upon pathological examination.

15.5 Familial dementia with other neurological features

- There are three clinical variants of inherited prion disease: familial Creutzfeltd–Jakob disease (CJD); Gerstmann–Sträussler–Scheinker (GSS); and fatal familial insomnia (FFI).
- Clinical phenotypes and penetrance vary between individual mutations.
- Huntington's disease (HD) is caused by a trinucleotide repeat expansion on the Huntingtin gene on chromosome 4; disease onset in both proband and offspring depends on the number of CAG repeats.
- Wilson's disease is a potentially treatable cause of dementia associated with a movement disorder; negative serum and urine biochemical studies do not absolutely exclude the disorder.
- Niemann–Pick disease type C (NPC), some of the spinocerebellar ataxia (SCA) subtypes, dentatorubropallidoluysian atrophy (DRPLA), CADASIL, and familial British/Danish dementia are rarer genetically determined causes of early-onset dementia.

Neurogenetic conditions are frequently associated with cognitive deficits. We have selected a few conditions commonly encountered in clinical practice and described our clinical approach.

15.5.1 Dementia with myoclonus

Myoclonus appearing early in the course of a dementing illness often raises the possibility of prion disease, although it is important to remember that this can also be a feature of other dementias such as familial AD (Godbolt *et al.* 2004).

Cellular prion proteins are membrane proteins of uncertain physiological function normally present in cells. Prions are pathogenic isoforms of cellular prion proteins that produce the pathognomonic protease-resistant residue. Prions are devoid of nucleic acids, but can become infective by converting normal cellular prion proteins into the pathogenic isoforms (Prusiner 2001). Alternatively, prions can also arise from mutations in the human prion gene. Prion disease has an incidence of 0.5–1 per million per year and about 8% of these cases are familial (Gibbons *et al.* 2000; Will *et al.* 1998).

Familial prion disease is caused by mutations in the prion gene on chromosome 20. It is inherited in an autosomal dominant manner. Over 30 mutations have been reported in this gene to date (Mead 2006). The phenotype of genetic prion disease falls into three broad categories, with some overlap: familial Creutzfeldt–Jakob disease (fCJD); Gerstmann–Sträussler–Scheinker disease (GSS); and fatal familial insomnia (FFI).

The fCJD subtype of inherited prion disease is the easiest to recognize. Similar to sporadic prion disease, these patients present with a rapidly progressive dementia with myoclonus and can also display periodic sharp waves on electroencephalography. On the other hand, patients with the GSS subtype of inherited prion disease typically present with a slowly progressive ataxia with late dementia, and may sometimes be missed if not tested for. The FFI subtype of inherited prion disease has a distinctive presentation including refractory insomnia and dysautonomia.

These three clinical subtypes are often associated with particular mutations, and genotype–phenotype correlation for inherited prion disease has been detailed in two recent reviews (Kovacs *et al.* 2002; Mead 2006). When counselling a family with inherited prion disease, it is often helpful to review the literature associated with the relevant mutation as phenotypes and penetrance both vary for different mutations.

Finally, polymorphisms in codon 129 of the prion gene have also been associated with prion disease risk. Methionine or valine homozygosity at codon 129 is associated with sporadic (non-familial) CJD (Palmer *et al.* 1991). Until recently, it was thought that all new variant CJD cases were methionine homozygotes, but two cases with valine homozygosity have since been identified from archival appendix samples (Ironside *et al.* 2006). However, the clinical status of these two patients is unknown at present.

15.5.2 Dementia with chorea

Typical Huntington's disease (HD), with chorea and cognitive and psychiatric features, is easily recognizable. It is worthwhile, however, to bear in mind the atypical forms including the Westphal variant, juvenile HD, and late-onset HD. The 'Westphal variant' refers to HD presenting with rigidity rather than chorea. This is not uncommon in the juvenile form of HD, but relatively rare in adult onset HD (Racette and Perlmutter 1998). Apart from a greater frequency of rigidity, patients with juvenile HD (onset < 20 years of age) are also more likely to have seizures and higher trinucleotide repeat numbers (Rasmussen *et al.* 2000). Patients with late-onset HD (onset > 50 years of age) typically present with a milder clinical picture, with predominantly motor and cognitive symptoms (James *et al.* 1994).

HD is caused by abnormal trinucleotide repeat expansion in the gene on chromosome 4 encoding for the huntingtin protein. Expanded trinucleotide repeats act in an autosomal dominant fashion, although rare cases with homozygous abnormal expansions did not appear to have more severe phenotypes (Wexler *et al.* 1987). A trinucleotide repeat count of < 27 has never been associated with HD. Among individuals with a repeat size of > 40, onset can be as late as the ninth decade, although to date there not been a documented person with > 40 repeats, normal lifespan, no symptoms, and no HD pathology upon autopsy (ACMG/ASHG 1998). The intervening repeat counts carry different risks for disease and different risks for CAG-repeat stability and thus transmission risk. These have been summarized in Table 15.2.

Mutations in a number of other genes may mimic Huntington's disease. These include prion, SCA3, SCA17, dentatorubropallidoluysian atrophy (DRPLA), neuroacanthocytosis, neuroferritinopathy, and junctophilin-3 mutations (Stevanin *et al.* 2003). Junctophilin-3 mutations have not been found in Caucasian or Asian populations to date. Benign hereditary chorea (BHC) is another form of autosomal dominant chorea, but its relatively mild motor phenotype and relative cognitive preservation make it easily distinguishable clinically (Breedveld *et al.* 2002). BHC may also be associated with infantile respiratory distress and hypothyroidism (Krude *et al.* 2002).

Table 15.2 Risk of developing HD as a function of number of trinucleotide CAG repeats

	Repeat count			
	< 2 (normal)	27–35 (intermediate)	36–3 (low defective)	> 3 (defective)
Can this person develop HD?	No	No	Yes but unlikely	Yes
Can this person's children develop HD?	No	Possibly	Yes	Yes

15.5.3 Dementia with ataxia

In addition to the GSS subtype of inherited prion disease described above, a number of other genetic ataxic conditions have traditionally been recognized to have significant cognitive involvement. These include spinocerebellar ataxia type 2 (Le Pira *et al.* 2002), spinocerebellar ataxia type 3 (Maruff *et al.* 1996), spinocerebellar ataxia type 17 (Koide *et al.* 1999), DRPLA (Kanazawa 1998), and neuroacanthocytosis. However, with increasing awareness of cognitive problems in neurogenetic diseases, this list is likely to grow.

15.5.4 Dementia with dystonia

The most important differential for dementia with a movement disorder is Wilson's disease because it is potentially treatable (Seniow *et al.* 2002). Wilson's disease is autosomal recessive in inheritance and the responsible gene has been cloned (ATP7B gene on chromosome 13). However, direct genetic testing remains difficult due to the large number of mutations and high number of compound heterozygotes (Ferenci 2004). Unfortunately, alternative methods of diagnosis (Kayser–Fleischer rings, serum ceruloplasmin, and 24-hour urinary copper excretion) can all be falsely negative (Ferenci *et al.* 2003). A liver biopsy with copper quantitation should be carried out if clinical suspicion is high.

Another condition presenting with dementia and dystonia in the cognitive clinic is Niemann–Pick type C (NPC). NPC is an autosomal recessive liposomal lipid storage disorder caused by mutations in either one of two genes (NPC1 on chromosome 18 and NPC2 on chromosome 14; Vanier and Millat 2003). Clinical clues to diagnosis include supranuclear palsy and hepatomegaly. First-line diagnostic procedures include liver biopsy and examination for foam cells on bone-marrow biopsy, although both can lead to false negatives. Functional essays on fibroblast culture (filipin and esterification tests) appear most sensitive.

15.5.5 Dementia with white matter changes on imaging

Cognitive impairment associated with white matter changes in a young person raises the possibility of a metabolic or mitochondrial condition. The differential diagnosis for this is broad (Kaye 2001), but the minimal work-up should include serum lactate, serum amino acid, and urinary organic acids.

Cerebral autosomal dominant arteriopathy with subcortical infarcts and leucoencephalopathy (CADASIL) can also present with cognitive symptoms and white matter changes on imaging (Buffon *et al.* 2006). CADASIL is inherited in an autosomal dominant manner and is caused by mutations in the Notch 3 gene on chromosome 19. Due to the size of the Notch 3 gene, direct sequencing has not been possible as a routine clinical test to date. Thus diagnosis by skin biopsy remains the reference standard for diagnosis—although judicious sequencing of a few exons may be sufficient to bring the sensitivity up to 90% (Peters *et al.* 2005).

15.5.6 Familial British dementia, familial Danish dementia

A single kindred in which presenile dementia is associated with spasticity and sometimes ataxia was first described in 1933 by Worster-Drought *et al.* By 1999 the kindred included over 200 individuals in seven generations (Vidal *et al.* 1999). Neuropathological features included striking white matter disease, non-neuritic amyloid plaque formation, and CAA. However, the biochemical identification of the amyloid peptide sequence showed that it was distinct from the Aβ peptide of AD. The condition has become known as familial British dementia, with the peptide now called ABri. The gene for the precursor protein of the ABri peptide was found to be on chromosome 13. A point mutation altered a stop codon and resulted in a mutant peptide

11 amino acids longer than the wild-type protein. The *C*-terminal 34 residues of this mutant peptide form the insoluble ABri deposits.

A duplication of 10 base pairs in this gene causes a similar peptide to be produced; this is the genetic lesion in familial Danish dementia, a phenotypically quite different condition involving cataracts, deafness, ataxia, and dementia in a single Danish kindred (Vidal *et al.* 2000).

15.6 **Genetic issues in clinical practice**

- A family history should always be explored in cases of early-onset dementia, but may also be relevant in elderly patients.
- No mutation in any of the known dementia genes is found in up to 30% of familial cases, though APP, PS-1, or PS-2 are highly likely to be detected in a patient with clinically clear-cut early-onset Alzheimer's disease and a convincing family history, particularly when disease onset is before 50.
- At-risk members of families with mutations should be referred for genetic counselling; differences in age of onset and penetrance between individual disease mutations should be taken into account.
- The rate of detection of mutations in apparently sporadic cases is low. Only one case attributable to a *de novo* mutation has been described.

Two main issues arise. Firstly, family members may ask about their risk of inheriting dementia. Secondly, the clinician needs to decide whether genetic issues are relevant and whether DNA screening is indicated. Family history should always be sought in a younger person with dementia. In some instances a family history of dementia may be concealed, because of the death of the mutation-carrying parent from other causes or because of family separation.

Family history may also be relevant in older patients, in that it may indicate a possible genetic influence on that person's illness, but it is unclear at this stage how important this is for offspring in terms of their lifetime risk of developing dementia. Evidence from numerous case-control studies suggests that they are at increased risk, but two large prospective studies using population-based samples did not find family history of dementia to be a risk factor for incident AD (Launer *et al.* 1999; Lindsay *et al.* 2002). It is possible that the cases ascertained in these studies were different from those typically involved in case-control studies in that some of them may not have presented for diagnosis, and hence may not have been recognized by their families as having dementia. Similarly, informants may not have remembered or recognized dementia in relatives. It is possible that the families of patients who present for treatment may be more likely to remember affected relatives as they try to seek reasons for the patient's condition (effort after meaning); this effect is a potential source of recall bias in case-control studies.

15.6.1 **Family history positive**

Most family history studies involve AD probands: much less information is available for FTD. About 25–50% of people seen at specialist clinics with AD will have a family history of dementia in a parent or sibling. This compares with 10.9% and 16.8% of incident cases identified in population-based samples (Launer *et al.* 1999; Lindsay *et al.* 2002). Where the family history reveals dementia inherited from one generation to the next with onset consistently before 55 years, dominant inheritance is probable, mutation screening is likely to be fruitful, and the risk to offspring is 50%. Detailed clinical description and neuropathological correlation are important, both for the family and for increasing our understanding of these rare conditions. Some members of such families may be reluctant to participate in clinical assessments, and may present late in their course, or only when management issues have become difficult. Until a disease-modifying treatment is available, this attitude must be respected.

At-risk family members who seek predictive testing should be referred for genetic counselling. Protocols developed for HD are readily applicable to other familial dementias. In familial AD with PS-1 mutations, the predicted phenotype could include spastic paraparesis with a later onset age, and it may be prudent to advise family members of the potential for this. In addition, the reported instances of possible incomplete penetrance of mutations in APP (V717I) and PS-1 (I143F) noted above should be borne in mind.

Where the family history is positive, but the onset age later or variable, DNA screening is much less rewarding and the risk to relatives, though probably increased, is less clearly quantifiable. One study estimated that the risk to relatives of AD patients was 52.8 ± 11.4% by age 94 compared with 22.1 ± 5.8% by age 90 years in relatives of controls (Wu *et al.* 1998). A large multi-centre clinic-based study found a cumulative risk to age 85 years of 26.9% in relatives of white probands, but 43.7% in relatives of African-American probands (Green *et al.* 2002). Most studies find that the risk to relatives decreases with increasing onset age of the proband (Silverman *et al.* 2005).

15.6.2 Frequency of mutations in familial cases

Most families with dominant inheritance of pathologically confirmed young-onset AD will be found to have a mutation in APP or PS-1. In a series of 65 families rigorously selected to have probable or definite AD with onset before 60 years in three generations, Raux *et al.* (2005) found mutations in all but 18%. Three of the families with mutations were found to have the E318G polymorphism, so the proportion with no known pathogenic mutation was about 22%. In a similar study from the UK, Janssen *et al.* (2003) found a pathogenic mutation in APP, PS-1, or PS-2 in 20 of 31 probands with AD, onset before 61 years, and family history in at least one first-degree relative. The probands without mutations were older at symptom onset than those in whom mutations had been found. Where at least one affected member developed symptoms before age 50, mutations were found in 17 of 19 families (89%); where the onset age was consistently above 50 years, mutations were found in only 3 of 12 families (25%).

15.6.3 Where family history is negative

Patients with no family history of dementia are more difficult to advise. Particularly where the onset age is young and concerns about heritability correspondingly great, it is hard to reassure patients and family members that the condition is unlikely to be genetic without screening for mutations, though the yield in this situation is very low. Even where mutation screening is negative, several possibilities remain. Since up to 30% of familial cases are also free of mutations in the known dementia genes, it is likely that more genes remain to be discovered, and new mutation events in these may explain at least some of the apparently non-familial cases. In addition, mosaicism may account for failure to detect mutations, as in the family reported by Beck *et al.* discussed below. Autosomal recessive inheritance is another possible means whereby a genetic mechanism can result in a disease without positive family history, but this has not so far been demonstrated in AD. Autosomal recessive inheritance could also be considered where siblings are affected but their parents are not, or where consanguinity (such as first cousin marriages) may be a factor.

Most of the known families with mutations are traceable for only a few generations. Whether this is because the mutation arose relatively recently or because of incomplete information about preceding generations is unknowable, but it is likely that at least some of today's apparently sporadic cases will be genetic founders.

Noted exceptions include the Volga German families (PS-2 N141I) and the large kindreds originating in Colombia (PS-1 E280A; Pastor *et al.* 2003) and Calabria (PS-1 M146L; Bruni 1998), where in each case many affected descendants can be traced to a single genetic founder.

15.6.4 **Frequency of mutations in apparently sporadic cases**

Where DNA screening for mutations in the known dementia genes has been carried out in apparently sporadic cases, mutations are found rarely, but the frequency is not nil. The most definitive study was the population-based study from The Netherlands. Of the 101 cases of AD with onset before age 65 screened for mutations in APP, PS-1, and PS-2 (Cruts *et al.* 1998; van Duijn *et al.* 1991), the authors found only one mutation in a patient without family history, R62H in PS-2, which has not been reported elsewhere. In their 1990 report of APP screening in this group, van Duijn *et al.* stated that 48 of the cases were sporadic; however in the 1998 report of presenilin screening of the same sample, only 34 were said to be sporadic, suggesting that affected relatives had been found for 14 of the originally sporadic cases. This gives a mutation frequency of 1 in 34 or 1 in 48.

Other studies are similar. In a French study of 13 patients with onset before 50 years and no family history of dementia, only one was found to carry a mutation, M139K in PS-1 (Dumanchin *et al.* 1998). Finckh *et al.* (2000) in a referral sample from five countries including 36 patients with presenile dementia, found only one mutation among the 17 patients with negative family history: this was T188K in PrP. Of three patients whose family history was unknown, two had mutations in APP.

The first report of a mutation in a proven non-familial case was by Tanahashi *et al.* (1996) who found a PS-1 mutation (H163R) in a 44-year-old man with symptoms beginning at 41 years. His parents (aged 82 and 76) and two siblings (53 and 47) were normal on neuropsychological assessment and did not carry the mutation. The authors confirmed the relationship between the patient and the family members by analysing the D1S80 VNTR marker. Other descriptions of apparently sporadic cases with mutations include those by Kwok *et al.* (1997), Goldman *et al.* (2004), and Pantieri *et al.* (2005).

In summary, mutations in the known AD genes are found rarely in apparently sporadic cases, even when the onset age is young. The case reported by Tanahashi *et al.* (1996) indicates that new mutations can occur, though most mutations are identified in familial cases. The relative rarity of familial cases with young onset but no identified mutation suggests that most causative genes have already been discovered. Together with the rarity of known mutations in sporadic cases, this further suggests that most sporadic young-onset cases will not be the founders of new AD kindreds.

One possible mechanism for the apparent paucity of detectable mutations could be somatic mosaicism. Beck *et al.* (2004) described a patient who died at 58 after 16 years of progressive parkinsonism, mild spastic paraparesis, and dementia. The neuropathology was AD. Family history was negative until the proband's daughter presented at 27 with a progressive cerebellar syndrome, spastic paraparesis, and dementia; she died after 12 years. The daughter was found to have a P436Q presenilin mutation, but this was not detectable in the mother by sequencing stored peripheral lymphocyte DNA extracted from peripheral blood. Further studies, including allele-specific oligonucleotide hybridization (ASOH), allowed the mutation to be detected faintly in peripheral blood; there was evidence of somatic mosaicism, with the mutation being detectable in more cells in the cerebral cortex than in peripheral blood. Mosaicism was also present in the mother's germ cell line: although the affected daughter inherited the P436Q mutation from her mother, two other siblings inherited the same allele but without the mutation.

15.6.5 When a mutation is found

When DNA studies reveal a putative mutation in a person with dementia, its significance needs to be assessed before offering advice to the family. Some mutations, such as the APP V717I London mutation, have been well studied and the clinician can rely on the published evidence. The history of the presenilin-1 E318G polymorphism as described above, however, shows that early conclusions can sometimes be proved wrong by later evidence.

The following checklist may be useful in evaluating the evidence that a particular mutation is pathogenic.

- Has the mutation been reported previously?
- If so, was it found in a family or in a sporadic case?
- Has there been autopsy confirmation in someone carrying the mutation, or at least in an affected relative?
- Have other family members undergone DNA testing and, if so, are the results consistent with segregation of the mutation with the disease?
- Has the mutation been found in a control group (which suggests that it may be a nonpathogenic polymorphism)?
- Is the nucleotide conserved in homologous genes (e.g. for PS-1, is it conserved in PS-2, or presenilins in other species such as the mouse or *C. elegans*)? If it is not conserved, it is less likely that a mutation would have functional significance.
- What is known about the likely functional consequences of the mutation? Have cell culture studies or transgenic animal studies been done and do they suggest that the mutation has an effect on Aβ isoforms or Aβ deposition (AD) or tau metabolism (FTD)?

Acknowledgement

The authors wish to thank Dr Anne Turner, Clinical Geneticist, Sydney Children's Hospital, for helpful comments.

References

ACMG/ASHG (1995). American College of Medical Genetics/ American Society of Human Genetics Working Group on ApoE and Alzheimer's Disease: statement on use of apolipoprotein E testing for Alzheimer's disease. *J. Am. Med. Assoc.* **274**, 1627–9.

ACMG/ASHG (1998). ACMG/ASHG statement. Laboratory guidelines for Huntington disease genetic testing. The American College of Medical Genetics/American Society of Human Genetics Huntington Disease Genetic Testing Working Group. *Am. J. Hum. Genet.* **62**, 1243–7.

Alzheimer's Disease Collaborative Group (1993). Apolipoprotein E genotype and Alzheimer's disease. *Lancet* **342**, 737–8.

Alzheimer's Disease Collaborative Group (1995). The structure of the presenilin 1 (S182) gene and identification of six novel mutations in early onset AD families. *Nat. Genet.* **11**, 219–22.

Ataka S., Tomiyama, T., Takuma, H., *et al.* (2004). A novel presenilin-1 mutation (Leu85Pro) in early-onset Alzheimer disease with spastic paraparesis. *Arch. Neurol.* **61**, 1773–6.

Baba, Y., Tsuboi, Y., Baker, M.C., *et al.* (2005). The effect of tau genotype on clinical features in FTDP-17. *Parkinsonism Relat. Disord.* **11**, 205–8.

Baker, M., Litvan, I., Houlden, H., *et al.* (1999). Association of an extended haplotype in the tau gene with progressive supranuclear palsy. *Hum. Mol. Genet.* **8**, 711–15.

Baker, M., Mackenzie, I.R., Pickering-Brown, S.M., *et al.* (2006). Mutations in progranulin cause tau-negative frontotemporal dementia linked to chromosome 17. *Nature* **442**, 916–19.

Beck, J.A., Poulter, M., Campbell, T.A., *et al.* (2004). Somatic and germline mosaicism in sporadic early-onset Alzheimer's disease. *Hum. Mol. Genet.* **13**, 1219–24.

Binetti, G., Signorini, S., Squitti, R., *et al.* (2003). Atypical dementia associated with a novel presenilin-2 mutation. *Ann. Neurol.* **54**, 832–6.

Bird, T.D., Lampe, T.H., Nemens, E.J., Miner, G.W., Sumi, S.M., and Schellenberg, G.D. (1988). Familial Alzheimer's disease in American descendants of the Volga Germans: probable genetic founder effect. *Ann. Neurol.* **23**, 25–31.

Bird, T.D., Levy-Lahad, E., Poorkaj, P., *et al.* (1996). Wide range in age of onset for chromosome 1–related familial Alzheimer's disease. *Ann. Neurol.* **40**, 932–6.

Brandt, R., Hundelt, M., and Shahani, N. (2005). Tau alteration and neuronal degeneration in tauopathies: mechanisms and models. *Biochim. Biophys. Acta* **1739**, 331–54.

Breedveld, G.J., van Dongen, J.W., Danesino, C., *et al.* (2002). Mutations in TITF-1 are associated with benign hereditary chorea. *Hum. Mol. Genet.* **11**, 971–9.

Brooks, W.S., Kwok, J.B., Halliday, G.M., *et al.* (2004). Hemorrhage is uncommon in new Alzheimer family with Flemish amyloid precursor protein mutation. *Neurology* **63**, 1613–17.

Bruni, A.C. (1998). Cloning of a gene bearing missense mutations in early onset familial Alzheimer's disease: a Calabrian study. *Funct. Neurol.* **13**, 257–61.

Buffon, F., Porcher, R., Hernandez, K., *et al.* (2006). Cognitive profile in CADASIL. *J. Neurol. Neurosurg. Psychiatry* **77**, 175–80.

Citron, M., Vigo-Pelfrey, C., Teplow, D.B., *et al.* (1994). Excessive production of amyloid beta-protein by peripheral cells of symptomatic and presymptomatic patients carrying the Swedish familial Alzheimer disease mutation. *Proc. Natl. Acad. Sci. USA* **91**, 11993–7.

Citron, M., Westaway, D., Xia, W., *et al.* (1997). Mutant presenilins of Alzheimer's disease increase production of 42-residue amyloid beta-protein in both transfected cells and transgenic mice. *Nat. Med.* **3**, 67–72.

Crook, R., Verkkoniemi, A., Perez-Tur, J., *et al.* (1998). A variant of Alzheimer's disease with spastic paraparesis and unusual plaques due to deletion of exon 9 of presenilin 1. *Nat. Med.* **4**, 452–5.

Cruts, M. and Van Broeckhoven, C. (1998). Presenilin mutations in Alzheimer's disease. *Hum. Mutat.* **11**, 183–90.

Cruts, M., van Duijn, C.M., Backhovens, H., *et al.* (1998). Estimation of the genetic contribution of presenilin-1 and -2 mutations in a population-based study of presenile Alzheimer disease. *Hum. Mol. Genet.* **7**, 43–51.

Cruts, M., Gijselinck, I., van der See, J., *et al.* (2006). Null mutations in progranulin cause ubiquitin-positive frontotemporal dementia linked to chromosome 17q21. *Nature* **442**, 920–4.

Dermaut, B., Cruts, M., Slooter, A.J., *et al.* (1999). The Glu318Gly substitution in presenilin 1 is not causally related to Alzheimer disease. *Am. J. Hum. Genet.* **64**, 290–2.

Dermaut, B., Kumar-Singh, S., Engelborghs, S., *et al.* (2004). A novel presenilin 1 mutation associated with Pick's disease but not beta-amyloid plaques. *Ann. Neurol.* **55**, 617–26.

Dermaut, B., Kumar-Singh, S., Rademakers, R., Theuns, J., Cruts, M., and Van Broeckhoven, C. (2005). Tau is central in the genetic Alzheimer–frontotemporal dementia spectrum. *Trends Genet.* **21**, 664–72.

Dumanchin, C., Brice, A., Campion, D., *et al.* (1998). De novo presenilin 1 mutations are rare in clinically sporadic, early onset Alzheimer's disease cases. French Alzheimer's Disease Study Group. *J. Med. Genet.* **35**, 672–3.

Ferenci, P. (2004). Pathophysiology and clinical features of Wilson disease. *Metab. Brain Dis.* **19**, 229–39.

Ferenci, P., Caca, K., Loudianos, G., *et al.* (2003). Diagnosis and phenotypic classification of Wilson disease. *Liver Int.* **23**, 139–42.

Finckh, U., Muller-Thomsen, T., Mann, U., *et al.* (2000). High prevalence of pathogenic mutations in patients with early-onset dementia detected by sequence analyses of four different genes. *Am. J. Hum. Genet.* **66**, 110–17.

Finckh, U., Kuschel, C., Anagnostouli, M., *et al.* (2005). Novel mutations and repeated findings of mutations in familial Alzheimer disease. *Neurogenetics* **6**, 85–9.

Forsell, C., Froelich, S., Axelman, K., *et al.* (1997). A novel pathogenic mutation (Leu262Phe) found in the presenilin 1 gene in early-onset Alzheimer's disease. *Neurosci. Lett.* **234**, 3–6.

Garrard, P. and Carroll, E. (2005). Presymptomatic semantic impairment in a case of fronto-temporal lobar degeneration associated with the +16 mutation in MAPT. *Neurocase* **11**, 371–83.

Gibbons, R.V., Holman, R.C., Belay, E.D., and Schonberger, L.B. (2000). Creutzfeldt–Jakob disease in the United States: 1979–1998. *J. Am. Med. Assoc.* **284**, 2322–3.

Goate, A., Chartier-Harlin, M.C., Mullan, M., *et al.* (1991). Segregation of a missense mutation in the amyloid precursor protein gene with familial Alzheimer's disease. *Nature* **349**, 704–6.

Godbolt, A.K., Cipolotti, L., Watt, H., Fox, N.C., Janssen, J.C., and Rossor, M.N. (2004). The natural history of Alzheimer disease: a longitudinal presymptomatic and symptomatic study of a familial cohort. *Arch. Neurol.* **61**, 1743–8.

Goldman, J.S., Miller, B.L., Safar, J., *et al.* (2004). When sporadic disease is not sporadic: the potential for genetic etiology. *Arch. Neurol.* **61**, 213–16.

Grabowski, T.J., Cho, H.S., Vonsattel, J.P., Rebeck, G.W., and Greenberg, S.M. (2001). Novel amyloid precursor protein mutation in an Iowa family with dementia and severe cerebral amyloid angiopathy. *Ann. Neurol.* **49**, 697–705.

Grasbeck, A., Horstmann, V., Nilsson, K., Sjobeck, M., Sjostrom, H., and Gustafson, L. (2005). Dementia in first-degree relatives of patients with frontotemporal dementia. A family history study. *Dement. Geriatr. Cogn. Disord.* **19**, 145–53.

Green, R.C., Cupples, L.A., Go, R., *et al.* (2002). Risk of dementia among White and African relatives of patients with Alzheimer's disease. *J. Am. Med. Assoc.* **287**, 329–36.

Greenberg, S.M., Shin, Y., Grabowski, T.J., *et al.* (2003). Hemorrhagic stroke associated with the Iowa amyloid precursor protein mutation. *Neurology* **60**, 1020–2.

Haan, J., Algra, P.R., and Roos, R.A. (1990). Hereditary cerebral hemorrhage with amyloidosis–Dutch type. Clinical and computed tomographic analysis of 24 cases. *Arch. Neurol.* **47**, 649–53.

Haan, J., Van Broeckhoven, C., van Duijn, C.M., *et al.* (1994). The apolipoprotein E epsilon 4 allele does not influence the clinical expression of the amyloid precursor protein gene codon 693 or 692 mutations. *Ann. Neurol.* **36**, 434–7.

Halliday, G.M., Song, Y.J., Lepar, G., *et al.* (2005). Pick bodies in a family with presenilin-1 Alzheimer's disease. *Ann. Neurol.* **57**, 139–43.

Hendriks, L., van Duijn, C.M., Cras, P., *et al.* (1992). Presenile dementia and cerebral haemorrhage linked to a mutation at codon 692 of the beta-amyloid precursor protein gene. *Nat. Genet.* **1**, 218–21.

Hodges, J.R., Davies, R.R., Xuereb, J.H., *et al.* (2004). Clinicopathological correlates in frontotemporal dementia. *Ann. Neurol.* **56**, 399–406.

Houlden, H., Baker, M., Morris, H.R., *et al.* (2001). Corticobasal degeneration and progressive supranuclear palsy share a common tau haplotype. *Neurology* **56**, 1702–6.

Hutton, M., Lendon, C.L., Rizzu, P., *et al.* (1998). Association of missense and 5′-splice-site mutations in tau with the inherited dementia FTDP-17. *Nature* **393**, 702–5.

Ironside, J., Bishop, M., Connolly, K., *et al.* (2006). Variant Creutzfeldt–Jakob disease: prion protein genotype analysis of positive appendix tissue samples from a retrospective prevalence study. *Br. Med. J.* **332**, 1164–5.

James, C.M., Houlihan, G.D., Snell, R.G., Cheadle, J.P., and Harper, P.S. (1994). Late-onset Huntington's disease: a clinical and molecular study. *Age Ageing* **23**, 445–8.

Janssen, J.C., Beck, J.A., Campbell, T.A., *et al.* (2003). Early onset familial Alzheimer's disease: Mutation frequency in 31 families. *Neurology* **60**, 235–9.

Jorm, A.F., Korten, A.E., and Henderson, A.S. (1987). The prevalence of dementia: a quantitative integration of the literature. *Acta Psychiatr. Scand.* **76**, 465–79.

Kamboh, M.I. (2004). Molecular genetics of late-onset Alzheimer's disease. *Ann. Hum. Gen.* **68**, 381–404.

Kamino, K., Orr, H.T., Payami, H., *et al.* (1992). Linkage and mutational analysis of familial Alzheimer disease kindreds for the APP gene region. *Am. J. Hum. Genet.* **51**, 998–1014.

Kanazawa, I. (1998). Dentatorubral-pallidsoluysian atrophy or Naito–Oyanagi disease. *Neurogenetics* **2**, 1–17.

Karlstrom, H., Brooks, W.S., Kwok, J.B., Kril, J.J., Halliday, G.M., and Schofield, P.R. (2005). Variable phenotype of Alzheimer's disease with spastic paraparesis. In *Genotype–proteotype–phenotype relationships in neurodegenerative diseases* (ed. J. Cummings, J. Hardy, M. Poncet, and Y. Christen), pp. 73–92. Springer-Verlag, Heidelberg.

Kaye, E.M. (2001). Update on genetic disorders affecting white matter. *Ped Neurol*, **24**, 11–24.

Klunemann, H.H., Fronhofer, W., Wurster, H., Fischer, W., Ibach, B., and Klein, H.E. (2002). Alzheimer's second patient: Johann F. and his family. *Ann. Neurol.* **52**, 520–3.

Koide, R., Kobayashi, S., Shimohata, T., *et al.* (1999). A neurological disease caused by an expanded CAG trinucleotide repeat in the TATA-binding protein gene: a new polyglutamine disease? *Hum. Mol. Genet.* **8**, 2047–53.

Kovacs, G.G., Trabattoni, G., Hainfellner, J.A., Ironside, J.W., Knight, R.S., and Budka, H. (2002). Mutations of the prion protein gene phenotypic spectrum. *J. Neurol.* **249**, 1567–82.

Krude, H., Schutz, B., Biebermann, H., *et al.* (2002). Choreoathetosis, hypothyroidism, and pulmonary alterations due to human NKX2–1 haploinsufficiency. *J. Clin. Invest.* **109**, 475–80.

Kwok, J.B., Taddei, K., Hallupp, M., *et al.* (1997). Two novel (M233T and R278T) presenilin-1 mutations in early-onset Alzheimer's disease pedigrees and preliminary evidence for association of presenilin-1 mutations with a novel phenotype. *Neuroreport* **8**, 1537–42.

Kwok, J.B., Li, Q.X., Hallupp, M., *et al.* (2000). Novel Leu723Pro amyloid precursor protein mutation increases amyloid beta42(43) peptide levels and induces apoptosis. *Ann. Neurol.* **47**, 249–53.

Kwok, J.B., Halliday, G.M., Brooks, W.S., *et al.* (2003). Presenilin-1 mutation L271V results in altered exon 8 splicing and Alzheimer's disease with non-cored plaques and no neuritic dystrophy. *J. Biol. Chem.* **278**, 6748–54.

Launer, L.J., Andersen, K., Dewey, M.E., *et al.* (1999). Rates and risk factors for dementia and Alzheimer's disease: results from EURODEM pooled analyses. EURODEM Incidence Research Group and Work Groups. European Studies of Dementia. *Neurology* **52**, 78–84.

Le Pira, F., Zappala, G., Saponara, R., *et al.* (2002). Cognitive findings in spinocerebellar ataxia type 2: genetic and clinical variables. *J. Neurol. Sci.* **201**, 53–7.

Levy, E., Carman, M.D., Fernandez-Madrid, I.J., *et al.* (1990). Mutation of the Alzheimer's disease amyloid gene in hereditary cerebral hemorrhage, Dutch type. *Science* **248**, 1124–6.

Levy-Lahad, E., Wasco, W., Poorkaj, P., *et al.* (1995*a*) Candidate gene for the chromosome 1 familial Alzheimer's disease locus. *Science* **269**, 973–7.

Levy-Lahad, E., Wijsman, E.M., Nemens, E., *et al.* (1995*b*) A familial Alzheimer's disease locus on chromosome 1. *Science* **269**, 970–3.

Lindsay, J., Laurin, D., Verreault, R., *et al.* (2002). Risk factors for Alzheimer's disease: a prospective analysis from the Canadian Study of Health and Aging. *Am. J. Epidemiol.* **156**, 445–53.

Lippa, C.F., Smith, T.W., Nee, L., *et al.* (1995). Familial Alzheimer's disease and cortical Lewy bodies: is there a genetic susceptibility factor? *Dementia* **6**, 191–4.

Mackenzie, I.R., Baker, M., West, G., *et al.* (2006). A family with tau-negative frontotemporal dementia and neuronal intranuclear inclusions linked to chromosome 17. *Brain* **129**, 853–67.

Marcon, G., Giaccone, G., Cupidi, C., *et al.* (2004). Neuropathological and clinical phenotype of an Italian Alzheimer family with M239V mutation of presenilin 2 gene. *J. Neuropathol. Exp. Neurol.* **63**, 199–209.

Martins, R.N., Turner, B.A., Carroll, R.T., *et al.* (1995). High levels of amyloid-beta protein from S182 (Glu246) familial Alzheimer's cells. *Neuroreport* **7**, 217–20.

Maruff, P., Tyler, P., Burt, T., Currie, B., Burns, C. and Currie, J. (1996). Cognitive deficits in Machado–Joseph disease. *Ann. Neurol.* **40**, 421–7.

Mattila, K.M., Forsell, C., Pirttila, T., *et al.* (1998). The Glu318Gly mutation of the presenilin-1 gene does not necessarily cause Alzheimer's disease. *Ann. Neurol.* **44**, 965–7.

Mead, S. (2006). Prion disease genetics. *Eur. J. Hum. Genet.* **14**, 273–81.

Mehta, N.D., Refolo, L.M., Eckman, C., *et al.* (1998). Increased Abeta42(43) from cell lines expressing presenilin 1 mutations. *Ann. Neurol.* **43**, 256–8.

Miravalle, L., Tokuda, T., Chiarle, R., *et al.* (2000). Substitutions at codon 22 of Alzheimer's abeta peptide induce diverse conformational changes and apoptotic effects in human cerebral endothelial cells. *J. Biol. Chem.* **275**, 27110–16.

Morita, M., Al-Chalabi, A., Andersen, P.M., *et al.* (2006). A locus on chromosome 9p confers susceptibility to ALS and frontotemporal dementia. *Neurology* **66**, 839–44.

Mullan, M., Crawford, F., Axelman, K., *et al.* (1992*a*). A pathogenic mutation for probable Alzheimer's disease in the APP gene at the N-terminus of beta-amyloid. *Nat. Genet.* **1**, 345–7.

Mullan, M., Houlden, H., Windelspecht, M., *et al.* (1992*b*). A locus for familial early-onset Alzheimer's disease on the long arm of chromosome **14**, proximal to the alpha 1-antichymotrypsin gene. *Nat. Genet.* **2**, 340–2.

Munch, C., Rosenbohm, A., Sperfeld, A.D., *et al.* (2005). Heterozygous R1101K mutation of the DCTN1 gene in a family with ALS and FTD. *Ann. Neurol.* **58**, 777–80.

Nacmias, B., Latorraca, S., Piersanti, P., *et al.* (1995). ApoE genotype and familial Alzheimer's disease: a possible influence on age of onset in APP717 Val → Ile mutated families. *Neurosci. Lett.* **183**, 1–3.

Natte, R., Maat-Schieman ML, Haan, J., Bornebroek, M., Roos, R.A., and van Duinen, S.G. (2001). Dementia in hereditary cerebral hemorrhage with amyloidosis–Dutch type is associated with cerebral amyloid angiopathy but is independent of plaques and neurofibrillary tangles. *Ann. Neurol.* **50**, 765–72.

Neary, D., Snowden J.S., Gustafson, L., *et al.* (1998). Frontotemporal lobar degeneration: a consensus on clinical diagnostic criteria. *Neurology* **51**, 1546–54.

Neary, D., Snowden, J., and Mann, D. (2005). Frontotemporal dementia. *Lancet Neurol.* **4**, 771–80.

Nicholl, D.J., Greenstone, M.A., Clarke, C.E., *et al.* (2003). An English kindred with a novel recessive tauopathy and respiratory failure. *Ann. Neurol.* **54**, 682–6.

Nilsberth, C., Westlind-Danielsson, A., Eckman, C.B., *et al.* (2001). The 'Arctic' APP mutation (E693G) causes Alzheimer's disease by enhanced Abeta protofibril formation. *Nat. Neurosci.* **4**, 887–93.

Nishimura, M., Yu, G., Levesque, G., *et al.* (1999). Presenilin mutations associated with Alzheimer disease cause defective intracellular trafficking of beta-catenin, a component of the presenilin protein complex. *Nat. Med.* **5**, 164–9.

Obici, L., Demarchi, A., de Rosa, G., *et al.* (2005). A novel AbetaPP mutation exclusively associated with cerebral amyloid angiopathy. *Ann. Neurol.* **58**, 639–44.

Palmer, M.S., Dryden, A.J, Hughes, J.T., and Collinge, J. (1991). Homozygous prion protein genotype predisposes to sporadic Creutzfeldt–Jakob disease. *Nature* **352**, 340–2.

Pantieri, R., Pardini, M., Cecconi, M., *et al.* (2005). A novel presenilin 1 L166H mutation in a pseudo-sporadic case of early-onset Alzheimer's disease. *Neurol. Sci.* **26**, 349–50.

Pastor, P., Roe, C.M., Villegas, A., *et al.* (2003). Apolipoprotein Eepsilon4 modifies Alzheimer's disease onset in an E280A PS1 kindred. *Ann. Neurol.* **54**, 163–9.

Pericak-Vance, M.A. and Haines, J.L. (2002). Alzheimer's disease. In *The genetic basis of common diseases*, 2nd edn (ed. R.A. King and J.I. Rotter), pp. Oxford University Press, Oxford.

Peters, N., Opherk, C., Bergmann, T., Castro, M., Herzog, J., and Dichgans, M. (2005). Spectrum of mutations in biopsy-proven CADASIL. *Arch. Neurol.* **62**, 1091–4.

Prelli, F., Castano, E.M., van Duinen, S.G., Bots, G.T., Luyendijk, W., and Frangione, B. (1988). Different processing of Alzheimer's beta-protein precursor in the vessel wall of patients with hereditary cerebral hemorrhage with amyloidosis–Dutch type. *Biochem. Biophys. Res. Commun.* **151**, 1150–5.

Prihar, G., Verkkoniem, A., Perez-Tur, J., *et al.* (1999). Alzheimer disease PS-1 exon 9 deletion defined. *Nat. Med.* **5**, 1090.

Prusiner, S.B. (2001). Shattuck lecture—neurodegenerative diseases and prions. *N. Engl. J. Med.* **344**, 1516–26.

Racette, B.A. and Perlmutter, J.S. (1998). Levodopa responsive parkinsonism in an adult with Huntington's disease. *J. Neurol. Neurosurg. Psychiatry* **65**, 577–9.

Rademakers, R., Cruts, M., Dermaut, B., *et al.* (2002). Tau negative frontal lobe dementia at 17q21: significant finemapping of the candidate region to a 4.8 cM interval. *Mol. Psychiatry* **7**, 1064–74.

Rademakers, R., Cruts, M., and Van Broeckhoven, C. (2004). The role of tau (MAPT) in frontotemporal dementia and related tauopathies. *Hum. Mutat.* **24**, 227–95.

Rasmussen, A., Macias, R., Yescas, P., Ochoa, A., Davila, G., and Alonso, E. (2000). Huntington disease in children: genotype–phenotype correlation. *Neuropediatrics* **31**, 190–4.

Raux, G., Guyant-Marechal, L., Martin, C., *et al.* (2005). Molecular diagnosis of autosomal dominant early onset Alzheimer's disease: an update. *J. Med. Genet.* **42**, 793–5.

Rogaev, E.I., Sherrington, R., Rogaeva, E.A., *et al.* (1995). Familial Alzheimer's disease in kindreds with missense mutations in a gene on chromosome 1 related to the Alzheimer's disease type 3 gene. *Nature* **376**, 775–8.

Rogaev, E.I., Sherrington, R., Wu, C., *et al.* (1997). Analysis of the 5′ sequence, genomic structure, and alternative splicing of the presenilin-1 gene (PSEN1) associated with early onset Alzheimer disease. *Genomics*, **40**, 415–24.

Rosso, S.M., Kamphorst, W., De Graaff, B., *et al.* (2001). Familial frontotemporal dementia with ubiquitin-positive inclusions is linked to chromosome 17q21–22. *Brain* **124**, 1948–57.

Rosso, S.M., Donker Kaat, L., Baks, T., *et al.* (2003). Frontotemporal dementia in The Netherlands: patient characteristics and prevalence estimates from a population-based study. *Brain* **126**, 2016–22.

Rossor, M.N., Fox, N.C., Beck, J., Campbell, T.C., and Collinge, J. (1996). Incomplete penetrance of familial Alzheimer's disease in a pedigree with a novel presenilin-1 gene mutation. *Lancet* **347**, 1560.

Rovelet-Lecrux, A., Hannequin, D., Raux, G., *et al.* (2006). APP locus duplication causes autosomal dominant early-onset Alzheimer disease with cerebral amyloid angiopathy. *Nat. Genet.* **38**, 24–6.

Sandbrink, R., Zhang, D., Schaeffer, S., *et al.* (1996). Missense mutations of the PS-1/S182 gene in German early-onset Alzheimer's disease patients. *Ann. Neurol.* **40**, 265–6.

Santacruz, K., Lewis, J., Spires, T., *et al.* (2005). Tau suppression in a neurodegenerative mouse model improves memory function. *Science* **309**, 476–81.

Schellenberg, G.D., Bird, T.D., Wijsman, E.M., *et al.* (1992). Genetic linkage evidence for a familial Alzheimer's disease locus on chromosome 14. *Science* **258**, 668–71.

Scheuner, D., Eckman, C., Jensen, M., *et al.* (1996). Secreted amyloid beta-protein similar to that in the senile plaques of Alzheimer's disease is increased in vivo by the presenilin 1 and 2 and APP mutations linked to familial Alzheimer's disease. *Nat. Med.* **2**, 864–70.

Seniow, J., Bak, T., Gajda, J., Poniatowska, R., and Czlonkowska, A. (2002). Cognitive functioning in neurologically symptomatic and asymptomatic forms of Wilson's disease. *Mov. Disord.* **17**, 1077–83.

Sherrington, R., Rogaev, E.I., Liang, Y., *et al.* (1995). Cloning of a gene bearing missense mutations in early-onset familial Alzheimer's disease. *Nature* **375**, 754–60.

Silverman, J.M., Ciresi, G., Smith, C.J., Marin, D.B., and Schnaider-Beeri, M. (2005). Variability of familial risk of Alzheimer disease across the late life span. *Arch. Gen. Psychiatry* **62**, 565–73.

Skibinski, G., Parkinson, N.J., Brown, J.M., *et al.* (2005). Mutations in the endosomal ESCRTIII-complex subunit CHMP2B in frontotemporal dementia. *Nat. Genet.* **37**, 806–8.

Smith, M.J., Kwok, J.B., McLean, C.A., *et al.* (2001). Variable phenotype of Alzheimer's disease with spastic paraparesis. *Ann. Neurol.* **49**, 125–9.

Sorbi, S., Nacmias, B., Forleo, P., Piacentini, S., Latorraca, S., and Amaducci, L. (1995). Epistatic effect of APP717 mutation and apolipoprotein E genotype in familial Alzheimer's disease. *Ann. Neurol.* **38**, 124–7.

St George-Hyslop, P., Haines, J., Rogaev, E., *et al.* (1992). Genetic evidence for a novel familial Alzheimer's disease locus on chromosome 14. *Nat. Genet.* **2**, 330–4.

St George-Hyslop, P., McLachlan, D.C., Tsuda, T., *et al.* (1994). Alzheimer's disease and possible gene interaction. *Science* **263**, 537.

Stanford, P.M., Halliday, G.M., Brooks, W.S., *et al.* (2000). Progressive supranuclear palsy pathology caused by a novel silent mutation in exon 10 of the tau gene: expansion of the disease phenotype caused by tau gene mutations. *Brain* **123** (5), 880–93.

Stanford, P.M., Brooks, W.S., Teber, E.T., *et al.* (2004). Frequency of tau mutations in familial and sporadic frontotemporal dementia and other tauopathies. *J. Neurol.* **251**, 1098–104.

Stevanin, G., Fujigasaki, H., Lebre, A.S., *et al.* (2003). Huntington's disease-like phenotype due to trinucleotide repeat expansions in the TBP and JPH3 genes. *Brain* **126**, 1599–603.

Tanahashi, H., Kawakatsu, S., Kaneko, M., Yamanaka, H., Takahashi, K., and Tabira, T. (1996). Sequence analysis of presenilin-1 gene mutation in Japanese Alzheimer's disease patients. *Neurosci. Lett.* **218**, 139–41.

Tang-Wai, D., Lewis, P., Boeve, B., *et al.* (2002). Familial frontotemporal dementia associated with a novel presenilin-1 mutation. *Dement. Geriatr. Cogn. Disord.* **14**, 13–21.

Tanzi, R.E. and Bertram, L. (2005). Twenty years of the Alzheimer's disease amyloid hypothesis: a genetic perspective. *Cell* **120**, 545–55.

Van Broeckhoven, C., Backhovens, H., Cruts, M., *et al.* (1992). Mapping of a gene predisposing to early-onset Alzheimer's disease to chromosome 14q24.3. *Nat. Genet.* **2**, 335–9.

Vance, C., Al-Chalabi, A., Ruddy, D., *et al.* (2006). Familial amyotrophic lateral sclerosis with frontotemporal dementia is linked to a locus on chromosome 9p13.2–21.3. *Brain* **129**, 868–76.

van Duijn, C.M., Hendriks, L., Cruts, M., Hardy, J.A., Hofman, A., and Van Broeckhoven, C. (1991). Amyloid precursor protein gene mutation in early-onset Alzheimer's disease. *Lancet* **337**, 978.

Van Herpen, T., Rosso, S.M., Serverijnen, L.A., *et al.* (2003). Variable phenotypic expression and extensive tau pathology in two families with the novel tau mutation L315R. *Ann. Neurol.* **54**, 573–81.

Vanier, M.T. and Millat, G. (2003). Niemann–Pick disease type C. *Clin. Genet.* **64**, 269–81.

Vidal, R., Frangione, B., Rostagno, A., *et al.* (1999). A stop-codon mutation in the BRI gene associated with familial British dementia. *Nature* **399**, 776–81.

Vidal, R., Revesz, T., Rostagno, A., *et al.* (2000). A decamer duplication in the 3′ region of the BRI gene originates an amyloid peptide that is associated with dementia in a Danish kindred. *Proc. Natl. Acad. Sci. USA* **97**, 4920–5.

Wakutani, Y., Watanabe, K., Adachi, Y., *et al.* (2004). Novel amyloid precursor protein gene missense mutation (D678N) in probable familial Alzheimer's disease. *J. Neurol. Neurosurg. Psychiatry* **75**, 1039–42.

Watts G.D., Wymer, J., Kovach, M.J., *et al.* (2004). Inclusion body myopathy associated with Paget disease of bone and frontotemporal dementia is caused by mutant valosin-containing protein. *Nat. Genet.* **36**, 377–81.

Wexler, N.S., Young, A.B., Tanzi, R.E., *et al.* (1987). Homozygotes for Huntington's disease. *Nature* **326**, 194–7.

Whitwell, J.L., Anderson, V.M., Scahill, R.I., Rossor, M.N., and Fox, N.C. (2004). Longitudinal patterns of regional change on volumetric MRI in frontotemporal lobar degeneration. *Dement. Geriatr. Cogn. Disord.* **17**, 307–10.

Wijsman, E.M., Daw, E.W., Yu, X., *et al.* (2005). APOE and other loci affect age-at-onset in Alzheimer's disease families with PS2 mutation. *Am. J. Med. Genet. B Neuropsychiatr. Genet.* **132**, 14–20.

Wilhelmsen, K.C., Forman, M.S., Rosen, H.J., *et al.* (2004). 17q- linked frontotemporal dementia-amyotrophic lateral sclerosis without tau mutations with tau and alpha-synuclein inclusions. *Arch. Neurol.* **61**, 398–406.

Will, R.G., Alperovitch, A., Poser, S., *et al.* (1998). Descriptive epidemiology of Creutzfeldt–Jakob disease in six European countries, 1993–1995. EU Collaborative Study Group for CJD. *Ann. Neurol.* **43**, 763–7.

Worster-Drought, C., Hill, T.R., and McMenemey, W.H. (1933). Familial presenile dementia with spastic paralysis. *J. Neurol. Psychopathol.* **14**, 27–34.

Wu, Z., Kinslow, C., Pettigrew, K.D., Rapoport, S.I., and Schapiro, M.B. (1998). Role of familial factors in late-onset Alzheimer disease as a function of age. *Alzheimer Dis. Assoc. Disord.* **12**, 190–7.

Xia, W., Zhang, J., Kholodenko, D., *et al.* (1997). Enhanced production and oligomerization of the 42-residue amyloid beta-protein by Chinese hamster ovary cells stably expressing mutant presenilins. *J. Biol. Chem.* **272**, 7977–82.

Zarranz, J.J., Ferrer, I., Lezcano, E., *et al.* (2005). A novel mutation (K317M) in the MAPT gene causes FTDP and motor neuron disease. *Neurology* **64**, 1578–85.

Part 4

Cognitive disorders in other neurological and psychiatric diseases

Chapter 16

Cognitive and behavioural disorders following traumatic brain injury

Anna Mazzucchi

16.1 **Introduction**

Traumatic brain injury (TBI) could be defined as an insult to the brain caused by an external force producing altered states of consciousness that result in impaired cognitive or physical functions.

The incidence of TBI in the Western world is about 1.5 to 2 cases per 1000 population. More than 70% of cases are due to motor vehicle accidents. Approximately 80% of TBI are classified as 'mild'; the remaining 20% as 'moderate' to 'severe'. Seventy per cent of total TBI is comprised of young people (15–30 years old), 75% of whom are males.

As well established both in scientific literature and medical practice, TBI, especially if severe, can produce structural and functional modifications of the brain, which in turn can result in a highly variable and complex interaction of symptoms depending on the motor, sensory, cognitive, emotional, behavioural, and autonomic spheres. The brain during traumatic collision is prone to insults due to a complex combination of acceleration and deceleration and translation and rotation forces causing contusions, diffuse axonal injuries (DAI), and haemorrhages. Moreover, damages to neurons may occur as a consequence of biochemical modifications (i.e. release of glutamate and aspartate, increase of free radicals, etc.), as a consequence of a drop in the levels of oxygen and glucose, and, finally, because of blood hypotension or increased intracranial pressure (Marmarou *et al.* 1991; Chestnut 1995; Teasdale 1995; Horn and Zasler 1996; Marion1996; Richardson 2000; Reider-Groswasser *et al.* 2002). This complex combination of and interaction among insults tends to produce a heterogeneous association of diffused and focalized damages that affect every possible area of the brain: cortical, subcortical, and midbrain. The contusions occur more frequently where the brain comes into contact with bony skull protuberances, i.e. in the basal and orbital-frontal regions and in the basal and polar temporal regions. Shearing strain occurs between tissues of different density where grey and white matter tracts meet causing lesions in basal ganglia, cerebellar peduncles, and reticular formation. Diffuse axonal injuries that occur as a consequence of axonal stretching (the latter very frequently caused by rotation forces) and from neurochemical causes (Gentleman 1999) generate the highest incidence of damages in the frontal and temporal regions (Scheid *et al.* 2003). In addition, mild TBI can produce cerebral damage whose severity is directly correlated with the length of loss of consciousness and of post-traumatic amnesia (see later sections).

16.2 **Neuropsychological disturbances following traumatic brain injury and their assessment**

The fast and progressive epidemiological increase of TBI recorded in the last 30 years has largely contributed to modifying the syndromic definition of the cognitive and behavioural disturbances that may appear following cerebral lesions. In fact, the cognitive and behavioural syndromes upon which the previous nosography was based are mainly those observed after cerebrovascular lesions, which are quite typically 'focal' and cause relatively circumscribed dysfunctions (aphasia, apraxia, acalculia, spatial neglect, etc.). On the contrary and as said above, cognitive–behavioural syndromes following concussion are caused by multiple lesions and dysfunctional after-effects characterized by being diffuse and by provoking the contemporaneous and interdependent dysfunction of several cerebral abilities. Therefore, since 1980, it has been felt necessary to also include in neurological and neuropsychological nosography cognitive and behavioural syndromes that specifically follow brain injury. These syndromes are mainly characterized by the contemporaneous impairment of the majority of neuropsychological faculties, especially those characterized by diffuse functional organization, such as attention, memory, and executive and behavioural functions. Not infrequently, though, symptomatologies depending on more focalized lesions such as circumscribed contusions, ischaemia, or intracerebral haemorrhages are also part of the syndrome. However, 'focal' symptomatologies appearing in the context of traumatic pathologies (i.e. aphasia or spatial neglect) tend to show less definite features than those occurring in consequence of lesions with cerebrovascular character and not infrequently tend to have more a favourable evolution.

For all these reasons and according to the features of each traumatic event (initial clinical severity, coma duration, distribution of contusive cerebral lesions, coexistence or not of complications in the acute and subacute phase), a great variability in the features, symptomatic combination, and evolution in time of cognitive and behavioural functions is to be expected. As a consequence, the clinical diagnostic assessment and the rehabilitative intervention for individuals who have suffered TBI have been radically rethought and operatively readjusted to suit a 'holistic' and strongly integrated vision (Ben-Yishay *et al.* 1982; Ben-Yishay and Diller 1993; Rattok *et al.* 1992; Prigatano 1999*a*; Sohlberg and Mateer 1989*a*, 2001*a*; Wilson 2003; Ponsford 2004; and many others). But this will be hinted at further on.

The clinical reference parameters that proved more valid and were therefore unanimously adopted for the syndromic definition of post-traumatic cognitive–behavioural outcomes are:

1 clinical severity of trauma;

2 clinical evolutional phase during which TBI is observed;

3 main dysfunctions affecting the individual.

As for TBI severity, this produces very variable clinical pictures that proceed along a syndromic continuum from mild TBI—causing circumscribed relatively mild dysfunctions of the most 'elevated' neuropsychological functions—to severe TBI. The latter produces variously combined deteriorations of the capacities of attention, memory, and communication, of the visual-perceptive faculties, and of the executive and behavioural functions. In consequence of that variability, the assessment and the rehabilitation of TBI patients always requires an individualized programme. Finally, very severe TBI trauma produces such marked deterioration of all neuropsychological functions as to make assessment and submission to a formal cognitive rehabilitation programme almost impossible.

The syndromic profile of cognitive impairments can also greatly vary according to the period when it is analysed, i.e. during an early post-traumatic evolutional phase, or during an intermediate or more advanced phase. In fact post-traumatic cognitive–behavioural outcomes tend to evolve positively over a long period of time, unlike those following cerebrovascular lesions. It happens thus that markedly pathological symptoms are observed in an early phase, following not only lesions of the brain, but also dysfunctions of the neurotransmitters and the temporary functional disconnection among cortical areas and between cortical and subcortical areas.

In a following phase that could be defined as intermediate, i.e. when the grossest dysfunctional phenomena are in partial remission, the cognitive–behavioural profile typical of TBI starts to take shape. This can be assessed by means of a formal neuropsychological examination that will help establish cognitive impairment hierarchy. It is thus possible to design a rehabilitative treatment customized to the patient's specific and prevailing problems and to establish the long-term prognosis and the guidelines on which to define the vocational goals. Only in a more advanced phase, which could be defined as the outcome phase and which usually coincides with the ending of the rehabilitation treatment, is it possible to define the specific 'cognitive–behavioural syndrome' that the subject will have to live with and that will determine his/her present and future quality of life (Webb *et al.* 1995).

Neuropsychological assessment also varies according to the post-traumatic phase and the clinical severity with which TBI comes to medical attention: in case of mild TBI neuropsychological assessment will be carried out a few weeks after the trauma. It will be mainly aimed at assessing the level of attention, memory, and executive functions and the emotion and personality profile. Patients with severe TBI are subject to neuropsychological assessment when they give proof of being aware and cooperative enough to be integrated into a rehabilitation programme aimed at correcting their special cognitive and behavioural dysfunctions. However, in case of severe TBI, it may prove necessary to submit the patient to further assessment at a later phase of his/her illness, so to evaluate the severity of the outcomes, the actual possibility for the patient to re-engage in his/her former social/work activities as well as the quality of life to be expected in the short and long term. In case of very severe TBI, because of the considerable cognitive and behavioural deterioration with which the patient presents, neuropsychological assessment is usually limited to the assessment of the basic capacities (attention and memory) and of the instrumental capacities (i.e. language, calculation). Occupational capacities are also evaluated: observation and questionnaires are used to assess the person's levels of autonomy in different everyday life activities.

It is worth noticing that neuropsychological assessment of a TBI, especially if aimed at rehabilitation, must be 'holistic' and 'integrated', even though it can be operatively carried out through the sequential analysis of function after function. In fact, as already said, each neuropsychological dysfunction influences and is influenced by the several coexisting others, as well as by emotional–behavioural aspects, sociocultural level, and the motivation of the subject. This is why a neuropsychological assessment is such a complicated thing to carry out and one that requires specific clinical and neuropsychological competence in brain traumatology to be used in a dynamic and creative way according to the different TBI cases to be tackled.

16.3 The 'mild' brain injury

Brain injury is defined as mild brain injury (MBI) when it causes loss of consciousness lasting less than 1 hour, a Glasgow Coma Score (GCS) of 14–15, and a post-traumatic amnesia lasting less than 24 hours (Kay *et al.* 1998). About 80% of brain injury can be classified as mild: the majority of cases recover without consequences 1–4 weeks after TBI. There is still a percentage of patients (about 20%) who may present with persistent symptoms. These symptoms sometimes fall within the so-called 'post-concussion syndrome', also defined as 'subjective mild concussion syndrome' (Rutherford 1989), and are connected with straining factors or the worsening of premorbid personality (Ponsford *et al.* 2000). At other times they are the expression of specific neuropsychological difficulties. The special feature of post-concussion syndrome consists in the discrepancy between the symptoms subjectively referred to by the patient (headache, vertigo, insomnia, sensitivity to noise and/or bright lights) and their objectively small significance at clinical or instrumental assessment. Among these symptoms, those with a cognitive–behavioural character are subjectively referred to by about half of the patients with mild TBI. They are irritability, swinging moods, depression, and concentration and memory problems. In the majority of cases such symptoms tend to remit spontaneously, but not infrequently and for some individuals they tend to become chronic. For a long time such a clinical picture was interpreted on a psychogenic and functional basis, but instrumental (Humayun *et al.* 1989; Montgomery *et al.* 1991; Hofman *et al.* 2001) and psychometric (Leininger *et al.* 1990; Ponsford and Kinsella 1992) anomalies have recently been found that support the idea of an organic basis for such disturbances. It is beginning to be accepted that their occurrence might be determined by the interaction of organic and psychogenic factors (Martelli *et al.* 1999; Sohlberg and Mateer 2001*b*).

Mild brain injury (MBI)

- Represents 80% of brain injury.
- Loss of consciousness: less than 1 hour.
- Glasgow Coma Score (GCS) score: 14–15.
- Post-traumatic amnesia: less than 24 hours.
- 80% recover without consequences 1 to 4 weeks after TBI.
- 20% may present persistent symptoms.
- Possible persistent neuropsychological symptoms: impaired attention and memory; slight disinhibition; diminished self-control; slight difficulty of judgement and of abstraction; difficulty of pragmatic speech organization; slightly impaired capacity of planning; impaired emotion and personality profile.

In a continuum with the MBI subjective syndrome are those syndromes that could be defined as truly neuropsychological, in that their organic nature is revealed by clinical investigations and formal tests. They especially affect middle-aged or elderly patients who complain of less efficiency in dealing and coping with everyday situations and of increased slowness in problem-solving. They also report the need for greater efforts of attention and concentration to obtain the same results as before the trauma when carrying out working or studying activities. In such cases it appears evident that not just isolated functions are damaged, but the executive functions in general (see further on), in particular the attentive supervision and the working memory that are connected to the frontal lobes (Kay 1986). Some patients, though, show the contemporaneous impairment of several functions and selective cognitive deficits such as memory deficit, slight disinhibition, diminished self-control, slight difficulty of judgement and of abstraction, difficulty in pragmatic speech organization, slightly impaired capacity of planning (Shapiro and Sacchetti 1993; Zasler and Martelli 2003).

Studies focusing on the social and working reintegration of patients subject to MBI (Kay *et al.* 1992; Zasler and Martelli 2003) show that the majority of individuals with TBI outcomes cannot go back to work in a short time or, if back, are less efficient than in premorbid time, while 10% end up by losing their job. Hence there is a need to provide specific rehabilitative treatment for MBI so as to help patients to overcome their difficulties and avoid consequences on their quality of life (Green *et al.* 1997).

When an individual with MBI becomes aware of his/her diminished efficiency in everyday life activities and in carrying out his/her job, he/she almost always experiences a complex emotional and behavioural reaction with prevailing feelings of inadequacy, uncertainty, depression, and diminished self-esteem. On the other hand, as there are usually good prospects for MBIs to resume their pre-traumatic activities, it is essential to design supporting strategies fit for solving the specific problems patients refer about. Reliable guidelines for the treatment of MBIs have been developing in recent years (Gronwall 1986; Cicerone 1992; Kay 1993; Liberto *et al.* 1993; Green *et al.* 1997). What follows is a list of the most agreed upon programmatic points.

All authors agree that, to prevent patients' excessive emotional reactions, it is first of all necessary to give them at an early stage exhaustive information about the pathogenic nature of their symptoms, reassuring them that these represent the 'normal' consequence of the trauma. Instructions must also be provided on how to improve efficiency, concentration capacity, exertion endurance, etc. as well as instructions about the most appropriate way to deal with everyday problems and situations (Sohlberg and Mateer 2001*b*).

Given the special emotional context surrounding MBIs, it is necessary for patients to establish a good 'therapeutic relationship' with their neuropsychologist, who can help them solve the conflict between recovery expectations and objective post-traumatic disturbances. A good neuropsychologist can also provide the MBI patient with better insight about the nature of his/her symptoms and more accurate self-evaluation and self-monitoring, helping him/her to fully accept his/her new situation. It is thus possible for MBIs to realistically reorganize their activities and carry out a critical analysis of their performances, enabling them to plan with adequate flexibility the necessary changes and adaptations to be brought about in their working and everyday activities and the best way to do so.

In those cases in which evident cognitive sequelae persist, formal cognitive rehabilitative treatment may prove necessary. As said above, MBIs can show concentration or attentive supervision deficits, working memory or/and prospective memory impairment, difficulty in learning complex material, judgement and problem-solving difficulties, and sometimes also difficulties in planning work. To remedy these disturbances, a targeted rehabilitative approach is required that will set out and make use of rehabilitative situations as similar as possible to those of the context where the patient will be re-integrated (Sohlberg and Mateer 2001*b*).

While treating MBIs, a therapists must also design special 'counselling programmes' for the patients' family members and/or 'significant others'. Very often people interacting with the patient find it difficult to understand and thus accept the cognitive and emotional modifications brought about by trauma. Such misunderstandings can cause tension in interpersonal relationships and foster depreciatory attitudes towards the patient who ends up by feeling uneasy not only at work but also within his/her family circle. It is the neurologist's or neuropsychologist's task to adequately inform the patient's family members while suggesting the best, i.e. most encouraging and reassuring, attitudes to adopt. The effectiveness of such guidelines in the rehabilitative treatment of mild TBI has been confirmed by recent publications (Tiersky *et al.* 2005) and by a just as recent Cochrane review (Turner-Stokes *et al.* 2005).

16.4 **The moderate brain injury and the correlated cognitive and behavioural disturbances**

Brain injury is defined 'moderate' when it scores 13 to 9 on the Glasgow Coma Scale (Kay *et al.* 1998). This category of patients with brain injury, which makes up 10–12% of all TBI, includes patients whose condition may rapidly (i.e. in the immediate days after trauma) evolve towards mild TBI, especially as regards cognitive symptoms but also patients whose condition worsens in the days immediately following hospitalization, especially as far as cognitive and behavioural outcomes are concerned, and who thus fall under severely brain-injured severe TBI (see further on). This category also includes patients (about a third of the total) who present with cognitive–behavioural outcomes that are a bit worse than mild TBI and a bit better than severe TBI, though they always basically show the same syndromic features because of the prevailing involvement of frontal and temporal lobes, i.e. attention, attentive supervision, concentration deficit; anterograde learning difficulty; working and prospective memory impairment; impairment of critical, self-critical, and judgement capacities; problem solving and pragmatic communication difficulties; relational and emotional behaviour impairment; limited endurance of stress and fatigue; regression of personality; diminished initiative and self-control.

Moderate brain injury

- Represents 10% of brain injury.
- Loss of consciousness: less than 24 hours.
- Glasgow Coma Score (GCS) score: 9–13.
- Post-traumatic amnesia: less than 7 days.
- 20% may recover without consequences 1–6 months after TBI.
- 80% present persistent symptoms.
- Persistent neuropsychological symptoms: attention, attentive supervision, and concentration deficit; anterograde learning difficulty; working and perspective memory impairment; impairment of critical, self-critical, and judgement capacities; problem-solving and pragmatic communication difficulties; relational and emotional behaviour impairment limited endurance of stress and fatigue; regression of personality; diminished initiative and self-control.

The rehabilitative cognitive and behavioural treatment of these subgroups of moderate TBI does not differ from that given in case of mild TBI (see above) or severe TBI (see further on). The cognitive models of reference are relatively similar, as are the treatment methodologies and their goal, i.e. the recovery of autonomies and the social and work reintegration.

16.5 The severe brain injury: a variable combination of cognitive and behavioural disturbances

TBI is classified as severe when it scores from 8 to 3 on the Glasgow Coma Scale. (Kay *et al.* 1998). Severe TBI makes up 8–10% of all concussions. Individuals with severe TBI who suffered from more or less long periods of coma all show relevant motor, sensorial, cognitive, and behavioural outcomes. They invariably need long and complex rehabilitative treatments based on team-integrated management of all disabilities. In clinical practice, within the syndromic categories of patients with severe TBI, variable combinations of cognitive and behavioural disturbances may be observed that depend on the intrinsic and overall TBI severity. In fact, we can be confronted by very different clinical pictures depending on the length of coma associated with the TBI (which can range from 1 week to one or several months), even though the international classification, based on the score on the Glasgow Coma Score during acute phase, tends to classify the cases under the same category.

The prevailing 'diffuse' character of neuropsychological syndromes and the prevalence within them of cognitive and behavioural symptoms that must be correlated with the severity of the lesions in the frontal and temporal areas has already been discussed. This accounts for the constant coexistence in severe TBI of memory, attention, executive function, and behaviour impairments, as well as impairments of the logical capacities, of abstract judgement, and of problem-solving (Luria 1973; Ben-Yishay and Diller 1983*a*, *b*; Goldstein and Levin 1987; Stuss and Benson 1987), which can be of such severity as to heavily influence the patient and his/her family's future quality of life. As repeatedly stated, such disturbances can appear in various ways and combinations as part of post-traumatic pathology. Whatever their aspect, they all require a 'holistic' clinical and neuropsychological approach. What follows is a description of the most frequent cognitive and behavioural features following severe TBI.

As for behavioural disorders, a patient with a severe TBI outcome may show, according to the prevailing dysfunction of the dopaminergic, serotoninergic, cholinergic, or noradrenergic system (see Fig. 16.1), disturbances of the executive functions (see further on), personality, temperament, and mood disturbances, and behavioural disorders. Behavioural disorders can be divided into two subgroups: (1) disorders of arousal, drive, and motivation; (2) disorders of inhibitory and regulatory control. A patient suffering from the former disorders looks inert, apathetic, lacks interests and motivation, is unable to take initiatives (akinetic–abulic syndrome), is prone to fatigue and easily distracted, overdependent on his/her environment and family, indifferent to affections, scarcely aware of his/her difficulties and of the changes following trauma. On the other hand, a patient suffering from disorders of inhibitory and regulatory control may appear socially and sexually disinhibited, irritable, aggressive, lacking control and self-criticism, hyperactive without precise goals, dysphoric, inappropriate in social intercourse, impoverished in affectivity, intolerant of environmental or family requests, frustrated by change of role and by

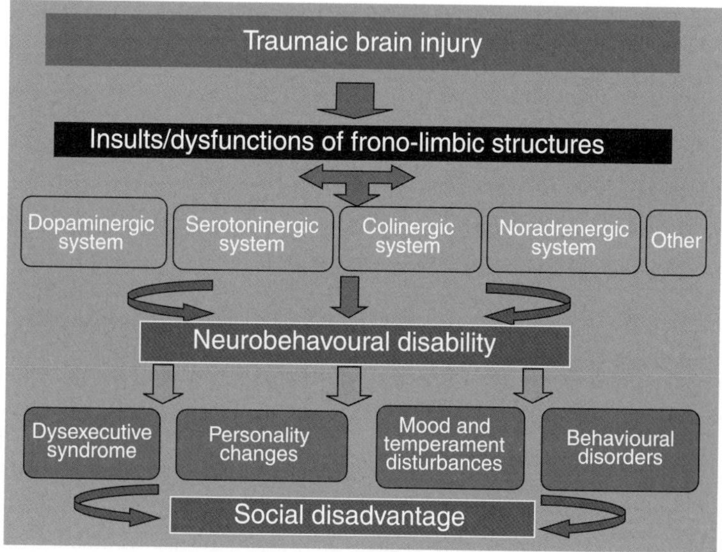

Fig. 16.1 The post-traumatic cascade from the traumatic event to the social disadvantage.

the necessity of being taken care of by others (Wood 2001). Both these behavioural situations heavily influence cognitive performance, but are in turn negatively influenced by the coexistence of cognitive disturbances such as attention and memory disorders and consequent unawareness of others, impulsivity, misinterpretation, misjudgements, social carelessness.

In clinical practice it is useful to bear in mind that post-traumatic behavioural disorders, especially the most severe, may represent the worsening evolution of a premorbid situation. It is also useful to bear in mind that behavioural disturbances may be negatively influenced by coexisting metabolic disturbances and sleep or mood disorders. They can also be the expression of epileptic activity (partial seizure-like phenomena) or be due to improper use of drugs (Glenn 2002).

Severe brain injury

- Represents 10% of brain injury.
- Loss of consciousness: more than 24 hours.
- Glasgow Coma Score (GCS) score: 3–8.
- Post-traumatic amnesia: more than 7 days.
- 100% present persistent more or less evident symptoms.
- Persistent neuropsychological symptoms: more or less* severe attention and concentration impairment; anterograde learning and recollection difficulties; working and prospective memory impairment; severe impairment of critical, self-critical, and judgement capacities; problem-solving and pragmatic communication deterioration; relational and emotional behaviour disturbances; regression of premorbid personality; loss of initiative and self-control.

*Severity of symptoms is highly correlated with coma length and post-traumatic amnesia length.

As for personality changes, those most frequently observed are the following: impoverishing or regression of premorbid personality to the point of adopting childish attitudes; a tendency to defer to or even depend on others; the development of obsessive–compulsive and stereotyped or ritualistic symptoms.

These four categories of disorders prompt the onset of a general neurobehavioural disability (see Fig. 16.1) leading, especially if rehabilitative treatment proves inadequate to patient's needs, to social disadvantage (Ben-Yishay and Lakin 1989; Prigatano, 1999*a*). This generates in turn, as the final event of the post-traumatic cascade, refusal of social activities, breakdown of relationships, isolation, emotional maladjustment and difficulty in keeping partners, friends, and jobs.

Attention disturbances are a typical feature of the syndrome following severe TBI: the individual, often due to scarce motivation, analyses information and context in a superficial or incomplete way; he/she doesn't adequately distinguish primary from secondary information; he/she submits situations to impulsive and incomplete analysis leading to incorrect conclusions. The patient is often unable to filter or inhibit interferences and his/her attention is thus easily distracted. Alternatively, he/she is unable to adequately distribute his/her attention over complex or articulate situations: he/she loses the reasoning or speech or action thread thus coming to rash conclusions or is unable to bring to an end what was started. The carrying out of the different praxic–procedural activities is too hasty or too slow, approximate, inaccurate in details, with frequent sequential mistakes. Lack of sensitivity to the needs of others and, more generally, social carelessness also fall within this category of disorders, even though they result from coexisting disorders of critical and self-critical faculties.

As for memory disturbances, they persist in almost all cases of severe TBI. Briefly, they may depend on two sets of problems that are often not easily distinguishable but that can partially coexist (see Fig. 16.2). The first set consists of difficulty/inability to adequately record information, which thus falls too quickly into oblivion and cannot be adequately retrieved after a while. This set of problems usually follows prevailing insults/dysfunctions of the hippocampo–mammillo–thalamic circuit and can produce, according to the severity of the lesions and the prevailing unilaterality or bilaterality of the same, either partial or global amnesia. Memory disturbances secondary to TBI are, however, more frequently due to a second set of problems having to do with the inability to inhibit interference during learning, to stick to the logical order of the events to be remembered, to adopt adequate learning strategies, to establish the correct logical sequence of the material to be learned, to plan a sequence of actions in the most convenient order, and, finally, to control the recalling of memories. These difficulties depend especially on a deficit of executive function and of working memory (Baddeley 1986) and are due in great part to insults/dysfunctions of the frontolimbic system.

Three sets of disorders can impair the linguistic functions: aphasic disorder (found only in 7% of TBI); ideational disorder with difficulty in generating discourse; and disorder of pragmatic communicative behaviour. As for the definition of the syndrome and the rehabilitative treatment, aphasic disorders only partially differ from aphasic disorders following cerebrovascular lesions. Disorders of verbal ideation and formulation mainly consist in the reduction of syntactic–grammatical–lexical flexibility. This makes it difficult to effectively find qualifying, synthetic, and abstract expression and generates an inability to keep thematic organization and 'global coherence' of language (Glosser and Deser 1990). Communicative behaviour disorders essentially correspond to the disorders of so-called 'pragmatic' competence, i.e. the competence that modulates language as an instrument of thought formulation, verbal organization, effectiveness in conveying information, and interpersonal and social interaction (Prutting and Kirchner 1983, 1987; Penn and Cleary 1988; Sohlberg and Mateer 1989*b*, 2001*c*; Hartley and Jensen 1991, 1992; Body *et al.* 1999; Togher *et al.* 1999). As a consequence, the patient uses matter-of-fact sentences

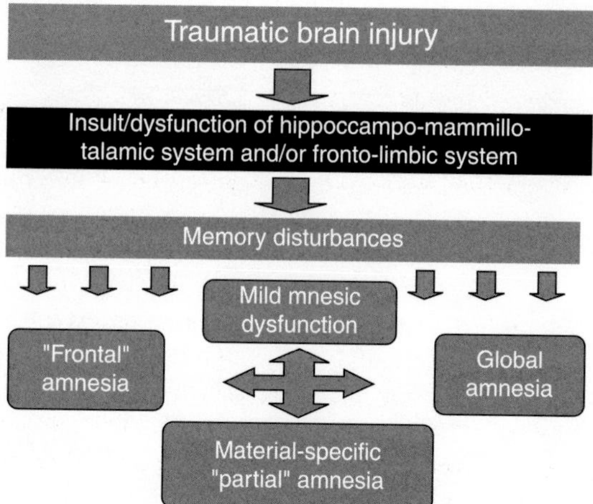

Fig. 16.2 Principal categories of memory disturbances following traumatic brain injury.

that are repetitive in their content, circumscribed to everyday reality, and scarcely informative; his/her reasoning is disorganized or redundant and limits itself to the most superficial aspects or to the scarcely relevant details of a matter (Togher *et al.* 1999). These latter two sets of problems both occur in cases of damage to the prefrontal areas and are closely connected to disorders of the executive functions.

The executive functions include a great part of the abilities required to plan, organize, initiate, and put into being voluntary behaviours in the correct sequence and in an adequate response to the social and environmental requirements, goals, and demands. The correct execution of an action, be it verbal or motor, is but the final part of a complex mental process. This process proves to be the more adequate to pre-set goals, the more it is preceded by mental judgements taking into consideration not only the feasibility of each single act leading to final goal, but also its effect on people and environment (Sohlber and Mateer 2001*d*). The executive functions, in fact, are inextricably intertwined with many aspects of operative, emotional, and relational behaviour. As we said above, the executive functions are correlated with the frontal areas, more specifically with the prefrontal areas. Following concussion, the prefrontal areas are almost always affected by contusion insults and diffuse axonal injury. This is why all severe TBI may present with more or less severe disorders of the executive functions. Very briefly, executive disorders generate two sets of difficulties (see Fig. 16.3). The first set is due to prevailing compromise of the interconnections between the two frontal lobes. This results in poor self-control, incapacity of insight, incapacity of self-monitoring leading to incapacity of bringing about the necessary changes when operational choices prove mistaken. On the other hand, the individual

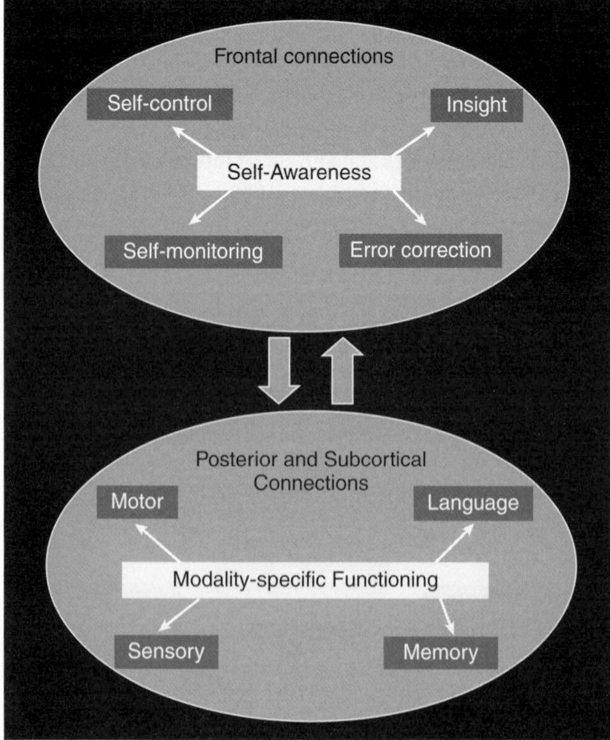

Fig. 16.3 The executive abilities and their anatomo-functional correlations.

with such difficulties tends to persevere in the use of a given strategy even when it proves unsuitable (Sohlberg and Mateer 2001*d*; Turner and Levine 2003). The second set of difficulties, due to prevailing compromise of the interconnections between the prefrontal areas of the encephalon and the most posterior and subcortical ones (Sohlberg and Mateer 2001*d*; Turner and Levine 2003), results in problem-solving difficulties, i.e. difficulties in correctly analysing and formulating problems and activities to be carried out. They may involve either the verbal or operative domain and consist in an incapacity to previously set the goals to be achieved. The choice of wrong learning or operative strategies, the choice of too practical or simplified solutions, and errors in planning or maintaining the action and language sequence are also cases of problem-solving difficulties (Luria and Tsveskova 1967; Benton 1968, Shallice 1982).

16.6 **Cognitive and behavioural rehabilitation following severe brain injury: a holistic and integrated methodological approach**

Rehabilitative care of people who suffer from TBI requires an ample background of integrated notions on clinical neurology, clinical neuropsychology, cognitive sciences, psychodynamic and behavioural sciences, and neuropsychological rehabilitation. They are not so much of use in the definition of general operative rules, as in tracing the outline of the rehabilitative intervention required in every single case (Levin *et al.* 1987; Sohlberg and Mateer 1989*a*, 2001*a*; Christensen and Uzzel 1994, 1999; Ponsford 1995, 2004; Mazzucchi and Avanzi 1998; Mazzucchi *et al.* 1999; Prigatano 1999*a*; and many others). Rehabilitative care cannot but be provided by a team of clinicians, experts, and therapists especially trained in this complex discipline. It is crucial that the clinical neuropsychologist and therapist be specially trained and in possession of a high degree of professional knowledge and experience in the field. As such training is rarely part of educational programmes, it not easy to find experts in the field (Mazzucchi and Parma 1999).

In addition, in planning the cognitive rehabilitative treatment of individuals with severe TBI disturbances, it is necessary, as anticipated above, to pay attention to the severity of post-traumatic sequelae, the post-traumatic evolutional phase at the moment of clinical/rehabilitative intervention, and the patient's symptomatic profile. Care must also be taken in the choice of the methods that seem appropriate in each case and in the definition of actually achievable goals.

TBI: cognitive rehabilitation

- Early post-traumatic phase: non-specific stimulation of simplest activities of daily life (ADL), reorientation techniques
- Intermediate post-traumatic phase: formal neuropsychological rehabilitative procedures for impaired cognitive abilities (memory, language, attention, information processing, etc.), occupational therapy, and behavioural conditioning
- Advanced post-traumatic phase: cognitive holistic approach (integrated rehabilitation of cognitive operative strategies and behaviour)
- Reintegration phase: advanced occupational therapy, vocational treatment, use of compensations, social and environmental reintegration
- Follow-up: TBI long-term support and backing programmes for the families

Rehabilitative procedures are selected according to the neuropsychological and behavioural features found. For instance, patients who have suffered very severe cognitive TBI consequences and who, as happens in the majority of these cases, can only produce minimal response to environmental stimuli can only be approached in an ecological way. In other words, the rehabilitative team and the family members have the task of stimulating the patient's residual capacities that can presumably be used in carrying out the simplest activities of daily life (ADL) or in establishing the best possible environmental relationship. The goal is to achieve, when possible, a more or less satisfactory degree of autonomy enabling the patient to carry out simple and routine activities (McNeny 1990). The same approach can be used when a patient with severe TBI is at an early post-traumatic phase and is confused, disoriented, not very cooperative, unable to concentrate attention for more than a few seconds. In this case, it is possible, also with the help of the family, to have recourse to 'non-specific' personal and environmental stimulation: the patient is given simple, easy-to-interpret stimuli and is required to carry out simple daily activities (washing, getting dressed, eating, tidying his/her things up, etc.).

The use of reorientation techniques may prove useful with patients at quite an early phase of the post-traumatic course, who nevertheless show partial awareness of their situation and a certain limited degree of cooperation, while still presenting with diffuse and relevant cognitive–behavioural deterioration. Reorientation techniques contribute to re-building an identity in the patient and improving his/her interaction with the environment. They also improve his/her degree of autonomy in ADL (reality orientation therapy; McNeny and Dise 1990; Sloan and Ponsford 1995). When a patient with severe TBI attains sufficient personal and environmental orientation and a degree of attention and cooperation such as to make possible formal and exhaustive neuropsychological assessment, it is then also possible to design a customized rehabilitative programme according to the diagnosed neuropsychological disturbances profile. This will be divided into special sessions aimed at treating attention and memory, linguistic, logical, and executive dysfunctions as well as behavioural abnormalities according to methodologies and procedures by now well-established in the scientific literature (Prigatano 1999*b*; Sohlberg and Mateer 2001*e*; Ponsford 2004; Wilson 2003).

In a more advanced phase, when the patient shows signs of having recovered the most elementary levels of cognitive elaboration, it may prove useful to try to recover operative strategies. Residual neuropsychological capacities, if left to the patient's spontaneous use, prove inefficient. Though this may depend on residual inertia or scarce motivation, it more usually depends, as has been proven, on lack of spontaneous activation of operating strategies aimed at obtaining the desired goals or at finishing what started. In this phase, then, the rehabilitative programme must be aimed at making the patient re-discover and spontaneously apply the most suitable strategies for analysing and processing information, planning and organizing target-oriented activities, activating adequate procedures of criticism and self-criticism in compliance with the different contexts and the different environmental and interpersonal interactions implied in every activity (Levin *et al.* 1987; Prigatano 1999*b*; Sohlberg and Mateer 1989*a*, 2001*d*; Christensen and Uzzel, 1994, 1999; Ponsford 1995, 2004.)

A phase habitually follows that could be defined as use of compensation. During this phase the patient tries to find ways of making up for those abilities that rehabilitative intervention could not further modify or bring to levels of functionality compatible with the patient's autonomy, e.g. the ability to use a computer, an electronic notebook, or other technology (Chute 2002; Wilson 2003; Gartland 2004). When a patient attains a still more advanced phase in which the residual cognitive capacities are not liable to further modification but are such as to allow renewal of productive, work, or study activities, the partly cognitive and partly 'occupational' rehabilitative intervention—according to the type of reintegration proving possible—will be

aimed at preparing socio-occupational reintegration. In such cases the rehabilitation programme will be customized, if possible, on the basis of the patient's previous job and previous social environment and of the still modifiable residual impairments that could jeopardize reintegration (Tate *et al.* 2003). If this goal appears inaccessible, the vocational programme will be adapted to the residual cognitive and behavioural resources relevant to the domestic and social environment.

For TBI patients with more or less severe neuropsychological and behavioural sequalae, it is also worth devising, after discharge from hospital and/or rehabilitative treatment, long-term support, either because of the domestic and socio-occupational reintegration difficulties that may occur or because of the patient's residual behavioural disturbances or because it is particularly hard for the patient to accept the changes brought about in his/her life by the traumatic event (Ben-Yishay and Lakin 1989; Prigatano 1999*a*).

16.7 **The involvement and role of the families in the post-traumatic treatment of brain-injured subjects**

In the several monographs by now available specializing in TBI and in particular in those devoted to rehabilitation treatment, chapters regarding TBI patients' families are systematically included (Ylvisaker 1985; Rosenthal *et al.* 1990; Williams and Kay 1996; Mazzucchi *et al.* 1999). Several articles about the matter are also found in scientific reviews (Solomon and Scherzer 1991; Cope and Wolfson 1994; Devany Serio *et al.* 1995; Blosser and De Pompei 1995). It is, in fact, commonly observed in clinical practice and is by now established that families can considerably influence the quality of post-traumatic course, the reaching of rehabilitative goals, as well as the long-term quality of social and vocational reintegration.

The experience of the last 20 years has suggested the creation of special back-up programmes for TBI patients' family members, running side-by-side with rehabilitation treatment of the patients themselves. Such programmes include meetings with the families to:

- adequately inform them about the characteristics of the post-traumatic outcomes and the short- and long-term prognosis;
- inform them about the therapeutic and rehabilitative treatment;
- teach families how to correctly interact with a patient with cognitive and/or behavioural disturbances, how to avoid inadequate behaviour (overprotective or overstimulating behaviour), or how to obtain from the patient better participation in everyday activities;
- give the families support during the difficult process of accepting outcomes that cannot be further modified;
- train families to manage patients with severe cognitive or behavioural outcomes once home;
- post-discharge, to psychologically support families and check that the attained goals are maintained.

References

Baddely, A. (1986). *Working memory*. Clarendon Press, Oxford.

Benton, A.L. (1968). Differential behavioural effects in frontal lobe disease. *Neuropsychologia* **6**, 53–60.

Ben-Yishay, Y. and Diller, L. (1983*a*). Cognitive deficits. In *Rehabilitation of the head injured adult* (ed. M. Rosenthal, E.R. Griffith. *et al.*), pp. 167–83. F.A. Davis Co, Philadelphia.

Ben-Yishay, Y. and Diller, L. (1983*b*). Cognitive remediation. In *Rehabilitation of the head injured adult* (ed. M. Rosenthal, E.R. Griffith. *et al.*), pp. 367–8. F.A. Davis Co, Philadelphia.

Ben-Yishay, Y. and Diller, L. (1993). Cognitive remediation in traumatic brain injury: update and issues. *Arch. Phys. Med. Rehabil.* **74**, 204–13.

Ben-Yishay, Y. and Lakin, P. (1989). Structured group treatment for brain injury survivors. In *Neuropsychological treatment after brain injury* (ed. D.W. Ellis and A. Christensen), pp. 271–96. Kluwer Academic Publishers, Boston.

Ben-Yishay, Y., Rattok, J., Ross, B., Lakin, P., Silver, S., Thomas, L., and Diller L. (1982). A rehabilitation-relevant system for cognitive, interpersonal and vocational rehabilitation of traumatically head injured persons. In *Working approaches to remediation of cognitive deficits in brain damaged persons*, Rehabilitation Monograph No. 64, pp. 1–15. New York University Medical Centre Institute of Rehabilitation Medicine, New York.

Blosser, J. and De Pompei, R. (1995). Fostering effective family involvement through mentoring. *J. Head Trauma Rehabil.* **10** (2), 46–56.

Body, R., Perkins, M., and McDonald, S. (1999). Pragmatics, cognition and communication in traumatic brain injury. In *Communication disorders following traumatic brain injury* (ed. S. McDonald, L. Togher, and C. Code), pp. 81–112. Psychology Press, Hove.

Chesnut, R.M. (1995). Secondary brain insults after head injury: clinical perspectives. *New Horiz.* **3**, 366–75.

Christensen, A. and Uzzell, B.P. (1994). *Brain injury and neuropsycholoical rehabilitation. International perspectives.* Lawrence Erlbaum Associates, Hillsdale, New Jersey.

Christensen, A. and Uzzel, B.P. (eds.) (1999). *International handbook of neuropsychological rehabilitation.* Plenum Press, New York.

Chute, D.L. (2002). Neuropsychological technologies in rehabilitation. *J. Head Inj. Rehabil.* **17**, 369–77.

Cicerone, K.D. (1992). Psychological management of post-concussive disorders. In *Rehabilitation of post-concussive disorders* (ed. J.L. Horn and N.D. Zasler), pp. 129–41. Hanley and Belfus, Inc, Philadelphia.

Cope, D.N. and Wolfson, B. (1994). Crisis intervention with the family in the trauma setting. *J. Head Trauma Rehabil.* **9**, 67–81.

Devany Serio, C., Kreitzer, J.S., *et al.* (1995). Predicting family needs after brain injury: implications for intervention. *J. Head Trauma Rehabil.* **10**, 32–45.

Gartland, D. (2004). Considerations in the selection and use of technology with people who have cognitive deficits following acquired brain injury. *Neuropsychol. Rehabil.* **14** (1–2), 61–75.

Gentleman, D. (1999). Improving outcome after traumatic brain injury—progress and challenges. *Br. Med. Bull.* **55** (4), 910–26.

Glenn, M.B. (2002). A differential diagnostic approach to the pharmacological treatment of cognitive, behavioural and affective disorders after traumatic brain injury. *J. Head Trauma Rehabil.* **17**, 273–83.

Glosser, G. and Deser, T. (1990). Patterns of discourse production among neurological patients with fluent language disorders. *Brain Lang.* **40**, 67–88.

Goldstein, F.L. and Levin, H.S. (1987). Disorders of reasoning and problem solving ability. In Neuropsychological Rehabilitation (ed. M. Manfred, A. Benton, *et al.*), pp. 327–54. Guilford Press, New York.

Green, B.S., Stevens, K.M., and Wolfe, T.D. (1997). *Mild traumatic brain injury. A therapy and resource manual.* Singular Publishing Group Inc, San Diego.

Gronwall, D. (1986). Rehabilitation programs for patients with mild head injury: components, problems, and evaluation. *J. Head Trauma Rehabil.* **1**, 53–62.

Hartley, L.L. and Jensen, P.J. (1991). Narrative and procedural discourse after closed head injury. *Brain Inj.* **5**, 267–85.

Hartley, L.L. and Jensen, P.J. (1992). Three discourse profiles of closed-head-injury speakers: theoretical and clinical implications. *Brain Inj.* **6**, 271–82.

Hofman, P.A.M., Stapert, S.Z., van Kroonenburgh, M.J.P.G., *et al.* (2001). MR imaging, single-photon emission CT and neurocognitive performance after mild traumatic brain injury. *Am. J. Neuroradiol.* **22**, 441–9.

Horn, L.J. and Zasler, N.D. (eds.) (1996). *Medical rehabilitation of traumatic brain injury*. Hanley and Belfus, Inc, Philadelphia.

Humayun, M.S., Presty, S.K., *et al.* (1989). Local cerebral glucose abnormalities in mild closed head injury patients with cognitive impairments. *Nucl. Med. Commun.* **10**, 335–44.

Kay, T.E. (1986). *Minor head injury: an introduction for professionals*. National Head Injury Publication 1–12.

Kay, T.E. (1993). Neuropsychological treatment of mild traumatic brain injury. *J. Head Trauma Rehabil.* **8**, 74–85.

Kay, T.E., Cavallo, M.M, *et al.* (1992). Minor head injury in the emergency room: an outcome study. *Arch. Phys. Med. Rehabil.* **73**, 955.

Kay, T., Harrington, D.E., Adams, R., *et al.* (1998). Definition of mild traumatic brain injury. *J. Head Trauma Rehabil.* 8, 86–7.

Leininger B. E. Gramling S.E., *et al.* (1990). Neuropsychological deficits in symptomatic head injury patients after concussion and mild concussion. *J. Neurol. Neurosurg. Psychiatry* **53**, 293–6.

Levin, H.S., Grafman, J., *et al.* (1987). *Neurobehavioral recovery from head injury*. Oxford University Press, Oxford.

Liberto, L., Tomlin, K., *et al.* (1993). Cognitive rehabilitation. In *Minor head trauma. Assessment, management and rehabilitation* (ed. S. Mandel, R. Thayer Sataloff, *et al.*), pp. 290–305. Springer-Verlag, New York.

Luria, A.R. (1973). *The working brain: an introduction for neuropsychology*. Basic Books, New York.

Luria, A.R. and Tesvetskova, L.S. (1967). *Les troubles de la résolution des problèmes. Analyse neuropsychologique*. Gautier-Villars, Paris.

Marion, D.W. (1996). Pathophysiology and initial neurosurgical care: future directions. In *Medical rehabilitation of traumatic brain injury* (ed. L.J. Horn and N.D. Zasler), pp. 29–52. Hanley and Belfus, Inc, Philadelphia.

Marmarou, A., Anderson, R.L., *et al.* (1991). Impact of ICP instability and hypotension on outcome in patients with severe head trauma. *J. Neurosurg.* **75**, 159–66.

Martelli, M.F., Zasler, N.D., Mancini, A.M., and MacMillan, P. (1999). Psychological assessment and application in impairments and disability evaluations. In *Guide to functional capacity evaluation with impairment rating applications* (ed. R.V. May and M.F. Martelli), pp. NADEP Publications, Richmond.

Mazzucchi, A. and Avanzi, S. (1998). Disturbi post-traumatici del linguaggio. In *La riabilitazione neuropsicologica dei traumatizzati cranici* (ed. A. Mazzucchi and R. Brianti), pp. 75–100. Masson, Milan.

Mazzucchi, A. and Parma, M. (1999). The neuropsychological rehabilitator: who are you? Neuropsychological rehabilitation calls for a specific professional qualification. *Eur. Medicophys.* **35**, 221–8.

Mazzucchi, A., Cattelani, R., Cavatorta, S. Parma, M., *et al.* (1999). TBI rehabilitation as an integrated task of clinicians and families: local and national experiences. In *International handbook of neuropsychological rehabilitation* (ed. A.L. Christensen and B. Uzzel), pp. 299–314. Plenum Press, New York.

McNeny, R. (1990). Deficits in activities of daily living. In *Rehabilitation of the adult and child with traumatic brain injury* (ed. M. Rosenthal, E.R. Griffith, *et al.*), pp. 193–205. F.A. Davis Company, Philadelphia.

McNeny, R. and Dise, J. (1990). Reality orientation therapy. In *Rehabilitation of the adult and child with traumatic brain injury* (ed. M. Rosenthal, E.R. Griffith, *et al.*), pp. 366–73. F.A. Davis Company, Philadelphia.

Montgomery, E.A., Fenton, G.W., *et al.* (1991). The psychobiology of minor head injury. *Psychol. Med.* **21**, 375–84.

Penn, C. and Cleary, J. (1988). Compensatory strategies in the language of closed head injured patients. *Brain Inj.* **2**, 3–18.

Ponsford, J. (1995). Mechanisms, recovery, and sequelae of traumatic brain injury: a foundation for the REAL approach. In *Traumatic brain injury: rehabilitation for everyday adaptive living* (ed. J. Ponsford, S. Sloan, and P. Snow), pp. 1–64. Lawrence Erlbaum Associates, Hove.

Ponsford, J. (2004). *Cognitive and behavioral rehabilitation*. The Guilford Press, New York.

Ponsford, J.L. and Kinsella, G. (1992). Attentional deficits following closed-head injury. *J. Clin. Exp. Neuropsychol.* **10**, 693–708.

Ponsford, J., Willmott, C., Rothwell, A., Cameron, P., Kelly, A.M., Nelms, R., *et al.* (2000). Factor sinfluencing outcome following mild traumatic brain injury in adults. *J. Int. Neuropsychol. Soc.* **6** (5), 568–79.

Prigatano, G.P. (1999*a*). Neuropsychological rehabilitation for cognitive and personality disorders after brain injury. In *Principles of neuropsychological rehabilitation* (ed. G.P. Prigatano), pp. 178–200. Oxford University Press, New York.

Prigatano, G.P. (1999*b*). Disorders of self awareness after brain injury. In *Principles of neuropsychological rehabilitation* (ed. G.P. Prigatano), pp. 265–93. Oxford University Press, New York.

Prutting, C.A. and Kirchner, D.M. (1983). Applied pragmatics. In *Pragmatics assessment and intervention issue in language* (ed. T. Gallagher and C. Prutting), pp. 26–68. College Hill Press, San Diego.

Prutting, C.A. and Kirchner, D.M. (1987). A clinical appraisal of the pragmatic aspects of language. *J. Speech Hearing Disord.* **52**, 105–19.

Rattok, J., Ben Yishai, Y., Lakin, P., Piasetsky, E., Ross, B., Silver, S., Vakil, E., Zide, E., and Diller, L. (1992). Outcome of different treatment mixes in a multidimensional neuropsychological rehabilitation program. *Neuropsychology* **6**, 3395–415.

Reider-Groswasser, I., Groswasser, Z., Ommaya, A., *et al.* (2002). Quantitative imaging in late traumatic brain injury. Part I: Late imaging parameters in closed and penetrating head injury. *Brain Inj.* **16**, 517–25.

Richardson, J.T.E. (2000). Definitions, epidemiology and causes. In *Clinical and neuropsychological aspects of closed head injury*, 2nd edn (ed. J.T.E. Richardson), pp. 1–38. Psychology Press, Hove.

Rosenthal, M., Griffith, E.R., *et al.* (1990). *Rehabilitation of the head injured adult*. F.A. Davis Company, Philadelphia.

Rutherford, W.H. (1989). Post-concussion symptoms: relationship to acute neurological indices, individual differences, and circumstances of injury. In *Mild head injury* (H.S. Levin, H.M. Eisenberg, *et al.*), pp. 217–28. Oxford University Press, Oxford.

Shallice, T. (1982). Specific impairments in planning. In *The neuropsychology of cognitive functions* (ed. D.E. Broadbent and L. Weiskrantz), pp. 199–209. The Royal Society Press, London.

Shapiro, S.R. and Sacchetti, T.S. (1993). *Neuropsychological sequelae of minor head trauma. In Minor head trauma. Assessment, management and rehabilitation* (ed. S. Mandel, R. Thayer Sataloff, *et al.*), pp. 86–110. Springer-Verlag, New York.

Scheid, R., Preol, C., Gruber, O., Wiggins, C., and von Cramon, D.Y. (2003). Diffuse axonal injury associated with chronic brain injury: evidence from T2-weighted gradient-echo imaging at 3T. *Am. J. Neuroradiol.* **24**, 1049–56.

Sloan, S. and Ponsford, J. (1995). Assessment of cognitive difficulties following TBI. In *Traumatic brain injury: rehabilitation for everyday adaptive living* (ed. J. Ponsford, S. Sloan, and P. Snow), pp. 65–102. Lawrence Erlbaum Associates, Hove.

Sohlberg, M.M. and Mateer, C.A. (eds) (1989*a*). *Introduction to cognitive rehabilitation. Theory and practice.* The Guilford Press, New York.

Sohlberg, M.M. and Mateer, C.A. (1989*b*). The remediation of language impairments associated with head injury'. In *Introduction to cognitive rehabilitation. Theory and practice* (ed. M.M. Sohlberg. and C.A. Mateer), pp. 212–31. The Guilford Press, New York.

Sohlberg, M.M. and Mateer, C.A. (eds.) (2001*a*). *Cognitive rehabilitation: an integrative neuropsychological approach.* The Guilford Press, New York.

Sohlberg, M.M. and Mateer, C.A. (2001*b*). Management strategies for mild traumatic brain injury. In *Cognitive rehabilitation: an integrative neuropsychological approach* (ed. M.M. Sohlberg. and C.A. Mateer), pp. 453–82. The Guilford Press, New York.

Sohlberg, M.M. and Mateer, C.A. (2001*c*). Communication issues. In *Cognitive rehabilitation: an integrative neuropsychological approach* (ed. M.M. Sohlberg. and C.A. Mateer), pp. 306–36. The Guilford Press, New York.

Sohlberg, M.M. and Mateer, C.A. (2001*d*). Management of dysexecutive syndrome. In *Cognitive rehabilitation: an integrative neuropsychological approach* (ed. M.M. Sohlberg. and C.A. Mateer), pp 230–68. The Guilford Press, New York.

Sohlberg, M.M. and Mateer, C.A. (2001*e*). The assessment and management of unawareness. In *Cognitive rehabilitation: an integrative neuropsychological approach* (ed. M.M. Sohlberg. and C.A. Mateer), pp. 269–305. The Guilford Press, New York.

Solomon, R.C. and Scherzer, B.P. (1991). Some guidelines for family therapists working with the traumatically brain injured and their families. *Brain Inj.* **5** (3), 253–66.

Stuss, D.T. and Benson, D.F. (1987). The frontal lobes and control of cognition and memory. In *The frontal lobes revisited* (ed. E. Perecman), pp. 141–58. The IRBN Press, New York.

Tate, R.L., Strettles, B., and Osoteo, T. (2003). Enhancing outcomes after traumatic brain injury: a social rehabilitation approach. In *Neuropsychological rehabilitation: theory and practice* (ed. B.A. Wilson), pp. 137–70. Swets, and Zeitlinger, Lisse.

Teasdale, G.M. (1995). Head injury. *J. Neurol. Neurosurg. Psychiatry* **58**, 526–39.

Tiersky, L.A., Anselmi, V., Johnston, M.V., Kurtyka, J., Roosen, E., Schwartz, T., and Deluca, J.A. (2005). Trial of neuropsychological rehabilitation in mild-spectrum traumatic brain injury. *Arch. Phys. Med. Rehabil.* **86** (8), 1565–74.

Togher, L., Hand, L., and Code, C. (1999). Exchanges of information in the talk of people with traumatic brain injury. In *Communication disorders following traumatic brain injuries* (ed. S. McDonald, L. Togher, and C. Code), pp. 113–46. Psychology Press, Hove.

Turner, G.R. and Levine, B. (2003). Disorders of executive functioning and self-awareness. In *Cognitive and behavioral rehabilitation* (ed. J. Ponsford), pp. 224–68. The Guilford Press, New York.

Turner-Stokes, L., Disler, P.B., Nair, A., and Wade, D.T. (2005). Multi-disciplinary rehabilitation for acquired brain injury in adults of working age. *Cochrane Database Syst. Rev.* (3), CD004170.

Webb, C.R., Wregley, M., Yoels, W., and Fine, P.R. (1995). Explaining quality of life for persons ith traumatic brain injury 2 years after injury. *Arch. Phys. Med. Rehabil.* **76**, 1113–19.

Williams, J.M. and Kay, T. (1996). Head injury: a family matter. Paul Brooks Publishing, Baltimore, Maryland.

Wilson, B.A. (ed.) (2003). *Neuropsychological rehabilitation: theory and practice.* Swets and Zeitlinger, Lisse.

Wood, R.Ll. (2001). Understanding neurobehavioural disability. In *Neurobehavioural disability and social handicap following traumatic brain injury* (ed. R.Ll. Wood and T. McMillan), pp. 3–28. Psychology Press, Hove.

Ylvisaker, M. (1985). *Head injury rehabilitation: children and adolescents.* Taylor and Francis, London.

Zasler, N.D. and Martelli, M.F. (2003). Mild traumatic brain injury: impairment and disability assessment caveats. *Neuropsychol. Rehabil.* **13**, 31–41.

Chapter 17

Neuropsychological problems: cognitive and affective disturbances in multiple sclerosis

Daniela Wyss and Jürg Kesselring

17.1 Introduction

The aim of this chapter is to describe the frequency, pattern, and natural history of cognitive and affective disorders associated with multiple sclerosis (MS) and to discuss possible ways of coping with the myriad of challenges the disease presents.

Clinicians throughout most of the twentieth century espoused a widely held view that intellectual and cognitive deficits as well as emotional problems were rare in MS and they therefore focused mainly on physical disability. It was assumed that cognitive dysfunction appeared very late in the disease course and that it only occurred in patients with significant physical disability. During the past two decades, however, research has shown that mental changes as well as emotional and behavioural disturbances in MS occur frequently and may be disabling.

Up to 65% of patients exhibit some neuropsychological dysfunction during the course of their disease. It is a major contributing factor to unemployment, impairment of daily functioning, even accidents, and loss of social activity in those affected by MS.

The areas of cognition typically impaired are memory, attention, information processing, executive function, and visuospatial skills. Cognitive dysfunction is independent of disease duration and level of disability, and cognitive decline may begin in the earliest stages of MS before patients become even mildly disabled physically.

Brain imaging studies show a positive correlation between the extent of brain atrophy and cognitive dysfunction. Despite its prevalence in MS, cognitive dysfunction often goes undiagnosed or is misdiagnosed as depression, stress, stubbornness, lack of intelligence, or psychosis.

Affective disorders present an important clinical challenge. In particular, clinical or subclinical depression may be present in up to 50% of MS patients and, in 20–25%, depression becomes so marked as to require treatment by a specialist. Clinicians should be sensitive to complaints such as irritability and sadness. The risk of suicide, particularly in earlier stages of the disease, is markedly higher than in general population.

Bipolar affective disorders are relatively rare, though they occur more frequently in MS than in the normal population. Frank psychosis in MS is even rarer. For decades, the mood of MS patients has been described as typically euphoric. More recent studies demonstrate, however, that euphoria in MS patients occurs only after long disease duration and together with very marked physical and cognitive deficits. Even then the prevalence rate does not exceed 10%. One in 10 patients is affected by so-called 'pathological laughing and crying', an uncontrollable laughing and/or crying neither induced by a specific stimulus nor corresponding to inner mood.

It often is difficult to differentiate which of the disturbances are due to organic disease and which are psychological reactions to a chronic disease with a still unknown cause, no secure prognosis, not yet established treatment standards, an unpredictable course, and a potential to lead to severe disability and handicap (Kesselring and Klement 2001; Taylor and Taylor 1998).

17.2 Premorbid personality

Retrospective investigations of patients already affected have repeatedly attempted to characterize a specific premorbid personality and to determine the personality characteristics that predispose to the disease. Such investigations (Paulley 1976) have claimed that the premorbid personality of MS patients is characterized by hysterical aspects, as notes on 'hysteria' are frequently found in case reports of MS patients. In fact, MS may manifest itself in earlier phases of the disease by various symptoms that may be found in hysterical ('histrionic') personalities: sensory disturbances; emotional instability; and particularly fatigue.

If, from such observations, the inference is made that hysterical personality characteristics may dispose to the development of MS, it only discloses a lack of ability to diagnose early manifestations of MS. 'In its infancy multiple sclerosis used to be called hysteria' said the famous Queen Square physician Farquhard Buzzard more than 100 years ago. Usually the term 'hysteria' is used imprecisely and includes conversion phenomena, dissociations, or only characteristics of individual personalities. Generally, it discloses more about the way in which physicians think about their patients than describing clinically relevant data (Kesselring 1997).

Though there is no specific 'MS personality', personality changes due to organic disease and changes of behaviour as a reaction to the illness are often observed. Difficult and threatening feelings such as fear, anger, sadness, despair, and aggression can occur. Papuc and Pawlowska (2005) showed that patients in relapse have a higher level of anxiety, a more negative attitude towards themselves, a lack of self-confidence, and they isolate themselves more from society as compared to MS patients in remission. Such reactions are to be expected in a disabling disease that can have a devastating effect on family and work.

17.3 Cognitive functions

The presence of intellectual impairment in MS has been known since the first studies of Charcot and Vulpain who described the weakening of memory in these patients. In contrast to Charcot's observations, clinicians throughout most of the twentieth century held the view that intellectual or cognitive deficits in MS were rare, occurring in less than 5% of patients. Furthermore, it was assumed that cognitive dysfunction appeared very late in the disease course and that it only occurred in patients with significant physical disability. During the past two decades, neuropsychological research has shown that these assumptions about the mental changes in MS were incorrect.

17.3.1 Frequency, pattern, and natural history of cognitive disturbances

Reports on the frequency of disturbances of cognitive functions in MS patients are very variable and depend on the methods used and on the type of patients examined. In about one-half of patients in whom no mental disturbances are found on routine neurological examination, cognitive deficits may be detected during detailed neuropsychological examination (Brassington and Marsh 1998; Prosiegel and Michael 1993; Engel *et al.* 2005). The common pattern of poor correlation between self-related and objective cognitive function (Maor *et al.* 2001;

Carone *et al.* 2005) thus appears to be a result of the patients' (adaptive or maladaptive) coping mechanisms rather than being due to inaccurate measurement (Gold *et al.* 2003; Randolph *et al.* 2004).

Clinicians who rely on self-reports in creating an evaluation and treatment plan should consider the patient's cognitive and emotional states. Goreover *et al.* (2005) demonstrated that the level of self-awareness of neurobehavioural symptoms is related to level of cognitive impairment. In addition, symptoms of depression and anxiety seem to reduce accurate self-reporting.

Studies using neuropsychological testing have shown that subtle or moderate impairments of cognitive functions may be found in 45–65% of MS patients with a disease duration of even less than 2 years (Lyon-Caen *et al.* 1986) without leading to disability in daily life. The prevalence rates are somewhat lower in community-based samples and higher among clinic attendees. This relatively narrow prevalence range is somewhat surprising given that these studies have used different neuropsychological tests. If such impairments are found, it is very likely that they will further decline over the next 3 years, whereas unimpaired cognitive functions indicate that they will remain stable over the next 3 years (Kujala *et al.* 1997).

As is known for all symptoms of MS, considerable interpatient variability is observed with regard to the pattern and severity of cognitive impairments. For 10% of MS patients, cognitive dysfunction is quite severe and is manifested by a widespread deterioration on measures of general intelligence and more specific measures of attention, memory, reasoning, language, and visuospatial processing. However, most patients experience mild to moderate degrees of cognitive dysfunction with relative sparing in many cognitive abilities. As a group, MS patients display relatively small declines on standardized measures of intelligence.

17.3.2 **Memory**

The cognitive function most frequently impaired in patients with MS is memory. In earlier phases of the disease disturbances of memory are found in a great proportion of MS patients when tested appropriately, but more subtle disturbances of memory may at least in part be due to depression and are frequently associated with personality changes (Good *et al.* 1992). Interestingly, according to Beck's negative cognitive schema notion, nondepressed MS patients significantly overestimated their everyday memory, whereas moderately depressed patients' everyday memory ratings mirrored their actual neuropsychological performance (Bruce and Arnett 2004).

Patients with MS often show problems involving working-memory tasks, while short-term memory—as assessed by memory-span tasks—remains unimpaired. In long-term memory—a relatively unlimited and permanent memory store—impairment is commonly observed if spontaneous and free recall is required. Recognition memory is normal or less impaired than free recall. Patients with MS are more easily distracted from tasks involving learning capabilities and memory, although learning capabilities remain intact in the absence of distraction (La Pointe *et al.* 2005). Disturbances in learning of verbal and non-verbal material become more frequent with longer duration of the disease.

Some authors consider this special pattern in memory deficits in MS patients as evidence that their encoding of information is unimpaired, but that they have problems in retrieving the stored information (Rao 1995). Beatty *et al.* (1996), however, have reported that only 53% of their MS patients exhibited a pattern of memory impairment in which the most marked feature was inconsistent retrieval. Thornton and Raz (1997) found in their quantitative review that MS patients show impairments across all memory domains, and that long-term memory dysfunctions are not only based on retrieval deficits (see also Thornton *et al.* 2002). Staffen *et al.* (2005) in their study of memory and magnetic resonance spectroscopy (MRS) of the frontal brain region in early MS suggest a general relationship between the metabolic status of the frontal lobes and memory functions.

17.3.3 Attention

Apart from memory, attention is one of the most frequently affected cognitive functions in MS. Attentional functions should be assessed in detail and treated selectively (Plohmann *et al.* 1998).

MS patients perform as well as controls as regards the accuracy but not the speed of tasks of divided or automatic attention; however, they perform significantly worse on more measures of attention that need more effort. MS thus appears to produce a general slowing of cognitive processes (Kail 1998; Archibald and Fisk 2000). Several studies have examined attention and information processing speed in MS patients using a variety of tests, including the Paced Auditory Serial Addition Test (PASAT). Patients with MS are significantly impaired relative to control subjects on both the easy and hard versions. There also seem to exist correlations between some measures of information processing speed and memory (Olivares *et al.* 2005).

Penner *et al.* (2006) analysed patterns of brain activation in MS patients with different grades of attentional deficits. MS patients with mild impairment showed increased and additional activation of brain areas that were in part not activated in normal subjects. Those were located mainly in the frontal cortex and posterior parietal cortex. This effect decreased with increasing task complexity and was strongest for alertness. In MS patients with severe impairment no additional activation was found in prefrontal structures and activation in the premotor cortex was not significantly different from that in controls. These findings suggest that compensation in MS patients is in part achieved by functional integration of frontal and parietal association areas. The extent of compensation seems to depend on the brain's capacity to access additional brain structures. Exhaustion of this capacity may finally lead to severe cognitive impairment and may be an explanation of fatigue.

17.3.4 Visuospatial processes and executive functions

Visuospatial processes and figure copying as well as motor speed and reaction time are also affected in MS patients when compared to normal individuals and patients with other neurological diseases.

Patients with MS may also have problems in executive functions and planning skills. On specialized tests of abstract or conceptual reasoning such as the Wisconsin Card Sorting Test or the Tower of London, patients with MS show perseveration errors and more problems in profiting from feedback.

Kleeberg *et al.* (2004) found a difference in decision-making and risk-taking between MS patients and a comparison group. MS patients persisted longer than the comparison group in making disadvantageous choices, suggesting significantly slower learning in MS. This slower learning was associated with impaired emotional reactivity in patients versus the comparison group, but not with executive dysfunction. Impaired emotional dimensions of behaviour also correlated with slower learning. Given the considerable consequences that impaired decision-making can have on daily life, this factor may contribute to handicap and altered quality of life secondary to MS and is dependent on emotional experience.

17.3.5 Language functions

MS patients perform normally or with relatively minor impairment on tests of general intelligence and language. Both expressive and receptive language functions are relatively preserved in

MS (Jonsdottir *et al.* 1998). It is likely that cognitive dysfunction was underappreciated by clinicians for many years because of the relative absence of communication deficits in MS patients.

Aphasia can occur in MS, but it is relatively rare and typically occurs in association with the appearance of large demyelinating lesions within the white matter of the left cerebral hemisphere.

17.3.6 Neuropsychological assessment

There is growing evidence indicating that cognitive impairment is amenable to effects of medication (Sormani *et al.* 2005) and behavioural counselling. In addition, neuropsychological tests could serve as early diagnostic tools to detect subtle disease progression (Haase *et al.* 2003; Pepping and Ehde 2005). Unfortunately, routine neuropsychological testing is rare in MS clinics because screening is ineffective and testing strategies are often too cumbersome or expensive (Benedict 2005).

Comprehensive neuropsychological testing can take 3–5 hours to complete. There is a considerable need for a brief assessment tool to screen for cognitive dysfunction in MS patients in the clinic setting. The Mini-Mental State Examination has been shown to be insensitive to detecting all but the most severely impaired patients with cognitive dysfunction. Several recently developed cognitive screening examinations (such as the Multiple Sclerosis Neuropsychological Screening Questionnaire as well as the Minimal Assessment of Cognitive Function in Multiple Sclerosis; Benedict 2005), taking 20–30 minutes, have demonstrated adequate sensitivity and specificity compared to more comprehensive neuropsychological tests. Such screening batteries, however, should be used mainly to identify patients in need of a more comprehensive assessment conducted by a trained clinical neuropsychologist. Information derived from such screening batteries is inadequate to address complicated issues regarding differential diagnosis, vocational assessment, and disability evaluation (Rao 1995).

17.3.7 Driving performance

Kotterba *et al.* (2003) pointed out the need to also focus on driving skills in MS patients. They assessed driving performance in patients with MS. Compared to controls, the accident rate and concentration faults of the patients using the driving simulator were increased.

While there was no correlation with the Expanded Disability Status Scale (EDSS) score, the accident rate was correlated with the Multiple Sclerosis Functional Composite (MSFC). Regarding the three dimensions of the MSFC, accidents were related to the number of correct answers and Z-scores in the Paced Auditory Serial Addition Test (PASAT) as a measure for cognitive functions. However, there are great interindividual differences.

In the MSFC, most deficits could be evaluated by using the PASAT. As there was a significant correlation between the accident rate in the driving simulator and the PASAT results, accidents seem to be influenced more by cognitive decline than by physical impairment. This indicates that the MSFC is a broader, more dimensional scale than the EDSS and should be preferred in the case of driving assessment. At the present time, the driving simulator seems to be a useful instrument to judge driving abilities, especially in cases with ambiguous neuropsychological results.

17.3.8 Subgroups and MRI

More recent studies in MS are devoted to the investigation of subgroups, e.g. primary versus secondary progressive MS (Camp *et al.* 1999; Comi *et al.* 1995) and clinically isolated syndromes suggestive of MS (Feinstein *et al.* 1992).

The degree and pattern of cognitive dysfunction is highly correlated with the amount and location of white matter disease within the cerebral hemispheres, as detected by neuroimaging studies (Tiberio *et al.* 2005). Natural history studies suggest that changes in cognitive test performance are correlated with increasing lesion load on MRI (Karlinska and Selmaj 2005; Lazeron *et al.* 2005; Morgen *et al.* 2006).

Attempts to relate the location of cerebral abnormalities to specific patterns of cognitive test performance have also been reported. In an MRI study, Rao (1995) found that MS patients with a higher percentage of frontal white matter lesions made more perseverative errors on the Wisconsin Card Sorting Test. There is also evidence of impaired interhemispheric communication. MS patients, particularly those with significant callosal atrophy on MRI, experience left ear suppression on a verbal dichotic listening task and prolonged naming latency in the left visual field on an object naming task.

Overall, macroscopic and microscopic brain damage is more important than the corresponding regional brain disease in determining deficits of selective cognitive domains (Rovaris and Filippi 1999). There seems to be a critical threshold for developing cognitive dysfunction depending on the amount of lesion load and atrophy. Adaptive cerebral plasticity may have an important influence on the relationship between MS pathology and its clinical expression (Cifelli and Matthews 2002).

In primary progressive MS, the disease process is more confined to the spinal cord and therefore leads to less cognitive impairment than the secondary progressive form in spite of comparable disability as determined on the EDSS.

Usually there is no or only a weak correlation between cognitive deficits and the degree of physical disability or the duration of illness or depression. Although there are differences in scientific opinion, most studies suggest that cognitive dysfunction and depression are not strongly correlated. Good *et al.* (1992), however, have suggested that even more discrete disturbances in memory are at least in part due to depression and are frequently associated with personality changes. Cognitive deficits are usually not correlated with anxiety symptoms, but sometimes they are connected with the experience of apathy, indifference, or euphoria. Such patients display behavioural symptoms similar to the ones observed in patients with focal frontal lobe damage.

Other authors have described correlations between cognitive dysfunctions in MS and the amount and location of white matter disease as determined by MRI (indices: total cerebral lesion load, cerebral metabolism, size of the lateral and third ventricles, size of the corpus callosum). Pathological studies indicate that virtually all definite MS patients have cerebral white matter lesions at autopsy. Atrophy of the corpus callosum and enlargement of the ventricles are also common.

17.3.9 **Quality of life**

Cognitive problems have a negative impact on the quality of life. For some patients with MS, deficits in comprehending emotional information may also contribute to their difficulties in maintaining effective social interactions (Beatty *et al.* 2003). MS patients with impaired cognitive functions are less likely to be working, are less engaged in social or vocational activities, and have a greater difficulty in performing household tasks. They are more frequently dependent on other persons in activities of daily living than are MS patients without cognitive deficits. A recent study shows that MS patients with impaired autobiographical memory are more content with their quality of life than are unimpaired patients (Kenealy *et al.* 2000).

Early detection of cognitive dysfunctions in MS patients by neuropsychological testing helps to determine the work status of MS patients and to adapt the work settings to their remaining abilities. This should enable a greater proportion of MS patients to keep their jobs. It is also important to inform family members about the relationship between MS and cognitive dysfunctions. Patients' cognitive problems are often incorrectly attributed to obstinacy or depression. This causes additional stress, which should be avoided.

17.4 **Affective disorders**

Psychiatric disorders have long been described in MS. However, these symptoms were only well evaluated in the last 15 years (Defer 2001). Affective disorders occur with increasing frequency in MS (Feinstein 2004). This is true in men and women and across all relevant age groups, although the association gets weaker with advancing age. Higher frequencies of affective disorder occur in women with MS than in men with MS. The highest frequency of affective disorders is found in MS patients between 25 and 44 years of age (Patten *et al.* 2005).

17.4.1 **Depression and suicide**

The most important affective disorder in MS patients is depression (Kesselring 1997; Minden and Schiffer 1990; Schubert and Foliart 1993; Ehde and Bombardier 2005; Siegert and Abernethy 2005). As many as 50% of MS patients experience clinical or subclinical depression during the course of their disease. It is characterized by an 'inability to mourn', loss of hope, and pessimism, and is often associated with general loss of energy, sleep disturbances, weight loss, and lack of interest. Such episodes may precede neurological manifestations in MS. They may occur in most patients at some stage of their disease and are occasionally considered a major symptom. Although depression is clinically relevant and frequent in MS, in contrast to cognition it is not related to physical disease progression (Haase *et al.* 2004). Risk factors for depression are female sex and severity of disability. In 20–25% of patients depression becomes so marked as to require treatment by a specialist (Schubert and Foliart 1993). The risk of suicide, particularly in the earlier stages of the disease, is markedly higher than in the general population (Stenager *et al.* 1992). Regular screening for depression in this population is appropriate (Galeazzi *et al.* 2005).

Clinicians should also be sensitive to complaints such as irritability and sadness in patients with MS, even when symptoms do not fulfil criteria for formal, psychiatric diagnoses. Feinstein and Feinstein (2001) found that such complaints are associated with levels of psychological distress that approach those experienced by patients with major depression. Given that these subsyndromes of affective instability respond well to pharmacological therapy, detection and adequate treatment can significantly reduce one important aspect of morbidity associated with MS.

In the study of Bombardier *et al.* (2004), 14% of a large community sample of persons with MS screened positive for possible alcohol abuse or dependence, and 7.4% reported misusing illicit drugs or prescription medication within the previous month. Possible alcohol abuse and drug misuse were associated with younger age, less severe MS-related disability, and being employed, as well as greater self-reported depressive symptomatology. Most persons with alcohol problems indicated interest in learning more about ways to stop or cut down. There may be greater risk of harm due to substance abuse in people with MS because of the potential magnification of motor and cognitive impairments. Comprehensive MS care should include substance abuse screening and advice to cut down or abstain (see also Quesnel and Feinstein 2004).

Depressive disturbances in MS are so frequent and of such importance that they must be analysed and treated with particular care, sympathy, and persistence.

17.4.1.1 Possible causes of depression

Depressive symptoms are as frequent in MS patients as in similarly disabled patients with muscular diseases, which suggests that they are a reaction to the disease and its consequences. On the other hand, the observation that depressive episodes in MS patients are often associated with 'endogenous signs' such as vegetative disturbances and diurnal changes in mood argues for an organic basis.

Feinstein *et al.* (2004) identified medial inferior prefrontal cortex T2 lesion volume and left anterior temporal cerebrospinal fluid (CSF) volume to be two independent predictors of depression accounting for 42% of the depression variance score. Although both lesion burden and atrophy are important in the pathogenesis of depression in MS, psychosocial influences should also be considered.

Drugs such as corticosteroids and possibly interferon (IFN) may also lead to depression (Loftis and Hauser 2004). Considering the uncertainty of a link between IFN-beta and depression and/or suicide, as well as the complete remission of psychiatric complications after IFN discontinuation and/or antidepressant treatment, physicians should closely monitor the psychiatric status of patients, but should not refrain from including them in IFN-beta treatment programmes, even when they have past or present depression (Goeb *et al.* 2006).

17.4.2 Bipolar affective disorder

Bipolar affective disorders (manic episodes) in association with MS occur more frequently than would be expected by chance (Feinstein *et al.* 2004). The possibility of a shared genetic diathesis could explain the association, although preliminary results need replication. Both MS and bipolar disorder are associated with white matter changes on MRI, although the pathogenesis of these lesions is likely to be different. There is MRI evidence suggesting that manic patients with psychosis have plaques that are distributed predominantly in temporal horn areas bilaterally.

MS patients who become hypomanic or manic on steroid therapy are more likely to have a family story of affective disorders and/or alcoholism or a premorbid psychiatric history of such disorders. This should not be a contraindication to treatment with steroids, although caution is advised. Lithium carbonate is an effective treatment for manic and hypomanic (including steroid-induced) episodes. Sodium valproate is an effective alternative treatment for patients unable to tolerate lithium. Should mania be accompanied by psychosis, neuroleptic medications may be required. Benzodiazepines are useful as an adjunct for sedation, but carry a high risk for addiction.

17.4.3 Psychosis

Psychosis associated with MS is a rare occurrence and probably does not exceed chance expectation. Feinstein *et al.* (1992) found a trend for psychotic MS patients to have a higher total lesion load, particularly in periventricular areas. In all cases, neurological symptoms preceded the onset of psychosis. The psychotic group also had a later age of onset of psychosis than psychotic patients without brain disease. These results point to an aetiological association between the pathological process of MS and psychosis.

There are data to suggest that MS-related psychosis is distinct from schizophrenia, namely, presenting with a later age of presentation, preservation of affective response, quicker reaction of symptoms, fewer psychotic relapses, better response to treatment, and more favourable outcome.

Neuroleptic drugs such as clozapine and risperidone, in small doses, are the treatment of choice, although reports of their efficacy are anecdotal.

17.4.4 Euphoria and pathological laughter and crying

For decades it was taken for granted that the mood of MS patients is typically euphoric, as described by many authors since Charcot. 'Euphoria' describes a type of mood characterized by inappropriate/inadequate serenity (in view of physical disability). Comparative investigations with patients with muscular disease and similar physical disabilities demonstrate that euphoria in MS patients occurs only after long disease duration and with very marked neurological deficits, and is part of an 'organic psycho-syndrome' caused by extensive cerebral lesions. Even in very disabled MS patients this type of mood does not occur in more than 10%.

Anosognosia (a lack of insight into the disease) may be a blessing for severely disabled patients and their caregivers. It is, however, as rare as euphoria in the early and middle phases of the disease.

So-called 'affect incontinence' (i.e. abruptly changing affective expressions that do not correspond to inner mood) may be very disabling for both patients and those around them. It may occur as paroxysmal phenomena and is considered to be due to organic lesions (Kesselring 1997). Many patients describe a type of 'internal disconnection' that does not allow them to express verbally or non-verbally affects that they feel interiorly. Pathological laughing and crying affect one in 10 patients with MS and are distinct from emotional lability. They occur more often in severely physically disabled patients with long-standing disease.

In the study of Feinstein *et al.* (1997) patients had a mean EDSS score of 6.5, had had MS for a mean of 10 years, and had entered a chronic progressive phase of their illness. Pathological laughing and crying were not associated with disease exacerbations. Compared with controls, patients were not more depressed or anxious, but had a greater decline in IQ. The presence of cognitive deficits in these cases relative to controls implies more extensive brain involvement (Lyon-Caen *et al.* 1986).

17.5 Stress and MS

17.5.1 Stress and coping

The scientific community offers different, partly contradictional theories about stress. Cognitive-transactional models (Lazarus 1993) explain stress as the result of complex feedback loops including subjective perception and appraisal based on perceived control over the environment. Successful coping is based less on objective presence of resources, but more on the subjective perception of them.

In the theory of Hobfoll (1989) stress is defined as loss of resources. Pre-standing resources can be exploited and may lead to additional gain (upward spiral), whereas the threat of or actual loss of resources leads to additional loss (downward spiral). If possibilites to get back or to restore resources are rare, a person gets stressed. In this theory cognitive appraisal is also very important. Consequences of coping are visible in health, quality of life, social contacts, work, or in other criteria.

17.5.2 Resources

In the 1980s social research shifted its focus from deficits to possible resources helping to cope with problems and critical life events. Coping literature mainly differentiates personal from social resources.

Personal resources are traits promising a health-conserving and/or a health-promoting influence. The most widely examined personal resources are dispositional optimism (a relatively stable and generalized expectation of positive events; Scheier and Carver 1992; see also de Ridder *et al.* 2004), self-efficacy (an optimistic expectation to influence the environment; Bandura 1996), and locus of control (Rotter 1966). The theory of locus of control differentiates inner versus outer locus of control. A person with an inner locus of control considers events to be a consequence of personal actions and not caused by fate, outer circumstances, etc.

House (1981) differentiates four kinds of social support: (1) emotional support (empathy, care, love); (2) practical or material support (e.g. giving a ride, organizing daily necessities, or helping financially); (3) information (see MacLean and Russell 2005); and (4) feedback.

An investigation of Wortman (1984) demonstrates that emotional support (especially listening) is of primary importantance (see also Cheung and Hocking 2004). When appropriate, support may have beneficial consequences (Pakeham 2005; Schwartz and Frohner 2005; Harrison *et al.* 2004). In the study of Clingerman *et al.* (2004) women with lower social support scores consistently perceived greater functional limitation than those with higher social support scores. In addition, Schwartz and Frohner (2005) showed that social support made a significant and unique contribution to the mental health dimension of quality of life in MS patients. But social support only has beneficial consequences when there is compatibility between needed and granted support (passform concepts). Inappropriate personal assistance may result in dependency, which detracts from personal control and worsens quality of life (King and Arnett 2005; Messmer *et al.* 2004). By recognizing the specific factors that link personal control to illness trajectory, appropriate and timely support can be negotiated.

17.5.3 **Efficiency of resources and coping**

In daily life, we see a richness of different reaction forms to cope with difficult situations, illness, and loss. There have been several attempts to categorize resources and to measure their efficacy.

Although many questions are still to be answered, we know that the effects of resources and coping cannot be generalized. They have to be assessed in front of the person dealing with a specific situation Bogle *et al.*1999; Reynolds and Prior 2003). The interaction between personal and social resources is difficult to clarify. In the model of Bodenmann (1997), social resources (family, friends, MS societies) mostly are employed only secondarily, when personal resources are exhausted.

17.5.4 **MS as a stress-induced illness?**

So-called 'life event research' examines the hypothesis that psychosocial factors induce or exacerbate emotional and physical illnesses. The assumption of an increased health risk when many or intensive stressors or critical life events are present is most important (see Mohr and Cox 2001).

Studies about MS patients and stress do not provide a consensus as to the relationship between stress and MS. Few studies have defined the critical features of these stressful situations or examined the role of stress-mediating and -moderating variables. Available evidence indicates that the relationship between life stress and relapse is complex, and is likely to depend on several factors such as stressor chronicity, frequency, severity, and type, and individual patient characteristics such as depression, health locus of control, and coping strategy use (see also Mohr and Pelletier 2006). Little is known about how these factors, individually or in combination, are related to MS disease activity. Viral infections are also likely to precipitate relapse in MS, and significant life stress may further enhance this relationship.

MS patients are particularly vulnerable to a deteriorating cycle of stressful life events, illness episodes, and disability. Timely multidisciplinary care interventions aimed at both minimizing psychological distress and physical symptoms may alter this downward reciprocal cycle. Little is known of the pathogenesis of these putative stress-induced changes in disease activity, and almost all stressor studies suffer from some biases or limitations.

17.5.5 Quality of life

Many people who live with long-lasting illnesses experience a decline in their quality of life. Health-related quality of life (HRQoL) has been more intensively studied in MS than in any other neurological disorder (Pollmann *et al.* 2005; Mitchell *et al.* 2005; Benedict *et al.* 2005). Traditional medical models of impairment and disability are an incomplete summary of disease burden. Quality of life can be thought of as the sum of all sources of satisfaction (including anticipated sources) minus all threats (including anticipated threats).

Being subjectively reasonably happy and as socially active as desired seems central to an acceptable quality of life for MS patients (Somerset *et al.* 2002). The extent of personal control and individual illness trajectory form a cornerstone to reach this aim.

Many psychosocial factors—including coping, mood, self-efficacy, and perceived support—influence the quality of life of patients with MS more than biological variables such as weakness or extent of MRI lesions. Pressures due to changed economic circumstances as well as coping with these pressures is important in the quality of life of people with MS (McCabew and DeJudicibus 2005). Neuropsychiatric complications such as cognitive impairment and fatigue are also important predictors, even in those patients in the early stages of the disease.

The issues that prevent people with MS from working tend to be disease-related as well as work-related (O'Connor *et al.* 2005; Smith and Arnett 2005). Ability to work depends partly on physical limitations or cognitive problems, but it cannot be based solely on these measures of function (Pompeii *et al.* 2005). Work ability among individuals extends beyond measures of impairment and includes level of education, job characteristics, and disease symptoms such as fatigue.

For persons with MS, employment has both costs and significant benefits. Accommodations in the workplace and modifications of roles and responsibilities at home can make it possible for individuals to continue working. Healthcare providers must consider the complexity and timing of decisions by people with MS to continue or leave employment before recommending either action (Johnson *et al.* 2004; Johnson and Fraser 2005). Identifying critical periods of intervention to stabilize this cost–benefit balance is a critical next step for understanding issues of employment and MS.

17.5.6 Support of health professionals and MS societies

Healthcare professionals influence the presence and are part of resources for those who are particularly vulnerable to resource loss so that they can participate successfully in work, recreational, and home environments. They can use presence, listening, and observational skills to identify verbal and non-verbal cues of resource depletion. People with MS often have multiple complex needs that require input from a wide range of services. New models of health promotion are being developed that integrate self-help and professional help. These approaches have been applied in other chronic diseases and should be adapted and studied among people with MS (Bombardier *et al.* 2005; Vitali 2004).

Besides family and healthcare professionals, national and international MS societies are of great help. They provide accurate, up-to-date information for individuals with MS, their families, and healthcare providers; they organize meetings and support research. Often there is a telephone hotline and the possibility of joining other patients in a network as well as professional support in medical and psychological questions.

References

Archibald, C.J. and Fisk, J.D. (2000). Information processing efficiency in patients with multiple sclerosis. *J. Clin. Exp. Neuropsychol.* **22** (5), 686–701.

Bandura, A. (1996). Ontological and epistemiological terrains revisited. *J. Behav. Ther. Exp. Psychiatry* **27** (4), 323–45.

Beatty, W.W., Goodkin, D.E., Hertsgaard, D., and Monson, N. (1996). Memory disturbance in multiple sclerosis: reconsideration of patterns of performance on the selective reminding test. *J. Clin. Exp. Neuropsychol.* **18**, 56–62.

Beatty, W.W., Orbelo, D.M., Sorocco, K.H., and Ross, E.D. (2003). Comprehension of affective prosody in multiple sclerosis. *Mult. Scler.* **9** (2), 148–53.

Benedict, R.H. (2005). Integrating cognitive function screening and assessment into the routine care of multiple sclerosis patients. *CNS Spec.* **10** (5), 384–91.

Benedict, R.H., Wahlig, E., Bakshi, R., Fishman, I., Munschauer, F., Zivadinov, R., and Weinstock-Guttmann, B. (2005). Predicting quality of life in multiple sclerosis, accounting for physical disability, fatigue, cognition, mood disorder, personality and behavior change. *J. Neurol. Sci.* **231** (1–2), 29–34.

Bodemann, G. (1997). Stress und Coping als Prozess. In *Psychologie der Bewältigung* (ed. C. Tesch-Römer, C. Salewski, and G. Schwarz), pp. 74–92. Psychologie Verlags Union, Weinheim.

Bogle, N., Percy, M., and Morrison, W. (1999). Will I make it through this choppy water? A psychological characteristic as a predeterminant factor to coping with multiple sclerosis. *Axone* **20** (3), 63–6.

Bombardier, C.H., Blake, K.D., Ehde, D.M., Gibbons, L.E., Moore, D., and Kraft, G.H. (2004). Alcohol and drug abuse among persons with multiple sclerosis. *Mult. Scler.* **10** (1), 35–40.

Bombardier, C.H., Wadhwani, R., and La Rotonda, C. (2005). Health promotion in people with multiple sclerosis. *Phys. Med. Rehabil. Clin. N. Am.* **16** (2), 557–70.

Brassington, J.C. and Marsh, N.V. (1998). Neuropsychological aspects of multiple sclerosis. *Neuropsychol. Rev.* **8**, 43–77.

Bruce, J.M. and Arnett, P.A. (2004). Self-reported everyday memory and depression in patients with multiple sclerosis. *J. Clin. Exp. Neuropsychol.* **26** (2), 200–14.

Camp, S.J., Stevenson, V.L., Thompson, A.J., Miller, D.H., Borras, C., Auriacombe, S., Brochet, B., Falautano, M., Filippi, M., Herisse-Dulo, L., Montalban, X., Parrcira, E., Polman, C.H., De Sa, J., and Langdon, D.W. (1999). Cognitive function in primary and transitional progressive multiple sclerosis: a controlled study with MRI correlates. *Brain* **122**, 1341–8.

Carone, D.A., Benedict, R.H., Munschauer, F.E. 3rd, Fishman, I., and Weinstock-Guttman, B. (2005). Interpreting patient/informant discrepancies of reported cognitive symptoms in MS. *J. Int. Neuropsychol. Soc.* **11** (5), 574–83.

Cheung, J. and Hocking, P. (2004). Caring as worrying: the experience of spousal carers. *J. Adv. Nurs.* **47**, 475–82.

Cifelli, A. and Matthews, P.M. (2002). Cerebral plasticity in multiple sclerosis: insights from fMRI. *Mult. Scler.* **8** (3), 193–9.

Clingerman, E., Stuifbergen, A., and Becker, H. (2004). The influence of resources on perceived functional limitations among women with multiple sclerosis. *J. Neurosci. Nurs.* **36** (6), 312–21.

Comi, G., Filippi, M., Martinelli, V., Campi, A., Rodegher, M., Alberoni, M., Siravian, G., and Canal, N. (1995). Brain MRI correlates of cognitive impairment in primary and secondary progressive multiple sclerosis. *J. Neurol. Sci.* **132**, 222–7.

Defer, G. (2001). Neuropsychological evaluation and psychopathology of multiple sclerosis. *Rev. Neurol. (Paris)* **157** (8–9, Pt. 2), 1128–34.

De Ridder, D., Fournier, M., and Bensing, J. (2004). Does optimism affect symptom report in chronic disease? What are its consequences for self-care behaviour and physical functioning? *J. Psychosom. Res.* **56** (3), 341–50.

Ehde, D.M. and Bombardier, C.H. (2005). Depression in persons with multiple sclerosis. *Phys. Med. Rehabil. Clin. N. Am.* **16** (2), 437–48, ix.

Engel, C., Greim, B., and Zettel, U.K. (2005). Cognitive dysfunctions in multiple sclerosis patients. *Nervenarzt* **76** (8), 943–4, 946–8, 951–3.

Feinstein, A. (2004). The neuropsychiatry of multiple sclerosis. *Can. J. Psychiatry* **49** (3), 157–63.

Feinstein, A. and Feinstein, K. (2001). Depression associated with multiple sclerosis. Looking beyond diagnosis to symptom expression. *J. Affect. Disord.* **66** (2–3), 193–8.

Feinstein, A., Kartsounis, L.D., Miller, D.H., Youl, B.D., and Ron, M.A. (1992). Clinically isolated lesions of the type seen in multiple sclerosis: a cognitive, psychiatric and MRI follow-up study. *J. Neurol. Neurosurg. Psychiatry* **55**, 869–76.

Feinstein, A., Feinstein, K., Gray, T., and O'Connor, P. (1997). Prevalence and neurobehavioral correlates of pathological laughing and crying in multiple sclerosis. *Arch. Neurol.* **54** (9), 1116–21.

Feinstein A., Roy, R., Lobaugh, N., Feinstein, M.A., O'Connor, P., and Black, S. (2004). Structural brain abnormalities in multiple sclerosis patients with major depression. *Neurology* **62**, 586–90.

Galeazzi, G.M., Ferrari, S., Giaroli, G., Mackinnon, A., Merelli, E., Motti, L., and Rigatelli, M. (2005). Psychiatric disorders and depression in multiple sclerosis outpatients: impact of disability and interferon beta therapy. *Neurol. Sci.* **26** (4), 255–62.

Goeb, J.L., Even, C., Nicolas, G., Gohier, B., Dubas, F., and Garre, J.B. (2006). Psychiatric side effects of interferon-beta in multiple sclerosis. *Eur. Psychiatry* **21**, 186–93.

Gold, S.M., Schulz, H., Monch, A., Schulz, K.H., and Heesen, C. (2003). Cognitive impairment in multiple sclerosis does not affect reliability and validity of self-report health measures. *Mult. Scler.* **9** (4), 404–10.

Good, D., Clark, C.M., Oger, J.L., Paty, D., and Klonoff, H. (1992). Cognitive impairment and depression in mild multiple sclerosis. *J. Nerv. Ment. Dis.* **180**, 730–2.

Goreover, Y., Chiaravalloti, N., and DeLuca, J. (2005). The relationship between self-awareness of neurobehavioral symptoms, cognitive functioning, and emotional symptoms in multiple sclerosis. *Mult. Scler.* **11** (2), 203–12.

Haase, C.G., Tinnefeld, M., Lienemann, M., Ganz, R.E., and Faustmann, P.M. (2003). Depression and cognitive impairment in disability-free early multiple sclerosis. *Behav. Neurol.* **14** (1–2), 39–45.

Haase, C.G., Tinnefeld, M., Daum, I., Ganz, R.E., Haupts, M., and Faustmann, P.M. (2004). Cognitive but not mood dysfunction develops in multiple sclerosis during 7 year of follow-up. *Eur. Neurol.* **52** (2), 92–5.

Harrison, T., Stuifbergen, A., Adachi, E., and Becker,, H. ((2004). Marrige, impairment and acceptance in persons wiht multiple sclerosis. *West. J. Nurs.* **26** (3), 266–85.

Hobfoll, S.E. (1989). *The ecology of stress.* Hemisphere, Washington DC.

House, J,S. (1981). *Work, stress and social support.* Addison Wesley, Reading.

Johnson, K.L. and Fraser, R.T. (2005). Mitigating the impact of multiple sclerosis on employment. *Phys. Med. Rehabil. Clin. N. Am.* **16** (2), 571–82.

Johnson, K.L., Yorkston, K.M., Klasner, E.R., Kuehn, C.M., Johnson, E., and Amtmann, D. (2004). The cost and benefits of employment: a qualitative study of experiences of persons with multiple sclerosis. *Arch. Phys. Med. Rehabil.* **85** (2), 201–9.

Jonsdottir, M.K., Magnusson, T., and Kjartansson, O. (1998). Pure alexia and word-meaning deafness in a patient with multiple sclerosis. *Arch. Neurol.* **55** (11), 1473–4.

Kail, R. (1998). Speed of information processing in patients with multiple sclerosis. *J. Clin. Exp. Neuropsychol.* **20**, 98–106.

Karlinska, I. and Selmaj, K. (2005). Cognitive impairment in multiple sclerosis. *Neurol. Neurochir. Pol.* **39** (2), 125–33.

Kenealy, P.M., Beaumont, J.G., Lintern, T., and Murell, R. (2000). Autobiographical memory, depression and quality of life in multiple sclerosis. *J. Clin. Exp. Neuropsychol.* **22**, 125–31.

Kesselring, J. (1997). *Multiple sclerosis*. Cambridge University Press, Cambridge.

Kesselring, J. and Klement, U. (2001). Cognitive and affective disturbances in MS: a review. *J. Neurol.* **248** (3), 180–3.

King, K.E. and Arnett, P.A. (2005). Predictors of dyadic adjustment in multiple sclerosis. *Mult. Scler.* **11** (6), 700–7.

Kleeberg, J., Bruggimann, L., Annoni, J-M., van Melle, G., Bogousslaysky, J., and Schluep, M. (2004). Altered decision-making in multiple sclerosis: a sign of impaired emotional reactivity? *Ann. Neurol.* **56**, 787–95.

Kotterba, S., Orth, M., Eren, E., Fangerau, T., and Sindern, E. (2003). Assessment of driving performance in patients with relapsing–remitting multiple sclerosis by a driving simulator. *Eur. Neurol.* **50** (3), 160–4.

Kujala, P., Portin, R., and Ruutiainen, J. (1997). The progress of cognitive decline in multiple sclerosis. A controlled 3-year follow-up. *Brain* **120**, 289–97.

LaPointe, L.L., Maitland, C.G., Blanchard, A.A., Kemker, B.E., Stierwalt, J.A., and Heald, G.R. (2005). The effects of auditory distraction on visual cognitive performance in multiple sclerosis. *J. Neuro-ophthalmol.* **25** (2), 92–4.

Lazarus, R.S. (1993). Coping theory and research: past, present and future. *Psychosom. Med.* **55**, 234–47.

Lazeron, R.H., Boringa, J.B., Schouten, M., Uitdehaag, B.M., Bergers, E., Lindeboom, J., Eikelenboom, M.I., Scheltens, P.H., Barkhof, F., and Polman, C.H. (2005). Brain atrophy and lesion load as explaining parameters for cognitive impairment in multiple sclerosis. *Mult. Scler.* **11** (5), 524–31.

Loftis, J.M. and Hauser, P. (2004). The phenomenology and treatment of interferon-induced depression. *J. Affect. Disord.* **82** (2), 175–90.

Lyon-Caen, O., Jouvent, R., Hauser, S., Chaunu, M.P., Benoit, N., Wildlocher, F., and Lhermitte, F. (1986). Cognitive functions in recent-onset demyelinating diseases. *Arch. Neurol.* **43**, 1138–41.

Mc Cabew, M.P. and De Judicibus, M. (2005). The effects of economic disadvantage on psychological well-being and quality of life among people with multiple sclerosis. *J. Health Psychol.* **10** (1), 163–73.

MacLean, R. and Russell, A. (2005). Innovative ways of responding to the information needs of people with MS. *Br. J. Nurs.* **14** (14), 754–7.

Maor Y., Olmer, L., and Mozes, B. (2001). The relation between objective and subjective impairment in cognitive function among multiple sclerosis patients—the role of depression. *Mult. Scler.* **7** (2), 131–5.

Messmer, M., Mancuso, L., Battaglia, M.A., Zagami, P., and Mohr, D.C. (2004). Peer support groups in multiple sclerosis, current effectiveness and future directions. *Mult. Scler.* **10** (1), 80–4.

Minden, S.L. and Schiffer, R.B. (1990). Affective disorders in multiple sclerosis. Review and recommendations for clinical research. *Arch. Neurol.* **47**, 98–104.

Mitchell, A.J., Benito-Leon, J., Gonzalez, J.M., and Rivera-Navarro, J. (2005). Quality of life and its assessment in multiple sclerosis: integrating physical and psychological components of wellbeing. *Lancet Neurol.* **4** (9), 556–66.

Mohr, D.C. and Cox, D. (2001). Multiple sclerosis: empirical literature for the clinical health psychologist. *J. Clin. Psychol.* **57** (4), 479–99.

Mohr, D.C. and Pelletier, D. (2006). A temporal framework for understanding the effects of stressful life events on inflammation in patients with multiple sclerosis. *Brain Behav. Immun.* **20** (1), 27–36.

Morgen, K., Sammer, G., Courtney, S.M., Wolters, T., Melchior, H., Blecker, C.R., Oschmann, P., Kaps, M., and Vaitl, D. (2006). Evidence for a direct association between cortical atrophy and cognitive impairment in relapsing–remitting MS. *Neuroimage* **30** (3), 891–8.

O'Connor, R.J., Cano, S.J., Ramio, I., Torrenta, L., Thompson, A.J., and Playford, E.D. (2005). Factors influencing work retention for people with multiple sclerosis: cross-sectional studies using qualitative and quantitative methods. *J. Neurol.* **252** (8), 892–6.

Olivares, T., Nieto, A., Sanchez, M.P., Wollmann, T., Hernandez, M.A., and Barroso, J. (2005). Pattern of neuropsychological impairment in the early phase of relapsing–remitting multiple sclerosis. *Mult. Scler.* **11** (2), 191–7.

Pakeham, K.I. (2005). The positive impact of multiple sclerosis (MS) on carers: associations between carer benefit finding and positive and negative adjustment domains. *Disabil. Rehabil.* **27** (17), 985–97.

Papuc, E. and Pawlowska, B. (2005). Personality features in multiple sclerosis patients with a relapsing–remitting course of the disease. *Psychiatr. Pol.* **39** (4), 669–78.

Patten, S.B., Svenson, L.W., and Metz, L.M. (2005). Descriptive epidemiology of affective disorders in multiple sclerosis. *CNS Spect.* **10** (5), 365–71.

Paulley, J.W. (1976). Psychological management of multiple sclerosis. *Psychother. Psychosom.* **727**, 26–40.

Penner, I.K., Kappos, L., Rausch, M. Opwis, K., and Radu, E.W. (2006). Therapy-induced plasticity of cognitive functions in MS patients: insights from fMRI. *J. Physiol. (Paris)* **99** (4–6), 455–62.

Pepping, M. and Ehde, D.M. (2005). Neuropsychological evaluation and treatment of multiple sclerosis: the importance of a neuro-rehabilitation focus. *Phys. Med. Rehabil. Clin. N. Am.* **16** (2), 411–36.

Plohmann, A.M., Kappos, L., Ammann, W., Thordai, A., Wittwer, A., Huber, S., Bellaiche, Y., and Lechner-Scott, J. (1998) Computer assisted retraining of attentional impairments in patients with multiple sclerosis. *J. Neurol. Neurosurg. Psychiatry* **64**, 455–62.

Pollmann, W., Busch, C., and Voltz, R. (2005). Quality of life in multiple sclerosis. Measures, relevance, problems, and perspectives. *Nervenarzt* **76** (2), 154–69.

Pompeii, L.A., Moon, S.D., and McCrory, D.C. (2005). Measures of physical and cognitive function and work status among individuals with multiple sclerosis: a review of the literature. *J. Occup. Rehabil.* **15** (1), 69–84.

Prosiegel, M. and Michael, C. (1993). Neuropsychology and multiple sclerosis: diagnostic and rehabilitative approaches. *J. Neurol. Sci. (Suppl.)* **115**, 51–4.

Quesnel, S. and Feinstein, A. (2004). Multiple sclerosis and alcohol: a study of problem drinking. *Mult. Scler.* **10** (2), 197–201.

Randolph, J.J., Arnett, P.A., and Freske, P. (2004). Metamemory in multiple sclerosis: exploring affective and executive contributors. *Arch. Clin. Neuropsychol.* **19** (2), 259–79.

Rao, S.M. (1995). Neuropsychology of multiple sclerosis. *Curr. Opin. Neurol.* **8**, 216–20.

Reynolds, F. and Prior, S. (2003). Sticking jewels in your life: exploring women's strategies for negotiating an acceptable quality of life with multiple sclerosis. *Qual. Health Res.* **13** (9), 1225–51.

Rotter, J.B. (1966). Generalized expectancies for internal versus external control of reinforcement. *Psychol. Monogr.* **80** (1), 1–28.

Rovaris, M. and Filippi, M. (1999). Magnetic resonance techniques to monitor disease evolution and treatment trial outcomes in multiple sclerosis. *Curr. Opin. Neurol.* **12** (3), 337–44.

Scheier, M.F. and Carver, C.S. (1992). Effects of optimism on psychological and physical well-being; theoretical overview and empirical update. *Cogn. Ther. Res.* **16**, 201–28.

Schubert, D.S. and Foliart, R.H. (1993). Increased depression in multiple sclerosis patients. A meta-analysis. *Psychosomatics* **34**, 124–30.

Schwartz, C. and Frohner, R. (2005). Contribution of demographic, medical, and social support variables in predicting the mental health dimension of quality of life among people with multiple sclerosis. *Health Soc. Work* **30** (3), 203–12.

Siegert, R.J. and Abernethy, D.A. (2005). Depression in multiple sclerosis: a review. *J. Neurol. Neurosurg. Psychiatry* **76** (4), 469–75.

Smith, M.M. and Arnett, P.A. (2005). Factors related to employment status changes in individuals with multiple sclerosis. *Mult. Scler.* **11** (5), 602–9.

Somerset, M., Sharp, D., and Campbell, R. (2002). Multiple sclerosis and quality of life: a qualitative investigation. *J. Health Serv. Res. Policy* **7** (3), 151–9.

Sormani, M.P., Bruzzi, P., Beckmann, K., Kappos, L., Miller, D.H., Polman, C., Pozzilli, C., Thompson, A.J., Wagner, K., and Filippi, M. (2005). The distribution of magnetic resonance imaging response to interferonbeta-1b in multiple sclerosis. *J. Neurol.* **252** (12), 1455–8.

Staffen, W., Zauner, H., Mair, A., Kutzelnigg, A., Kapeller, P., Stangl, H., Raffer, E., Niederhofer, H., and Ladurner, G. (2005). Magnetic resonance spectroscopy of memory and frontal brain region in early multiple sclerosis. *J. Neuropsychiatry Clin. Neurosci.* **17** (3), 357–63.

Stenager, E.N., Szenager, E., Koch Henrikson, N., Brønnum-Hansen, H., Hyllested, K., Jensen, K., *et al.* (1992). Suicide and multiple sclerosis: an epidemiological investigation. *J. Neurol. Neurosurg. Psychiatry* **55**, 542–5.

Taylor, A. and Taylor, R.S. (1998). Neuropsychologic aspects of multiple sclerosis. *Phys. Med. Rehabil. Clin. N. Am.* **9** (3), 643–57.

Thornton, A.E. and Raz, N. (1997). Memory impairment in multiple sclerosis. A quantitative review. *Neuropsychology* **B11**, 357–66.

Thornton, A.E., Raz, N., and Tucke, K.A. (2002). Memory in multiple sclerosis: contextual encoding deficits. *J. Int. Neuropsychol. Soc.* **8** (3), 395–409.

Tiberio, M., Chard, D.T., Altmann, D.R., Davies, G., Griffin, C.M., Rashid, W., Sastre-Garriga, J., Thompson, A.J., and Miller, D.H. (2005). Gray and white matter volume changes in early RRMS. A 2-year longitudinal study. *Neurology* **64** (6), 1001–7.

Vitali, S. (2004). Paraclinical support of the person diagnosed with multiple sclerosis. *Int. Mult. Scler. J.* **11** (1), 2.9.

Wortman, C.B. (1984). Social support and the cancer patient: conceptual and methodological issues. *Cancer* **53**, 2339–60.

Chapter 18

Neuropsychology of epilepsy

Christoph Helmstaedter

18.1 Introduction

With a prevalence of 1%, a cumulative incidence of 2–4%, and more than 40 million affected persons worldwide, epilepsy is one of the most common diseases affecting the central nervous system (Engel 2004). Epilepsy is defined by the repetitive and unprovoked occurrence of epileptic seizures (i.e. by the occurrence of internal or external behavioural changes that go along with pathological paroxysmal hypersynchronous rhythmic electric discharges in larger neuronal networks). In most patients, these electrophysiological changes can be assessed during seizures (ictally) via electroencephalographic (EEG) recordings from the surface of the head. However, epileptic activity, which in and of itself does not attest to epilepsy, can also be observed interictally in the time between seizures. The risk of a relapse after the first unprovoked seizure is 37%. This relapse risk decreases as the seizure-free time increments increase. However, the relapse rate can increase up to 73% after a second unprovoked seizure occurs (Hauser *et al.* 1998). Epilepsy can be successfully treated in most cases but, apart from seizures, the cognitive, psychiatric, and psychosocial consequences must also be considered with this disease. Epilepsy is a disease at the edge between neurology and psychiatry. Because of this and because multiple disciplines (neurophysiology, neuropathology, neuroradiology, neurosurgery, and neuropsychology) are concerned with this disease, research in epileptology was interdisciplinary from the very beginning of the understanding that the source of epilepsy must be the brain. Since the early beginnings of epilepsy surgery back in the 1930s in Montreal, Canada, neuropsychology, cognitive neuroscience, and clinical epileptology have all been found to be strongly interwoven and they still stimulate each other. Milestones in epilepsy research include Jasper and Penfield's electrocortical functional mapping, which to this day represents a valuable tool in epilepsy surgery (Penfield and Jasper 1954; Ojemann 1982), and Scoville and Milner's (2000) lessons about memory from bilateral temporomesial resections for seizure control. From Sperry's split brain studies or June Wada's intracarotidal amobarbital procedure we were able to learn about hemisphere dominance and plasticity (Wada and Rasmussen 1960; Gazzaniga 2005). The introduction of chronic invasive EEG recordings and structural and functional magnetic resonance imaging (MRI) allowed for quantitative and qualitative structure function correlations with high spatial and temporal resolution. This standard and selective epilepsy surgery allowed for cross-sectional and longitudinal lesional neuropsychological research (Wieser 1986). Finally, recent attempts to apply deep brain stimulation for seizure control must be mentioned, even though the effects of this procedure on behaviour cannot yet be determined (Kanner 2004). Within the context of epilepsy surgery there is hardly a diagnostic tool that has not yet been systematically applied in order to improve patient selection, the surgical approach, or outcome prediction and that did not allow for the correlation of the brain and its functions to cognition and behaviour. Quantitative and qualitative structural and functional MRI, positron emission tomography (PET), single photon emission computerized tomography (SPECT), magnetoencephalography (MEG), intracranial

EEG, electrocortical stimulation, and event-related potentials (ERPs) belong to the diagnostic repertoire in epileptology.

Traditionally, neuropsychology in epilepsy involves localization diagnostics in terms of the lateralization and intrahemispheric localization of impairments. Because of improved imaging and EEG techniques, questions of outcome and quality control of medical and surgical treatment of epilepsy are currently of major interest (Trenerry 1996). This development is in full accordance with a qualitative change in the treatment of epilepsy, which not only aims at seizure control, but also at the preservation or even improvement of the patient's cognitive performance, his or her psychosocial situation, and his or her subjectively experienced quality of life.

The neurocognitive and behavioural findings in epilepsy will be outlined along with the different types of epilepsies. The effects of disease and treatment on cognition in epilepsy will be considered as well as the question of how epilepsy and its treatment can interact with mental development and mental decline. The extent to which the findings of the respective areas serve for modelling normal brain functions will be of secondary interest.

18.2 Classification

In general, seizures are categorized as either generalized or focal (partial) seizures This classification is based on whether the pathological hypersynchronous EEG activity is recorded widely distributed or focally over the cortical surface. Seizures are labelled 'secondarily generalized' when they have a focal origin with a subsequent spread into the hemispheres. Focal seizures can coincide with loss of consciousness (= complex partial seizure) or without loss of consciousness (= simple partial seizure). This seizure classification is strongly influenced by the classification of epilepsies, which follows their aetiology and localization. Accordingly, idiopathic and symptomatic or cryptogenic focal epilepsies are differentiated. The first has a strong genetic component with no known underpinning lesions and the second is due to a definitive pathology or to an assumed and not yet known pathology. Most, but not all, idiopathic epilepsies are characterized by generalized seizures. In some idiopathic epilepsies, epileptic activity shows a preference for certain frontal or centrotemporal locations (Commission on Terminology and Classification of the International League against Epilepsy 1989). It is important to note that, with the progress being made in imaging, electroencephalography, neuropsychology, and genetics technology, the definitions and classifications of generalized versus focal, partial versus complex partial, or idiopathic versus symptomatic are constantly changing (Engel 2001). Recognition of autosomal dominant frontal lobe epilepsy, for example, contradicts the separation of focal symptomatic versus idiopathic generalized epilepsies. Another example is that with invasive EEG recordings there is evidence that behaviourally generalized seizures do not necessarily have a generalized electrophysiological correlate. Also the definition of complex partial seizures as being seizures with a loss of consciousness must be questioned. Active testing during seizures shows that complex partial seizures can go along with selective impairment of language functions that can be misunderstood as a loss of consciousness.

18.3 Aetiology

In contrast to most other CNS diseases, epilepsy is characterized by the fact that not only structural morphological lesions, but also dynamic epileptic dysfunction, affect cognition and behaviour. Treatment affects epilepsy and, in the case of surgery, it also affects the brain structure. In contrast to lesions and surgical defects, the influence of epilepsy and its medication is potentially reversible (see Fig. 18.1).

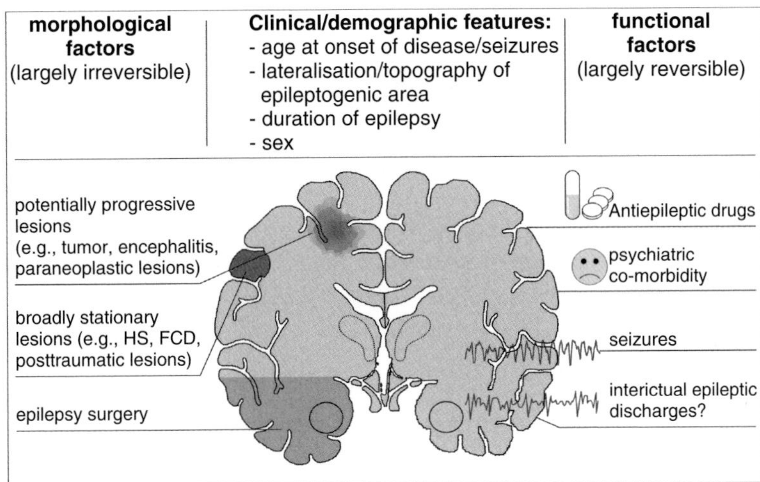

Fig. 18.1 Aetiological model comprising the more static and the dynamic underpinnings of cognitive impairement in epilepsy. (Taken from Elger *et al.* 2004.)

Psychiatric comorbidity must be considered as the third dynamic factor in epilepsy (Elger *et al.* 2004). Thus, the cognitive condition in a patient with epilepsy is the result of the complex interaction of more stable and dynamic factors. With this, we must also consider that epilepsy not only results from altered brain structures or functions, but that epilepsy itself can also exert an influence upon brain maturation and functional organization. Many patients with early onset epilepsies show atypical hemispheric dominance patterns that appear to be not genuine, but rather lesion- and epilepsy-driven (Helmstaedter *et al.* 1997*d*). Because of this and since epilepsy has its natural peak in childhood and later on in adulthood, the constant and dynamic determinants of cognitive impairments must be set into a developmental neuropsychological framework that considers the interactions of epilepsy with the maturing and ageing brain.

18.4 **Types of epilepsy**

Epilepsies differ with regard to aetiology, genetic determination, severity, chronic course, and their response to treatment. Depending on the type of epilepsy, onset, and duration, the epileptic activity and seizures can have a different impact on the course of cognitive development with maturation or ageing. Table 18.1 provides an overview over the different types of epilepsy, their initial conditions, and their cognitive prognosis. More detailed information about the neuropsychological aspects of these different types of epilepsy will be provided in the following sections.

18.4.1 **Idiopathic epilepsies**

Idiopathic epilepsies are most notably characterized by a genetic predisposition and the absence of significant brain lesions. Idiopathic generalized epilepsies are additionally characterized by generalized EEG patterns that cover the whole cortex. In contrast, idiopathic partial epilepsies show preferences of epileptic activity over certain brain regions (i.e. centrotemporal or rolandic epilepsy). It is a commonly held assumption that idiopathic epilepsies are easier to treat and that they are associated with less severe cognitive impairments. This is true in many respects, but this could result in an underestimation of the cognitive and behavioural problems found with idiopathic epilepsies.

Table 18.1 Cognition in different types of epilepsy

Type of epilepsy	Manifestation	Precipitating situation	Cognitive development
Idiopathic epilepsies			
Early childhood epilepsy with GTCS & hemi grand mal	Age 5–15	Normal	Unfavourable/dementia
Benign myoclonic epilepsy	Until age 3.	Normal	Positive/retardation possible
Severe myoclonic epilepsy (mitochondirial defects)	Age 1	Normal	Unfavourable/dementia
Myoclonic–astatic epilepsy	Until age 5	Mostly normal	Ranges depending on course from partial deficits to dementia
Absence epilepsy			
Early onset	Age 1–4	Normal	Partial deficits possible
Pyknolepsia	age 5–8	Normal	Partial deficits possible
Juvenile	age 9–12.	Normal	Partial deficits possible
Juvenile myoclonic epilepsy	Age 12–25	Normal	Partial deficits (frontal?)
Juvenile epilepsy with GTCS	Age 12–25	Normal	Partial deficits (frontal?)
Symptomatic or cryptogenic epilepsies			
Focal epilepsies	Every age	Normal or impaired	Onset- and localization-dependent partial deficits and low IQ
Frontal lobe	Every age	Normal or impaired	Predominant impairment of executive functions
Temporal lobe	Every age, often early	Normal or impaired	Predominant episodic memory impairment (material-specific)
Parieto- occipital	Every age, often early	Normal or impaired	Frontal or temporal like rather than classic parietal dysfunctions
E. partialis continua, Rasmussen encephalitis	Every age	Mostly impaired	Often one hemisphere affected; unfavourable/dementia
Encephalopathy/catastrophic epilepsy			
West syndrome	Age 1	Mostly impaired	Unfavourable/retardation
Lennox Gastaut syndrome	Age 2–7	Mostly impaired	Unfavourable/retardation
Benign partial epilepsies and related syndromes			
Rolando epilepsy	Age 2–12	Maturation disorder (hereditary)	Partial deficits
Pseudo-Lennox syndrome	Age 2–7	Maturation disorder (hereditary)	Impaired language development & other partial deficits
Bioelectric status epilepticus during sleep (ESES)	Age 2–10	Maturation disorder (hereditary)	Onset- and course-dependent retardation and dementia

Table 18.1 (continued) Cognition in different types of epilepsy

Type of epilepsy	Manifestation	Precipitating situation	Cognitive development
Landau–Kleffner syndrome	Age 4–10	Maturation disorder (hereditary)	Auditory agnosia and aphasia predominant/retardation

GTCS, Generalized tonic-clonic seizure.

18.4.1.1 Idiopathic generalized epilepsy

Traditionally, epilepsies are divided into two major groups. The first group consists of idiopathic epilepsies which include the generalized epilepsies (IGE; e.g. epilepsies with tonic-clonic seizures, juvenile absence epilepsy, or myoclonic epilepsy) and the benign partial epilepsies (e.g. benign epilepsy with centrotemporal spikes; BECTS). The second group is comprised of the symptomatic or probably symptomatic focal epilepsies (e.g. mesial temporal lobe epilepsy and neocortical epilepsies). The term generalized epilepsy and the fact that, in these epilepsies, generalized epileptic activity can be recorded over cortical areas may misleadingly suggest that cognitive impairments must also be generalized. On the contrary, patients with IGE show only minor problems with respect to global intelligence, but display rather significant problems in the areas of attention, psychomotor speed, visuospatial skills, and non-verbal memory. Language and verbal memory appear to be unaffected (Pavone *et al.* (2001). Mirsky *et al.* (2001). Hommet *et al.* 2006).

The close relationship between epileptic discharges and cognitive dysfunction is fundamental for the understanding of cognitive impairment in IGE (see the example of an absence in Fig. 18.2).

Because no underlying lesion can be discerned in idiopathic epilepsies, IGE has been thought to be the best model for studying the relationship of epilepsy and cognition. Interestingly enough, cognition and epilepsy in IGE appear to be related in both directions. Impairments become evident as a function of epileptic activity, but activities can also activate epileptic discharges and even seizures. In a large study, Matsuoka *et al.* (2000) showed such activation during cognitive tasks involving motor (e.g. writing) or higher cognitive functions (e.g. calculating, reading). Comparable observations have also been made in those patients with symptomatic temporal lobe epilepsy where seizures occurring particularly during memory evaluations indicated activation of the temporal lobe epileptic focus (Helmstaedter *et al.* 1992). However, in the Matsuoka study, patients with IGE appeared to be much more prone to showing neuropsychological EEG activation than those patients with focal epilepsies.

In IGE, the negative effects of spike–wave bursts on sensory and executive functions can be noted. Therefore, visual and auditory continuous performance tasks that require sustained attention appear best suited to diagnose the specific dysfunctions for this group of patients (Mirsky *et al.* 2001). In this type of epilepsy, it appears more likely that impairment in these latter functions secondarily affects other functions of intelligence rather than that mental retardation is a primary feature of the disease. This, however, does not exclude the possibility of developmental delay and retardation when IGE interferes with basal cognitive functions over a long period of time. Earlier absence epilepsies with an onset in early childhood or at school age are at greater risk for a worse outcome than juvenile absence epilepsies.

18.4.1.2 Benign childhood epilepsy with centrotemporal spikes

Benign childhood epilepsy with centrotemporal spikes (BECTS) is a frequently diagnosed epilepsy (10–15%), which starts between ages 5 and 9 and extends into adolescence. It has a comparatively good prognosis, in that most patients become seizure-free after puberty. However,

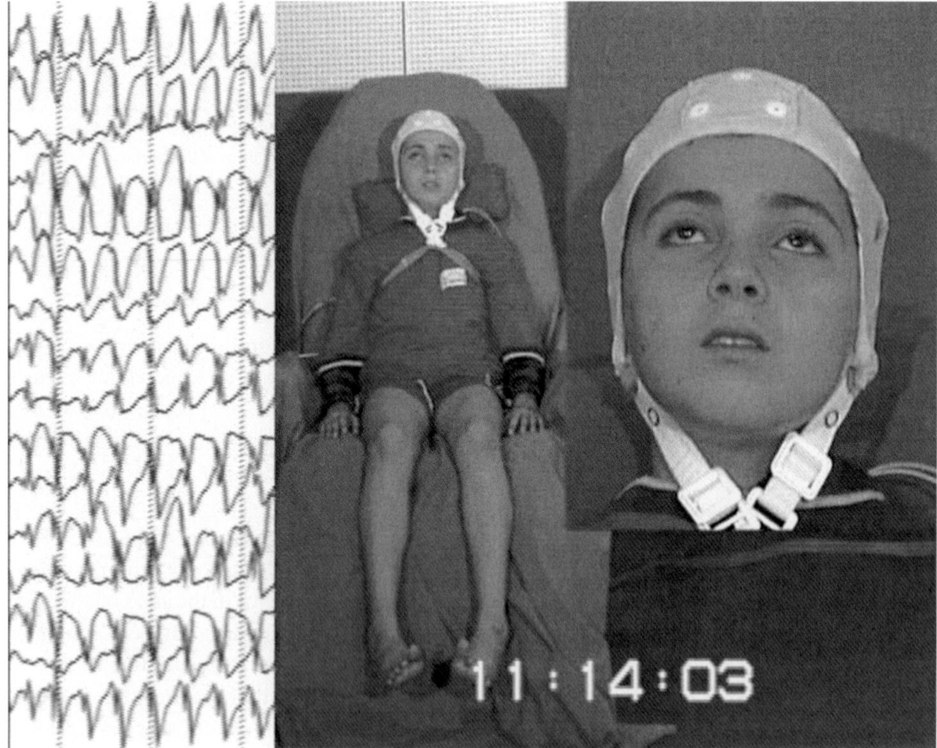

Fig. 18.2 Absence with typical 3/s spike wave pattern going along with a momentary loss of consciousness.

with regard to cognitive functioning, the benign nature of this type of epilepsy must be doubted. Particularly during its active phase, neuropsychological deficits have been reported in various domains including attention, motor functions, short-term memory, and visual and perceptive abilities. However, language problems relating to the interictal dysfunction of perisylvian language areas appear to be a major characteristic of BECTS (Hommet *et al.* 2006). Abnormality of auditory evoked potentials (P85–120) and the absence of mismatch negativity raise evidence that patients with BECTS have abnormal processing of auditory information at a sensory level ipsilateral to the hemisphere evoking spikes during sleep (Liasis *et al.* 2006). According to a recent study, educational problems are met in about half of the patients, most of them with neuropsychological and language problems suggestive of a developmental learning disability (Vinayan *et al.* 2005). This study also supports an earlier observation made in a very large population; the absence of temporofrontal dipole discharges can be taken as an indicator for a learning disability (Gregory and Wong 1992). BECTS does not appear to be progressive. In contrast, with the remission of epilepsy, children catch up and develop normally. Minor persisting problems in executive functions and verbal comprehension in children in remission suggest possible long-term effects (Monjauze *et al.* 2005; Lindgren *et al.* 2004). A complete absence of seizures and complete remission of epileptic activity appear essential for a good cognitive outcome.

As with language problems in patients with centrotemporal spikes, visual information processing appears particularly affected in benign partial epilepsy with occipitally located discharges (Wolff *et al.* 2005).

Very special conditions are met in the Landau–Kleffner syndrome (LKS) or the 'continuous spikes and waves during slow wave sleep' syndrome (CSWS; Roulet Perez *et al.* 1993). Particularly with respect to BECTS it might be of interest that these conditions are also associated with language problems. However, here a progressive loss and decline of already acquired functions is observed, which can result in severe mental retardation. Children with CSWS show autistic features as well as features of a frontal lobe syndrome, and the mental retardation in these children is believed to result from extensive and continuing epileptic dysfunction affecting the frontal lobes (Roulet Perez *et al.* 1993; Scholtes *et al.* 2005). It should be mentioned that epilepsy or epileptic activity is frequently found in children with autistic spectrum disorders. Gabis *et al.* (2005) found that 40% of the 56 autistic children studied were diagnosed with epilepsy. Thus, EEG should be performed in such children and recordings taken during the night should also be included. Very recent findings suggest a significant role of early thalamic lesions in the aetiology of CSWS (Guzzetta *et al.* 2005). In contrast to BECTS, where in the first line expressive language functions appear affected, the Landau–Kleffner syndrome is characterized by a sequential and sometimes hierarchical loss of language functions beginning with sensory aphasia, followed by auditory agnosia and finally word deafness as the disease progresses (Kaga 1999). A dissociation between the discrimination of environmental sounds and phonological auditory discrimination indicates problems particularly in the auditory phonological domain (Korkman *et al.* 1998). Characteristic and presumably also predictive for mental decline is the phenomenon of the non-convulsive 'electrical status epilepticus in sleep' (ESES). Since there is an overlap between BECTS, LKS, and CSWS, transitions between the more benign condition in BECTS and the severe encephalopathic conditions in LKS and CSWS seem possible (Galanopoulou *et al.* 2000).

18.4.1.3 Juvenile myoclonus epilepsy

Juvenile myoclonus epilepsy (JME) starts predominantly between the ages of 12 and 18 years and is characterized by neuropsychological and behavioural features suggesting the presence of a frontal dysexecutive syndrome (Janz 1985, 2002; Hommet *et al.* 2006). This is indicated by neuropsychological findings that suggest problems with reasoning, concept formation, mental speed and flexibility, or problems in visual working memory (Devinsky *et al.* 1997; Sonmez *et al.* 2004; Swartz *et al.* 1996). However, frontal lobe dysfunction does not appear to be specific to JME. It can be observed in other patients with IGE as well and is also a common feature of symptomatic frontal lobe epilepsies (Helmstaedter 2001). Whether frontal lobe cognitive dysfunction together with personality change (e.g. limited self-control, elevated suggestibility, indifference, rapid mood changes) form a syndrome characteristic of JME needs to be proven (Janz 1985). It should be noted that the aetiological model of 'generalized' epilepsy is weakening, provided that partial rather than global impairments are found in IGE. In accordance with the neuropsychological findings there is evidence from EEG and from histological, structural, and functional imaging studies supporting a particular involvement of the frontal lobes, the thalamus, and thalamo-cortical loops in IGE (Meencke and Janz 1985; Woermann *et al.* 1999; Salek-Haddadi *et al.* 2003; Aghakhani *et al.* 2004; Koepp 2005).

By summarizing the findings in idiopathic epilepsies a wide range of rather mild impairments can be discerned in idiopathic generalized and partial epilepsies. The conditions represented in encephalopathies LKS and CSWS are the exception. In addition to diffuse impairment and learning disorders, characteristic impairments have been observed and can be related to the brain sites involved in the respective syndrome. The impairments can be best understood on the basis of the close relationship between active epileptic processes interfering with cognitive networks of more basal activating, perceptive and executive functions. Within a developmental framework the time during which epilepsy interferes with critical periods of cognitive development is of major importance (i.e. before, at, or after language acquisition, or at the time before or when frontal executive functions develop). Frontal executive functions develop last and may therefore represent a common endpoint of the impairments seen in the idiopathic generalized or partial epilepsies. With remission of epilepsy, recovery from acute epilepsy-driven impairment can be observed, but some long-term residual deficits cannot be excluded, particularly when epilepsy has previously interfered with mental development to a significant degree. Because no morphological cortical damage could be demonstrated with BECTS, LKS, or CSWS until now, these epilepsies provide a very interesting insight into cognitive development. Previously acquired skills can be irreversibly lost without visible damage if the disease starts early, if it affects significant brain areas, and if it lasts long enough. 'Use it or lose it' is obviously only one scenario of mental retardation; the loss of cortical functions due to the continuous reception of erratic nonsense input is probably another. Aetiologically, the thalamus and thalamo-cortical networks come into focus and future research will show whether focal lesions will also become evident in these epilepsies.

18.4.2 **Focal symptomatic epilepsies**

In contrast to idiopathic epilepsies in which the impact of epileptic dysfunction on cognition is the prevailing factor, the nature of focal symptomatic epilepsies is more decisively determined by the location and aetiology of epilepsy. As for the location of the epilepsy, the International Classification of Epilepsies differentiates localization-related epilepsies according to the cerebral lobes (frontal, temporal, parietal, occipital). However, the temporal lobes and the temporomesial structures represent particularly vulnerable structures, which are susceptible to becoming epileptogenic.

18.4.2.1 Temporal lobe epilepsies

With a diagnosis rate of 70%, temporal lobe epilepsy (TLE) represents the majority of the chronic symptomatic epilepsies; about half of these epilepsies show hippocampal sclerosis and/or atrophy. Whether mesial TLE represents a nosological entity or a syndrome is still a matter of debate (Wieser 2004). Neuropsychologically, mesial temporal lobe epilepsy is characterized by impaired declarative memory, often accompanied with low levels of global intelligence (Hermann *et al.* 1997). The latter finding requires special attention since poor intelligence in TLE is often associated with an early onset of epilepsy and can thus be indicative of mental retardation (Helmstaedter 2005; Hermann *et al.* 2002). Consideration of the course of cognitive development and the educational level of siblings or parents can support this diagnosis. Memory impairment is evident in TLE independent of the age at the onset of epilepsy (Helmstaedter 2005).

The technical facilities available for the presurgical evaluation of epilepsy patients have significantly contributed to our understanding of the close relationship between the morphological and functional integrity of the temporal lobe structures and declarative episodic memory (i.e. the acquisition and later recall of time- and context-dependent information). This has been demonstrated by correlating memory function to intracranially recorded evoked potentials which were assessed by old/new differentiation in a N400 word recognition paradigm. The better the mesial structures can be recruited during such a memory task, the better the memory will also be in memory tasks outside of the experimental setting (Elger *et al.* 1997; Helmstaedter *et al.* 1997*b*). With the same procedure, it was also possible to demonstrate the relevance of NMDA-receptor activity for memory formation. Application of ketamine, an NMDA-receptor antagonist that is most likely seen within the hippocampal CA1 subregion, completely suppressed memory formation and the respective electrophysiological correlates within the hippocampus proper (Grunwald *et al.* 1999). This strong relation has also been demonstrated by cell count methods, which showed that neuron loss in certain hippocampal subregions can be related to memory performance (Zaidel *et al.* 1998; Sass *et al.* 1994). Even a correlation of memory performance to long-term potentiation as assessed on a cellular level in human hippocampal slices be demonstrated (see Fig. 18.3; Beck *et al.* 2000). With electrophysiological coherence measures from depth electrodes, it is possible to directly relate cortico-mesial phase synchronization between the rhinal cortex and the hippocampus to the formation of declarative memories in the awake state and even during sleep (Fell *et al.* 2001, 2006).

Since episodic memory is largely a function of the language dominant hemisphere, left temporal and left temporo-mesial epilepsies are very often associated with material-specific impairment of verbal learning and memory. Mesial and neocortical structures differentially contribute to verbal memory in that mesial structures serve consolidation and retrieval, while neocortical structures process the content. Therefore, impaired performance in delayed recall measures is highly indicative for left mesial pathology (Helmstaedter *et al.* 1997*b*). Impairment of verbal learning, verbal short-term memory, and semantic memory are less specific markers, which can be indicative of left infero-temporal or temporo-lateral lesions or foci (Helmstaedter 2002; Seidenberg *et al.* 2005; Hamberger *et al.* 2005; Helmstaedter *et al.* 1997*a*; Ojemann *et al.* 1988). Category-specific impairments in semantic word fluency have been suggested in lateralized temporal lobe epilepsies, but this is still a matter of debate (Jokeit *et al.* 1998; Gleissner and Elger 2001). Differing from left TLE, in right TLE only a quantitatively but not a qualitatively different performance in figural memory has been observed dependent on the presence/absence of hippocampal sclerosis (Gleissner *et al.* 1998). Furthermore, the relation between figural visual spatial memory impairment and right temporal lobe epilepsy is far less consistent than that between verbal memory and the left temporal lobe. While there are studies that clearly indicate such a relation by showing specific deficits in design learning (Gleissner *et al.* 1998), in spatial memory

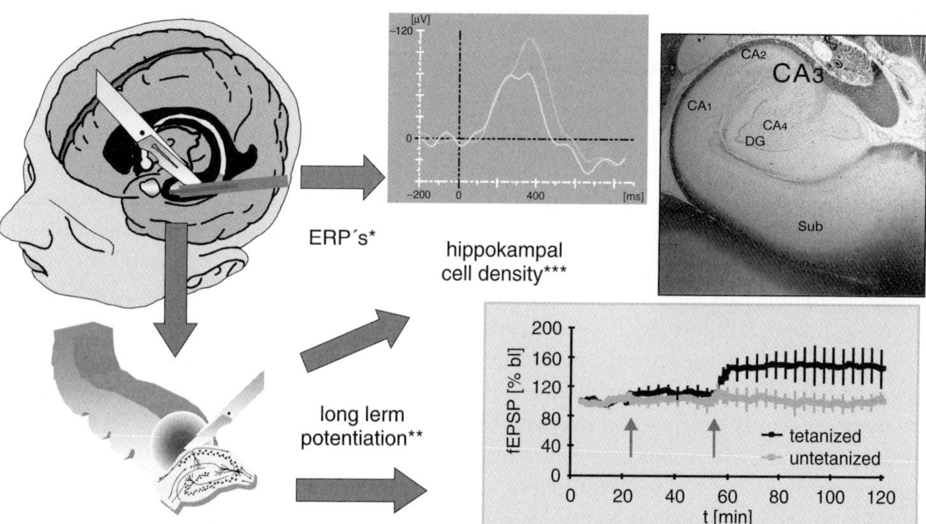

** Beck et al. 2000 J. Neuroscience ** Elger et al. 2000 Neuropsychologia *** Zentner et al. 1999 J Neurosurgery*

Fig. 18.3 Approaches to human memory in surgical patients with temporal lobe epilepsy. Episodic memory is related to: ∗ ERPs recorded from intrahippocampal electrodes (published by Elger *et al.* 1997); ∗∗ cell counts from intrahippocampal electrodes (published by Zentner *et al.* 1999); ∗∗∗ long-term potentiation recorded from human hippocampal slices (published by Beck *et al.* 2000).

(Breier *et al.* 1996), in the identification of famous faces (Glosser *et al.* 2003), or the recognition of emotional facial expression (Meletti *et al.* 2003), false lateralizing figural memory deficits are nevertheless very common. In right TLE, lack of impairment has been attributed to a more bilateral cerebral organization of non-verbal memory networks, covert verbalization, or the type of the test and test materials (e.g. abstractness, complexity) (Helmstaedter *et al.* 1995; Helmstaedter 2002). False lateralizing figural memory impairment in left TLE is rather due to atypical language dominance and gender differences (Helmstaedter *et al.* 1999). Frontal lobe dysfunctions are also common in TLE, particularly when generalized tonic clonic seizures are reported (Jokeit *et al.* 1997). There is a tight interaction between temporal and prefrontal areas in memory processes (Buckner and Wheeler 2001; Fernandez and Tendolkar 2001) and frontal impairments in TLE appear to be due to irradiating epileptic dysfunction or diachisis phenomena, which can be controlled after successful seizure control. After successful TLE surgery in patients with PET signs of prefrontal hypometabolism before surgery, functional neuroimaging may show normalization of metabolism. This parallels the improvement seen in non-temporal functions after successful surgery (Spanaki *et al.* 2000; Helmstaedter *et al.* 2003).

18.4.2.2 Frontal lobe epilepsies

With a rate of approximately 10–20%, frontal lobe epilepsies (FLE) represent the second largest group of symptomatic epilepsies (Kellinghaus and Luders 2004). They form a much less consistent neuropsychological entity than temporal lobe epilepsy. In contrast to TLE, in which hippocampal sclerosis is a predominant and quite homogeneous morphological feature, more heterogeneous aetiological factors are involved in frontal lobe epilepsy. The frontal lobes are comprised of regions that are involved in various functions. These functions include working memory (prefrontal), social and moral behaviour (orbitofrontal), initiation and organization of behaviour (prefrontal and supplementary motor area), processing of emotions and reward (basal forebrain and cingulum), language (Broca's area), or motor control (precentral). There are multiple connections of the frontal lobes to other brain areas, but whether epileptic dysfunction in FLE has a distant effect on nonfrontal areas as is seen in TLE with respect to frontal areas needs to be established. For example, postoperative recovery in temporal lobe functions does not appear as impressive as the recovery of frontal functions after temporal lobe surgery (Helmstaedter *et al.* 1998; Lendt *et al.* 2002). In any case, frontal lobe executive functions reach into most other cognitive functions. Diffuse and non-specific impairments can be the consequence. Therefore, frontal lobe dysfunction in FLE is rarely diagnosed by a single dysfunction or test, but rather in terms of a cognitive profile (Helmstaedter 2001; Risse 2006). Cognitive impairments characteristic for FLE largely resemble those described within the lesion-related literature, but in this respect it is important to note that most literature on patients with FLE also refers to patients with lesions. Neuropsychological differences between lesional and nonlesional (cryptogenic) FLE have not yet been described. An important technical aspect of the evaluation of patients with FLE is that, independently of the presence or absence of lesions, impairments might be missed because test situations are mostly clearly structured with clear cut demands. This reduces the level of freedom for the patient and can help him or her to overcome particular problems associated with behavioural control. Patients may nevertheless appear normal or they may primarily suffer from behavioural and emotional problems. Most consistent are problems with attention, short-term or working memory, mental flexibility, response inhibition, anticipation, or planning and decision-making. Motor coordination tests have been found to be particularly sensitive with respect to frontal lobe epilepsy.

One can summarize the various cognitive and behavioural problems in FLE by suggesting a 'frontal dysexecutive syndrome' with problems in the selection, initiation, execution, and inhibition of responses in different domains (e.g. attention, motor function, emotion, reasoning, language). No systematic problems have yet been described as dependent on the lateralization of FLE, nor have special neurocognitive problems been associated with frontal subregions (Helmstaedter 2001; Upton and Thompson 1997; Exner *et al.* 2002; Shulman 2000).

18.4.2.3 Parietal and occipital lobe epilepsies

Posterior epilepsies are rare with a 10% rate and the neuropsychological characteristics of parietal and occipital lobe epilepsies have thus not yet been described with larger groups of patients. Test batteries for epilepsy patients may cover visual attention, language, or praxia, but rarely do the tests address somatosensory processes, astereognosis, perceptual thresholds, or transmodal functions that would tap functions of the posterior cortices (Jones-Gotman *et al.* 1987). Acute parietal or occipital neuropsychological symptoms mostly become manifest only in seizure semiology or in postictal states. Since most of the patients have chronic epilepsies on the basis of early lesions or malformations the classic posterior symptoms of aphasia, alexia, agraphia, acalculia, agnosia, optic ataxia, neglect, etc. are very rare. Primary or secondary perceptive and sensory problems often appear well compensated on a behavioural level because epilepsy and lesions fall into a time window during which the brain is still functionally plastic and able to cope with the lesions. The resulting impairments are mostly diffuse and mental retardation is seen quite often in parietal epilepsies, presumably because early epilepsy interferes with functions of the input system (Helmstaedter and Lendt 2001). The brain matures from posterior to anterior and negative effects of early damage of posterior functions can well be suggested to influence the maturation and functional development of structures and functions that become fully developed later on. Furthermore, as has also been described for seizure semiology and EEG, the cognitive impairments in posterior epilepsies often mimic those of frontal or temporal lobe epilepsies (Helmstaedter and Lendt 2001; Kasowski *et al.* 2003). Whether this reflects distant effects of posterior foci on frontal and temporal lobe functions by irradiation of epileptic dysfunction via the ventral and dorsal stream needs to be shown. For the neuropsychological diagnosis of parietal epilepsies, tests of stereognosis or haptic search appear to be sensitive tests (Salanova *et al.* 1995; Jones-Gotman *et al.* 2005).

18.5 **Lesions**

Aetiologically, no specific causes for cognitive impairments can be discerned in focal symptomatic epilepsy. Major lesions in focal epilepsies are mostly stationary defects such as developmental malformations, hippocampal sclerosis or atrophy, head trauma, or vascular malformations (see Fig. 18.3). Potentially progressive defects such as neoplastic and paraneoplastic tumours, CNS infections, inflammatory and autoimmunological processes appear to be less common. These aetiologies alone can lead to cognitive impairments ranging from mild impairment in circumscribed domains to severe mental retardation or mental decline. In this respect, it is important to know that the cognitive impairments in symptomatic epilepsies are not lesion-specific, but that they differ due to differences in age at the time of the onset of the lesion (early onset lesions interfere with brain maturation), differences in functionality of the affected tissues (epileptogenic regions can also be functional), differences in the course and dynamics of the underlying disease (neoplastic, encephalitis), and finally because of a different lateralization and localization (Elger *et al.* 2004).

Lesions normally are not involved in function, but this cannot always be excluded as has been demonstrated for dysplasias, glioneural tumours, or heterotopic grey matter in an intracranial ERP study or in fMRI activation studies (Kirschstein *et al.* 2003; Jirsch *et al.* 2006; Richardson *et al.* 1998).

18.6 Epileptic activity and seizures

As for epileptic activity and epileptic dysfunction, seizures, pre- and postictal states, and interictal epileptic activity/dysfunction are differentiated. Ictal, peri-, and interictal dysfunction can add to the impairments that are already present due to morphological/structural pathology in symptomatic epilepsies. Cognitive impairment becomes most evident during a seizure. Seizures not only produce positive symptoms (e.g. staring, automatisms, dystonic posturing, etc.), which are subsumed under the term 'seizure semiology', but also negative symptoms in terms of impairment or loss of functions (e.g. language, consciousness, motor control, memory, etc.; see Fig. 18.4).

Both types of symptoms can provide valuable clues about the localization and lateralization of the involved brain structures. However, in contrast to seizure semiology, which can be observed, negative symptoms only become evident with testing (Luders *et al.* 1999; Lux *et al.* 2002). A more direct relation between the localization of seizure activity and behaviour is given when primary sensory or motor areas are affected. This relation is lost when seizures originate or spread into secondary or tertiary association areas, mesial fronto-limbic, or midbrain structures. Then, seizure semiology appears less as a direct correlate of excitatory activity in the respective areas but rather as the expression of a disinhibition of atavistic and, in part, very complex templates of behaviour. Very special neuropsychological conditions are met during nonconvulsive status epilepticus, which means ongoing, electophysiologically assessed, seizure-like epileptic activity without loss of consciousness and without the overt motor signs of a simple partial or complex partial seizure. A nonconvulsive status may become overtly manifest in a psychiatric condition but in a condition with predominantly cognitive dysfunctions as well. However, with invasive depth electrode recordings quite asymptomatic states can also be observed. Systematic observations are rare (Walker *et al.* 2005). EEG-monitored bedside testing of consciousness, responsivity, reactivity, memory, and higher functions in verbal and non-verbal modes can be helpful for diagnosing this condition, particularly when repeated testing after medical cessation of the assumed status indicates recovery. One might get a picture of such states by observing frontal

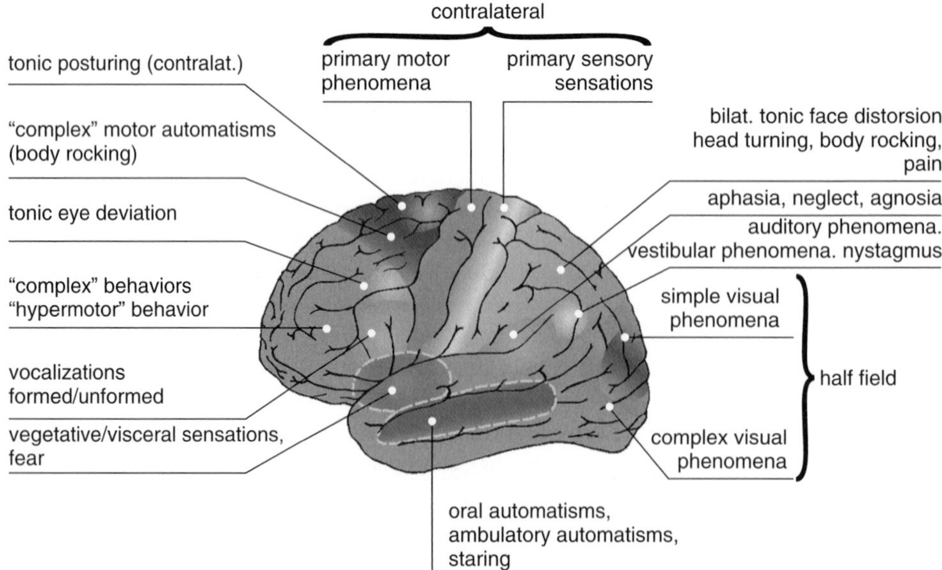

Fig. 18.4 Seizure semiology can provide valuable information for seizure localization.

lobe nonconvulsive seizures as they occur. Patients in such states showed largely preserved, low-level reactive and reflexive behaviour, strongly varying attention levels, severe impairment of self-initiated planned behaviour, behavioural loops with stereotyped and perseverative responses, idiomotoric apraxia, and generally impaired higher cognitive functions (reasoning, calculating; Helmstaedter 2001). Behaviourally, the patients appear irritated and dysphoric. They may react in a repulsing manner, but not with directed aggression. Other special conditions are short-lasting amnestic attacks, which may be recurrent, which are mainly observed in temporal lobe epilepsy, and which appear due to circumscribed bilateral temporo-mesial dysfunction. These can be correlates of ictal or postictal states. Periods may last from minutes up to an hour. Consciousness and purposeful behaviour are preserved but the patients may be irritated about the disturbance (Gallassi *et al.* 1992; Kapur 1993).

Depending on the severity of the seizure, postictal impairments can last for hours (see Fig. 18.5). The impaired functions reconstitute hierarchically with the distance to the most affected structures and the type of continuing impairment can be indicative of the site of the seizure origin (Helmstaedter *et al.* 1994*b*).

A very interesting recent development is concerned with online seizure prediction. This is based on particular EEG characteristics that appear indicative of a seizure and that, in part, can be observed long before a seizure occurs (Lehnertz and Litt 2005). Neuropsychologically, one may thus raise the question as to whether there are cognitive changes or mood changes going along with such phases of an increased readiness to seizures. As for interictal epileptic activity in symptomatic focal epilepsies, an impact on cognition and behaviour is assumed to be similar to that discussed with the idiopathic epilepsies. However, the relation between epileptic activity and behavioural change appears much less reliable than in the idiopathic epilepsies. At present we do not know under what conditions interictal epileptic activity will or will not have an effect on cognition or behaviour (Aldenkamp *et al.* 1996). The existence of a sustained, rather than acute, impact of active epilepsy on cognition in focal epilepsies can be estimated with functional recovery of cognitive functions, behavioural disorders, and mood after successful epilepsy surgery (Helmstaedter *et al.* 2003; Lendt *et al.* 2000; Reuber *et al.* 2004).

To sum up the findings so far in focal symptomatic epilepsies, their cognitive and behavioural consequences depend to a lesser degree on the type of underlying lesion (developmental malformation, hippocampal sclerosis, tumor, etc.) than on localization and lateralization of the epileptogenic region and the age at the lesion/epilepsy onset. Structure–function relations commonly known from the lesion literature do not apply for early onset focal epilepsies.

Dependent on localization and lateralization, early onset focal epilepsies interfere with brain maturation on the one hand and have an effect on the interhemispheric organization of dominance patterns on the other hand. Diffuse and non-specific or atypical patterns of cognitive impairment are the consequence. Severe seizures can additionally lead to irreversible damage but the effect of seizures on cognition is mostly dynamic and reversible as is the impact of the medical treatment on cognition and behaviour (see Fig. 18.6).

18.7 **Treatment**

18.7.1 **Medical treatment**

Ictogenesis in focal epilepsy decisively depends on the intrinsic paroxysmal depolarization of the nerve cell. Therefore, anti-epileptic drugs (AEDs) aim at the prevention of repetitive action potentials: by blocking the natrium flow at the cell membrane; by augmentation of deficient gamma aminobutyric acid (GABA)ergic inhibitory processes; or by reduction of pathological glutamatergic excitation. In idiopathic generalized epilepsies, AEDs aim at receptors

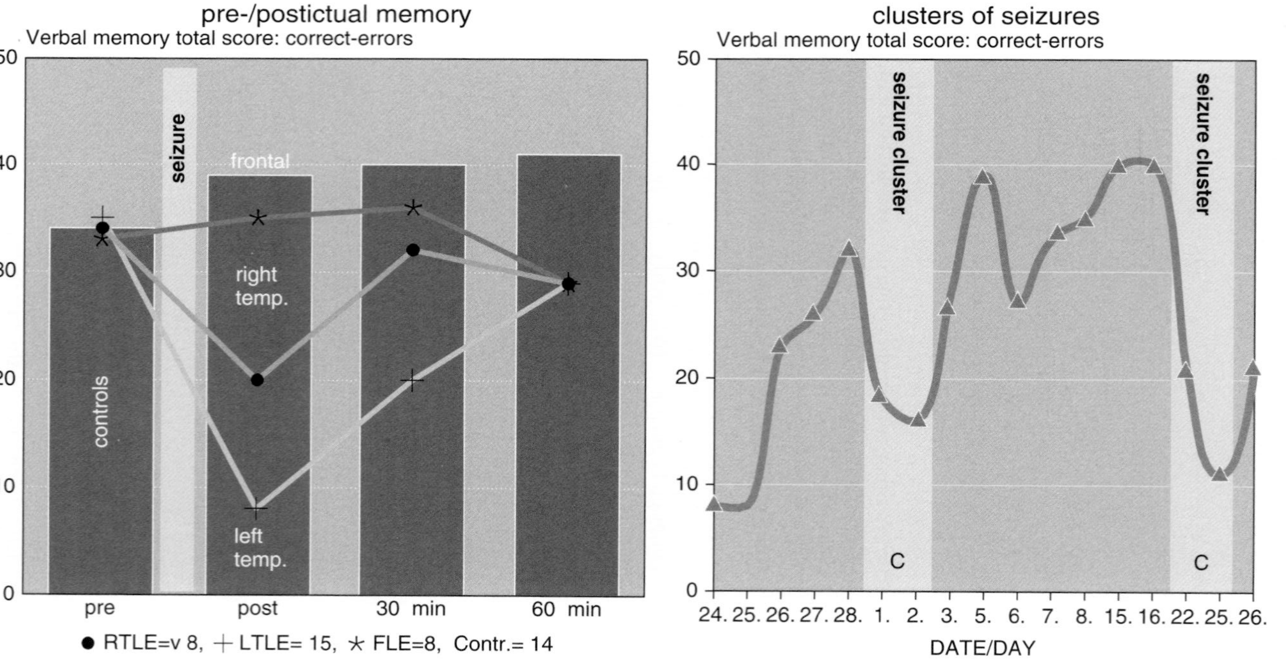

Fig. 18.5 Postictal impairment and recovery of verbal memory after a single seizure (left). Verbal memory breaks down on days with clusters of seizures (right). RTLE, right temporal lobe epilepsy; LTLE, left temporal lobe epilepsy; FLE, frontal lobe epilepsy; Contr., controls. The left-hand graph is taken from Helmstaedter *et al.* (1994*a*); the right-hand graph represents an unpublished single case.

early damage: "interference with maturation"
- the earlier the damage, the worse the outcome
- greater functional plasticity & reserves
- hindrance of development, retardation, global impairment [IQ]
late damage:
"interaction with age/ing"
- the later the damage, the worse
- decreasing plasticity & reserve capacities
- losses > retardation (partial > global impairments)

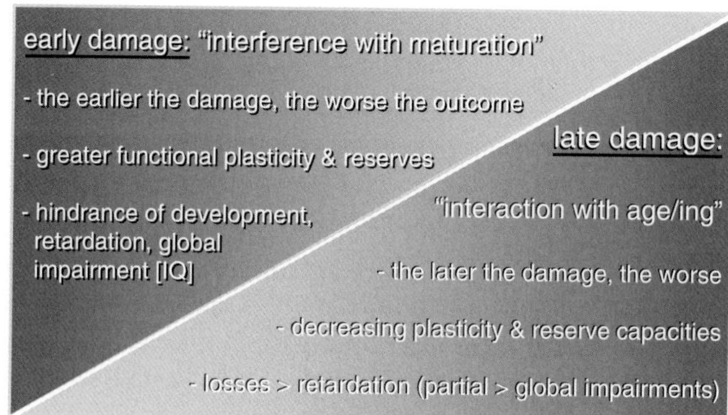

Fig. 18.6 Cognition in epilepsy in a neurodevelopmental context.

and ion-channels (e.g. T-calcium channels, GABA A/-B receptors), which are causative for synchronized bursts.

According to community-based studies, the majority of people with newly diagnosed epilepsy enter long-term remission. However, for about 40% of the patients the seizures will remain resistant to treatment. The success of the medical treatment depends on the number of seizures before treatment. This may reflect the severity of the disease or aetiology (idiopathic versus symptomatic and developmental or not), on the response to the first drug applied, and on psychiatric comorbidity (Kwan and Brodie (2004). Semah *et al.* 1998). The selection of the AED depends on the seizure type, syndrome diagnosis, half-life, and the effect of the AED on metabolism.

Anti-epileptic drugs control seizures and seizure reduction may have beneficial effects on cognition. Anti-epileptic treatment in and of itself, however, may have positive or negative psychotropic effects on cognition and behaviour. Cognitive side-effects of AEDs depend on the substance, the number of AEDs, the dose, the titration speed, and their efficacy with regard to seizure control. Therefore, neurocognitive evaluations should be preferentially performed when patients are on stable medication and within a steady state. Withdrawal of an AED can cause unwanted dynamics in this steady state, particularly when there are interactions between different AEDs. Withdrawal can furthermore negatively change the epileptic situation in terms of a provocation of (generalized-) seizures. As for cognitive and behavioural side-effects of AEDs, these can be idiosyncratic; this means that they are part of the action of the substance or they depend on titration speed and/or dose (blood serum concentration). Most of the AEDs induce dose-dependent diffuse signs of intoxication, which become evident with sedation, somnolence, dizziness, psychomotor slowing, ataxia, and ocular symptoms. Greater risks of dose-dependent adverse effects occur with polytherapy, and particularly when hepatic enzyme inducing or inhibiting drugs cause unwanted metabolic changes (Kwan and Brodie 2001).

The adverse effects of AEDs on cognitive functions may be due to the suppression of neuronal excitability or the enhancement of inhibitory neurotransmission in certain brain areas. Theoretically, this may be different in epileptogenic or non-epileptogenic tissues (Durwen and Elger 1993; Jokeit *et al.* 2001). Furthermore, AEDs may exert a different action depending on the degree of pre-existing morphological damage (Helmstaedter *et al.* 1993). As for the AEDs in use, there is converging evidence that the so-called older AEDs (phenobarbital, phenytoin, carbamazepine, and valproate) are more problematic with respect to cognition and behaviour than the so-called newer AEDs (lamotrigine, gabapentine, levitiracetam, topiramate, zonegran, etc.; see Table 18.2; Loring and Meador 2004; Ortinski and Meador 2004). However, one should keep in mind that the older drugs have been in use for a much longer period of time. Certain aspects of AEDs often become evident a long time after their introduction.

In general, no particular pattern of impairment is observed with different AEDs. According to Ketter *et al.* (1999), one can differentiate sedating effects that are evident in AEDs with a potentiation of GABA inhibitory neurotransmission (e.g. barbiturates, benzodiazepines, valproate, gabapentin, tiagabine, and vigabatrin) and stimulating and possibly anxiogenic effects with AEDs that attenuate glutamate excitatory neurotransmission (e.g. felbamate and lamotrigine). This scheme, however, is an oversimplification and does not apply equally well to all AEDs (Roberts *et al.* 2005). Preferential targets of AEDs include the attention and executive functions, but memory and language functions can also be affected (Aldenkamp *et al.* 2003).

From behavioural evaluations alone it is difficult to determine which aspects of cognitive processing are particularly affected and which sites of action can be discerned. This can be demonstrated with the negative cognitive side-effects of one of the newer generation AEDs, topiramate (TPM). This drug attracted attention when significant language problems were first seen in patients and then later in healthy control subjects (Martin *et al.* 1999). This raised the question as to whether TPM might specifically affect the language system in the left hemisphere. These language problems were mainly seen with respect to verbal fluency and later studies indicated that verbal fluency in this context represents only a striking and easily recognized marker for a more global frontal lobe dysfunction (Kockelmann *et al.* 2003). Side-effects of AEDs may also result from interactive effects between mood and cognition. Lamotrigine (LTG) was thought to have had a positive effect on cognition. This presumably results from its strong mood-stabilizing effect, which eventually led to its successful application in the treatment of patients with major

Table 18.2 Cognitive and behavioural side-effects of common anti-epileptic drugs*

Drug	Cognitive effects†	Behavioural effects†
Lamotrigine	0	–
Levetiracetam	0	+/–
Gabapentin	0	0
Tigabine	0	0
Oxcarbazepine	0	0
Pregabalin	(?)	(?)
Vigabatrin	0	+
Phenytoin	+	0
Carbamazepine	+	0
Sodium valproate	+	0
Zonisamide	(+)	(+)
Clobazam	+	+
Topiramate	+ (+)	+
Clonazepam	++	++
Phenobarbital	++	++

* Modified and extended according to Kwan and Brodie (2001).

† 0, No significant effect; +, negative effect; -, positive effect; (), preliminary result.

depression (Aldenkamp *et al.* (2002). Gajwani *et al.* 2005). Levitiracetam (LEV), another new AED, has arousal-activating effects that can result in better cognitive performance, but can also negatively affect behavioural control (e.g. aggression; Dinkelacker *et al.* 2003). Presumably, pharmaco-fMRI will become a useful tool in evaluating such hypotheses. Jokeit *et al.* (2001) showed reduction of temporo-mesial activation patterns during a memory task in patients with temporal lobe epilepsy under carbamazepine (VBZ).

Two studies recently gained interest in the epileptological community. They showed the negative effects of valproic acid (VPA) on the verbal IQ of children who were exposed to this drug in utero (Adab *et al.* 2004; Gaily *et al.* 2004). It is well known that developmental malformations (e.g. spina bifida and fetal anti-epileptic syndromes) can result from intrauterine exposition to anti-epileptic drugs (Moore *et al.* 2000; Morrow *et al.* 2006). This can be treated with counselling, folic acid prophylaxis, and early prenatal diagnostics. With intellectual impairment or mental retardation, the situation becomes more difficult although a certain overlap between malformations and intellectual retardation can be assumed. It is important to note that almost all studies stress the significant impact of the mother's IQ on the outcome and that impairments become less obvious in the presence of more intelligent mothers (Hirano *et al.* 2004). The pathomechanism by which the verbal IQ in particular becomes affected under VPA is not yet known. It is important to note that the current discussion leans toward VPA but that there are other drugs that we do not know much about. Further research in this area is critically needed. Effects of in utero exposition to AED are not uniform and we neither know the mechanism of damage nor which processes of brain maturation become affected.

18.7.2 **Surgery**

Surgery can be a very successful treatment option for patients with focal symptomatic epilepsies. Surgery is recommended when patients are pharmacoresistant, when they have a resectable epileptogenic region, and when surgery in the affected brain structures will not to lead to any serious negative side-effects (Engel 1987). In such cases, surgery can be curative. Surgery is resective in most cases but, when epilepsy originates in eloquent cortex, subpial transections are an option of choice. By this surgical method the horizontal transmission of epileptic activity between neighbouring parts of the brain is prevented without seriously harming language or motor functions. Another option is palliative surgery, which does not strive for complete seizure control but rather for seizure reduction or for the control of drop attacks. This is the case in patients with multiple foci or in patients in whom rapid interhemispheric seizure spread is controlled by transections of the corpus callosum.

According to a first randomized trial of surgical versus medical treatment, surgery was successful in 58% of operated versus 8% of medically treated patients (Wiebe *et al.* 2001). This outcome parallels what was reported in a recent longitudinal study on medical versus surgical treatment, in which large and homogeneous groups of patients with temporal lobe epilepsy were evaluated (Helmstaedter *et al.* 2003). Seizure outcome can vary with different baseline conditions (temporal/extratemporal localization, presence and type of a lesion, onset/duration of epilepsy, electroencephalographic focus consistent with lesion and seizure semiology, consistent neuropsychology, seizure severity, psychiatric comorbidity, etc). Successful seizure control improves the quality of life and coincides with a reduction of behavioural problems and improvement of mood (Helmstaedter *et al.* 2003; Reuber *et al.* 2004; Lendt *et al.* 1999). However, apart from seizure control, brain surgery can have both positive and negative effects on cognition and behaviour. This requires a careful preoperative evaluation of the site from where seizures take their origin and the functionality of the affected and nonaffected tissues (Helmstaedter 2004; Kral *et al.* 2002).

Methods of achieving this include EEG (extracranial/intracranial, interictal/ictal; Rosenow and Lüders 2004); structural and functional imaging techniques (Koepp and Woermann 2005); angiography optional with intracarotidal application of amobarbital or methohexital (brevital) (Trennery and Loring 1995; Buchtel *et al.* 2002); electrocortical stimulation (Ojemann 2003). From a neuropsychological point of view these diagnostic tools provide optimal conditions for validation of behavioural measures and for establishing relationships between structure, brain function, and behaviour (see Fig. 18.7).

From temporal lobe surgery on the language dominant side, one can propose an outcome prediction model that includes three main factors. These factors might also apply to other types of surgery. Thereafter, the outcome is first of all determined by the functional adequacy of the tissue to be resected. This is reflected by the facts that the resection of unimpaired tissue leads to greater losses and that greater losses in specific functions are observed in those patients with a better baseline performance (Helmstaedter *et al.* 1997*b*, 2004*a*; Chelune *et al.* 1991; Helmstaedter and Elger 1996).

In this regard Fig. 18.8 shows the example of two groups of patients with left temporal lobe epilepsy who had hippocampal sclerosis as the sole pathology and of one group of patients who had a left temporo-lateral pathology. All groups showed comparable verbal memory impairment before surgery. In the lateral lesionectomy group only the lesion was removed without causing additional problems in verbal memory. In the groups with mesial pathology a two-thirds temporal

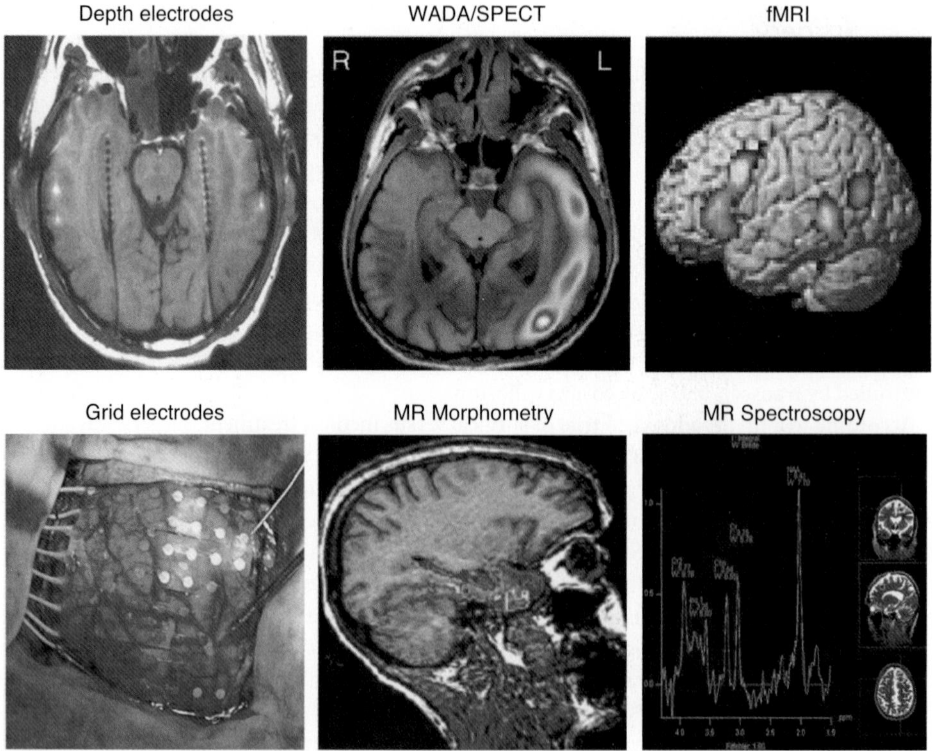

Fig. 18.7 Selection of diagnostic approaches to the brain and their function in presurgical evaluation of patients with pharmacoresistant epilepsy. Information from these tools can serve for correlation/ validation of behavioural neuropsychological data. This is a black and white version of Plate 17.

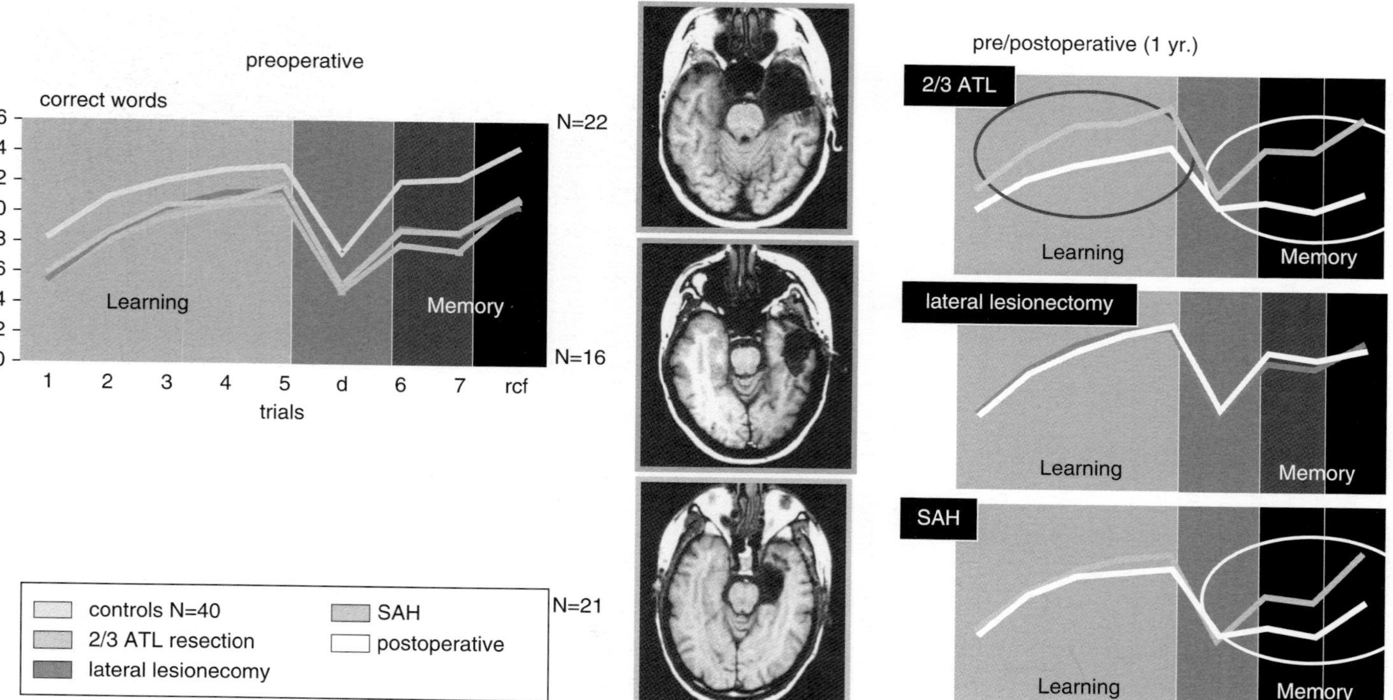

Fig. 18.8 Verbal learning and memory after different types of temporal lobe surgery. SAH, Selective amygdalohippocampectomy; ATL, anterior temporal lobe lobectomy.

lobe resection including the mesial structures led to problems in verbal learning and memory, and selective resection of the mesial structures to problems in memory.

The second factor is the patient's mental reserve capacities: these are reflected by the fact that the outcome is better for those patients with a better baseline performance, IQ, educational status, and for patients with a younger age at the time of surgery (e.g. whether or not the surgery is done within periods critical for plasticity or mental decline; Helmstaedter 1999; Helmstaedter *et al.* 2002, 2003; Lendt *et al.* 1999; Hermann *et al.* 1995; Gleissner *et al.* 2002*b*; Clusmann *et al.* 2002). The third predictive factor is seizure control: sucessful seizure control can lead to the aforementioned release effects and long-term recovery (Helmstaedter 2005).

In summarizing these findings, a poorer cognitive outcome becomes more likely with persistent seizures, with good preoperative memory performance, with an older age at the onset of epilepsy, with an older age at the time of surgery, with a larger extent of the resection, with greater collateral brain damage due to surgery, and with lower reserve capacities. For surgery this means that it should be considered as soon as patients turn out to be pharmacoresistant and that it should be successful in seizure control and restricted enough not to add additional impairment.

18.7.3 Gamma knife and deep brain stimulation

Because postoperative cognitive loss is a function of the damage of functional tissues due to surgery, radiosurgery and gamma knife surgery (GKS) in particular have been suggested as an alternative to resective surgery. GKS does not require craniotomy, and structural damage and subsequent necrosis are believed to be restricted to small target areas. This method has been applied in patients with hypothalamic hamartomas. The first results of a prospective but not randomized multicentre study of 21 patients with mesial TLE are now available. They indicate that 65% of the patients are seizure-free after 2 years with no neuropsychological deterioration (Regis *et al.* 2004*a*, *b*). However, categorical neuropsychological data have been used in this study and categorical data are often subject to a bottom effect (i.e. the patients could hardly become significantly worse). A recent report shows three cases that point in another direction (McDonald *et al.* 2004). A randomized controlled trial with elaborate neuropsychology would be necessary in order to compare the outcomes of resective surgery versus radiosurgery.

For the sake of completeness deep brain stimulation for seizure control in patients with refractory epilepsy must be mentioned. If resective surgery cannot be performed because the epileptogenic zone is within eloquent cortex and when significant neuropsychological consequences must be expected, then deep brain stimulation via an implanted pulse generator may be an option. High frequency electrical stimulation of thalamic nuclei obviously modulates neuronal excitability and can lead to significant seizure reduction and decrease of interictal epileptiform activity. Comparable results have been obtained with unilateral hippocampal stimulation with refractory mesial TLE. Up to now, whether stimulation indeed preserves function or whether it interferes with the functionality of the stimulated area has not been evaluated (Velasco *et al.* 1995; Benabid *et al.* 2002; Vonck *et al.* 2005). The ultimate goal of such an approach is the development of devices that combine seizure prediction and stimulation methods and allow for EEG-triggered suppression of epileptic activity by deep brain stimulation (Schwartz 2005).

18.7.4 Vagal nerve stimulation

In recent years, the electrical stimulation of the vagal nerve (VNS) has turned out to be something of a 'third way' for treating pharmacoresistant epilepsies (other than medical and surgical treatment; Schachter and Schmidt 2001).

Since its approval in 1997, this cardiac pacemaker-like impulse generator has been implanted in more than 25 000 patients worldwide. The device stimulates the vagal nerve via a spiral electrode and has also been approved for the treatment of very severe depression. Depending on the individual settings, the intermittent electrical pulses are applied to the vagal nerve (current, 0.25–3.00 mA; pulsewidth, 200–300 ms; pulse frequency, 20–30 Hz; cycles, ON-duration 7–30 s, OFF-duration: 15–300 s). With regard to efficacy and the suggested influence on cognitive functioning, it is important to know that the afferent projections of the vagal nerve either directly or indirectly approach brain areas that are also relevant to epilepsy (e.g. locus ceruleus, thalamus, hippocampus, and amygdalae). The clinical efficacy of the vagus nerve stimulator has been demonstrated with double-blind, dose-controlled studies. In about 40–50% of the patients, a seizure reduction of at least 50% can be obtained. The efficacy appears to increase with the duration of the treatment, but absolute seizure control is rare. From a neuropsychological standpoint, this instrument is of major interest since its intermittent and programmable stimulation condition allows for an experimental evaluation of the modulatory effects of peripheral vagal stimulation on CNS functions. Indeed, positive psychotropic effects in terms of improved attention, decision-making, or word recognition have been reported in addition to a negative effect on figural memory (Helmstaedter *et al.* 2001; Martin *et al.* 2004; Clark *et al.* 1999; Hassert *et al.* 2004). Apart from its acute effects, no persisting changes as assessed with a neuropsychological test battery have yet been demonstrated (Hoppe *et al.* 2001).

18.7.5 **Behavioural therapy**

Behaviour modification and neurofeedback are treatment options that have mainly arisen from three observations.

1 Seizures in reflex epilepsies can be suppressed by sensory stimulation.

2 Seizures often start with an aura as a first sign of an evolving seizure. This can be taken as a warning sign.

3 The EEG can be taken to visualize pathological and non-pathological brain activity (Dahl *et al.* 1992; Rockstroh *et al.* 1984; Lubar 1998; Sterman 2000).

On a superordinate level, a reduction of seizure-supporting behaviour (e.g. sleep deprivation and alcohol) and an increase of health-related behaviour (e.g. compliance) can have a positive effect on seizure frequency. A good example of how compliance can be improved has been demonstrated with the introduction of an electronic pill box (Rosen *et al.* 2004).

More interesting from a neuropsychological point of view is the self-control of seizures by counteracting measures in the presence of an aura or the interictal training of conditions that are incompatible with seizures via EEG biofeedback. EEG biofeedback explicitly or implicitly relies on the individual's cognitive, emotional, and imaginative processes, by which the patients try to modify their EEG activity, e.g. slow DC shifts, sensorimotor rhythm (see Fig. 18.9).

Both approaches, the neurofeedback and behavioural countermeasures, seem more effective in patients with an aura. As for the control mechanism, the neurophysiological principle of 'recruitment and availability' may serve as a common explanation for both approaches. This principle proposes that a spread of epileptic activity is most likely when focus-surrounding tissues have a medium activity level. Functional occupation of non-affected brain tissues as well as their inactivation prevents their recruitment by epilepsy (Speckmann 1986). A patient with an occipital focus and a fixation-off epilepsy (repetitive spike activity occurring with eye closure) may serve as an example. In this patient a linear relation could be shown between epileptic spike activity and graded variations of the visual input, and training of the control of epileptic activity in this

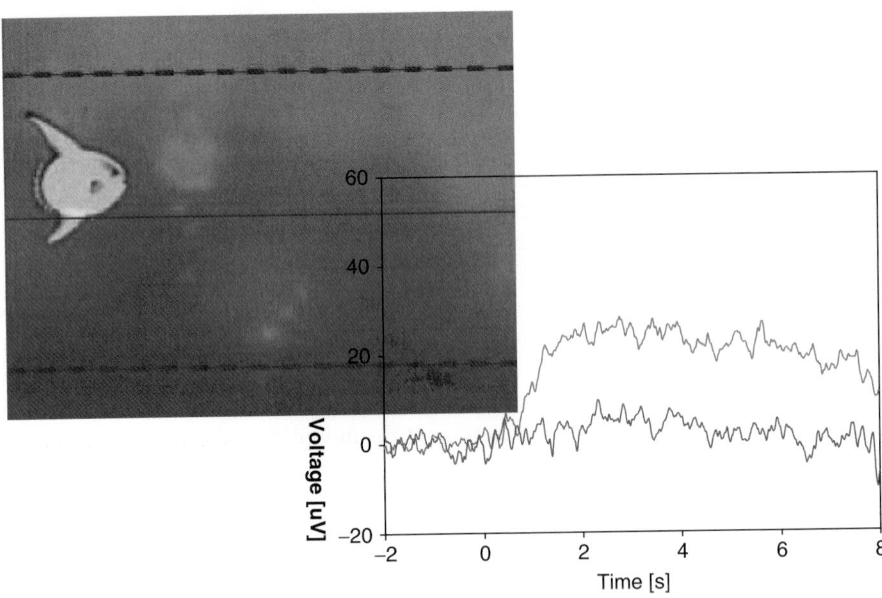

Fig. 18.9 Biofeedback of slow cortical potentials for control of epilepsy (task taken from NEURO PRAX®).

patient was able to reduce seizure frequency (Helmstaedter *et al.* 1988). Control mechanisms aim at weakly epileptic or non-epileptic tissues rather than strong epileptic tissues. This has been demonstrated with the evaluation of the effects of attending behaviour on seizure activity in the alumina-gel monkey model of focal epilepsy (Lockard and Wyler 1979). The strong local negative correlation between mental activation and epilepsy can also be shown with nonlinear analyses of EEG intrahippocampal depth recordings performed during memory and non-memory tasks that do or do not involve the mesial temporal lobe structures (Lehnertz *et al.* 1997).

Although the possibility of self-control has been known for a long time, the boom was in the 1970s and 1980s. Even though incredible effects on seizure frequency (up to 70% seizure reduction) and responder rates (up to 82%) have been described, these methods remained largely experimental and did not become a clinical standard. A critical point with regard to feedback and self-control techniques may be that, from a theoretical point of view, cerebral activation may not only suppress but also elicit seizures (Matsuoka *et al.* 2000; Helmstaedter *et al.* 1992). However, a recent study that used the feedback of galvanic skin response in order to increase the tonic level of peripheral sympathetic arousal achieved a 49% seizure reduction (median 59%). This shows that the issue of self-control via feedback is still under evaluation (Nagai *et al.* 2004). Prospective randomized and placebo-controlled studies of homogeneous patient groups that evaluate the sustained efficacy of behavioural interventions in epilepsy would be very valuable.

At present, educational modular programmes for patients and their relatives or caregivers that include teachings about epilepsy appear much more promising than applying self-control techniques alone. Such programmes also consider diagnostic issues, treatment, psychosocial aspects, and coping with epilepsy. Such teaching programmes improve quality of life and they can also lead to a reduction in seizure frequency (Snead *et al.* 2004; May and Pfafflin 2002).

18.8 **Chronic epilepsy and cognitive development**

18.8.1 **Mental decline?**

A point of major importance with regard to the impact of seizures and the impact of seizure activity on cognition in epilepsy is whether or not chronic epilepsy damages the brain (Sutula and Pitkänen 2002). As already described within the epilepsy seizure section, seizures and severe seizures in particular can result in irreversible damage. However, this appears to be an individual condition rather than the rule. According to a recent review on this issue, the cumulative effect of seizures on cognition appears less severe that might be expected (Dodrill 2004).

Cross-sectional studies in chronic, uncontrolled temporal lobe epilepsy indicate a significant decline in intelligence after intervals greater than three decades (Jokeit and Ebner 2002). However, those studies that cross-sectionally correlate cognitive performance with duration of epilepsy suffer from a shortcoming: since most epilepsies start early, their duration is largely synonymous with chronological age. A comparison of age regressions of performance in healthy subjects and patients puts such findings into perspective (see Fig. 18.10; Helmstaedter and Elger 1999).

Verbal memory decline, which is indicated by age regression in left mesial TLE, runs largely in parallel to the age regression observed in controls. Nevertheless, there is a memory decline

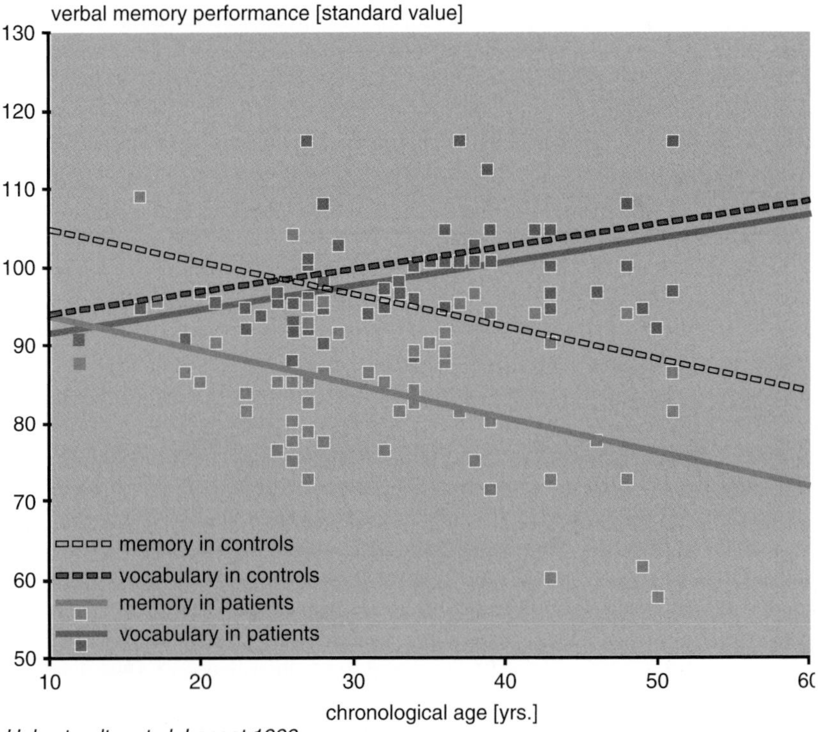

Fig. 18.10 Age regression of verbal memory (list learning) and vocabulary (semantic memory) in patients with left mesial temporal lobe epilepsy contrasted to age regressions in healthy controls. (Adapted from Helmstaedter and Elger 1999.)

in chronic uncontrolled TLE when patients are evaluated in a longitudinal study design. In summary, a very slow and individually progressing cognitive decline can be suggested (Rausch *et al.* 2003; Helmstaedter *et al.* 2003). Presumably this applies to chronic focal epilepsies in general, but this remains to be seen. It also remains to be demonstrated whether different domains are affected in other epilepsies or whether such a decline is specific or non-specific. Most of the impairments met in patients with symptomatic focal epilepsies seem to exist at, or even prior to, the onset of epilepsy, i.e. they result from the interference of lesions/epilepsy with brain maturation and mental development. As for chronic epilepsy, the impact of additional, later acquired lesions and their interaction with processes of ageing appear to be much more relevant for the individual cognitive development than the accumulation of seizures (Elger *et al.* 2004*a*; Helmstaedter 2005). This view would be in line with recent cross-sectional and longitudinal MRI volumetric evaluations in patients with chronic epilepsy, which do not suggest accelerated atrophy or volume loss with longer-lasting epilepsies (Liu *et al.* 2005).

No longitudinal studies that span time intervals longer than 10 years are available. Therefore, the impact of epilepsy on cognitive development must be deduced from a mixture of findings regarding epilepsies in children versus adults, retrospective evaluations of patients with early versus late onset of epilepsy, and an evaluation of patients who underwent epilepsy surgery at a younger versus older age. When epilepsy hits the maturing brain, then the underlying lesion, epileptic dysfunction, or negative treatment effects can cause developmental delay or retardation, even if the latter two factors are controlled. Global intellectual retardation is often the consequence. This is reflected by the fact that mental retardation is more likely to occur in early childhood epilepsies than in those epilepsies with an onset in adolescence or later. The more deleterious effect of earlier onset epilepsies on cognitive development is also indicated when evaluated in a mostly homogeneous group of patients with temporal lobe epilepsies. Childhood TLE displays more diffuse impairment than adult TLE. In particular, language functions are impaired more often in children, but material-specific memory deficits are similar in both groups (Helmstaedter and Lendt 2001; Nolan *et al.* 2004; Culhane-Shelburne *et al.* 2002). Retrospective evaluations in adult patients with TLE reveal that patients with earlier onset (> 15 years) show memory plus intellectual impairment, whereas patients with later onset epilepsies show primarily memory impairment. Comparable intellectual impairment is a rare condition in patients with untreated late diagnosed epilepsies (Helmstaedter 2005).

18.8.2 **Functional plasticity and reserve capacities**

18.8.2.1 Early onset epilepsy

The fact that early onset epilepsies lead to more severe and diffuse impairment than late onset epilepsies is irritating, given the fact that childhood also represents a period during which the brain can be assumed to be still highly functionally plastic. Indeed, there are astonishing cases of formerly left-hemisphere, language-dominant patients who underwent a left-sided hemispherectomy for seizure control (mostly patients with Rasmussen's encephalitis). Later on, they displayed at least partial contralateral language reorganization if the surgery was performed early enough. Such reorganization has been observed even in older children of up to 9 years of age (Hertz-Pannier *et al.* 2002; Vargha-Khadem *et al.* 1997; Boatman *et al.* 1999; Loddenkemper *et al.* 2003). However, as impressive as such case reports may be, it is a myth to believe that the loss of a total hemisphere can be completely compensated. The children will not achieve the performance level they would have shown had both hemispheres been fully functional and intact, even if the surgery had been realized at a very early age (Bayard and Lassonde 2001). This is consistent with the general finding in atypical language dominant patients with left hemisphere epilepsies: right hemisphere language restitution is not synonymous with better language functions (Helmstaedter *et al.* 1997*d*). Moreover, right hemisphere preservation and restitution of language is often achieved only at the cost of functions normally mediated by the right hemisphere (Ogden 1988, 1989; Mariotti *et al.* 1998). This negative effect of language restitution at the cost of non-language functions has been called the 'crowding' or 'suppression' effect. It becomes most obvious with respect to material- specific memory and should be understood in terms of an incompatibility of different modes of information processing rather than a struggle of functions for space (Helmstaedter *et al.* 1994*a*).

Studies based on results from separate unilateral short-term anaesthesia (WADA test; Wada and Rasmussen 1960) of the hemispheres suggest that more than one-third of the patients with focal symptomatic epilepsies show patterns of atypical hemispheric language dominance (see Fig. 18.11).

The presence and the degree of right-hemispheric participation in language are significantly correlated with an earlier age at onset of left-hemisphere epilepsy (Helmstaedter *et al.* 1997*d*; Saltzman-Benaiah *et al.* 2003). Apart from an early onset of epilepsy, children and adults with atypical language dominance are often left-handed, show lesions close by or within language-relevant structures, and display neuropsychological 'suppression effects' with distinct non-verbal memory deficits (Helmstaedter *et al.* 1997*d*; Gleissner *et al.* 2003). Atypical hemisphere dominance, however, is not an 'all or nothing' phenomenon and graded patterns of right hemisphere dominance can be observed as well as distinctive patterns of interhemispheric dissociations of expressive and receptive language or handedness and language (Kurthen *et al.* 1992; Baciu *et al.* 2003; Lee *et al.* 2005). Dissociation of memory and language can also be found (Wood *et al.* 1999; Jokeit *et al.* 1996). In contrast to widespread left-hemispheric damage which leads to contralateral reorganization, circumscribed epileptogenic lesions can lead to ipsilateral perilesional language reorganization (Liegeois *et al.* 2004). Whether ipsilateral reorganization depends on the type of lesion or on lesion onset is a matter for discussion (Duchowny *et al.* 1996; Ojemann *et al.* 1989, 2003). The presence of atypical dominance is not necessarily fixed to the presence of lesions close to or within the cortex normally relevant for language. It is observed as well with circumscribed lesions or foci not overlapping with language areas, indicating distant effects of

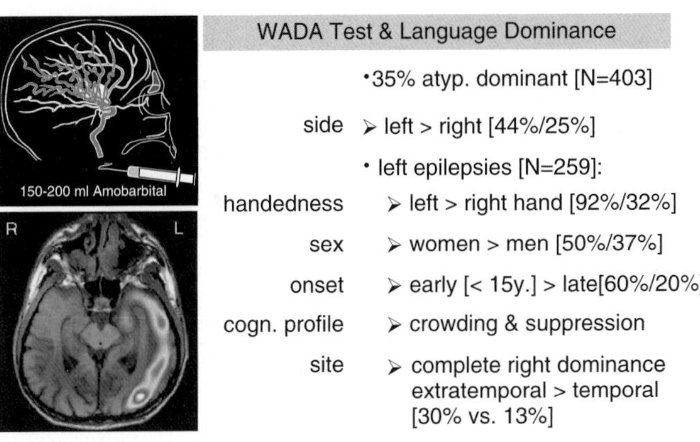

Fig. 18.11 Results from Wada tests in patients with focal epilepsies. (Based on unpublished data from the Bonn series of Wada tests; see also Helmstaedter *et al.* 1994*a*, 1997*d*, 1999*a*, 2004*b*.)

focal epilepsies on regions outside the epileptogenic area (Saltzman-Benaiah *et al.* 2003). That atypical dominance in epilepsy is not only 'lesion-driven' but also 'epilepsy-driven' has recently been shown by a correlation of atypical language dominance with left hemisphere epileptic activity in TLE (Janszky *et al.* 2003). This observation raises the interesting hypothesis that, if atypical language dominance can be epilepsy-driven, control of epilepsy might result in a reversal of language dominance (Helmstaedter *et al.* 2006).

It is important to note that there is a clinical bias in lateralization research, which focuses on left hemisphere epilepsies and considers right hemisphere epilepsies only when the seizure semiology indicates right hemisphere language or when the patients are left-handed. Evaluation of larger series of consecutive, nonselected patients with left and right epilepsies indicates, firstly, that 24% of patients with right hemispheric epilepsies also show a pattern of atypical language dominance and, secondly, that the possibility of a transfer of language functions from the right to the left hemisphere can be suggested (Helmstaedter *et al.* 1997*d*). The findings in right hemisphere epilepsies mirror those in left epilepsies in that atypical language dominance occurs more frequently in late-onset, right-sided epilepsies than in early-onset, right hemisphere epilepsies. This indicates that in the early-onset group, right-sided epilepsy forced predisposed right-sided language functions to be 'transferred' to the left hemisphere, or that early right-sided epilepsy prevented the establishment of language representation in that hemisphere (Helmstaedter *et al.* 1997*c*).

18.8.2.2 Later onset epilepsy

If epilepsy affects the mature brain, greater partial impairment is observed. When compared to adults, children show a greater functional plasticity and reserve capacity (Helmstaedter and Lendt 2001). For example, this can be demonstrated with recovery from epilepsy surgery (Gleissner *et al.* 2005). Patients with adult onset epilepsy experience irreversible impairment of fully acquired functions rather than retarded development. This can also be demonstrated within the context of epilepsy surgery. In this case surgery stands for an acquired lesion, which is very similar in children and adults and which allows for the evaluation of compensation and restitution capacities at different ages. In left TLE patients, there is a clear relationship between increased risks of postoperative verbal memory decline following anterior temporal lobectomy and increasing age at the onset of epilepsy (Helmstaedter 1999). When compared to adult TLE patients, TLE children below the age of 16 show a lower risk of postsurgical memory deterioration (Helmstaedter 1999; Lendt *et al.* 1999) and, within a 3–12 month follow-up, the postoperative memory decline appears to be more reversible in children than in adults (Gleissner *et al.* 2002). Although additionally acquired damage can add to the pre-existing damage and this might result in an accelerated mental decline (Helmstaedter *et al.* 2002), there is nevertheless evidence for processes of plasticity in the adult brain as well. Again, the respective knowledge mostly stems from TLE. With fMRI, for example, it could be demonstrated that verbal memory involves the right temporal lobe in left TLE (Golby *et al.* 2002) and that intracranially recorded, event-related potentials within the right hippocampus predict verbal memory outcome after left temporal surgery (Grunwald *et al.* 1998). There is also clinical evidence of adult memory reorganization from observations showing that, in preoperatively atypically dominant patients, the so-called 'suppression or crowding effect' was reversed after surgery (Gleissner *et al.* 2002*a*).

The question of whether patients with chronic epilepsy are at a greater risk for becoming demented as they age has rarely been addressed. A recent study on older patients found cognitive impairments comparable to those in patients with mild cognitive impairment (MCI). Patients with epilepsy on AED polytherapy displayed the worst performance (Griffith *et al.* 2006). Even when the epilepsy does not turn out to be a progressively dementing disease, the fact that the starting condition for physiological mental ageing is much worse than in healthy subjects suggests a larger portion of demented patients and a much earlier onset of dementia in patients with epilepsy (see Fig. 18.10; Helmstaedter and Elger 1999; Helmstaedter *et al.* 2002*b*).

For intelligence, a postponed decline in patients with a better education versus patients with a poorer education has been found. This indicates greater reserve capacities for those with a better education (Jokeit and Ebner 2002). Future research must address the question as to whether certain types of epilepsy (e.g. temporal lobe epilepsy with memory impairment or frontal lobe epilepsy with impaired executive functions, psychiatric comorbidity, and genetic predispositions for accelerated mental decline) are risk factors. These factors should be considered in patient counselling, particularly when surgical interventions that bear the risk of additional cognitive impairment are planned.

In conclusion it was a major aim of this chapter to show that a developmental neuropsychological approach is essential for the understanding of the impact of epilepsy and its treatment on cognition and behaviour. Epilepsy can serve to model neurodevelopmental impairments in childhood, the interaction of a chronic disease with physiological processes of ageing, and the brain's capacities to restitute and compensate with early versus late lesions. Finally, epilepsy provides a model to study the differential impact of lesions versus neuronal dysfunction on cognition.

References

Adab, N., Kini, U., Vinten, J., Ayres, J., Baker, G., Clayton-Smith, J., Coyle, H., Fryer, A., Gorry, J., Gregg, J., Mawer, G., Nicolaides, P., Pickering, L., Tunnicliffe, L., and Chadwick, D.W. (2004). The longer term outcome of children born to mothers with epilepsy. *J. Neurol. Neurosurg. Psychiatry* **75** (11), 1575–83.

Aghakhani, Y., Bagshaw, A.P., Benar, C.G., Hawco, C., Andermann, F., Dubeau, F., and Gotman, J. (2004). fMRI activation during spike and wave discharges in idiopathic generalized epilepsy. *Brain* **127** (5), 1127–44.

Aldenkamp, A.P., Overweg, J., Gutter, T., Beun, A.M., Diepman, L., and Mulder, O.G. (1996). Effect of epilepsy, seizures and epileptiform EEG discharges on cognitive function. *Acta Neurol. Scand.* **93** (4), 253–9.

Aldenkamp, A.P., Arends, J., Bootsma, H.P., Diepman, L., Hulsman, J., Lambrechts, D., Leenen, L., Majoie, M., Schellekens, A., and de Vocht, J. (2002). Randomized double-blind parallel-group study comparing cognitive effects of a low-dose lamotrigine with valproate and placebo in healthy volunteers. *Epilepsia* **43** (1), 19–26.

Aldenkamp, A.P., De Krom, M., and Reijs, R. (2003). Newer antiepileptic drugs and cognitive issues. *Epilepsia* **44** (Suppl. 4), 21–9.

Baciu, M.V., Watson, J.M., McDermott, K.B., *et al.* (2003). Functional MRI reveals an interhemispheric dissociation of frontal and temporal language regions in a patient with focal epilepsy. *Epilepsy Behav.* **4**, 776–80.

Bayard, S. and Lassonde, M. (2001). Cognitive, sensory and motor adjustment to hemispherectomy. In *Neuropsychology of childhood epilepsy* (ed. I. Jambaque), pp. 229–44. Kluwer Academic, New York.

Beck, H., Goussakov, I.V., Lie, A., Helmstaedter, C., and Elger, C.E. (2000). Synaptic plasticity in the human dentate gyrus. *J. Neurosci.* **20** (18), 7080–6.

Benabid, A.L., Minotti, L., Koudsie, A., de Saint Martin, A., and Hirsch, E. (2002). Antiepileptic effect of high-frequency stimulation of the subthalamic nucleus (corpus luysi) in a case of medically intractable epilepsy caused by focal dysplasia: a 30-month follow-up: technical case report. *Neurosurgery* **50** (6), 1385–91; discussion 1391–2.

Boatman, D., Freeman, J., Vining, E., *et al.* (1999). Language recovery after left hemispherectomy in children with late-onset seizures. *Ann. Neurol.* **46**, 579–86.

Breier, J.I., Plenger, P.M., Castillo, R., *et al.* (1996). Effects of temporal lobe epilepsy on spatial and figural aspects of memory for a complex geometric figure. *J. Int. Neuropsychol. Soc.* **2**, 535–40.

Buchtel, H.A., Passaro, E.A., Selwa, L.M., Deveikis, J., and Gomez-Hassan, D. (2002). Sodium methohexital (brevital) as an anesthetic in the Wada test. *Epilepsia* Sep **43** (9), 1056–61.

Buckner, R.L. and Wheeler, M.E. (2001). The cognitive neuroscience of remembering. *Nat. Rev. Neurosci.* **2**, 624–34.

Chelune, G.J., Naugle, R.I., Luders, H., and Awad, I.A. (1991). Prediction of cognitive change as a function of preoperative ability status among temporal lobectomy patients seen at 6-month follow-up. *Neurology* **41**, 399–404.

Clark, K.B., Naritoku, D.K., Smith, D.C., Browning, R.A., and Jensen, R.A. (1999). Enhanced recognition memory following vagus nerve stimulation in human subjects. *Nat. Neurosci.* **2** (1), 94–8.

Clusmann, H., Schramm, J., Kral, T., *et al.* (2002). Prognostic factors and outcome after different types of resection for temporal lobe epilepsy. *J. Neurosurg.* **97**, 1131–41.

Commission on Classification and Terminology of the International League Against Epilepsy (1989). Proposal for revised classification of epilepsies and epileptic syndromes. Commission on Classification and Terminology of the International League Against Epilepsy. *Epilepsia* **30** (4), 389–99.

Culhane-Shelburne, K., Chapieski, L., Hiscock, M., and Glaze, D. (2002). Executive functions in children with frontal and temporal lobe epilepsy. *J. Int. Neuropsychol. Soc.* **8**, 623–32.

Dahl, J., Brorson, L.O., and Melin, L. (1992). Effects of a broad-spectrum behavioral medicine treatment program on children with refractory epileptic seizures: an 8-year follow-up. *Epilepsia* **33** (1), 98–102.

Devinsky, O., Gershengorn, J., Brown, E., Perrine, K., Vazquez, B., and Luciano, D. (1997). Frontal functions in juvenile myoclonic epilepsy. *Neuropsychiatry Neuropsychol. Behav. Neurol.* **10** (4), 243–6.

Dinkelacker, V., Dietl, T., Widman, G., Lengler, U., and Elger, C.E. (2003). Aggressive behavior of epilepsy patients in the course of levetiracetam add-on therapy: report of 33 mild to severe cases. *Epilepsy Behav.* **4** (5), 537–47.

Dodrill, C.B. (2004). Neuropsychological effects of seizures. *Epilepsy Behav.* **5** (Suppl. 1), S21–4.

Duchowny, M., Jayakar, P., Harvey, A.S., *et al.* (1996). Language cortex representation: effects of developmental versus acquired pathology. *Ann. Neurol.* **40**, 31–8.

Durwen, H.F. and Elger, C.E. (1993). Verbal learning differences in epileptic patients with left and right temporal lobe foci–a pharmacologically induced phenomenon? *Acta Neurol. Scand.* **87** (1), 1–8.

Elger, C.E., Grunwald, T., Lehnertz, K., Kutas, M., Helmstaedter, C., Brockhaus, A., Van Roost, D., and Heinze, H.J. (1997). Human temporal lobe potentials in verbal learning and memory processes. *Neuropsychologia* **35** (5), 657–67.

Elger, C.E., Helmstaedter, C., and Kurthen, M. (2004). Chronic epilepsy and cognition. *Lancet Neurol.* **3** (11), 663–72.

Engel, J. Jr. (Ed.) (1987). *Surgical treatment of the epilepsies.* Raven Press, New York.

Engel, J. Jr. (2001). A proposed diagnostic scheme for people with epileptic seizures and with epilepsy: report of the ILAE Task Force on Classification and Terminology. *Epilepsia* **42**, 796–803.

Engel, J. Jr. (2004). The goal of epilepsy therapy: no seizures, no side effects, as soon as possible. *CNS Spectr.* **9** (2), 95–7.

Exner, C., Boucsein, K., Lange, C., Winter, H., Weniger, G., Steinhoff, B.J., and Irle, E. (2002). Neuropsychological performance in frontal lobe epilepsy. *Seizure* **11** (1), 20–32.

Fell, J., Klaver, P., Lehnertz, K., Grunwald, T., Schaller, C., Elger, C.E., and Fernandez, G. (2001). Human memory formation is accompanied by rhinal–hippocampal coupling and decoupling. *Nat. Neurosci.* **4** (12), 1259–64.

Fell, J., Fernandez, G., Lutz, M.T., Kockelmann, E., Burr, W., Schaller, C., Elger, C.E., and Helmstaedter, C. (2006). Rhinal–hippocampal connectivity determines memory formation during sleep. *Brain* **129**, 108–14.

Fernandez, G. and Tendolkar, I. (2001). Integrated brain activity in medial temporal and prefrontal areas predicts subsequent memory performance: human declarative memory formation at the system level. *Brain Res. Bull.* **55**, 1–9.

Gabis, L., Pomeroy, J., and Andriola, M.R. (2005). Autism and epilepsy: cause, consequence, comorbidity, or coincidence? *Epilepsy Behav.* **7**, 652–6.

Gaily, E., Kantola-Sorsa, E., Hiilesmaa, V., Isoaho, M., Matila, R., Kotila, M., Nylund, T., Bardy, A., Kaaja, E., and Granstrom, M.L. (2004). Normal intelligence in children with prenatal exposure to carbamazepine. *Neurology* **62** (1), 28–32.

Gajwani, P., Forsthoff, A., Muzina, D., Amann, B., Gao, K., Elhaj, O., Calabrese, J.R., and Grunze, H. (2005). Antiepileptic drugs in mood-disordered patients. *Epilepsia* **46** (Suppl. 4), 38–44. Review.

Galanopoulou, A.S., Bojko, A., Lado, F., and Moshe, S.L. (2000). The spectrum of neuropsychiatric abnormalities associated with electrical status epilepticus in sleep. *Brain Dev.* **22** (5), 279–95.

Gallassi, R., Morreale, A., Di Sarro, R., and Lugaresi, E. (1992). Epileptic amnesic syndrome. *Epilepsia* **33** (Suppl. 6), S21–5.

Gazzaniga, M.S. (2005). Forty-five years of split-brain research and still going strong. *Nat. Rev. Neurosci.* **6** (8), 653–9.

Gleissner, U. and Elger, C.E. (2001). The hippocampal contribution to verbal fluency in patients with temporal lobe epilepsy. *Cortex* **37** (1), 55–63.

Gleissner, U., Helmstaedter, C., and Elger, C.E. (1998). Right hippocampal contribution to visual memory: a presurgical and postsurgical study in patients with temporal lobe epilepsy. *J. Neurol. Neurosurg. Psychiatry* **65** (5), 665–9.

Gleissner, U., Helmstaedter, C., and Elger, C.E. (2002*a*). Memory reorganization in adult brain: observations in three patients with temporal lobe epilepsy. *Epilepsy Res.* **48**, 229–34.

Gleissner, U., Sassen, R., Lendt, M., Clusmann, H., Elger, C.E., and Helmstaedter, C. (2002*b*). Pre- and postoperative verbal memory in pediatric patients with temporal lobe epilepsy. *Epilepsy Res.* **51** (3), 287–96.

Gleissner, U., Kurthen, M., Sassen, R., Kuczaty, S., Elger, C.E., Linke, D.B., Urbach, H., and Helmstaedter, C. (2003). Clinical and neuropsychological characteristics of pediatric epilepsy patients with atypical language dominance. *Epilepsy Behav.* **4** (6), 746–52.

Gleissner, U., Sassen, R., Schramm, J., Elger, C.E., and Helmstaedter, C. (2005). Greater functional recovery after temporal lobe epilepsy surgery in children. *Brain* **128** (12), 2822–9.

Glosser, G., Salvucci, A.E., and Chiaravalloti, N.D. (2003). Naming and recognizing famous faces in temporal lobe epilepsy. *Neurology* **61**, 81–6.

Golby, A.J., Poldrack, R.A., Illes, J., *et al.* (2002). Memory lateralization in medial temporal lobe epilepsy assessed by functional MRI. *Epilepsia* **43**, 855–63.

Gregory, D.L. and Wong, P.K. (1992). Clinical relevance of a dipole field in rolandic spikes. *Epilepsia* **33** (1), 36–44.

Griffith, H.R., Martin, R.C., Bambara, J.K., Marson, D.C., and Faught, E. (2006). Older adults with epilepsy demonstrate cognitive impairments compared with patients with amnestic mild cognitive impairment. *Epilepsy Behav.* **8** (1), 161–8.

Grunwald, T., Lehnertz, K., Helmstaedter, C., *et al.* (1998). Limbic ERPs predict verbal memory after left-sided hippocampectomy. *Neuroreport* **9**, 3375–8.

Grunwald, T., Beck, H., Lehnertz, K., Blumcke, I., Pezer, N., Kurthen, M., Fernandez, G.,Van Roost, D., Heinze, H.J., Kutas, M., and Elger, C.E. (1999). Evidence relating human verbal memory to hippocampal N-methyl-D-aspartate receptors. *Proc. Natl. Acad. Sci. USA* **96** (21), 12085–9.

Guzzetta, F., Battaglia, D., Veredice, C., Donvito, V., Pane, M., Lettori, D., Chiricozzi, F., Chieffo, D., Tartaglione, T., and Dravet, C. (2005). Early thalamic injury associated with epilepsy and continuous spike–wave during slow sleep. *Epilepsia* **46** (6), 889–900.

Hamberger, M.J., Seidel, W.T., McKhann, G.M. 2nd, Perrine, K., and Goodman, R.R. (2005). Brain stimulation reveals critical auditory naming cortex. *Brain* **128** (11), 2742–9.

Hassert, D.L., Miyashita, T., and Williams, C.L. (2004). The effects of peripheral vagal nerve stimulation at a memory-modulating intensity on norepinephrine output in the basolateral amygdala. *Behav. Neurosci.* **118** (1), 79–88.

Hauser, W.A., Rich, S.S., Lee, J.R., Annegers, J.F., and Anderson, V.E. (1998). Risk of recurrent seizures after two unprovoked seizures. *N. Engl. J. Med.* **338** (7), 429–34.

Helmstaedter, C. (1999). Prediction of memory reserve capacity. *Adv. Neurol.* **81**, 271–9.

Helmstaedter, C. (2001). Behavioral aspects of frontal lobe epilepsy. *Epilepsy Behav.* **2** (5), 384–95.

Helmstaedter, C. (2002). Effects of chronic epilepsy on declarative memory systems. *Prog. Brain Res.* **135**, 439–53.

Helmstaedter, C. (2004). Neuropsychological aspects of epilepsy surgery. *Epilepsy Behav.* **5** (Suppl. 1), S45–55.

Helmstaedter, C. (2005). Effects of chronic temporal lobe epilepsy on memory functions. In *Cognitive dysfunction in children with temporal lobe epilepsy*, Progress in Epileptic Disorders Vol.1 (ed. A. Arzimanoglou, A. Aldenkamp, H. Cross, M. Lassonde, S.L. Moshé, and B. Schmitz), pp. 13–30. John Libbey Eurotext, Paris.

Helmstaedter, C. and Elger, C.E. (1996). Cognitive consequences of two-thirds anterior temporal lobectomy on verbal memory in 144 patients: a three-month follow-up study. *Epilepsia* **37** (2), 171–80.

Helmstaedter, C. and Elger, C.E. (1999). The phantom of progressive dementia in epilepsy. *Lancet* **354** (9196), 2133–4.

Helmstaedter, C. and Lendt, M. (2001). Neuropsychological outcome of temporal end extratemporal lobe resection in children. In *Neuropsychology of childhood epilepsy* (ed. I. Jambaque, M. Lassond, and O. Dulac), pp. 215–27. Academic/Plenum Press, New York:.

Helmstaedter, C., Riedel, R., and Stefan, H. (1988). [Treatment of drug-resistant focal epilepsy using visual orientation activity]. *EEG EMG Z. Elektroenzephalogr. Elektromyogr. Verwandte Geb.* **19** (2), 92–5. [In German.]

Helmstaedter, C., Hufnagel, A., and Elger, C.E. (1992). Seizures during cognitive testing in patients with temporal lobe epilepsy: possibility of seizure induction by cognitive activation. *Epilepsia* **33** (5), 892–7.

Helmstaedter, C., Wagner, G., and Elger, C.E. (1993). Differential effects of first antiepileptic drug application on cognition in lesional and non-lesional patients with epilepsy. *Seizure* **2** (2), 125–30.

Helmstaedter, C., Kurthen, M., Linke, D.B., and Elger, C.E. (1994*a*). Right hemisphere restitution of language and memory functions in right hemisphere language-dominant patients with left temporal lobe epilepsy. *Brain* **117** (4), 729–37.

Helmstaedter, C., Elger, C.E., and Lendt, M. (1994*b*). Postictal courses of cognitive deficits in focal epilepsies. *Epilepsia* **35** (5),1073–8.

Helmstaedter, C., Pohl, C., and Elger, C.E. (1995). Relations between verbal and nonverbal memory performance: evidence of confounding effects particularly in patients with right temporal lobe epilepsy. *Cortex* **31** (2), 345–55.

Helmstaedter, C., Gleissner, U., Di Perna, M., and Elger, C.E. (1997*a*). Relational verbal memory processing in patients with temporal lobe epilepsy. *Cortex* **33** (4), 667–78.

Helmstaedter, C., Grunwald, T., Lehnertz, K., Gleissner, U., and Elger, C.E. (1997*b*). Differential involvement of left temporolateral and temporomesial structures in verbal declarative learning and memory: evidence from temporal lobe epilepsy. *Brain Cogn.* **35** (1), 110–31.

Helmstaedter, C., Kurthen, M., Gleissner, U., Linke, D.B., and Elger, C.E. (1997*c*). Natural atypical language dominance and language shifts from the right to the left hemisphere in right hemisphere pathology. *Naturwissenschaften* **84**, 250–2.

Helmstaedter, C., Kurthen, M., Linke, D.B., and Elger, C.E. (1997*d*). Patterns of language dominance in focal left and right hemisphere epilepsies: relation to MRI findings, EEG, sex, and age at onset of epilepsy. *Brain Cogn.* **33** (2), 135–50.

Helmstaedter, C., Gleissner, U., Zentner, J., and Elger, C.E. (1998). Neuropsychological consequences of epilepsy surgery in frontal lobe epilepsy. *Neuropsychologia* **36** (7), 681–9.

Helmstaedter, C., Kurthen, M., and Elger, C.E. (1999). Sex differences in material-specific cognitive functions related to language dominance: an intracarotid amobarbital study in left temporal lobe epilepsy. *Laterality* **4** (1), 51–63.

Helmstaedter, C., Hoppe, C., and Elger, C.E. (2001). Memory alterations during high-intensity vagus nerve stimulation. *Epilepsy Res.* **47**, 37–42.

Helmstaedter, C., Reuber, M., and Elger, C.E. (2002). Interaction of cognitive aging and memory deficits related to epilepsy surgery. *Ann. Neurol.* **52** (1), 89–94.

Helmstaedter, C., Kurthen, M., Lux, S., Reuber, M., and Elger, C.E. (2003). Chronic epilepsy and cognition: a longitudinal study in temporal lobe epilepsy. *Ann. Neurol.* **54**, 425–32.

Helmstaedter, C., van Roost, D., Clusmann, H., *et al.* (2004*a*). Collateral brain damage, a potential source of cognitive impairment after selective surgery for control of mesial temporal lobe epilepsy. *J. Neurol. Neurosurg. Psychiatry* **75**, 323–6.

Helmstaedter, C., Brosch, T., Kurthen, M., and Elger, C.E. (2004*b*). The impact of sex and language dominance on material-specific memory before and after left temporal lobe surgery. *Brain* **127** (7), 1518–25.

Helmstaedter, C., Fritz, N.E., Gonzalez Perez, P.A., Elger, C.E., and Weber, B. (2006). Shift-back of right into left hemisphere language dominance after control of epileptic seizures: evidence for epilepsy driven functional cerebral organization. *Epilepsy Res.* **70** (2–3), 257–62.

Hermann, B.P., Seidenberg, M., Haltiner, A., and Wyler, A.R. (1995). The relationship of age at onset, chronological age, and adequacy of preoperative performance to verbal memory change following anterior temporal lobectomy. *Epilepsia* **36**, 137–45.

Hermann, B.P., Seidenberg, M., Schoenfeld, J., and Davies, K. (1997). Neuropsychological characteristics of the syndrome of mesial temporal lobe epilepsy. *Arch. Neurol.* **54** (4), 369–76.

Hermann, B.P., Seidenberg, M., and Bell, B. (2002). The neurodevelopmental impact of childhood onset temporal lobe epilepsy on brain structure and function and the risk of progressive cognitive effects. *Prog. Brain Res.* **135**, 429–38.

Hertz-Pannier, L., Chiron, C., Jambaque, I., *et al.* (2002). Late plasticity for language in a child's non-dominant hemisphere: a pre- and post-surgery fMRI study. *Brain* **125**, 361–72.

Hirano, T., Fujioka, K., Okada, M., Iwasa, H., and Kaneko, S. (2004). Physical and psychomotor development in the offspring born to mothers with epilepsy. *Epilepsia* **45** (Suppl. 8), 53–7.

Hommet, C., Sauerwein, H.C., De Toffol, B., and Lassonde, M. (2006). Idiopathic epileptic syndromes and cognition. *Neurosci. Biobehav. Rev.* **30** (1), 85–96.

Hoppe, C., Helmstaedter, C., Scherrmann, J., and Elger, C.E. (2001). No evidence for cognitive side effects after 6 months of vagus nerve stimulation in epilepsy patients. *Epilepsy Behav.* **2** (4), 351–6.

Janszky, J., Jokeit, H., Heinemann, D., Schulz, R., Woermann, F.G., and Ebner, A. (2003). Epileptic activity influences the speech organization in medial temporal lobe epilepsy. *Brain* **126** (9), 2043–51.

Janz, D. (1985). Epilepsy with impulsive petit mal (juvenile myoclonic epilepsy). *Acta Neurol. Scand.* **72** (5), 449–59.

Janz, D. (2002). The psychiatry of idiopathic generalized epilepsy. In *The neuropsychiatry of epilepsy* (ed. M. Trimble and B. Schmitz), pp. 41–61. Cambridge University Press, Cambridge.

Jirsch, J.D., Bernasconi, N., Villani, F., Vitali, P., Avanzini, G., and Bernasconi, A. (2006). Sensorimotor organization in double cortex syndrome. *Hum. Brain Mapp.* **26** (6), 535–43.

Jokeit, H. and Ebner, A. (2002). Effects of chronic epilepsy on intellectual functions. *Prog. Brain Res.* **135**, 455–63.

Jokeit, H., Ebner, A., Holthausen, H., Markowitsch, H.J., and Tuxhorn, I. (1996). Reorganization of memory functions after human temporal lobe damage. *Neuroreport* **7**, 1627–30.

Jokeit, H., Seitz, R.J., Markowitsch, H.J., *et al.* (1997). Prefrontal asymmetric interictal glucose hypometabolism and cognitive impairment in patients with temporal lobe epilepsy. *Brain* **120**, 2283–94.

Jokeit, H., Heger, R., Ebner, A., and Markowitsch, H.J. (1998). Hemispheric asymmetries in category-specific word retrieval. *Neuroreport* **9** (10), 2371–3.

Jokeit, H., Okujava, M., and Woermann, F.G. (2001). Carbamazepine reduces memory induced activation of mesial temporal lobe structures: a pharmacological fMRI-study. *BMC Neurol.* **1**, 6.

Jones-Gotman, M., Smith, M.L., and Zatorre, R.J. (1987). Neuropsychological testing for localizing and lateralizing the epileptogenic region. In *Surgical treatment of the epilepsies* (ed. J. Engel Jr.), pp. 245–62. Raven Press, New York.

Jones-Gotman, M., Francis, L., Iordanova-Maximov, M., and Sziklas, V. (2005). Haptic search: sensitive to subtle parietal-lobe lesions in epilepsy. *Epilepsia* **46** (Suppl. 6), 151.

Kaga, M. (1999). Language disorders in Landau–Kleffner syndrome. *J. Child Neurol.* **14** (2), 118–22.

Kanner, A.M. (2004). Deep brain stimulation for intractable epilepsy: which target and for which seizures? *Epilepsy Curr.* **4** (6), 231–2.

Kapur, N. (1993). Transient epileptic amnesia—a clinical update and a reformulation. *J. Neurol. Neurosurg. Psychiatry* **56** (11), 1184–90.

Kasowski, H.J., Stoffman, M.R., Spencer, S.S., and Spencer, D.D. (2003). Surgical management of parietal lobe epilepsy. *Adv. Neurol.* **93**, 347–56.

Kellinghaus, C. and Luders, H.O. (2004). Frontal lobe epilepsy. *Epileptic Disord.* **6** (4), 223–39.

Ketter, T.A., Post, R.M., and Theodore, W.H. (1999). Positive and negative psychiatric effects of antiepileptic drugs in patients with seizure disorders. *Neurology* **53** (5 Suppl. 2), S53–67.

Kirschstein, T., Fernandez, G., Grunwald, T., Pezer, N., Urbach, H., Blumcke, I., Van Roost, D., Lehnertz, K., and Elger, C.E. (2003). Heterotopias, cortical dysplasias and glioneural tumors participate in cognitive processing in patients with temporal lobe epilepsy. *Neurosci. Lett.* **338** (3), 237–41.

Kockelmann, E., Elger, C.E., and Helmstaedter, C. (2003). Significant improvement in frontal lobe associated neuropsychological functions after withdrawal of topiramate in epilepsy patients. *Epilepsy Res.* **54** (2–3), 171–8.

Koepp, M.J. (2005). Juvenile myoclonic epilepsy—a generalized epilepsy syndrome? *Acta Neurol. Scand. Suppl.* **181**, 57–62.

Koepp, M.J. and Woermann, F.G. (2005). Imaging structure and function in refractory focal epilepsy. *Lancet Neurol.* **4** (1), 42–53.

Korkman, M., Granstrom, M.L., Appelqvist, K., and Liukkonen, E. (1998). Neuropsychological characteristics of five children with the Landau–Kleffner syndrome: dissociation of auditory and phonological discrimination. *J. Int. Neuropsychol. Soc.* **4** (6), 566–75.

Kral, T., Clusmann, H., Urbach, J., Schramm, J., Elger, C.E., Kurthen, M., and Grunwald, T. (2002). Preoperative evaluation for epilepsy surgery (Bonn algorithm). *Zentralbl. Neurochir.* **63** (3), 106–10.

Kurthen, M., Helmstaedter, C., Linke, D.B., Solymosi, L., Elger, C.E., and Schramm, J. (1992). Interhemispheric dissociation of expressive and receptive language functions in patients with complex-partial seizures: an amobarbital study. *Brain Lang.* **43**, 694–712.

Kwan, P. and Brodie, M.J. (2001). Neuropsychological effects of epilepsy and antiepileptic drugs. *Lancet* **357** (9251), 216–22.

Kwan, P. and Brodie, M.J. (2004). Drug treatment of epilepsy: when does it fail and how to optimize its use? *CNS Spectr.* **9** (2), 110–19.

Lee, G.P., Westerveld, M., Blackburn, L.B., Park, Y.D., and Loring, D.W. (2005). Prediction of verbal memory decline after epilepsy surgery in children: effectiveness of Wada memory asymmetries. *Epilepsia* **46** (1):97–103.

Lehnertz, K. and Litt, B. (2005). The First International Collaborative Workshop on Seizure Prediction: summary and data description. *Clin. Neurophysiol.* **116** (3), 493–505.

Lehnertz, K., Weber, B., Helmstaedter, C., Wieser, H.G., and Elger C.E. (1997). Alterations in neuronal complexity during verbal memory task index recruitment potency in temporo-mesial structures *Epilepsia Suppl.* **3**, 238.

Lendt, M., Helmstaedter, C., and Elger, C.E. (1999). Pre- and postoperative neuropsychological profiles in children and adolescents with temporal lobe epilepsy. *Epilepsia* **40** (11), 1543–50.

Lendt, M., Helmstaedter, C., Kuczaty, S., Schramm, J., and Elger, C.E. (2000). Behavioural disorders in children with epilepsy: early improvement after surgery. *J. Neurol. Neurosurg. Psychiatry* **69** (6), 739–44.

Lendt, M., Gleissner, U., Helmstaedter, C., Sassen, R., Clusmann, H., and Elger, C.E. (2002). Neuropsychological outcome in children after frontal lobe epilepsy surgery. *Epilepsy Behav.* **3** (1), 51–9.

Liasis, A., Bamiou, D.E., Boyd, S., and Towell, A. (2005). Evidence for a neurophysiologic auditory deficit in children with benign epilepsy with centro-temporal spikes. *J. Neural Transm.* **42** (10), 378–89.

Liegeois, F., Connelly, A., Cross, J.H., *et al.* (2004). Language reorganization in children with early-onset lesions of the left hemisphere: an fMRI study. *Brain* **127** (6), 1229–36.

Lindgren, S., Kihlgren, M., Melin, L., Croona, C., Lundberg, S., and Eeg-Olofsson, O. (2004). Development of cognitive functions in children with rolandic epilepsy. *Epilepsy Behav.* **5** (6), 903–10.

Liu, R.S., Lemieux, L., Bell, G.S., Sisodiya, S.M., Bartlett, P.A., Shorvon, S.D., Sander, J.W., and Duncan, J.S. (2005). Cerebral damage in epilepsy: a population-based longitudinal quantitative MRI study. *Epilepsia* **46** (9), 1482–94.

Lockard, J.S. and Wyler, A.R. (1979). The influence of attending on seizure activity in epileptic monkeys. *Epilepsia* **20** (2), 157–68.

Loddenkemper, T., Wyllie, E., Lardizabal, D., *et al.* (2003). Late language transfer in patients with Rasmussen encephalitis. *Epilepsia* **44**, 870–1.

Loring, D.W. and Meador, K.J. (2004). Cognitive side effects of antiepileptic drugs in children. *Neurology* **62**, 872–7.

Lubar, J.F. (1998). Electroencephalographic biofeedback methodology and the management of epilepsy. *Integr. Physiol. Behav. Sci.* 33 (2),176–207.

Luders, H., Acharya, J., Baumgartner, C., Benbadis, S., Bleasel, A., Burgess, R., Dinner, D.S., Ebner, A., Foldvary, N., Geller, E., Hamer, H., Holthausen, H., Kotagal, P., Morris, H., Meencke, H.J., Noachtar, S., Rosenow, F., Sakamoto, A., Steinhoff, B.J., Tuxhorn, I., and Wyllie, E. (1999). A new epileptic seizure classification based exclusively on ictal semiology. *Acta Neurol. Scand.* **99** (3), 137–41.

Lux, S., Kurthen, M., Helmstaedter, C., Hartje, W., Reuber, M., and Elger, C.E. (2002). The localizing value of ictal consciousness and its constituent functions: a video-EEG study in patients with focal epilepsy. *Brain* **125** (12), 2691–8.

Mariotti, P., Iuvone, L., Torrioli, M.G., and Silveri, M.C. (1998). Linguistic and non-linguistic abilities in a patient with early left hemispherectomy. *Neuropsychologia* **36**, 1303–12.

Martin, C.O., Denburg, N.L., Tranel, D., Granner, M.A., and Bechara, A. (2004). The effects of vagus nerve stimulation on decision-making. *Cortex* **40** (4–5), 605–12.

Martin, R., Kuzniecky, R., Ho, S., Hetherington, H., Pan, J., Sinclair, K., Gilliam, F., and Faught, E. (1999). Cognitive effects of topiramate, gabapentin, and lamotrigine in healthy young adults. *Neurology* **52** (2), 321–7.

Matsuoka, H., Takahashi, T., Sasaki, M., Matsumoto, K., Yoshida, S., Numachi, Y., Saito, H., Ueno, T., and Sato, M. (2000). Neuropsychological EEG activation in patients with epilepsy. *Brain* **123** (2), 318–30.

May, T.W. and Pfafflin, M. (2002). The efficacy of an educational treatment program for patients with epilepsy (MOSES): results of a controlled, randomized study. Modular Service Package Epilepsy. *Epilepsia* **43** (5), 539–49.

McDonald, C.R., Norman, M.A., Tecoma, E., Alksne, J., and Iragui, V. (2004). Neuropsychological change following gamma knife surgery in patients with left temporal lobe epilepsy: a review of three cases. *Epilepsy Behav.* **5** (6), 949–57.

Meencke, H.J. and Janz, D. (1985). The significance of microdysgenesia in primary generalized epilepsy: an answer to the considerations of Lyon and Gastaut. *Epilepsia* **26** (4), 368–71.

Meletti, S., Benuzzi, F., Rubboli, G., *et al.* (2003). Impaired facial emotion recognition in early-onset right mesial temporal lobe epilepsy. *Neurology* **60**, 426–31.

Mirsky, A., Duncan, C., and Levav, M. (2001). Neuropsychological studies in idiopathic generalized epilepsies. In *Neuropsychology of childhood epilepsy* (ed. I. Jambaque, M. Lassonde, and O. Dulac), pp. 141–9. Plenum Press, New York.

Monjauze, C., Tuller, L., Hommet, C., Barthez, M.A., and Khomsi, A. (2005). Language in benign childhood epilepsy with centro-temporal spikes abbreviated form: rolandic epilepsy and language. *Brain Lang.* **92** (3), 300–8.

Moore, S.J., Turnpenny, P., Quinn, A., Glover, S., Lloyd, D.J., Montgomery, T., and Dean, J.C. (2000). A clinical study of 57 children with fetal anticonvulsant syndromes. *J. Med. Genet.* **37** (7),489–97.

Morrow, J.I., Russell, A., Gutherie, E., Parsons, L., Robertson, I., Waddell, R., Irwin, B., Morrison, P., McGivern, C.R., and Craig, J. (2006). Malformation risks of anti-epileptic drugs in pregnancy: A prospective study from the UK Epilepsy and Pregnancy Register. *J. Neurol. Neurosurg. Psychiatry* **77**, 193–8.

Nagai, Y., Goldstein, L.H., Fenwick, P.B., and Trimble, M.R. (2004). Clinical efficacy of galvanic skin response biofeedback training in reducing seizures in adult epilepsy: a preliminary randomized controlled study. *Epilepsy Behav.* **5** (2), 216–23.

Nolan, N.A., Redoblado, M.A., Lah, S., *et al.* (2004). Memory function in childhood epilepsy syndromes. *J. Paediatr. Child Health* **40**, 20–7.

Ogden, J.A. (1988). Language and memory functions after long recovery periods in left-hemispherectomized subjects. *Neuropsychologia* **26**, 645–59.

Ogden, J.A. (1989). Visuospatial and other 'right-hemispheric' functions after long recovery periods in left-hemispherectomized subjects. *Neuropsychologia* **27**, 765–76.

Ojemann, G.A. (1982). Models of the brain organization for higher integrative functions derived with electrical stimulation techniques. *Hum. Neurobiol.* **1** (4), 243–9.

Ojemann, G.A. (2003). The neurobiology of language and verbal memory: observations from awake neurosurgery. *Int. J. Psychophysiol.* **48** (2), 141–6.

Ojemann, G.A., Creutzfeldt, O., Lettich, E., and Haglund, M.M. (1988). Neuronal activity in human lateral temporal cortex related to short-term verbal memory, naming and reading. *Brain* **111** (6), 1383–403.

Ojemann, G., Ojemann, J., Lettich, E., and Berger, M. (1989). Cortical language localization in left, dominant hemisphere. An electrical stimulation mapping investigation in 117 patients. *J. Neurosurg.* **71** (3), 316–26.

Ojemann, S.G., Berger, M.S., Lettich, E., and Ojemann, G.A. (2003). Localization of language function in children: results of electrical stimulation mapping. *J. Neurosurg.* **98** (3), 465–70.

Ortinski, P. and Meador, K.J. (2004). Cognitive side-effects of antiepileptic drugs. *Epilepsy Behav.* **5**, S60–5.

Pavone, P., Bianchini, R., Trifiletti, R.R., Incorpora, G., Pavone, A., and Parano, E. (2001). Neuropsychological assessment in children with absence epilepsy. *Neurology* **56** (8), 1047–51.

Penfield, W. and Jasper, H. (1954). *Epilepsy and the functional anatomy of the brain.* Little Brown and Co, Boston.

Rausch, R., Kraemer, S., Pietras, C.J., *et al.* (2003). Early and late cognitive changes following temporal lobe surgery for epilepsy. *Neurology* **60**, 951–9.

Regis, J., Hayashi, M., Eupierre, LP., Villeneuve, N., Bartolomei, F., Brue, T., and Chauvel, P. (2004*a*). Gamma knife surgery for epilepsy related to hypothalamic hamartomas. *Acta Neurochir. Suppl.* **91**, 33–50.

Regis, J., Rey, M., Bartolomei, F., Vladyka, V., Liscak, R., Schrottner, O., and Pendl, G. (2004*b*). Gamma knife surgery in mesial temporal lobe epilepsy: a prospective multicenter study. *Epilepsia* **45** (5), 504–15.

Reuber, M., Andersen, B., Elger, C.E., and Helmstaedter, C. (2004). Depression and anxiety before and after temporal lobe epilepsy surgery. *Seizure* **13** (2), 129–35.

Richardson, M.P., Koepp, M.J., Brooks, D.J., Coull, J.T., Grasby, P., Fish, D.R., and Duncan, J.S. (1998). Cerebral activation in malformations of cortical development. *Brain* **121** (7), 1295–304.

Risse, G.L. (2006). Cognitive outcomes in patients with frontal lobe epilepsy. *Epilepsia* **47**, 87–9.

Roberts, G.M., Majoie, H.J., Leenen, L.A., Bootsma, H.P., Kessels, A.G., Aldenkamp, A.P., and Leonard, B.E. (2005). Ketter's hypothesis of the mood effects of antiepileptic drugs coupled to the mechanism of action of topiramate and levetiracetam. *Epilepsy Behav.* **6** (3), 366–72.

Rockstroh, B., Birbaumer, N., Elbert, T., and Lutzenberger, W. (1984). Operant control of EEG and event-related and slow brain potentials. *Biofeedback Self Regul.* **9** (2),139–60.

Rosen, M.I., Rigsby, M.O., Salahi, J.T., Ryan, C.E., and Cramer, J.A. (2004). Electronic monitoring and counseling to improve medication adherence. *Behav. Res. Ther.* **42** (4), 409–22.

Rosenow, F. and Lüders, H. (Eds.) (2004). *Presurgical assessment of the epilepsies with clinical neurophysiology and functional imaging. Handbook of clinical neurophysiology.* Elsevier, Amsterdam.

Roulet Perez, E., Davidoff, V., Despland, P.A., and Deonna, T. (1993). Mental and behavioural deterioration of children with epilepsy and CSWS: acquired epileptic frontal syndrome. *Dev. Med. Child Neurol.* **35** (8), 661–74.

Salanova, V., Andermann, F., Rasmussen, T., Olivier, A., and Quesney, L.F. (1995). Parietal lobe epilepsy. Clinical manifestations and outcome in 82 patients treated surgically between 1929 and 1988. *Brain* **118** (3), 607–27.

Salek-Haddadi, A., Lemieux, L., Merschhemke, M., Friston, K.J., Duncan, J.S., and Fish, D.R. (2003). Functional magnetic resonance imaging of human absence seizures. *Ann. Neurol.* **53** (5), 663–7.

Saltzman-Benaiah, J., Scott, K., and Smith, M.L. (2003). Factors associated with atypical speech representation in children with intractable epilepsy. *Neuropsychologia* **41**, 1967–74.

Sass, K.J., Westerveld, M., Buchanan, C.P., Spencer, S.S., Kim, J.H., and Spencer, D.D. (1994). Degree of hippocampal neuron loss determines severity of verbal memory decrease after left anteromesiotemporal lobectomy. *Epilepsia* **35** (6), 1179–86.

Schachter, S.C. and Schmidt, D. (2001). *Vagus nerve stimulation.* Martin Dunitz Verlag, London.

Scholtes, F.B., Hendriks, M.P., and Renier, W.O. (2005). Cognitive deterioration and electrical status epilepticus during slow sleep. *Epilepsy Behav.* **6** (2), 167–73.

Schwartz, T.H. (2005). The terminal man—from science fiction to therapy. *Epilepsy Curr.* **5**, 207–9.

Scoville, W.B. and Milner, B. (2000). Loss of recent memory after bilateral hippocampal lesions. 1957. *J. Neuropsychiatry Clin. Neurosci.***12** (1), 103–13.

Seidenberg, M., Geary, E., and Hermann, B. (2005). Investigating temporal lobe contribution to confrontation naming using MRI quantitative volumetrics. *J. Int. Neuropsychol. Soc.* **11** (4), 358–66.

Semah, F., Picot, M.C., Adam, C., Broglin, D., Arzimanoglou, A., Bazin, B., Cavalcanti, D., and Baulac, M. (1998). Is the underlying cause of epilepsy a major prognostic factor for recurrence? *Neurology* **51** (5), 1256–62.

Shulman, M.B. (2000). The frontal lobes, epilepsy, and behavior. *Epilepsy Behav.* **1** (6), 384–95.

Snead, K., Ackerson, J., Bailey, K., Schmitt, M.M., Madan-Swain, A., and Martin, R.C. (2004). Taking charge of epilepsy: the development of a structured psychoeducational group intervention for adolescents with epilepsy and their parents. *Epilepsy Behav.* **5** (4), 547–56.

Sonmez, F., Atakli, D., Sari, H., Atay, T., and Arpaci, B. (2004). Cognitive function in juvenile myoclonic epilepsy. *Epilepsy Behav.* **5** (3), 329–36.

Spanaki, M.V., Kopylev, L., DeCarli, C., *et al.* (2000). Postoperative changes in cerebral metabolism in temporal lobe epilepsy. *Arch. Neurol.* **57**, 1447–52.

Speckmann, E.J. (1986). *Experimentelle Epilepsieforschung.* Wissenschaftliche Buchgesellschaft, Darmstadt.

Sterman, M.B. (2000). Basic concepts and clinical findings in the treatment of seizure disorders with EEG operant conditioning. *Clin. Electroencephalogr.* **31** (1), 45–55.

Sutula, T. and Pitkänen, A. (ed.) (2002). *Do seizures damage the brain*? Progress in Brain Research, Vol. 135. Elsevier Science, Amsterdam.

Swartz, BE., Simpkins, F., Halgren, E., Mandelkern, M., Brown, C., Krisdakumtorn, T., and Gee, M. (1996). Visual working memory in primary generalized epilepsy: an 18FDG-PET study. *Neurology* **47** (5), 1203–12.

Trenerry, M.R. (1996). Neuropsychologic assessment in surgical treatment of epilepsy. *Mayo Clin. Proc.* **71** (12), 1196–20.

Trenerry, M.R. and Loring, D.W. (1995). Intracarotid amobarbital procedure. The Wada test. *Neuroimaging Clin. N. Am.* **5** (4), 721–8.

Upton, D. and Thompson, P.J. (1997). Neuropsychological test performance in frontal-lobe epilepsy: the influence of aetiology, seizure type, seizure frequency and duration of disorder. *Seizure* **6** (6), 443–7.

Vargha-Khadem, F., Carr, LJ., Isaacs, E., *et al.* (1997). Onset of speech after left hemispherectomy in a nine-year-old boy. *Brain* **120**, 159–82.

Velasco, F., Velasco, M., Velasco, A.L., Jimenez, F., Marquez, I., and Rise, M. (1995). Electrical stimulation of the centromedian thalamic nucleus in control of seizures: long-term studies. *Epilepsia* **36** (1), 63–71.

Vinayan, K.P., Biji, V., and Thomas, S.V. (2005). Educational problems with underlying neuropsychological impairment are common in children with benign epilepsy of childhood with centrotemporal spikes (BECTS). *Seizure* **14** (3), 207–12.

Vonck, K., Boon, P., Claeys, P., Dedeurwaerdere, S., Achten, R., and Van Roost, D. (2005). Long-term deep brain stimulation for refractory temporal lobe epilepsy. *Epilepsia* **46** (Suppl. 5), 98–9.

Wada, J. and Rasmussen, T. (1960). Intracarotid injection of sodium amytal for the lateralization of cerebral speech dominance: experimental and clinical observations. *J. Neurosurg.* **17**, 266–82.

Walker, M., Cross, H., Smith, S., Young, C., Aicardi, J., Appleton, R., Aylett, S., Besag, F., Cock, H., Delorenzo, R., Drislane, F., Duncan, J., Ferrie, C., Fujikawa, D., Gray, W., Kaplan, P., Koutroumanidis, M., O'Regan, M., Plouin, P., Sander, J., Scott, R., Shorvon, S., Treiman, D., Wasterlain, C., and Wieshmann, U. (2005). Nonconvulsive status epilepticus: Epilepsy Research Foundation Workshop Reports. *Epileptic Disord.* **7** (3), 253–96.

Wiebe, S., Blume, W.T., Girvin, J.P., and Eliasziw, M. (2001). Effectiveness and efficiency of surgery for temporal lobe epilepsy study group. A randomized, controlled trial of surgery for temporal-lobe epilepsy. *N. Engl. J. Med.* **345** (5), 311–18.

Wieser, H.G. (1986). Selective amygdalohippocampectomy: indications, investigative technique and results. In *Advances and technical standards in neurosurgery*, Vol 13 (ed. L. Symon *et al.*), pp. 39–133. Springer-Verlag, Vienna.

Wieser, H.G.; ILAE Commission on Neurosurgery of Epilepsy (2004). ILAE Commission Report. Mesial temporal lobe epilepsy with hippocampal sclerosis. *Epilepsia* **45** (6), 695–714.

Woermann, F.G., Free, S.L., Koepp, M.J., Sisodiya, S.M., and Duncan, J.S. (1999). Abnormal cerebral structure in juvenile myoclonic epilepsy demonstrated with voxel-based analysis of MRI. *Brain* **122** (11), 2101–8.

Wolff, M., Weiskopf, N., Serra, E., Preissl, H., Birbaumer, N., and Kraegeloh-Mann, I. (2005). Benign partial epilepsy in childhood: selective cognitive deficits are related to the location of focal spikes determined by combined EEG/MEG. *Epilepsia* **46** (10), 1661–7.

Wood, A.G., Saling, M.M., O'Shea, M.F., Jackson, G.D., and Berkovic, S.F. (1999). Reorganization of verbal memory and language: a case of dissociation. *J. Int. Neuropsychol. Soc.* **5**, 69–74.

Zaidel, D.W., Esiri, M.M., and Beardsworth, E.D. (1998). Observations on the relationship between verbal explicit and implicit memory and density of neurons in the hippocampus. *Neuropsychologia* **36** (10), 1049–62.

Zentner, J., Wolf, H.K., Helmstaedter, C., Grunwald, T., Aliashkevich, A.F., Wiestler, O.D., Elger, C.E., and Schramm, J. (1999). Clinical relevance of amygdala sclerosis in temporal lobe epilepsy. *J. Neurosurg.* **91** (1), 59–67.

Chapter 19

Cognition in schizophrenia

Jennifer H. Barnett and Paul C. Fletcher

19.1 Introduction

In this chapter, we review the nature of cognitive deficits in schizophrenia and related psychoses. We consider the patterns of cognitive deficits that characterize the illness and review evidence that such deficits may be observed even before the onset of symptoms. We trace the course of cognitive deficits across phases of the illness and consider the extent to which cognition, over and above symptoms, may account for some of the profound disability and suffering that characterizes schizophrenia. The relevance of findings from cognitive studies is also considered with respect to neurodevelopmental models of schizophrenia and to the potential importance of early treatment. In closing, we examine the importance of careful assessments of specific cognitive deficits in shaping the patterns of symptoms that an individual with schizophrenia may experience, considering in particular the extent to which specific types of delusions may be explicable in terms of models of normal and disrupted cognition.

19.2 Historical perspective

The current chapter is influenced by a growing interest in the nature of cognition in schizophrenia and related psychoses. In this respect, it follows a current trend that emphasizes the importance of research into the nature and implications of cognitive deficits in schizophrenia (Marder *et al.* 2004). However, it must be acknowledged that the study of schizophrenia has followed many trends and the current chapter should first be set against a historical perspective. There is little scope here to review the historical development of current ideas about schizophrenia and we strongly recommend the brief overview provided by Berrios (2000) who points out that we must remind ourselves that the concept of schizophrenia has evolved and is, perhaps, continuing to evolve. Schizophrenia does not appear, at any, point, to have been 'discovered'. Rather it has been nudged in various directions, losing and gaining theoretical constructions and, at any given instant, being shaped by the language of its time. While it is impossible to do his arguments justice here, two of Berrios's points are worth highlighting in advance of defining the illness and reviewing its cognitive characteristics. First, the evolution of our concepts of schizophrenia has not followed a linear or logical progression. It would be wrong to assume that each successive conceptualization is a step beyond the preceding one since it very often involves neither an extension nor a refutation. Second, in recognizing this, we must put aside the idea that previous observations and formulations have necessarily been about the same thing.

19.3 **What is schizophrenia?**

- Schizophrenia has a lifetime prevalence of about 1%, though rates differ according to diagnostic criteria.
- Genetic and environmental factors, and their interactions, are implicated in the aetiology of schizophrenia.
- Men have higher rates of schizophrenia than women.
- Men have a younger mean age of onset than women and a worse prognosis.

Schizophrenia is a condition defined primarily by the existence of key symptoms: delusions (abnormal beliefs, held with conviction and difficult to equate with an individual's cultural background); hallucinations (percepts in the absence of stimuli); and disordered thinking, together with an array of negative symptoms. So, despite the caveats raised above, a diagnosis of schizophrenia has a fairly specific meaning to a clinician. Current DSM-IV (American Psychiatric Association 1994) diagnostic criteria for schizophrenia are given in Table 19.1. Despite these guidelines, at first presentation it is often unclear whether schizophrenia is the appropriate diagnosis, partly because of the importance of duration in diagnosis and partly because phenomenology can evolve or resolve. In addition to schizophrenia-spectrum disorders such as delusional disorder and schizoaffective disorder, psychosis can be produced by organic causes or drug use, or may arise during affective disorders such as major depressive disorder or bipolar disorder. Diagnostic criteria for psychotic disorders other than schizophrenia are given in Table 19.2. Despite some qualms about the extent to which the diagnostic structure truly represents the nature of the disease, we should reassure ourselves that the positive predictive value of a diagnosis of schizophrenia over a 10 year period from onset is above 90% (Bromet *et al.* 2005).

Table 19.1 DSM-IV diagnostic criteria for schizophrenia (American Psychiatric Association 1994)

Characteristic symptoms

- Two or more of the following: delusions, hallucinations; disorganized speech; grossly disorganized or catatonic behaviour; negative symptoms
- Only one symptom required if delusions are bizarre or hallucinations consist of a voice keeping up a running commentary on the person's behaviour or thoughts, or two or more voices conversing with one another

Social/occupational dysfunction

- One or more major areas of functioning such as work, interpersonal relations, or self-care are markedly below the level achieved prior to the onset; *or*
- Where onset is in childhood or adolescence, failure to achieve expected level of interpersonal, academic, or occupational achievement

Duration

Continuous signs of the disturbance persist for at least 6 months, including at least 1 month of active-phase symptoms (or less if successfully treated). This may include periods of prodromal or residual symptoms when the signs of the disturbance may be manifested by only negative symptoms or two or more symptoms present in an attenuated form

Table 19.1 (continued) DSM-IV diagnostic criteria for schizophrenia (American Psychiatric Association 1994)

Schizoaffective and mood disorder exclusion

Schizoaffective disorder and mood disorder with psychotic features have been ruled out because:

- either no major depressive, manic, or mixed episodes have occurred concurrently with the active-phase symptoms; *or*
- if mood episodes have occurred during the active-phase symptoms, their total duration has been brief relative to the duration of the active and residual periods

Substance/general medical exclusion

The disturbance is not due to the direct physiological effects of a substance or a general medical condition

Relationship to a pervasive developmental disorder

If there is a history of autistic disorder or another pervasive developmental disorder, the additional diagnosis of schizophrenia is made only if prominent delusions or hallucinations are also present for at least a month (or less if successfully treated)

Classification of longitudinal course

Can be applied only after at least 1 year has elapsed since the initial onset of active-phase symptoms

- Episodic with interepisode residual symptoms
- Episodic with no interepisode residual symptoms
- Continuous
- Single episode in partial remission
- Single episode in full remission
- Other or unspecified pattern

Schizophrenia subtypes

- Paranoid type
- Disorganized type
- Catatonic type
- Undifferentiated type
- Residual type

Table 19.2 DSM-IV diagnostic criteria for other psychotic disorders (American Psychiatric Association 1994). Exclusion criteria not described

Schizophreniform disorder

- Symptom and exclusion criteria for schizophrenia are met
- An episode of the disorder, including prodromal, active, and residual phases, lasts at least 1 month but less than 6 months

Schizoaffective disorder

- An uninterrupted period of illness during which, at some time, there is a major depressive episode, a manic episode, or a mixed episode concurrent with symptoms that meet criteria for schizophrenia
- During the same period of illness, there must have been delusions or hallucinations for at least 2 weeks in the absence of prominent mood symptoms. Symptoms that meet criteria for a mood episode are present for a substantial portion of the total duration of the active and residual periods of the illness
- Subtypes: bipolar type; depressive type

Table 19.2 (continued) DSM-IV diagnostic criteria for other psychotic disorders (American Psychiatric Association 1994). Exclusion criteria not described

Delusional disorder

- Non-bizarre delusions of at least 1 month's duration
- Symptom criteria for schizophrenia have never been met
- Apart from the impact of the delusions, functioning is not obviously impaired and behaviour is not odd or bizarre
- If mood episodes have occurred concurrently with delusions, their total duration has been brief relative to the duration of the delusional periods

Brief psychotic disorder

- Presence of one or more of: delusions; hallucinations; disorganized speech; grossly disorganized or catatonic behaviour
- Duration of episode at least 1 day but less than 1 month
- Subtypes: with marked stressors; without marked stressors; with postpartum onset.

Substance-induced psychotic disorder

- Prominent delusions or hallucinations without insight that they are substance-induced
- Evidence that the symptoms developed during or within a month of substance intoxication or withdrawal, *or* that medication use is aetiologically related to the disturbance

Psychotic disorder not otherwise specified

- Postpartum psychosis that does not meet criteria for other psychotic disorders
- Psychotic symptoms that have lasted for less than a month
- Persistent auditory hallucinations in the absence of any other features
- Persistent non-bizarre delusions with periods of overlapping mood episodes
- Situations where a psychotic disorder is present but the clinician is unable to determine whether it is primary, due to a general medical condition, or substance-induced

Mood disorders—specifiers for psychotic features

Mood-congruent psychotic features:

- delusions or hallucinations whose content is entirely consistent with the typical depressive or manic themes

Mood-incongruent psychotic features:

- delusions or hallucinations whose content does not involve typical depressive or manic themes, such as persecutory delusions, thought insertion, thought broadcasting, and delusions of control

19.3.1 Epidemiology

Schizophrenia has a lifetime prevalence of around 1% and an annual incidence of 2–4 per 10 000 (Jablensky 1997). More men than women are diagnosed with schizophrenia (McGrath 2005). The incidence is largely consistent across all nations, developed and developing (Sartorius *et al.* 1972), although the rates differ considerably depending on the exact criteria used for diagnosis (McGrath 2005). Furthermore, risk for schizophrenia is increased in many groups of immigrants, especially second-generation immigrants in the UK (Sharpley *et al.* 2001; Cooper 2005).

19.3.2 Heritability

Compared with the approximately 1% lifetime risk for schizophrenia in the general population, first-degree relatives of people with schizophrenia have a greatly increased risk—around 10% for siblings, 6% for parents, and 13% for children (Gottesman and Shields 1982). More recent studies, with stricter diagnostic criteria, find pooled risks of 4.8% for first-degree relatives, compared with 0.5% in first-degree relatives of controls (Kendler and Diehl 1993). Concordance rates in twins range from 42% to 50% in monozygotic twins and from 0 to 14% in dizygotic twins (Cardno and Murray 2003). However, environmental factors also play a substantial role with adoption studies demonstrating the importance of both genetic and environmental factors (Heston 1966; Kety *et al.* 1971; Rosenthal *et al.* 1971). At least some of the familial risk is non-genetic; gene–environment interactions have been demonstrated in children of schizophrenic parents adopted into good versus disturbed adoptive families (Wahlberg *et al.* 1997). We will consider below the impact of genes on cognitive deficits in schizophrenia.

19.3.3 Disease onset and progression

Schizophrenia typically has an onset in late adolescence or early adulthood. Men have a younger mean age of onset (Hafner *et al.* 1993) and a worse prognosis (Angermeyer *et al.* 1990). The mean age of female schizophrenia patients at first contact with psychiatric services is around 3.5–6 years older than in male patients (Riecher-Rossler and Hafner 2000). This age difference appears in almost all cultures (Jablensky *et al.* 1992), suggesting that is not primarily due to culture-specific psychosocial factors. Some researchers have suggested that women are to some extent protected from schizophrenia between puberty and the menopause by high levels of oestrogen production (Hafner *et al.* 1993). This hypothesis may explain the second peak in age of onset that occurs in women around the time of the menopause as well as findings that symptom levels in women are modulated by oestradiol blood levels (Riecher-Rossler *et al.* 1994).

19.4 Cognition in schizophrenia

19.4.1 General considerations and problems in charting cognitive impairment in schizophrenia

- Assessment of the nature and development of cognitive deficits in schizophrenia is highly complex.
- There is a wide range of severity and type of cognitive impairment seen in schizophrenia.

Assessing cognition in psychotic disorders is difficult. As well as those difficulties inherent in all neuropsychological assessment (problems with reliability and validity of chosen tests), additional considerations include the suitability of assessment batteries for patients with acute psychosis or prominent negative symptoms. Longitudinal studies such as those aiming to assess cognitive change throughout the course of the disorder are associated with additional difficulties such as the effects of practice and of normal and abnormal age-related cognitive change. It can be peculiarly difficult to establish test–retest reliability in patients because of the possibility that some patients with schizophrenia experience cognition decline (see below). Most neuropsychological instruments used in schizophrenia have been validated, and their reliability assessed, in healthy volunteers and/or patients with known and static neurological injury. Moreover, the functional neuroanatomical implications of test failure in patients with schizophrenia may be different to those in neurological patients since, if schizophrenia involves aberrant neurodevelopment, neural circuitry may well be affected.

Tests that are specifically validated for use in schizophrenia must take into account the wide range of levels of cognitive function present in schizophrenia, from patients who are apparently neuropsychologically normal to those with apparent premature dementia (Kremen *et al.* 2000). Related to this is the selection of normative data or an appropriate control group. Most neuropsychological tests show some effect of IQ so comparisons with patients with schizophrenia must be matched on IQ. However, IQ assessment takes time, and a commonly used alternative, years of education, also presents difficulties since the onset of schizophrenia around late adolescence may well disrupt education and lead to lower than expected achievement. In addition to these basic difficulties in experimental design, the practicalities of neuropsychological assessment in psychotic disorders tend to depend heavily on the level of symptoms and cooperation of the patient: it may be impossible to complete demanding neuropsychological assessments during acute psychotic phases, and prominent negative symptoms such as avolition and slowing of thought may excessively affect performance on some tests. These should be taken into account both in the design of neuropsychological studies of schizophrenia and when assessing the performance of individual patients for clinical or research purposes.

Assessing cognitive change over time, while critical, ultimately, to understanding the nature and progression of cognitive impairment in the disorder, brings specific problems. Repeated attempts at the same test are likely to improve performance, and it can be difficult to distinguish between these practice effects and genuine change in cognitive function. Practice effects may also be confounded with other variables of interest, such as IQ, age, and initial cognitive function: patients who perform very well may be less likely to benefit from practice than those who score initially poorly. Another problem in longitudinal studies of schizophrenia is dropout of participants (Kurtz 2005). As well as reducing power, it may also lead to biased results because patients who remain in longitudinal studies may differ systematically from those who do not.

One other point worth noting about studies of cognition in schizophrenia is that cross-sectional studies have often focused predominantly on established schizophrenia and have largely concentrated on patients with chronic illness (either outpatients or inpatients). More recently, attempts have been made to focus on those in their first episode of illness. Attempts to study cognition longitudinally have concentrated on following patients from first episode, or prior to that by identifying individuals at high genetic risk or showing the earliest ('prodromal') symptoms. As a consequence, while cross-sectional studies have produced more evidence with respect to the established condition and to the specific diagnosis, follow-up studies have incorporated a number of related diagnostic groupings. Data from both approaches will be reviewed here and, in a number of instances, we will report findings on people with early psychotic illness who will not necessarily have gone on to develop schizophrenia. Nevertheless, we feel it is important to consider these data despite the diagnostic uncertainty.

Finally, the following review of cognitive impairments should be set against an important observation: that the sheer range of cognitive impairments, and therefore cognitive function, seen in groups of psychotic patients means that there are many individuals who do not experience noticeable cognitive problems. Furthermore, the majority of cognitive impairment will already have occurred by the time of first onset, and most patients do not worsen significantly after this point. In fact, over the first few years, cognitive function improves in many people, at least in those whose symptoms are adequately treated with antipsychotic drugs. Finally, although cognitive impairments can significantly impact on daily functioning, effective psychological (Greenwood *et al.* 2005) and pharmacological (Turner *et al.* 2004) treatments for cognitive impairment are currently being identified.

19.4.2 General aspects of cognition in schizophrenia and related psychotic disorders

Cognitive impairments are especially notable in:

- general IQ;
- executive function;
- memory;
- attention.

Patients with schizophrenia tend to show impairments on almost all neuropsychological tests. Heinrichs and Zakzanis (1998) undertook a meta-analysis of cognitive studies in schizophrenia, comparing 22 cognitive variables from 204 studies published between 1980 and 1997. They found evidence of deficits in all 22 variables, with the largest effect sizes in global verbal memory, motor skills, performance and full-scale IQ, continuous performance tests, word fluency, and the Stroop test.

19.4.2.1 General IQ deficits

Impairment in generalized cognitive function (compared with both school peers and with siblings), as measured by IQ tests, has been consistently associated with schizophrenia (Aylward *et al.* 1984). It may be that higher IQ is protective against schizophrenia; for example, superior cognitive function may enable patients to maintain a higher level of functioning despite schizophrenic symptoms (Munro *et al.* 2002). Alternatively, higher IQ may protect against the cognitive failures that underpin cognitive theories of schizophrenia (see below), such as aberrant self-monitoring (Frith 1992), data-gathering biases (Garety and Freeman 1999), or attributional biases (Baker and Morrison 1998), and so prevent symptoms. Alternatively, lower IQ may be a risk factor for schizophrenia because it is evidence of impaired neurodevelopment or early brain insult. Lower IQ is found in children and adolescents who will later develop schizophrenia when compared with their healthy peers in population samples from birth cohorts (Jones *et al.* 1994; Cannon *et al.* 2002), and army conscripts (David *et al.* 1997; Davidson *et al.* 1999; Gunnell *et al.* 2002; Reichenberg *et al.* 2002). Whatever the aetiology of the association, verbal IQ appears to be less affected than performance IQ (Amminger *et al.* 2000) and male patients more impaired than females (Aylward *et al.* 1984). Despite some suggestions of continuing intellectual decline in schizophrenia (Eberhard *et al.* 2003), there is little reliable evidence of decline in IQ after the onset of the disorder (Aylward *et al.* 1984; Russell *et al.* 1997).

19.4.2.2 Executive function

Executive function is a frustratingly vague term, In the current setting, we use it to refer to processes generally invoked by novel or non-routine situations and necessitating the control and shifting of attention, cognitive flexibility and abstraction, and the ability to hold and manipulate information 'online'. These various facets of executive function involve the partially segregated frontal-subcortical networks that have been identified connecting areas of frontal cortex, basal ganglia, and thalamus (Alexander *et al.* 1986; DeLong *et al.* 1990).

Patients with schizophrenia show widespread deficits in tests of executive function. The Wisconsin Card Sorting Test (WCST; Berg 1948) is the most common test of abstraction and attention shifting and its impairment is associated with dorsolateral prefrontal cortex damage. Poor performance on the WCST task in schizophrenia is associated with a specific failure, in functional imaging studies, to activate the dorsolateral prefrontal cortex (Weinberger *et al.* 1986). Studies in schizophrenia have found that patients often persevere in making incorrect responses despite feedback (Stuss *et al.* 1983; Abbruzzese *et al.* 1996), although some patients also have difficulty learning and maintaining the original response set, and the difference in ratio between perseverative and non-perseverative errors in patients and controls on the WCST may be marginal (Li 2004). Coaching and incentives improve the performance of patients characterized by psychomotor poverty or reality distortion, but not patients with symptoms of disorganization (Rowe and Shean 1997), and patients often return to their previous poor performance immediately after coaching is withdrawn (Goldberg *et al.* 1987).

19.4.2.3 Memory

It has been suggested that memory impairment in schizophrenia may be so severe as to constitute an amnesic syndrome (McKenna *et al.* 1990). Although many facets of memory seem impaired in schizophrenia, there are differences in the magnitude of impairment between different types of memory. Episodic memory (the memory for particular events or episodes) is characteristically impaired. A general finding that emerges is of particular deficits when the chosen memory task requires a richer retrieval of encoded items than when simple recognition tasks are used (in which case a simple feeling of familiarity may suffice to produce a correct response) though this general rule is not without exceptions (for a review see Fletcher and Honey 2006). Heinrichs and Zakzanis's (1998) meta-analysis found deficits in both verbal memory for non-verbal memory. A second meta-analysis (Aleman *et al.* 1999) found larger effect sizes for measures of recall than recognition memory, with similar effect sizes across verbal and non-verbal domains. A further meta-analysis of recognition memory found evidence for greater impairment in visual recognition than verbal recognition (Pelletier *et al.* 2005). Another useful distinction in episodic memory is between tasks that tap basic recognition of items and those that require a judgement about the source (e.g. previous location or temporal ordering) of those items. It may be argued that the latter tasks also require a richer recollection and it is noteworthy that their performance is impaired in schizophrenia (Brebion *et al.* 2005).

Working memory, the ability to hold and manipulate information 'online', is, under many circumstances, dependent upon executive function. This is especially so when tasks require that subjects not merely hold information on-line but also manipulate that information (e.g. being required to reorder it in their mind). While there is clear evidence of working memory deficits in schizophrenia even when such manipulation processes are not, apparently, engaged (Aleman *et al.* 1999), it appears that tasks with manipulation requirements show greater impairments than tasks requiring simple maintenance of information (Perry *et al.* 2001; Kim *et al.* 2004). Indeed, such deficits have also been observed in non-psychotic relatives of people with schizophrenia (Conklin *et al.* 2005).

19.4.2.4 Attention

Attention is not a single entity but includes a range of functions, such as orienting to novel stimuli, selective filtering of information, and sustained vigilance, involving different brain systems (Posner 1988). Patients with schizophrenia perform poorly on these tasks, tending to miss targets and to respond inappropriately to non-targets (Orzack and Kornetsky 1966; Kurtz *et al.* 2001). Deficits are present both when acutely ill and in remission (Asarnow and MacCrimmon 1978), and are also present in the unaffected relatives of patients with schizophrenia (Cornblatt and Keilp 1994), leading to suggestions that visual attention deficits may be endophenotypic markers of schizophrenia (Cornblatt and Malhotra 2001); this is discussed in more detail below. It is possible that deficits are due to difficulties encoding the stimuli (Elvevag *et al.* 2000) and this is supported by findings that patients perform particularly poorly on tests using degraded stimuli (Liu *et al.* 2002).

19.4.3 Cognition in first-episode psychosis

Research efforts have recently turned to detecting and assessing cognitive function in patients during their first psychotic episode, preferably before treatment has commenced. The logic behind such studies is that cognition in these patients should be unaffected by antipsychotic treatment and any potential long-term neurotoxic effects of psychosis. In general, findings largely support those of the literature in chronic schizophrenia: patients with first-episode psychosis (FEP) are also impaired in almost all cognitive domains, including executive function, verbal and non-verbal memory, and attention (Saykin *et al.* 1994; DeLisi *et al.* 1995; Hutton *et al.* 1998; Mohamed *et al.* 1999; Bilder *et al.* 2000; Townsend *et al.* 2001; Joyce *et al.* 2002; Addington *et al.* 2003; Giovannetti *et al.* 2003). Many of these studies assess only first-episode schizophrenia patients; others include mixed groups of patients with non-affective and/or affective psychoses. Inconsistent results have shown patients in first-episode psychosis performing at the same level as or, alternatively, better than groups of chronic patients with schizophrenia (Bilder *et al.* 1992; Moritz *et al.* 2002). These conflicting results may be attributable to the possibility that some patients who experience a first episode of schizophrenia do not continue into a chronic illness and therefore 'escape' studies of chronically ill patients.

19.4.4 Cognition in prodromal or at-risk mental states (ARMS)

There is some evidence that cognitive impairments are also present during what may be a prodromal phase of schizophrenia. Such phases are complex and subtle: clinical features are summarized in Table 19.3. Such studies are generally small and often include both people who later do make the transition to psychosis and those who have not, and may never do so. Nevertheless, they may provide critical clues to the cognitive changes that herald the onset of the disease. The Basel study (Gschwandtner *et al.* 2003) found significant differences between ARMS patients and age-matched healthy controls on measures of executive function, working memory, and attention, in fine motor function, and in eye movements. Hawkins *et al.* (2004) compared ARMS patients, healthy controls, and patients with schizophrenia across a battery of tests of attention, memory, and executive function. The ARMS patients showed normal IQ and cognitive performance that was worse than that of controls but better than that of the schizophrenia patients. A small study of 11 patients, nine of whom were psychotic 1 year later, showed impaired performance on sustained attention and spatial memory tasks, but no impairments on tests of executive function or on pattern recognition (Bartok *et al.* 2005).

It is predictable that ARMS patients will perform worse than healthy controls since, to meet the criteria for an 'at-risk mental state', they must have experienced a recent decline in function. A better design is therefore to compare those patients who meet ARMS criteria who do and do not later become psychotic. These studies are currently rare because of the difficulty in collecting adequate sample sizes. Nonetheless, results from the Melbourne PACE clinic (*www.pace-clinic.org*) have shown deficits in measures of working memory (Wood *et al.* 2003) in those who have transitioned into psychosis compared with those who have not. Brewer *et al.* (2005) found significantly lower IQ in the group in general when compared with controls, and also lower (estimated premorbid) IQ scores, and visual and verbal learning tasks. Patients who later became psychotic performed more poorly on two indices of immediate memory from the

Table 19.3 Melbourne criteria for the psychosis prodrome (adapted from Yung *et al.* 2003)

Group 1: Attenuated psychotic symptoms

- Presence of at least one of the following: ideas of reference; odd beliefs or magical thinking; perceptual disturbance; paranoid ideation; odd thinking and speech; odd behaviour and appearance *at attenuated levels*
- Frequency of symptoms: at least several times per week. Change in mental state present for at least 1 week and not longer than 5 years

Group 2: Brief limited intermittent psychotic (BLIP) symptoms

- Transient psychotic symptoms. Presence of at least one of the following: ideas of reference; magical thinking; perceptual disturbance; paranoid ideation; odd thinking and speech
- Duration of episode less than 1 week; symptoms resolve spontaneously;
- BLIP occurred within the past year.;

Group 3: Trait and state risk factors

- First-degree relative with a DSM-IV psychotic disorder or schizotypal personality disorder
- Significant decrease in mental state or functioning (30+ point reduction in Global Assessment of Functioning (GAF) scale)—maintained for at least a month and not longer than 5 years
- Decrease in functioning occurred within the last year

Acute psychosis threshold

- Presence of at least one of the following: ideas of reference; magical thinking; perceptual disturbance; paranoid ideation; odd thinking and speech
- Frequency of symptoms at least several times a week
- Duration of mental state change is longer than 1 week

Weschler Memory Scale. However, there were no differences in sustained attention between those who do and do not become psychotic (Francey *et al.* 2005), suggesting that it may be a stable, trait-like impairment. Despite methodological difficulties, studies like this may be crucial in improving our ability to detect which patients presenting with non-specific but potentially prodromal symptoms are most at risk for psychosis.

19.4.5 How does cognition change across time?

Much is unknown about how cognition changes across time in schizophrenia. This is important because there appear to be two clear cognitive outcomes in schizophrenia: a fairly stable impairment in long-term outpatients and a major decline in cognition in elderly inpatients (Rund 1998; Kurtz 2005). The current generation of studies including individuals with first psychotic episode or prodromal symptoms should shed light on the precursors of these two outcomes. In addition, ongoing longitudinal assessments both in general population cohorts and in high-risk samples may help to identify cognitive differences between patients who do and do not develop a psychotic disorder. The biggest studies of patients with first episode psychosis (Bilder *et al.* 2000; Addington *et al.* 2003) find cognitive deficits of similar magnitude to those found in studies of chronic schizophrenia (Heinrichs and Zakzanis 1998). Studies examining school records or army conscription tests have established that there is some decrement in cognitive functioning prior to the onset of psychosis (Aylward *et al.* 1984; Reichenberg *et al.* 2002). However, there is relatively little evidence for the nature and timing of cognitive change. Fuller *et al.* (2002) studied standardized scholastic test performance in 70 children who later developed schizophrenia. They found little cognitive decrement prior to age 13, but a significant decline in test scores, particularly language scores, between ages 13 and 16 in the pre-schizophrenic children relative to their peers. Caspi *et al.* (2003) compared the performance of people who were healthy at the time of conscription into the Israeli army (age 16–17 years) and then retested them after the first hospitalization for schizophrenia. While significant within-subject changes were found over time in the future schizophrenia patients, the schizophrenia patients did not show the improvement that controls showed on the second assessment; indeed, there was some minimal decline in function. The patients worsened on measures of concentration and mental speed, and of abstract reasoning, while verbal reasoning and arithmetic appeared preserved. However this decline was small compared with the large decrement in cognitive function present at the earlier assessment

19.4.6 **Neurodevelopmental or neurodegenerative impairment?**

While there is some evidence of worsening cognitive impairment across time (favouring a neurodegenerative model of schizophrenia), observations more generally support a neurodevelopmental model in which most of the impairment occurs prior to the onset of symptoms.

Neurodevelopmental models of schizophrenia (Murray and Lewis 1987; Weinberger 1987) assert that schizophrenia involves subtle abnormalities in neurodevelopment arising from a number of possible prenatal and perinatal factors, the consequences of which do not fully manifest until adolescence or early adulthood. Suggested risk factors include winter birth, prenatal influenza and other prenatal or neonatal infections, prenatal famine, and obstetric complications (Jones *et al.* 1998; Cannon *et al.* 2003). Several versions of the model exist. Some (Murray and Lewis 1987) emphasize the role of environmental factors and propose a neurodevelopmental subgroup of schizophrenia, while others (Weinberger 1987) emphasize a continuum of pathology and the importance of normal developmental processes such as puberty. Recently, several researchers have suggested theories involving multiple developmental 'hits', including both the period immediately before or after birth, and further periods of risk around puberty, where the brain may once again be vulnerable (e.g. Pantelis *et al.* 2003*b*). One study assessing structural change before and after a transition to psychosis (Pantelis *et al.* 2003*a*) found significant bilateral reduction in the cingulate gyri, left orbitofrontal cortex, and left parahippocampal regions. Further studies are needed in patients this early in the disorder before conclusions can be drawn, but it seems likely that significant structural brain change does occur during this stage.

Neurodevelopmental models explain consistent findings that children who will later develop schizophrenia show poorer cognitive performance. Jones *et al.* (1994) compared participants in the 1946 British Birth Cohort who had developed schizophrenia ($n = 30$) with those who had not by the age of 36 years ($n = 4716$). They found multiple differences between the groups: cases were slower to attain developmental milestones such as walking and talking and performed more poorly on cognitive tests at ages 8, 11, and 15 years. These findings of poorer cognition in pre-schizophrenic children have been replicated in other birth cohorts in Britain (Crow *et al.* 1995) and Finland (Isohanni *et al.* 1998; Cannon *et al.* 1999). Neuropathological evidence for neurodevelopmental models of schizophrenia includes findings of abnormal brain asymmetries (normally formed in the second trimester of pregnancy), relatively little evidence of progressive structural change after the onset of the disorder, the presence of cortical changes without gliosis, and cytoarchitectural abnormalities suggestive of a defect in neuronal migration (Weinberger 1995). There is also evidence of premorbid functional abnormalities. For example, children who will later develop schizophrenia show more motor abnormalities than their unaffected siblings (Walker *et al.* 1994) and delays in the attainment of developmental milestones such as walking and talking (Fish 1960; Fish *et al.* 1992; Jones *et al.* 1994).

A neurodegenerative hypothesis on the other hand would suggest progressive cognitive decline. Since both stable and declining cognitive courses are seen in individual patients (Rund 1998; Kurtz 2005) the picture is not a clear one. On the whole, while there is some evidence for worsening of cognition in patients with chronic schizophrenia, observations generally support a neurodevelopmental model where the majority of cognitive impairment occurs prior to the onset of psychosis, and where normal developmental processes such as puberty interact with genetic or other vulnerability to increase cognitive impairment prior to onset.

19.5 **What is the importance of cognitive impairment in schizophrenia?**

- Cognitive impairment may be a major factor in determining the limitations in day-to-day functioning in schizophrenia.
- Cognition may be critical in both determining and shaping symptoms of psychosis and may interact with symptoms in contributing to functional outcomes.
- Is cognitive decline related to the duration of untreated illness?

Clearly, there are cognitive deficits that accompany and perhaps precede the onset of schizophrenia. It becomes pertinent to consider what this actually means to the patient in terms of the impact upon daily function and upon the prevailing clinical picture.

19.5.1 **Relation of cognitive deficits to daily function**

It is now well established that cognitive performance in schizophrenia is predictive of functional outcome (Green 1996; Green *et al.* 2000*a*), a development that has implications for treatment (Green *et al.* 2004). The functional consequences of cognitive impairment in schizophrenia may be of substantial personal, social, and economic importance. Cognitive deficits are a further barrier to employment and social functioning for patients who may be already struggling to cope with chronic symptoms and treatment side-effects.

In outpatients, vocational functioning is a useful outcome measure. Patients who are able to maintain employment or study tend to perform better on cognitive tasks (Bellack *et al.* 1999; McGurk and Meltzer 2000). Moreover, cognitive function predicts performance on work rehabilitation programmes (Bryson *et al.* 1998; Bell and Bryson 2001; Gold *et al.* 2002; Evans *et al.* 2004). Community social function shows less consistent associations with cognitive function (Addington *et al.* 1998; Prouteau *et al.* 2004), but social problem-solving paradigms show associations with verbal memory and executive function (Addington and Addington 1999) that remain reliable over several years (Addington and Addington 2000).

These results establish that cognition can be a 'rate-limiting' factor in functional outcome in schizophrenia, but they do not explain how. It is in one sense obvious that a patient who has difficulty concentrating and a poor memory may find both his or her work and social life suffering. It is also possible that some other factor mediates the link between cognition and function; for example, affect perception may link cognitive and social deficits (Green *et al.* 2000*b*). More obviously, persistent symptoms might independently impair both cognitive performance and functional outcome.

One important concept in evaluating the impact of cognition is 'quality of life', which often includes measures of subjective well-being as well as aspects of social and occupational function and the impact of residual symptoms. Like other measures of functioning, aspects of quality of life are predicted by memory (McDermid Vaz and Heinrichs 2002) and other cognitive scores (Fujii *et al.* 2004; Sota and Heinrichs 2004) as well as negative symptoms (Browne *et al.* 1996; Galletly *et al.* 1997). Norman and colleagues (2000) have argued, however, that subjective well-being is related more to positive than negative symptoms.

19.5.2 **Relationship between cognition and symptoms**

The link between symptoms and cognitive function in schizophrenia is complex. Negative symptoms such as avolition may lower cognitive test scores, while florid psychosis can make assessment impossible. As a result, relatively little is known about the relationship of symptoms and cognition during acute phases of schizophrenia. One study (McGrath *et al.* 2001) assessed patients on a visuospatial working memory task during acute and subacute phases (on admission to a psychiatric unit, and then 4 weeks later). They found substantial working memory impairment in both acute and subacute phases, with significant associations between negative symptom level and working memory performance. The relationship to positive symptoms was not strong, in keeping with findings in patients in remission or with stable symptom levels that show little evidence of an association between cognitive impairment and positive symptoms. However, the association between negative symptoms and cognitive impairments has been recognized for 20 years (Addington 2000). Recently, negative symptoms have been associated with memory, executive function, sustained attention, and general intelligence (Harvey *et al.* 1996; Voruganti *et al.* 1997; Basso *et al.* 1998; Nieuwenstein *et al.* 2001; Hughes *et al.* 2003; Pantelis *et al.* 2004). Thought-disorder has also been associated with cognitive deficits (Bilder *et al.* 1985; Basso *et al.* 1998; Nieuwenstein *et al.* 2001; Pantelis *et al.* 2004).

19.5.3 **Relationship between cognition, symptoms, and function**

There are a number of ways in which symptoms and cognition could affect function, directly or indirectly and with differing degrees of independence. Evans *et al.* (2004) studied the associations between cognition, symptoms and vocational outcome in outpatients taking part in one of two vocational rehabilitation schemes. McGurk *et al.* (2000) studied social and adaptive function in elderly inpatients. In both studies, cognition predicted outcome more than did symptoms, although significant correlations were found between negative (but not positive) symptoms and function. A third study (Velligan *et al.* 1997) also found a greater predictive effect of cognition. The data were actually consistent with a model in which cognition influenced function both directly and indirectly, by mediating the effects of symptoms. However, the opposite pattern of results, supporting greater predictive effects of negative symptoms than cognition, has also been reported (Norman *et al.* 1999). Clearly, further data are required to resolve these inconsistencies.

19.5.4 **Cognition in relatives of patients with schizophrenia**

Healthy relatives of people with schizophrenia do show cognitive impairments. Compared with volunteers who have no family history of psychosis, parents, children, and siblings of patients with schizophrenia show impairments in executive function (Faraone *et al.* 2000;

Laurent *et al.* 2000; Staal *et al.* 2000; Egan *et al.* 2001; Rybakowski and Borkowska 2002; Gochman *et al.* 2004), sustained attention (Egan *et al.* 2000; Chen *et al.* 2004), and aspects of verbal (Sponheim *et al.* 2004) and non-verbal (Byrne *et al.* 1999) memory. A recent meta-analysis (Sitskoorn *et al.* 2004) found the largest effect sizes in verbal recall and executive function, with smaller effects on attention.

This research has been enhanced by findings from 'high-risk' studies that follow up the children of psychiatric patients, including those with schizophrenia. These prospective studies have all the methodological advantages of longitudinal studies including an ability to detect change and to follow up the apparently healthy relatives who later become psychotic. The New York High Risk Project has shown that children who later developed schizophrenia show relatively specific deficits in verbal memory, attention, and motor skills (Erlenmeyer-Kimling *et al.* 2000). Individuals in the Edinburgh High Risk study who have experienced some psychotic symptoms showed significantly worse verbal memory and executive function than those who have not (Cosway *et al.* 2000).

In healthy relatives, greater familial risk is associated with greater cognitive impairment, suggesting an effect of genetic loading. People with one schizophrenic relative showed less cognitive impairment than those with two affected relatives (Faraone *et al.* 2000; Johnstone *et al.* 2002). Patients with greater cognitive impairment have healthy relatives with greater cognitive impairment too (Egan *et al.* 2000), though this may reflect the general heritability of cognition and not schizophrenia.

19.5.5 **The impact of duration of untreated psychosis**

Many samples of individuals with a first episode of psychosis actually comprise a number of people with a long history of untreated psychosis (Larsen *et al.* 1996; Barnes *et al.* 2000; Hoff *et al.* 2000). There is some evidence that a longer duration of untreated psychosis (DUP) is deleterious to cognitive function (Joyce *et al.* 2002; Tyson *et al.* 2004). It is not clear whether this might indicate that psychosis has a neurotoxic effect or whether individuals with longer DUP at presentation tend to be the ones with schizophrenia rather than, say, affective disorders. Furthermore, other studies have failed to find an association between cognitive function and DUP (Hoff *et al.* 2000) (Heydebrand *et al.* 2004; Ho *et al.* 2003; Norman *et al.* 2001). Perhaps, DUP is a marker, rather than determinant of course (McGlashan 1999).

Poor premorbid functioning in schizophrenia may be an important factor; it is associated with more severe symptoms and more severe cognitive impairment (Rabinowitz *et al.* 2002) as well as increased DUP (Verdoux *et al.* 2001). Patients with longer DUP were more likely to be unemployed, living alone, or homeless (Barnes *et al.* 2000), factors that could conceivably result from untreated psychotic symptoms. Longer DUP may be on a multifactorial pathway between poor premorbid function and poor outcome. Munro *et al.* (2002) found that lower childhood IQ predicted both poor social outcome and reduced service utilization once schizophrenia had developed.

Does this tentative, though unproven link between DUP and cognitive performance point to the importance of early intervention in schizophrenia? Despite widespread interest in such early intervention, there is no clear evidence of its clinical benefits in terms of early treatment of people in prodromal states or first psychotic episodes (Marshall and Lockwood 2004). Some studies comparing clinical outcome of treatment with duration of untreated illness have found no association over 6 month (Ho *et al.* 2000) or 24 month (Craig *et al.* 2000) periods, although others (e.g. Loebel *et al.* 1992) have found associations between DUP and outcome. A recent review (Norman *et al.* 2005) suggested that DUP is correlated with better treatment outcome, especially with respect to positive symptoms over the first year. However both the aetiological mechanism, and its longer-term effects, remain unclear.

The situation may be slightly different in patients who have received long-term treatment for chronic schizophrenia. One study of 48 inpatients, many of whom had been admitted before the widespread use of antipsychotic drugs (Scully *et al.* 1997), compared the effects of DUP and subsequent duration of treatment symptoms, general cognitive function, and executive function. DUP was associated with both negative symptoms and general cognitive function, but not positive symptoms or executive function. Duration of antipsychotic treatment was not associated with any outcome measures. This study strongly supports the idea that schizophrenia may involve a progressive decline that is halted by adequate antipsychotic treatment. Wyatt *et al.* (1997) studied the records of first-admission schizophrenia patients from the 1950s and 1960s and compared the long-term outcomes of those who were randomized to receive or not receive antipsychotic medication. They found that patients who were initially treated with antipsychotics had fewer readmissions during the second year after discharge and functioned at a higher level 6–7 years after discharge. The relationship between DUP and outcome may therefore differ according to treatment generations.

19.6 Do the symptoms of psychosis have a cognitive basis?

- Can cognitive models of symptoms develop our understanding of how and why those symptoms arise?
- Can such models provide a key to linking complex psychopathology to underlying neurobiology?

An important question is whether we might understand symptoms in terms of aberrant cognitive processes. Specifically, could it be that hallucinations, delusions, thought disorder, and negative symptoms are manifestations of deficits in cognition? The importance and currency of this question has been reflected in the developments of 'cognitive neuropsychology' (Frith 1992) or 'cognitive neuropsychiatry' (Halligan and David 2001). In essence, these approaches consider symptoms in terms of models of normal processing and of defects in this processing. Importantly, they seek to make testable predictions that could serve to refute these models. Furthermore, in embedding descriptions of psychopathology in models of healthy cognitive processing, they offer ways of uniting descriptions at the neurobiological, cognitive, and psychopathological levels. Studies of schizophrenia have suffered from a lack of such a synthesis and, for this reason, we feel that it is important to conclude this chapter by considering certain specific cognitive deficits in schizophrenia/psychosis and how these may explain and predict the different symptoms. This is not intended as an exhaustive review of cognitive neuropsychological/neuropsychiatric accounts of symptoms but rather to draw attention to a burgeoning field of study and to illustrate, with brief examples, how useful this field may be. We will consider briefly certain key symptoms occurring in schizophrenia and other psychotic illnesses: delusions; passivity phenomena; and delusional misidentification. We point out that other key symptoms of schizophrenia, perhaps most notably auditory hallucinations and negative symptoms, have also been the subjective of detailed cognitive assessments. While space constraints prohibit an examination of these latter phenomena, we draw the attention of an interested reader to other sources of information (Frith 1992; Halligan and David 2001; David 2004).

19.6.1 Cognitive models of delusions

From their earliest formulations, ideas about schizophrenia have emphasized changes in association formation. This is manifest, perhaps most clearly, in delusions—fixed, irrational beliefs often held with unshakeable conviction. In the frame of a cognitive neuropsychological approach, since understanding learning mechanisms and subsequent inferences is critical to understanding the formation of associations (and hence beliefs about the world) and since delusions may be described in terms of the formation of bizarre and inappropriate associations, it is reasonable that delusions should be considered in terms of associative learning and inference. The notion of such a disturbance has also been implicit in accounting for the odd perception and attention that occur during the early stages of schizophrenia (Mcghie and Chapman 1961; Chapman 1966). In this respect, Gray and Hemsley speculate that a key feature of schizophrenia lies in a failure to integrate stored material with current perceptual input (Gray *et al.* 1991; Hemsley 1994). The consequence of such an abnormality, they suggested, would be changes in novelty processing, in attentional allocation, and, ultimately, in associative learning. Such a mechanism, though it is certainly incomplete with respect to understanding delusions, has the advantage of framing ideas about this symptom in terms of neuroscientific work on attentional and perceptual experiences of the world. For example, it may expressed in terms of a mismatch between actual and expected outcomes—in other words, prediction error, a key component of learning (Schultz and Dickinson 2000). It also provides a framework for relating them to underlying neurochemistry given the suggestion that dopaminergic disturbance in basal ganglia would disrupt association formation and attentional allocation (Miller 1976, 1993). These theoretical frameworks have been developed and extended in a more recent model of delusion formation that has, at its core, the suggestion that mesolimbic dopamine firing is disrupted, altering the ways in which salience is allocated both to external events, people, and objects and to internal representations (Kapur 2003; Kapur *et al.* 2005).

Kapur's work, and preceding models on which it draws, represent a systematic attempt to ground cognitive models in neurobiology and to show how they may relate to higher behaviours and experiences. They make a number of predictions about profiles of cognition in individuals with, or vulnerable to, delusions. If these models are correct, then it should be possible to observe, in illness characterized by delusions, some evidence of abnormal associative learning and of abnormal behavioural responses to conditions engaging association formation. In this respect, it is of clear, though indirect, relevance that learning and memory are demonstrably abnormal in schizophrenia (Aleman *et al.* 1999; Pelletier *et al.* 2005). Furthermore, there may also be disturbances under circumstances where prior exposure to stimuli should render test stimuli either more or less predictable. For example, in a mismatch negativity (MMN) paradigm, brain responses to 'deviant' stimuli (stimuli that constitute a mismatch in the context of those that preceded them) have been noted to be reliably different in schizophrenia (Light and Braff 2005*b*) in a way that is related to general functioning (Light and Braff 2005*a*) and may be diagnostically specific (Umbricht *et al.* 2003). Conversely, prepulse inhibition (PPI) of the startle response, in which a prior stimulus attenuates the effects of a subsequent more intense stimulus, is attenuated in schizophrenia (Braff *et al.* 2001). These two sets of findings suggest that there is a failure in the normal response to a stimulus that stands out from its surroundings (attenuated MMN) and a failure of a predictive stimulus to attenuate the response to a subsequent stimulus (loss of PPI). Additionally, negative priming, whereby prior experience of ignoring a stimulus makes one slower to respond when that stimulus must no longer be ignored, is also attenuated in schizophrenia (e.g. Mcqueen *et al.* 2003). All of these findings are compatible with the notion that delusional belief formation is associated with abnormal learning (possibly through abnormal prediction error signalling), although this statement is made cautiously since the findings are also compatible with other accounts. More direct assessments in the setting of associative learning tasks have suggested that schizophrenia may be associated with changes in two phenomena: blocking and latent inhibition (LI). Both depend upon prior exposure reducing either prediction error signal (blocking) or attentional allocation to test stimuli (LI). The consequence is that, under normal circumstances, test stimuli are relatively resistant to association formation, an effect that may be reduced in people with schizophrenia (Jones *et al.* 1992). That is, under these circumstances, people with the illness may learn more quickly as a result of changes both in associative learning and in the concomitant attentional allocation. While this is highly consistent with the model described above, it should be noted that findings are variable with respect to both blocking (Oades *et al.* 1996) and latent inhibition (Swerdlow *et al.* 2005) and are perhaps strongly related to symptom profile, medication status, and other variables.

The above represents little more than an initial attempt to explain a component of delusions and it is set out to illustrate the potential importance and value of relating cognition directly to symptoms in psychotic illness. We point out that more complete models of delusion formation have been proposed. A delusional belief is frequently accompanied by emotional changes, by anxiety, and by internal–external confusions. The model above does not encompass these characteristics, nor does it exclude them. In this respect, it is important to note that other models of delusions have identified multiple factors more directly applicable to these other characteristics of delusions (e.g. Freeman *et al.* 2002). Such models evoke pre-existing beliefs, cognitive styles, and reasoning biases (Garety and Freeman 1999), for example, individuals' perceptions of their own vulnerability and cognitive biases such as a tendency to 'jump to conclusions' (Garety *et al.* 1991), together with erroneous internal–external biases (Peters and Garety 2006).

19.6.2 **Cognitive models of passivity phenomena**

Passivity phenomena refer to a subject's belief that he or she is under control of an external agent and, while these phenomena can occur in a number of domains (movements, thinking, emotion), for illustrative purposes we shall here confine our discussion to delusions of motor control. In these delusions, the sufferer has the compelling belief that his movements are generated by an external agent. Again, it is a challenge to understand such an unusual and complex phenomenon in terms of underlying cognitive process. Frith (2005) has suggested that we explore this phenomenon in terms of a model of normal movement control. In brief, he proposed that a sense of agency arises because the generation of a movement, under normal circumstances, is associated with an accurate prediction of the sensory changes that result from that movement. There is behavioural and functional neuroimaging evidence that people tend to suppress the sensory consequences of their actions (Blakemore *et al.* 1998*a*; Blakemore and Frith 2003; Shergill *et al.* 2003) and Frith proposes that delusions of motor control arise when there is an error in this prediction such that the sensory consequences remain unsuppressed and the normal sense of agency is disrupted.

If this view of delusions of motor control is correct, it makes a number of testable predictions about other deficits in schizophrenia. First, it has been suggested (Claxton 1975; Blakemore *et al.* 1998*b*, 2000*b*) that one of the consequences of a suppression of the sensory consequences of one's own movements is that we are unable to tickle ourselves since the essence of the tickle sensation is its unpredictability. If, as the model suggests, this suppression is lost in delusions of control then they should find self-generated movements more ticklish than control subjects do. Tentative evidence has emerged suggesting that it is indeed the case that people with passivity phenomena (and, interestingly, auditory hallucinations) do indeed find stimulation by themselves more ticklish (Blakemore *et al.* 2000*a*). It has also been shown that people with schizophrenia appear less likely to dampen down the sensory consequences of their actions when making a simple pressing movement (Shergill *et al.* 2005). In addition, predicting the consequences of actions would be necessary to successful imagining of a movement. If one is asked to imagine performing a series of movements, then one is able to show a degree of accuracy, with imagining difficult or complex movements taking longer than imagining simple, easy ones. If people with delusions of control have a problem in making necessary predictions, it would follow that they may be worse at imagining movements. Recent work has shown that this may indeed be the case (Maruff *et al.* 2003). Finally, normal ability to predict an outcome of movements would allow for anticipatory motor changes: if I move a weight up and down, the force of my grip must change (greater when moving the weight up, less when moving it down). Generally, we can do this very well and can make the necessary adjustments with a precision of timing that suggests that these adjustments are not secondary to sensory feedback but, rather, must be anticipatory. Here the findings are somewhat at odds with the predictions of the model. It has been shown that people with schizophrenia appear to have problems, not when automatic, anticipatory adjustments are required, but rather when conscious control is required (Delevoye-Turrell *et al.* 2002). Furthermore, more recent work has suggested that anticipatory responses to lifting, hitting, or resisting tasks are unimpaired in schizophrenia (Delevoye-Turrell *et al.* 2003). Overall, therefore, the evidence in favour of this model of delusions of control is contradictory. Nevertheless, this field illustrates the value of a cognitive neuropsychological approach in generating and testing models of psychopathology.

19.6.3 Cognition and delusional misidentification

> Who is that person who drives my family up to the hospital every evening? It is a cheek. He stays at home and opens all my husband's letters. Anyway at least he pays the bills…He does look very like my husband only perhaps a little fatter.'
>
> [Female in patient on psychiatric ward, quoted in Sims 1988]

There are two main types of delusional misidentification of persons. I will focus on the one known as Capgras syndrome, which is more common. In Capgras syndrome the sufferer believes that a person known to him/her has been replaced by a double, as illustrated in the quotation above. The occurrence of Capgras spans ethnicity, age, and gender (it may be a little more common in women). It has been estimated to occur in up to 4% of patients with psychosis. It is usually associated with schizophrenia (although not just with mental illness and can occur in association with many physical illnesses; Forstl *et al.* 1991).

Once again, the cognitive neuropsychological approach to understanding this complex phenomenon lies in relating it to the normal cognitive processing that would, usually, uphold the function thought to be aberrant—in this case, face recognition. Ellis and Young (1990) suggested that Capgras syndrome could be understood in terms of a two-route model of face processing in which a facial identity is recognized explicitly (I know who this person is) and at a more implicit/affective level (this person feels familiar). In patients with Capgras, they asserted, there would be normal overt recognition of a familiar face but an absence of the covert recognition. This would produce, they suggested, a strange experience: conscious recognition without the affective response that would normally accompany such recognition. In the context of a general state of suspiciousness, the odd experience becomes a delusional misidentification (this person looks like the someone I know but they don't feel right). They contrasted this with prosopagnosia in which explicit recognition is impaired in the face of preserved implicit recognition. Two subsequent studies provided evidence in support of this model (Ellis *et al.* 1997; Hirstein and Ramachandran 1997). In each, subjects with Capgras syndrome showed an absence of the normal skin conductance response accompanying faces that they explicitly recognized. It was, as predicted by Ellis and Young, the mirror image of prosopagnosia and provides evidence that the Capgras delusion, though complex, may be understood and explored in the setting of a simple model of face recognition.

Acknowledgement

P.C. Fletcher is supported by the Wellcome Trust. J. Barnett was supported by the MRC during the completion of this work.

References

Abbruzzese, M., Ferri, S., and Scarone, S. (1996). Performance on the Wisconsin Card Sorting Test in schizophrenia: perseveration in clinical subtypes. *Psychiatry Res.* **64**, 27–33.

Addington, J. (2000). Cognitive functioning and negative symptoms in schizophrenia. In *Cognition in schizophrenia: impairments, importance and treatment strategies* (ed. P. Harvey), pp. 193–209. Oxford: Oxford University Press.

Addington, J. and Addington, D. (1999). Neurocognitive and social functioning in schizophrenia. *Schizophr. Bull.* **25**, 173–82.

Addington, J. and Addington, D. (2000). Neurocognitive and social functioning in schizophrenia: a 2.5 year follow-up study. *Schizophr. Res.* **44**, 47–56.

Addington, J., McCleary, L., and Munroe-Blum, H. (1998). Relationship between cognitive and social dysfunction in schizophrenia. *Schizophr. Res.* **34**, 59–66.

Addington, J., Brooks, B.L., and Addington, D. (2003). Cognitive functioning in first episode psychosis: initial presentation. *Schizophr. Res.* **62**, 59–64.

Aleman, A., Hijman, R., de Haan, E.H., and Kahn, R.S. (1999). Memory impairment in schizophrenia: a meta-analysis. *Am. J. Psychiatry* 156,1358–66.

Alexander, G.E., DeLong, M.R., and Strick, P.L. (1986). Parallel organization of functionally segregated circuits linking basal ganglia and cortex. *Annu. Rev. Neurosci.* **9**, 357–81.

American Psychiatric Association (1994). *Diagnostic and statistical manual of mental disorders*, 4th edn (DSM-IV). APA, Washington DC.

Amminger, G.P., Schlogelhofer, M., Lehner, T., Looser Ott, S., Friedrich, M.H., and Aschauer, H.N. (2000). Premorbid performance IQ deficit in schizophrenia. *Acta Psychiatr. Scand.* **102**, 414–22.

Angermeyer, M.C., Kuhn, L., and Goldstein, J.M. (1990). Gender and the course of schizophrenia: differences in treated outcomes. *Schizophr. Bull.* **16**, 293–307.

Asarnow, R.F. and MacCrimmon, D.J. (1978). Residual performance deficit in clinically remitted schizophrenics: a marker of schizophrenia? *J. Abnorm. Psychol.* **87**, 597–608.

Aylward, E., Walker, E., and Bettes, B. (1984). Intelligence in schizophrenia: meta-analysis of the research. *Schizophr. Bull.* **10**, 430–59.

Baker, C.A. and Morrison, A.P. (1998). Cognitive processes in auditory hallucinations: attributional biases and metacognition. *Psychol. Med.* **28**, 1199–208.

Barnes, T.R., Hutton, S.B., Chapman, M.J., Mutsatsa, S., Puri, B.K., and Joyce, E.M. (2000). West London first-episode study of schizophrenia. Clinical correlates of duration of untreated psychosis. *Br. J. Psychiatry* **177**, 207–11.

Bartok, E., Berecz, R., Glaub, T., and Degrell, I. (2005). Cognitive functions in prepsychotic patients. *Prog. Neuropsychopharmacol. Biol. Psychiatry* **29**, 621–5.

Basso, M.R., Nasrallah, H.A., Olson, S.C., and Bornstein, R.A. (1998). Neuropsychological correlates of negative., disorganized and psychotic symptoms in schizophrenia. *Schizophr. Res.* **31**, 99–111.

Bell, M.D. and Bryson, G. (2001). Work rehabilitation in schizophrenia: does cognitive impairment limit improvement? *Schizophr. Bull.* **27**, 269–79.

Bellack, A.S., Gold, J.M., and Buchanan, R.W. (1999). Cognitive rehabilitation for schizophrenia: problems, prospects, and strategies. *Schizophr. Bull.* **25**, 257–74.

Berg, E.A. (1948). A sample objective test for measuring flexibility in thinking. *J. Gen. Psychol.* **39**, 15–22.

Berrios, G.E. (2000). Schizophrenia: a conceptual history. In *New Oxford textbook of psychiatry* (ed. M.G. Gelder, J.J. Lopez-Ibor, and N.C. Andreasen), pp. 567–71. Oxford University Press, Oxford.

Bilder, R.M., Mukherjee, S., Rieder, R.O., and Pandurangi, A.K. (1985). Symptomatic and neuropsychological components of defect states. *Schizophr. Bull.* **11**, 409–19.

Bilder, R.M., Turkel, E., Lipschutz-Broch, L., and Lieberman, J.A. (1992). Antipsychotic medication effects on neuropsychological functions. *Psychopharmacol. Bull.* **28**, 353–66.

Bilder, R.M., Goldman, R.S., Robinson, D., Reiter, G., Bell, L., Bates, J.A., Pappadopulos, E., Willson, D.F., Alvir, J.M., Woerner, M.G., Geisler, S., Kane, J.M., and Lieberman, J.A. (2000). Neuropsychology of first-episode schizophrenia: initial characterization and clinical correlates. *Am. J. Psychiatry* **157**, 549–59.

Blakemore, S.J. and Frith, C.D. (2003). Self-awareness and action. *Curr. Opin. Neurobiol.* **13** (2), 219–24.

Blakemore, S.J., Rees, G., and Frith, C.D. (1998*a*). How do we predict the consequences of our actions? A functional imaging study. *Neuropsychologia* **36** (6), 521–9.

Blakemore, S.J., Wolpert, D.M., and Frith, C.D. (1998*b*). Central cancellation of self-produced tickle sensation. *Nat. Neurosci.* **1** (7), 635–40.

Blakemore, S.J., Smith, J., Steel, R., Johnstone, C.E., and Frith, C.D. (2000*a*). The perception of self-produced sensory stimuli in patients with auditory hallucinations and passivity experiences: evidence for a breakdown in self-monitoring. *Psychol. Med.* **30** (5), 1131–9.

Blakemore, S.J., Wolpert, D., and Frith, C. (2000*b*). Why can't you tickle yourself? *Neuroreport* **11** (11), R11–16.

Braff, D.L., Geyer, M.A., and Swerdlow, N.R. (2001). Human studies of prepulse inhibition of startle: normal subjects., patient groups., and pharmacological studies. *Psychopharmacology (Berl.)* **156** (2–3), 234–58.

Brebion, G., Gorman, J.M., Malaspina, D., and Amador, X. (2005). A model of verbal memory impairments in schizophrenia: two systems and their associations with underlying cognitive processes and clinical symptoms. *Psychol. Med.* **35** (1), 133–42.

Brewer, W.J., Francey, S.M., Wood, S.J., Jackson, H.J., Pantelis, C., Phillips, L.J., Yung, A.R., Anderson, V.A., and McGorry, P.D. (2005). Memory impairments identified in people at ultra-high risk for psychosis who later develop first-episode psychosis. *Am. J. Psychiatry* **162**, 71–8.

Bromet, E.J., Naz, B., Fochtmann, L.J., Carlson, G.A., and Tanenberg-Karant, M. (2005). Long term diagnostic stability and outcome in recent first-episode cohort studies of schizophrenia. *Schizophr. Bull.* **31**, 639–49.

Browne, S., Roe, M., Lane, A., Gervin, M., Morris, M., Kinsella, A., Larkin, C., and Callaghan, E.O. (1996). Quality of life in schizophrenia: relationship to sociodemographic factors., symptomatology and tardive dyskinesia. *Acta Psychiatr. Scand.* **94**, 118–24.

Bryson, G., Bell, M.D., Kaplan, E., and Greig, T. (1998). The functional consequences of memory impairments on initial work performance in people with schizophrenia. *J. Nerv. Ment. Dis.* **186**, 610–15.

Byrne, M., Hodges, A., Grant, E., Owens, D.C., and Johnstone, E.C. (1999). Neuropsychological assessment of young people at high genetic risk for developing schizophrenia compared with controls: preliminary findings of the Edinburgh High Risk Study (EHRS). *Psychol. Med.* **29**, 1161–73.

Cannon, M., Jones, P., Huttunen, M.O., Tanskanen, A., Huttunen, T., Rabe-Hesketh, S., and Murray R.M. (1999). School performance in Finnish children and later development of schizophrenia: a population-based longitudinal study. *Arch. Gen. Psychiatry* **56**, 457–63.

Cannon, M., Caspi, A., Moffitt, T.E., Harrington, H., Taylor, A., Murray, R.M., and Poulton, R. (2002). Evidence for early-childhood., pan-developmental impairment specific to schizophreniform disorder: results from a longitudinal birth cohort. *Arch. Gen. Psychiatry* **59**, 449–56.

Cannon, M., Kendell, R., Susser, E., and Jones, P. (2003). Prenatal and perinatal risk factors for schizophrenia. In *The epidemiology of schizophrenia* (ed. R.M. Murray, P.B. Jones, E. Susser, J. van Os., and M. Cannon), pp. 74–99. Cambridge University Press, Cambridge.

Cardno, A. and Murray, R.M. (2003). The 'classical' genetic epidemiology of schizophrenia. In *The epidemiology of schizophrenia* (ed. R.M. Murray, P.B. Jones, E. Susser, J. van Os., and M. Cannon), pp. 199–219. Cambridge University Press, Cambridge.

Caspi, A., Reichenberg, A., Weiser, M., Rabinowitz, J., Kaplan, Z., Knobler, H., Davidson-Sagi, N., and Davidson, M. (2003). Cognitive performance in schizophrenia patients assessed before and following the first psychotic episode. *Schizophr. Res.* **65**, 87–94.

Chapman, J. (1966). The early symptoms of schizophrenia. *Br. J. Psychiatry* **112**, 225–51.

Chen, W.J., Chang, C.H., Liu, S.K., Hwang, T.J., and Hwu, H.G. (2004). Sustained attention deficits in nonpsychotic relatives of schizophrenic patients: a recurrence risk ratio analysis. *Biol. Psychiatry* **55**, 995–1000.

Claxton, G. (1975). Why can't we tickle ourselves? *Percept. Mot. Skills* **41** (1), 335–8.

Conklin, H.M., Curtis, C.E., Calkins, M.E., and Iacono, W.G. (2005). Working memory functioning in schizophrenia patients and their first-degree relatives: cognitive functioning shedding light on etiology. *Neuropsychologia* **43**, 930–42.

Cooper, B. (2005). Immigration and schizophrenia: the social causation hypothesis revisited. *Br. J. Psychiatry* **186**, 361–3.

Cornblatt, B.A. and Keilp, J.G. (1994). Impaired attention., genetics., and the pathophysiology of schizophrenia. *Schizophr. Bull.* **20**, 31–46.

Cornblatt, B.A. and Malhotra, A.K. (2001). Impaired attention as an endophenotype for molecular genetic studies of schizophrenia. *Am. J. Med. Genet.* **105**, 11–15.

Cosway, R., Byrne, M., Clafferty, R., Hodges, A., Grant, E., Abukmeil, S.S., Lawrie, S.M., Miller, P., and Johnstone, E.C. (2000). Neuropsychological change in young people at high risk for schizophrenia: results from the first two neuropsychological assessments of the Edinburgh High Risk Study. *Psychol. Med.* **30**, 1111–21.

Craig, T.J., Bromet, E.J., Fennig, S., Tanenberg-Karant, M., Lavelle, J., and Galambos, N. (2000). Is there an association between duration of untreated psychosis and 24-month clinical outcome in a first-admission series? *Am. J. Psychiatry* **157**, 60–6.

Crow, T.J., Done, D.J., and Sacker, A. (1995). Childhood precursors of psychosis as clues to its evolutionary origins. *Eur. Arch. Psychiatry Clin. Neurosci.* **245**, 61–9.

David, A.S. (2004). The cognitive neuropsychiatry of auditory hallucinations: an overview. *Cogn. Neuropsychiatry* **9** (1–2), 107–23.

David, A.S., Malmberg, A., Brandt, L., Allebeck, P., and Lewis, G. (1997). IQ and risk for schizophrenia: a population-based cohort study. *Psychol. Med.* **27**, 1311–23.

Davidson, M., Reichenberg, A., Rabinowitz, J., Weiser, M., Kaplan, Z., and Mark, M. (1999). Behavioral and intellectual markers for schizophrenia in apparently healthy male adolescents. *Am. J. Psychiatry* **156**, 1328–35.

Delevoye-Turrell, Y., Giersch, A., and Danion, J.M. (2002). A deficit in the adjustment of grip force responses in schizophrenia. *Neuroreport* **13** (12), 1537–9.

Delevoye-Turrell, Y., Giersch, A., and Danion, J.M. (2003). Abnormal sequencing of motor actions in patients with schizophrenia: evidence from grip force adjustments during object manipulation. *Am. J. Psychiatry* **160** (1), 134–41.

DeLisi, L.E., Tew, W., Xie, S., Hoff, A.L., Sakuma, M., Kushner, M., Lee, G., Shedlack, K., Smith, A.M., and Grimson, R. (1995). A prospective follow-up study of brain morphology and cognition in first-episode schizophrenic patients: preliminary findings. *Biol. Psychiatry* **38**, 349–60.

DeLong, M.R., Alexander, G.E., Miller, W.C., and Crutcher, M.D. (1990). Anatomical and functional aspects of basal ganglia-thalamocortical circuits. In *Function and dysfunction in the basal ganglia* (ed. A.J. Franks, J.W. Ironside, H.S. Mindham, R.J. Smith, E.G.S. Spokes, and W. Winlow), pp. 3–32. Manchester University Press, Manchester.

Eberhard, J., Riley, F., and Levander, S. (2003). Premorbid IQ and schizophrenia. Increasing cognitive reduction by episodes. *Eur. Arch. Psychiatry Clin. Neurosci.* **253**, 84–8.

Egan, M.F., Goldberg, T.E., Gscheidle, T., Weirich, M., Bigelow, L.B., and Weinberger, D.R. (2000). Relative risk of attention deficits in siblings of patients with schizophrenia. *Am. J. Psychiatry* **157**, 1309–16.

Egan, M.F., Goldberg, T.E., Gscheidle, T., Weirich, M., Rawlings, R., Hyde, T.M., Bigelow, L., and Weinberger, D.R. (2001). Relative risk for cognitive impairments in siblings of patients with schizophrenia. *Biol. Psychiatry* **50**, 98–107.

Ellis, H.D. and Young, A.W. (1990). Accounting for delusional misidentifications. *Br. J. Psychiatry* **157**, 239–48.

Ellis, H.D., Young, A.W., Quayle, A.H., and De Pauw, K.W. (1997). Reduced autonomic responses to faces in Capgras delusion. *Proc. R. Soc. Lond. B* **264** (1384), 1085–92.

Elvevag, B., Weinberger, D.R., Suter, J.C., and Goldberg, T.E. (2000). Continuous performance test and schizophrenia: a test of stimulus–response compatibility, working memory, response readiness, or none of the above? *Am. J. Psychiatry* **157**, 772–80.

Erlenmeyer-Kimling, L., Rock, D., Roberts, S.A., Janal, M., Kestenbaum, C., Cornblatt, B., Adamo, U.H., and Gottesman, I.I. (2000). Attention, memory, and motor skills as childhood predictors of schizophrenia-related psychoses: the New York High-Risk Project. *Am. J. Psychiatry* **157**, 1416–22.

Evans, J.D., Bond, G.R., Meyer, P.S., Kim, H.W., Lysaker, P.H., Gibson, P.J., and Tunis, S. (2004). Cognitive and clinical predictors of success in vocational rehabilitation in schizophrenia. *Schizophr. Res.* **70**, 331–42.

Faraone, S.V., Seidman, L.J., Kremen, W.S., Toomey, R., Pepple, J.R., and Tsuang, M.T. (2000). Neuropsychologic functioning among the nonpsychotic relatives of schizophrenic patients: the effect of genetic loading. *Biol. Psychiatry* **48**, 120–6.

Fish, B. (1960). Involvement of the central nervous system in infants with schizophrenia. *Arch. Neurol.* **2**, 115–21.

Fish, B., Marcus, J., Hans, S.L., Auerbach, J.G., and Perdue, S. (1992). Infants at risk for schizophrenia: sequelae of a genetic neurointegrative defect. A review and replication analysis of pandysmaturation in the Jerusalem Infant Development Study. *Arch. Gen. Psychiatry* **49**, 221–35.

Fletcher, P.C. and Honey, G.D. (2006). Schizophrenia, ketamine and cannabis: evidence of overlapping memory deficits. *Trends Cogn. Sci.* **10** (4), 167–74.

Forstl, H., Almeida, O.P., Owen, A.M., Burns, A., and Howard, R. (1991). Psychiatric, neurological and medical aspects of misidentification syndromes: a review of 260 cases. *Psychol. Med.* **21** (4), 905–10.

Francey, S.M., Jackson, H.J., Phillips, L.J., Wood, S.J., Yung, A.R., and McGorry, P.D. (2005). Sustained attention in young people at high risk of psychosis does not predict transition to psychosis. *Schizophr. Res.* **79**, 127–36.

Freeman, D., Garety, P.A., Kuipers, E., Fowler, D., and Bebbington, P.E. (2002). A cognitive model of persecutory delusions. *Br. J. Clin. Psychol.* **41**, 331–47.

Frith, C. (1992). *The cognitive neuropsychology of schizophrenia.* Lawrence Erlbaum, Hove.

Frith, C. (2005). The self in action: lessons from delusions of control. *Conscious. Cogn.* **14**, 752–70.

Fujii, D.E., Wylie, A.M., and Nathan, J.H. (2004). Neurocognition and long-term prediction of quality of life in outpatients with severe and persistent mental illness. *Schizophr. Res.* **69**, 67–73.

Fuller, R., Nopoulos, P., Arndt, S., O'Leary, D., Ho, B.C., and Andreasen, N.C. (2002). Longitudinal assessment of premorbid cognitive functioning in patients with schizophrenia through examination of standardized scholastic test performance. *Am. J. Psychiatry* **159**, 1183–9.

Galletly, C.A., Clark, C.R., McFarlane, A.C., and Weber, D.L. (1997). Relationships between changes in symptom ratings, neurophysiological test performance and quality of life in schizophrenic patients treated with clozapine. *Psychiatry Res.* **72**, 161–6.

Garety, P.A. and Freeman, D. (1999). Cognitive approaches to delusions: a critical review of theories and evidence. *Br. J. Clin. Psychol.* **38** (2), 113–54.

Garety, P.A., Hemsley, D.R., and Wessely, S. (1991). Reasoning in deluded schizophrenic and paranoid patients: biases in performance on a probabilistic inference task. *J. Nerv. Ment. Dis.* **179**, 194–201.

Giovannetti, T., Goldstein, R.Z., Schullery, M., Barr, W.B., and Bilder, R.M. (2003). Category fluency in first-episode schizophrenia. *J. Int. Neuropsychol. Soc.* **9**, 384–93.

Gochman, P.A., Greenstein, D., Sporn, A., Gogtay, N., Nicolson, R., Keller, A., Lenane, M., Brookner, F., and Rapoport, J.L. (2004). Childhood onset schizophrenia: familial neurocognitive measures. *Schizophr. Res.* **71**, 43–7.

Gold, J.M., Goldberg, R.W., McNary, S.W., Dixon, L.B., and Lehman, A.F. (2002). Cognitive correlates of job tenure among patients with severe mental illness. *Am. J. Psychiatry* **159**, 1395–402.

Goldberg, T.E., Weinberger, D.R., Berman, K.F., Pliskin, N.H., and Podd, M.H. (1987). Further evidence for dementia of the prefrontal type in schizophrenia? A controlled study of teaching the Wisconsin Card Sorting Test. *Arch. Gen. Psychiatry* **44**, 1008–14.

Gottesman, I.I. and Shields, J. (1982). *Schizophrenia: the epigenetic puzzle.* Cambridge University Press, Cambridge.

Gray, J.A., Feldon, J., Rawlins, J.N.P., Hemsley, D.R., and Smith, A.D. (1991). The neuropsychology of schizophrenia. *Behav. Brain Sci.* **14**, 1–20.

Green, M.F. (1996). What are the functional consequences of neurocognitive deficits in schizophrenia? *Am. J. Psychiatry* **153**, 321–30.

Green, M.F., Kern, R.S., Braff, D.L., and Mintzm J, (2000*a*). Neurocognitive deficits and functional outcome in schizophrenia: Are we measuring the 'right stuff'? *Schizophr. Bull.* **26**, 119–36.

Green, M.F., Kern, R.S., Robertson, M.J., Sergi, M.J., and Kee, K.S. (2000*b*). Relevance of neurocognitive deficits for functional outcome in schizophrenia. In *Cognition in schizophrenia: impairments, importance and treatment strategies* (ed. T. Sharma and P. Harvey), pp. 178–92. Oxford University Press, Oxford.

Green, M.F., Nuechterlein, K.H., Gold, J.M., Barch, D.M., Cohen, J., Essock, S., Fenton, W.S., Frese, F., Goldberg, T.E., Heaton, R.K., Keefe, R.S., Kern, R.S., Kraemer, H., Stover, E., Weinberger, D.R., Zalcman, S., and Marder, S.R. (2004). Approaching a consensus cognitive battery for clinical trials in schizophrenia: the NIMH-MATRICS conference to select cognitive domains and test criteria. *Biol. Psychiatry* **56**, 301–7.

Greenwood, K.E., Landau, S., and Wykes, T. (2005). Negative symptoms and specific cognitive impairments as combined targets for improved functional outcome within cognitive remediation therapy. *Schizophr. Bull.* **31**, 910–21.

Gschwandtner, U., Aston, J., Borgwardt, S., Drewe, M., Feinendegen, C., Lacher, D., Lanzarone, A., Stieglitz, R.D., and Riecher-Rossler, A. (2003). Neuropsychological and neurophysiological findings in individuals suspected to be at risk for schizophrenia: preliminary results from the Basel early detection of psychosis study—Fruherkennung von Psychosen (FEPSY). *Acta Psychiatr. Scand.* **108**, 152–5.

Gunnell, D., Harrison, G., Rasmussen, F., Fouskakis, D., and Tynelius, P. (2002). Associations between premorbid intellectual performance, early-life exposures and early-onset schizophrenia. Cohort study. *Br. J. Psychiatry* **181**, 298–305.

Hafner, H., Maurer, K., Loffler, W., and Riecher-Rossler, A. (1993). The influence of age and sex on the onset and early course of schizophrenia. *Br. J. Psychiatry* **162**, 80–6.

Halligan, P.W. and David, A.S. (2001). Cognitive neuropsychiatry: towards a scientific psychopathology. *Nat. Rev. Neurosci.* **2** (3), 209–15.

Harvey, P.D., Lombardi, J., Leibman, M., White, L., Parrella, M., Powchik, P., and Davidson, M. (1996). Cognitive impairment and negative symptoms in geriatric chronic schizophrenic patients: a follow-up study. *Schizophr. Res.* **22**, 223–31.

Hawkins, K.A., Addington, J., Keefe, R.S., Christensen, B., Perkins, D.O., Zipurksy, R., Woods, S.W., Miller, T.J., Marquez, E., Breier, A., and McGlashan, T.H. (2004). Neuropsychological status of subjects at high risk for a first episode of psychosis. *Schizophr. Res.* **67**, 115–22.

Heinrichs, R.W. and Zakzanis, K.K. (1998). Neurocognitive deficit in schizophrenia: a quantitative review of the evidence. *Neuropsychology* **12**, 426–45.

Hemsley, D.R. (1994). Perceptual and cognitive abnormalities as the bases for schizophrenic symptoms. In *The neuropsychology of schizophrenia* (ed. A. David and J. Cutting), pp. 97–116. Psychology Press, Hove.

Heston, L.L. (1966). Psychiatric disorders in foster home reared children of schizophrenic mothers. *Br. J. Psychiatry* **112**, 819–25.

Heydebrand, G., Weiser, M., Rabinowitz, J., Hoff, A.L., DeLisi, L.E., and Csernansky, J.G. (2004). Correlates of cognitive deficits in first episode schizophrenia. *Schizophr. Res.* **68**, 1–9.

Hirstein., W. and Ramachandran., V. S. (1997) Capgras syndrome: a novel probe for understanding the neural representation of the identity and familiarity of persons. *Proc. R. Soc. Lond. B* **264** (1380), 437–44.

Ho, B.C., Andreasen, N.C., Flaum, M., Nopoulos, P., and Miller, D. (2000). Untreated initial psychosis: its relation to quality of life and symptom remission in first-episode schizophrenia. *Am. J. Psychiatry* **157**, 808–15.

Ho, B.C., Alicata, D., Ward, J., Moser, D.J., O'Leary, D.S., Arndt, S., and Andreasen, N.C. (2003). Untreated initial psychosis: relation to cognitive deficits and brain morphology in first-episode schizophrenia. *Am. J. Psychiatry* **160**, 142–8.

Hoff, A.L., Sakuma, M., Razi, K., Heydebrand, G., Csernansky, J.G., and DeLisi, L.E. (2000). Lack of association between duration of untreated illness and severity of cognitive and structural brain deficits at the first episode of schizophrenia. *Am. J. Psychiatry* **157**, 1824–8.

Hughes, C., Kumari, V., Soni, W., Das, M., Binneman, B., Drozd, S., O'Neil, S., Mathew, V., and Sharma, T. (2003). Longitudinal study of symptoms and cognitive function in chronic schizophrenia. *Schizophr. Res.* **59**, 137–46.

Hutton, S.B., Puri, B.K., Duncan, L.J., Robbins, T.W., Barnes, T.R., and Joyce, E.M. (1998). Executive function in first-episode schizophrenia. *Psychol. Med.* **28**, 463–73.

Isohanni, I., Jarvelin, M.R., Nieminen, P., Jones, P., Rantakallio, P., Jokelainen, J., and Isohanni, M. (1998). School performance as a predictor of psychiatric hospitalization in adult life. A 28-year follow-up in the Northern Finland 1966 Birth Cohort. *Psychol. Med.* **28**, 967–74.

Jablensky, A. (1997). The 100-year epidemiology of schizophrenia. *Schizophr. Res.* **28**, 111–25.

Jablensky, A., Sartorius, N., Ernberg, G., Anker, M., Korten, A., Cooper, J.E., Day, R., and Bertelsen, A. (1992). Schizophrenia: manifestations., incidence and course in different cultures. A World Health Organization ten-country study. *Psychol. Med. Monogr. Suppl.* **20**, 1–97.

Johnstone, E.C., Lawrie, S.M., and Cosway, R. (2002). What does the Edinburgh high-risk study tell us about schizophrenia? *Am. J. Med. Genet.* **114**, 906–12.

Jones, P., Rodgers, B., Murray, R., and Marmot, M. (1994). Child development risk factors for adult schizophrenia in the British 1946 birth cohort. *Lancet* **344**, 1398–402.

Jones, P.B., Rantakallio, P., Hartikainen, A.L., Isohanni, M., and Sipila, P. (1998). Schizophrenia as a long-term outcome of pregnancy, delivery, and perinatal complications: a 28-year follow-up of the 1966 north Finland general population birth cohort. *Am. J. Psychiatry* **155**, 355–64.

Jones, S.H., Gray, J.A., and Hemsley, D.R. (1992). Loss of the Kamin blocking effect in acute but not chronic schizophrenics. *Biol. Psychiatry* **32** (9), 739–55.

Joyce, E., Hutton, S., Mutsatsa, S., Gibbins, H., Webb, E., Paul, S., Robbins, T., and Barnes, T. (2002). Executive dysfunction in first-episode schizophrenia and relationship to duration of untreated psychosis: the West London Study. *Br. J. Psychiatry Suppl.* **43**, s38–44.

Kapur, S. (2003). Psychosis as a state of aberrant salience: a framework linking biology., phenomenology and pharmacology in schizophrenia. *Am. J. Psychiatry* **190**, 13–23.

Kapur, S., Mizrahi, R., and Li, M. (2005). From dopamine to salience to psychosis—linking biology, pharmacology and phenomenology of psychosis. *Schizophr. Res.* **79**, 59–68.

Kendler, K.S. and Diehl, S.R. (1993). The genetics of schizophrenia: a current, genetic–epidemiologic perspective. *Schizophr. Bull.* **19**, 261–85.

Kety, S.S., Rosenthal, D., Wender, P.H., and Schulsinger, F. (1971). Mental illness in the biological and adoptive families of adopted schizophrenics. *Am. J. Psychiatry* **128**, 302–6.

Kim, J., Glahn, D.C., Nuechterlein, K.H., and Cannon, T. (2004). Maintenance and manipulation of information in schizophrenia: further evidence for impairment in the central executive component of working memory. *Schizophr. Res.* **68**, 173–87.

Kremen, W.S., Seidman, L.J., Faraone, S.V., Toomey, R., and Tsuang, M.T. (2000). The paradox of normal neuropsychological function in schizophrenia. *J. Abnorm. Psychol.* **109**, 743–52.

Kurtz. M.M. (2005). Neurocognitive impairment across the lifespan in schizophrenia: an update. *Schizophr. Res.* **74**, 15–26.

Kurtz, M.M., Ragland, J.D., Bilker, W., Gur, R.C., and Gur, R.E. (2001). Comparison of the continuous performance test with and without working memory demands in healthy controls and patients with schizophrenia. *Schizophr. Res.* **48**, 307–16.

Larsen, T.K., McGlashan, T.H., Johannessen, J.O., and Vibe-Hansen, L. (1996). First-episode schizophrenia: II. Premorbid patterns by gender. *Schizophr. Bull.* **22**, 257–69.

Laurent, A., Biloa-Tang, M., Bougerol, T., Duly, D., Anchisi, A.M., Bosson, J.L., Pellat, J., d'Amato, T., and Dalery, J. (2000). Executive/attentional performance and measures of schizotypy in patients with schizophrenia and in their nonpsychotic first-degree relatives. *Schizophr. Res.* **46**, 269–83.

Li, C.S. (2004). Do schizophrenia patients make more perseverative than non-perseverative errors on the Wisconsin Card Sorting Test? A meta-analytic study. *Psychiatry Res.* **129**, 179–90.

Light, G.A. and Braff, D.L. (2005*a*). Mismatch negativity deficits are associated with poor functioning in schizophrenia patients. *Arch. Gen. Psychiatry* **62** (2), 127–36.

Light, G.A. and Braff, D.L. (2005*b*). Stability of mismatch negativity deficits and their relationship to functional impairments in chronic schizophrenia. *Am. J. Psychiatry* **162** (9), 1741–3.

Liu, S.K., Chiu, C.H., Chang, C.J., Hwang, T.J., Hwu, H.G., and Chen, W.J. (2002). Deficits in sustained attention in schizophrenia and affective disorders: stable versus state-dependent markers. *Am. J. Psychiatry* **159**, 975–82.

Loebel, A.D., Lieberman, J.A., Alvir, J.M., Mayerhoff, D.I., Geisler, S.H., and Szymanski, S.R. (1992). Duration of psychosis and outcome in first-episode schizophrenia. *Am. J. Psychiatry* **149**, 1183–8.

Marder, S.R., Fenton, W., and Youens, K. (2004). Schizophrenia., IX: Cognition in Schizophrenia—the MATRICS initiative. *Am. J. Psychiatry* **161** (1), 25.

Marshall, M. and Lockwood, A. (2004). Early intervention for psychosis. *Cochrane Database Syst. Rev.* CD004718.

Maruff, P., Wilson, P., and Currie, J. (2003). Abnormalities of motor imagery associated with somatic passivity phenomena in schizophrenia. *Schizophr. Res.* **60** (2–3), 229–38.

McDermid Vaz, S.A. and Heinrichs, R.W. (2002). Schizophrenia and memory impairment: evidence for a neurocognitive subtype. *Psychiatry Res* **113**, 93–105.

Mcghie, A. and Chapman, J. (1961). Disorders of attention and perception in early schizophrenia. *Br. J. Med. Psychol.* **34**, 103–16.

McGlashan, T.H. (1999). Duration of untreated psychosis in first-episode schizophrenia: marker or determinant of course? *Biol. Psychiatry* **46**, 899–907.

McGrath, J.J. (2005). Myths and plain truths about schizophrenia epidemiology—The NAPE lecture 2004. *Acta Psychiatr. Scand.* **111**, 4–11.

McGrath, J., Chapple, B., and Wright, M. (2001). Working memory in schizophrenia and mania: correlation with symptoms during the acute and subacute phases. *Acta Psychiatr. Scand.* **103**, 181–8.

McGurk, S.R. and Meltzer, H.Y. (2000). The role of cognition in vocational functioning in schizophrenia. *Schizophr. Res.* **45**, 175–84.

McGurk, S.R., Moriarty, P.J., Harvey, P.D., Parrella, M., White, L., and Davis, K.L. (2000). The longitudinal relationship of clinical symptoms, cognitive functioning, and adaptive life in geriatric schizophrenia. *Schizophr. Res.* **42**, 47–55.

McKenna, P.J., Tamlyn, D., Lund, C.E., Mortimer, A.M., Hammond, S., and Baddeley, A.D. (1990). Amnesic syndrome in schizophrenia. *Psychol. Med.* **20**, 967–72.

Mcqueen, G., Galway, T., Goldberg, J.O., and Tipper, S.P. (2003). Impaired distractor inhibition in patients with schizophrenia on a negative priming task. *Psychol. Med.* **33**, 121–9.

Miller, R. (1976). Schizophrenic psychology, associative learning and forebrain dopamine. *Med. Hypotheses* **2**, 203–11.

Miller, R. (1993). Striatal dopamine in reward and attention: a system for understanding the symptomatology of acute schizophrenia and mania. *Int. Rev. Neurobiol.* **35**, 161–278.

Mohamed, S., Paulsen, J.S., O'Leary, D., Arndt, S., and Andreasen, N. (1999). Generalized cognitive deficits in schizophrenia: a study of first-episode patients. *Arch. Gen. Psychiatry* **56**, 749–54.

Moritz, S., Andresen, B., Perro, C., Schickel, M., Krausz, M., and Naber, D. (2002). Neurocognitive performance in first-episode and chronic schizophrenic patients. *Eur. Arch. Psychiatry Clin. Neurosci.* **252**, 33–7.

Murray, R.M. and Lewis, S.W. (1987). Is schizophrenia a neurodevelopmental disorder? *Br. Med. J. (Clin. Res. Ed.)* **295**, 681–2.

Munro, J.C., Russell, A.J., Murray, R.M., Kerwin, R.W., and Jones, P.B. (2002). IQ in childhood psychiatric attendees predicts outcome of later schizophrenia at 21 year follow-up. *Acta Psychiatr. Scand.* **106**, 139–42.

Nieuwenstein, M.R., Aleman, A., and de Haan, E.H. (2001). Relationship between symptom dimensions and neurocognitive functioning in schizophrenia: a meta-analysis of WCST and CPT studies. Wisconsin Card Sorting Test. Continuous Performance Test. *J. Psychiatr. Res.* **35**, 119–25.

Norman, R.M., Malla, A.K., Cortese, L., Cheng, S., Diaz, K., McIntosh, E., McLean, T.S., Rickwood, A., and Voruganti, L.P. (1999). Symptoms and cognition as predictors of community functioning: a prospective analysis. *Am. J. Psychiatry* **156**, 400–5.

Norman, R.M.G., Malla, A.K., McLean, T., Voruganti, L.P.N., Cortese, L., McIntosh, E., Cheng, S., and Rickwood, A. (2000). The relationship of symptoms and level of functioning in schizophrenia to general wellbeing and the Quality of Life Scale. *Acta Psychiat. Scand.* **102**, 303–9.

Norman, R.M., Townsend, L., and Malla, A.K. (2001). Duration of untreated psychosis and cognitive functioning in first-episode patients. *Br. J. Psychiatry* **179**, 340–5.

Norman, R.M., Lewis, S.W., and Marshall, M. (2005). Duration of untreated psychosis and its relationship to clinical outcome. *Br. J. Psychiatry Suppl.* **48**, s19–23.

Oades, R.D., Zimmerman, B., and Eggers, C. (1996). Conditioned blocking in patients with paranoid, non-paranoid psychosis or obsessive compulsive disorder: associations with symptoms, personality and monoamine metabolism. *J. Psychiatr. Res.* **30** (5), 369–90.

Orzack, M.H. and Kornetsky, C. (1966). Attention dysfunction in chronic schizophrenia. *Arch. Gen. Psychiatry* **14**, 323–6.

Pantelis, C., Velakoulis, D., McGorry, P.D., Wood, S.J., Suckling, J., Phillips, L.J., Yung, A.R., Bullmore, E.T., Brewer, W., Soulsby, B., Desmond, P., and McGuire, P.K. (2003*a*). Neuroanatomical abnormalities before and after onset of psychosis: a cross-sectional and longitudinal MRI comparison. *Lancet* **361**, 281–8.

Pantelis, C., Yucel, M., Wood, S.J., McGorry, P.D., and Velakoulis, D. (2003*b*). Early and late neurodevelopmental disturbances in schizophrenia and their functional consequences. *Aust. NZ J. Psychiatry* **37**, 399–406.

Pantelis, C., Harvey, C.A., Plant, G., Fossey, E., Maruff, P., Stuart, G.W., Brewer, W.J., Nelson, H.E., Robbins, T.W., and Barnes, T.R. (2004). Relationship of behavioural and symptomatic syndromes in schizophrenia to spatial working memory and attentional set-shifting ability. *Psychol. Med.* **34**, 693–703.

Pelletier, M., Achim, A.M., Montoya, A., Lal, S., and Lepage, M. (2005). Cognitive and clinical moderators of recognition memory in schizophrenia: a meta-analysis. *Schizophr. Res.* **74**, 233–52.

Perry, W., Heaton, R.K., Potterat, E., Roebuck, T., Minassian, A., and Braff, D.L. (2001). Working memory in schizophrenia: transient 'online' storage versus executive functioning. *Schizophr. Bull.* **27** (1), 157–76.

Peters, E. and Garety, P. (2006). Cognitive functioning in delusions: a longitudinal analysis. *Behav. Res. Ther.* **44**, 481–514.

Posner, M.I. (1988). Structures and functions of selective attention. In *Master lectures in clinical neuropsychology and brain function: research, measurement and practice* (ed. T. Boll and B. Bryant), pp. 171–202. American Psychological Association, Washington, DC.

Prouteau, A., Verdoux, H., Briand, C., Lesage, A., Lalonde, P., Nicole, L., Reinharz, D., and Stip, E. (2004). The crucial role of sustained attention in community functioning in outpatients with schizophrenia. *Psychiatry Res.* **129**, 171–7.

Rabinowitz, J., De Smedt, G., Harvey, P.D., and Davidson, M. (2002). Relationship between premorbid functioning and symptom severity as assessed at first episode of psychosis. *Am. J. Psychiatry* **159**, 2021–6.

Reichenberg, A., Weiser, M., Rabinowitz, J., Caspi, A., Schmeidler, J., Mark, M., Kaplan, Z., and Davidson, M. (2002). A population-based cohort study of premorbid intellectual., language., and behavioral functioning in patients with schizophrenia., schizoaffective disorder, and nonpsychotic bipolar disorder. *Am. J. Psychiatry* **159**, 2027–35.

Riecher-Rossler, A. and Hafner, H. (2000). Gender aspects in schizophrenia: bridging the border between social and biological psychiatry. *Acta Psychiatr. Scand. Suppl.* **407**, 58–62.

Riecher-Rossler, A., Hafner, H., Stumbaum, M., Maurer, K., and Schmidt, R. (1994). Can estradiol modulate schizophrenic symptomatology? *Schizophr. Bull.* **20**, 203–14.

Rosenthal, D., Wender, P.H., Kety, S.S., Welner, J., andSchulsinger, F. (1971). The adopted-away offspring of schizophrenics. *Am. J. Psychiatry* **128**, 307–11.

Rowe, E.W. and Shean, G. (1997). Card-sort performance and syndromes of schizophrenia. *Genet. Soc. Gen. Psychol. Monogr.* **123**, 197–209.

Rund, B.R. (1998). A review of longitudinal studies of cognitive functions in schizophrenia patients. *Schizophr. Bull.* **24**, 425–35.

Russell, A.J., Munro, J.C., Jones, P.B., Hemsley, D.R., and Murray, R.M. (1997). Schizophrenia and the myth of intellectual decline. *Am. J. Psychiatry* **154**, 635–9.

Rybakowski, J.K. and Borkowska, A. (2002). Eye movement and neuropsychological studies in first-degree relatives of schizophrenic patients. *Schizophr. Res.* **54**, 105–10.

Sartorius, N., Shapiro, R., Kimura, M., and Barrett, K. (1972). WHO international pilot study of schizophrenia. *Psychol. Med.* **2**, 422–5.

Saykin, A.J., Shtasel, D.L., Gur, R.E., Kester, D.B., Mozley, L.H., Stafiniak, P., and Gur, R.C. (1994). Neuropsychological deficits in neuroleptic naive patients with first-episode schizophrenia. *Arch. Gen. Psychiatry* **51**, 124–31.

Schultz, W. and Dickinson, A. (2000). Neuronal coding of prediction errors. *Annu. Rev. Neurosci.* **23**, 473–500.

Scully, P.J., Coakley, G., Kinsella, A., and Waddington, J.L. (1997). Psychopathology, executive (frontal) and general cognitive impairment in relation to duration of initially untreated versus subsequently treated psychosis in chronic schizophrenia. *Psychol. Med.* **27**, 1303–10.

Sharpley, M., Hutchinson, G., McKenzie, K., and Murray, R.M. (2001). Understanding the excess of psychosis among the African-Caribbean population in England. Review of current hypotheses. *Br. J. Psychiatry Suppl.* **40**, s60–8.

Shergill, S.S., Bays, P.M., Frith, C.D., and Wolpert, D.M. (2003). Two eyes for an eye: the neuroscience of force escalation. *Science* **301**, 187.

Shergill, S.S., Samson, G., Bays, P.M., Frith, C.D., and Wolpert, D.M. (2005). Evidence for sensory prediction deficits in schizophrenia. *Am. J. Psychiatry* **162** (12), 2384–2386.

Sims, A. (1988). *Symptoms in the mind.* Bailliere, London.

Sitskoorn, M.M., Aleman, A., Ebisch, S.J., Appels, M.C., and Kahn, R.S. (2004). Cognitive deficits in relatives of patients with schizophrenia: a meta-analysis. *Schizophr. Res.* **71**, 285–95.

Sota, T.L. and Heinrichs, R.W. (2004). Demographic, clinical, and neurocognitive predictors of quality of life in schizophrenia patients receiving conventional neuroleptics. *Compr. Psychiatry* **45**, 415–21.

Sponheim, S.R., Steele, V.R., and McGuire, K.A. (2004). Verbal memory processes in schizophrenia patients and biological relatives of schizophrenia patients: intact implicit memory, impaired explicit recollection. *Schizophr. Res.* **71**, 339–48.

Staal, W.G., Hijman, R., Hulshoff Pol, H.E., and Kahn, R.S. (2000). Neuropsychological dysfunctions in siblings discordant for schizophrenia. *Psychiatry Res.* **95**, 227–35.

Stuss, D.T., Benson, D.F., Kaplan, E.F., Weir, W.S., Naeser, M.A., Lieberman, I., and Ferrill, D. (1983). The involvement of orbitofrontal cerebrum in cognitive tasks. *Neuropsychologia* **21**, 235–48.

Swerdlow, N.R., Stephany, N., Wasserman, L.C., Talledo, J., Sharp, R., Minassian, A., and Auerbach, P.P. (2005). Intact visual latent inhibition in schizophrenia patients in a within-subject paradigm. *Schizophr. Res.* **72** (2–3), 169–83.

Townsend, L.A., Malla, A.K., and Norman, R.M. (2001). Cognitive functioning in stabilized first-episode psychosis patients. *Psychiatry Res.* **104**, 119–31.

Turner, D.C., Clark, L., Pomarol-Clotet, E., McKenna, P., Robbins, T.W., and Sahakian, B.J. (2004). Modafinil improves cognition and attentional set shifting in patients with chronic schizophrenia. *Neuropsychopharmacology* **29**, 1363–73.

Tyson, P.J., Laws, K.R., Roberts, K.H., and Mortimer, A.M. (2004). Stability of set-shifting and planning abilities in patients with schizophrenia. *Psychiatry Res.* **129**, 229–39.

Umbricht, D., Koller, R., Schmid, L., Skrabo, A., Gruebel, C., Huber, T., and Stassen, H. (2003). How specific are deficits in mismatch negativity generation to schizophrenia? *Biol. Psychiatry* **53**, 1120–31.

Velligan, D.I., Mahurin, R.K., Diamond, P.L., Hazleton, B.C., Eckert, S.L., and Miller, A.L. (1997). The functional significance of symptomatology and cognitive function in schizophrenia. *Schizophr. Res.* **25**, 21–31.

Verdoux, H., Liraud, F., Bergey, C., Assens, F., Abalan, F., and van Os, J. (2001). Is the association between duration of untreated psychosis and outcome confounded? A two year follow-up study of first-admitted patients. *Schizophr. Res.* **49**, 231–41.

Voruganti, L.N., Heslegrave, R.J., and Awad, A.G. (1997). Neurocognitive correlates of positive and negative syndromes in schizophrenia. *Can. J. Psychiatry* **42**, 1066–71.

Wahlberg, K.E., Wynne, L.C., Oja, H., Keskitalo, P., Pykalainen, L., Lahti, I., Moring, J., Naarala, M., Sorri, A., Seitamaa, M., Laksy, K., Kolassa, J., and Tienari, P. (1997). Gene–environment interaction in vulnerability to schizophrenia: findings from the Finnish Adoptive Family Study of Schizophrenia. *Am. J. Psychiatry* **154**, 355–62.

Walker, E.F., Savoie, T., and Davis, D. (1994). Neuromotor precursors of schizophrenia. *Schizophr. Bull.* **20**, 441–51.

Weinberger, D.R. (1987). Implications of normal brain development for the pathogenesis of schizophrenia. *Arch. Gen. Psychiatry* **44**, 660–9.

Weinberger, D.R. (1995). From neuropathology to neurodevelopment. *Lancet* **346**, 552–7.

Weinberger, D.R., Berman, K.F., and Zec, R.F. (1986). Physiologic dysfunction of dorsolateral prefrontal cortex in schizophrenia. I. Regional cerebral blood flow evidence. *Arch. Gen. Psychiatry* **43**, 114–24.

Wood, S.J., Pantelis, C., Proffitt, T., Phillips, L.J., Stuart, G.W., Buchanan, J.A., Mahony, K., Brewer, W., Smith, D.J., and McGorry, P.D. (2003). Spatial working memory ability is a marker of risk-for-psychosis. *Psychol. Med.* **33**, 1239–47.

Wyatt, R.J., Green, M.F., and Tuma, A.H. (1997). Long-term morbidity associated with delayed treatment of first admission schizophrenic patients: a re-analysis of the Camarillo State Hospital data. *Psychol. Med.* **27**, 261–8.

Yung., A.R., Phillips., L.J., Yuen., H.P., *et al.* (2003). Psychosis prediction: 12-month follow up of a high-risk ('prodromal') group. *Schizophrenia Res.* **60**, 21–32.

Chapter 20

Neurocognition of depression

Belinda Lennox

People ought to know that the brain is the sole origin of pleasure and joy, laughter and jests, sadness and worry, as well as dysphoria and crying. Through the brain we can think, see, hear, and differentiate between feeling ashamed, good, bad, happy ... Through the brain we become insane, enraged, we develop anxiety and fear, which can come in the night or during the day, we suffer from sleeplessness, we make mistakes and have unfounded worries, we lose the ability to recognize reality, we become apathetic, and we cannot participate in social life. We suffer all those things mentioned.

[Hippocrates 400 BC; translation from Marneros and Goodwin 2005]

20.1 What is depression?

- Depression is a disorder of mood, cognition, and behaviour with associated disturbance of brain structure and function.
- Psychomotor retardation reflects ventral striatum-cortico-thalamic network dysfunction and is associated with severe depression.
- There is decreased hippocampal volume and disturbed memory and learning in depression.
- Amygdala–anterior cingulate networks normally responsible for emotion regulation are disturbed in depression.
- Cognitive distortions seen in depression have associated abnormalities in prefrontal regions.
- Neurocognitive characteristics can distinguish between unipolar and bipolar depressive disorders.

It can be claimed that there is an epidemic of depression. Lifetime prevalence estimates for major depressive disorder range from 15% to 17% (95% confidence interval (CI); American Psychiatric Association 1994). There is an associated huge global burden of morbidity, ranking second only to ischaemic heart disease (WHO; *http://www.who.int/healthinfo/bodgbd2002revised/en/index.html*). However, in spite of the disorder being recognized since ancient times, we still have few clues as to the aetiology of the disorder. It is known to have a moderate genetic heritability (Kendler *et al.* 2006), more so in women than men. Specific genes have not been identified, and it is improbable that there is a single gene of major effect.

Within this diagnostic label there is marked heterogeneity. The milder end of the spectrum appears to be a different type of disorder to more moderate depressive disorder, with a natural history that tends to resolve over time, and with poor response to antidepressant medication. At the other end of the spectrum severe depression with psychotic symptoms seems a different disorder again, with shared genetic associations with other psychotic illness, and treatment and outcome also more akin to those of psychotic disorders than moderate depressive disorders. The current diagnostic system adopts a 'pick and mix' system of symptoms, with no particular symptom type having more diagnostic importance than another, although depressed mood or anhedonia has to be present in all cases (Table 20.1).

A different approach to the definition of disorder is by taking a dimensional, symptom-based approach. Depression is a combination of affective, cognitive, and behavioural symptoms. Each of these symptom types is probably related to different brain processes that are altered in the depressed state. A further line of investigation is in the exploring of these brain processes. Even if the symptoms presenting in the patients are not able to discriminate between the underlying aetiologies, it is possible that associated neurocognitive deficits do. This so-called endophenotypic approach to investigation is an exciting new direction for psychiatric research.

20.2 **Endophenotypes**

Endophenotypes are hidden markers of the disorder that are detectable by neuropsychological testing, structural, or functional magnetic resonance imaging (fMRI) investigation. They form a

Table 20.1 DSM-IV symptom criteria for major depressive disorder (American Psychiatric Association 1994)

Five (or more) of the following symptoms have been present during the same 2 week period and represent a change from previous functioning. At least one of the symptoms is either: (1) depressed mood; or (2) loss of interest or pleasure.

1 Depressed mood most of the day, nearly every day, as indicated by either subjective report (e.g. feels sad or empty) or observation made by others (e.g. appears tearful). Note: In children and adolescents, can be irritable mood

2 Markedly diminished interest or pleasure in all or almost all activities most of the day, nearly every day (as indicated by either subjective account or observation made by others)

3 Significant weight loss when not dieting or weight gain (e.g. a change of more than 5% of body weight in a month) or decrease or increase in appetite nearly every day. Note: In children, consider failure to make expected weight gains

4 Insomnia or hypersomnia nearly every day

5 Psychomotor agitation or retardation nearly every day (observable by othersnot merely subjective feelings of restlessness or being slowed down)

6 Fatigue or loss of energy nearly every day

7 Feelings of worthlessness or excessive or inappropriate guilt (which may be delusional) nearly every day (not merely self-reproach or guilt about being sick)

8 Diminished ability to think or concentrate, or indecisiveness, nearly every day (either by subjective account or as observed by others)

9 Recurrent thoughts of death (not just fear of dying), recurrent suicidal ideation without a specific plan, or a suicide attempt, or a specific plan for committing suicide

bridge between clinical symptomatology and underlying genetic aetiology. They are quantifiable trait manifestations of the disorder, are continuous variables within the population that are defined both by fewer genes than the clinical phenotype, and are less removed from the site of gene action. (Gottesman and Shields 1973). This approach has been utilized successfully in other medical and psychiatric disorders, but has so far not been developed in the study of psychiatric disorders (Gottesman and Gould 2003). Criteria used to identify endophenotypes are that they must be associated with illness in the population, they must be state-independent, they must be heritable, they must co-segregate with illness within families, and they must be found in non-affected family members at a higher rate than in the general population.

Possible candidates for endophenotypic markers for depression are now discussed, grouped together by functional association.

20.3 **Psychomotor symptoms and the basal ganglia**

> He is apparently unable to move and express himself freely. This very circumstance, that the answers come slowly, even on matters of indifference, shows that in this patient we have not to deal with a fear of expressing himself but with some general obstacle to the utterance of speech. Indeed, not only speech but all action of the will is extremely difficult to him. This constraint is by far the most obvious clinical feature of the disease and compared with this, the sad, oppressed mood has but little prominence.
>
> Kraepelin 1904

Psychomotor retardation is the characteristic feature of melancholic depression. Objective measures of motor responsiveness and levels of motor activity are reduced.

Psychomotor retardation is a key clinical feature of major depressive disorder, with slowed reaction times, decreased motor activity, and slowed speech consistently being demonstrated. Retardation is associated with global severity of depression and, in particular, with psychotic depression. It is a predictor of response to some antidepressant treatment. In previous diagnostic systems, motor retardation was thought to be a useful discriminator between so-called endogenous and neurotic subgroups of depressed patients. In addition, psychomotor symptoms have discriminatory value in separating out patients not meeting the criteria for major depressive disorder, unlike other so-called biological symptoms, such as disturbed sleep, appetite loss, or loss of energy (Sobin and Sackheim 1997).

'Psychomotor retardation' as referred to by psychiatrists is the same phenomenon as the neurologists' 'bradykinesia', where it is viewed as an indication of nigrostriatal dopamine loss as part of the clinical phenotype of Parkinson's disease. There is a close relationship between depressive illness and Parkinson's disease, with depression predisposing to Parkinson's disease and Parkinson's disease predisposing to depression. A direct illustration of this close association of mood and movement can be seen in patients with Parkinson's disease who experience fluctuations in motor state (on and off periods). These fluctuations occur on a daily basis and have a direct relationship to the dopaminergic system, in that they respond to dopaminergic treatment. Associated with these motor fluctuations are fluctuations in mood, with slowness of thinking, fatigue, and depression described. These on–off phenomena demonstrate the ability to directly influence mood state with neurochemical fluctuation. Unlike many of the neurocognitive abnormalities associated with depression that are described below, these rapidly changing states of depression associated with basal ganglia dysfunction cannot be thought of as secondary to negative automatic thoughts or distorted perception, or other higher cognitive functions. Instead, they seem to be subcortical in origin (Lennox and Lennox 2002).

It is therefore not surprising that functional imaging studies have demonstrated basal ganglia dysfunction in primary depressive disorder. However, there have been very few studies to separate out the motor symptoms of depression and relate them to specific functional imaging deficits. One positron emission tomography (PET) study associated high scores on psychomotor retardation factor with reduced blood flow in left dorsolateral prefrontal cortex and angular cortex (Bench *et al.* 1993) and another single photon emission computerized tomography (SPECT) study associated psychomotor slowing with hypoperfusion of the inferior frontal and anterior temporal cortex and anterior cingulate cortex (Mayberg *et al.* 1994) Another line of association is the finding of white matter hyperintenisities, particularly in more elderly depressed groups. Subcortical hyperintensities, particularly in the caudate, are associated with a poor prognosis in those with a late onset depression and no family history of depressive illness. These findings indicate that ischaemic changes in basal ganglia and subcortical structures can act as a cause for depression in this group.

These findings therefore indicate a ventral striatum–cortical-thalamic circuit in the association of slowed movement and depressed mood that has particular prognostic and treatment indications in depression.

20.4 **Memory dysfunction and the hippocampus**

There have been many studies clearly demonstrating impairments in all aspects of memory and learning in depression (visual and verbal, short- as well as long-term) Clinically, patients have distorted memory for negative experiences and a hazy recollection of events when unwell. Decreased hippocampal volume in depression is the most consistent finding from structural imaging studies in depression.

The hippocampus is smaller in volume in depression than in age- and sex-matched controls. It also appears as though hippocampal volume directly relates to performance on memory tasks. There is an indication that this level of cognitive impairment on memory tasks increases with number of episodes of depression, which would be compatible with the notion that episodes of illness have a toxic effect upon memory regions. In support of this the hippocampal volume loss may be more prominent in those with recurrent or chronic illness (Videbech and Ravnkilde 2004) and in older patients.

The direct association between clinical symptom, cognitive abnormality, and structural deficit is an attractive model for evolution of depression. The mechanism for this atrophy is assumed to be the effects of glucocorticoids. Raised levels of corticosteroids have been shown to impair both learning and memory. The hippocampus also has a role in regulating the hippocampal–pituitary–adrenal (HPA) axis. There is therefore a mechanistic link with other risk factors for depressive illness such as early life stresses as well as later chronic stress, which all affect circulating glucocorticoid levels The fact that these anatomical changes are also seen in children indicates that the effect of glucocorticoids in early life, and even prenatally, can affect brain development and possibly a later susceptibility to depressive illness.

It is proposed that antidepressants can reverse this atrophy. It is not known whether this improvement in hippocampal size on treatment is directly related to improvement in episodic memory, however, or how this relates to longer-term prognosis. More work needs to be done on the aetiological significance of memory disturbance and hippocampal abnormality.

20.5 **Emotion processing and the amygdala**

Depressed people have distorted perceptions of emotional stimuli. Studies show that, when depressed, people tend to perceive neutral information as more negative and are biased towards negatively intoned information. They will react more quickly when shown negative words or pictures than when shown neutral or positive material. Studies have tried to separate out the cognitive stage at which this bias occurs. Is it that depressed people only take in information that is congruent with their mood state? Or is it that there isn't a bias at the level of attention, but rather that, at a higher level, negatively intoned information is prefentially processed and laid down in memory or, at an even later stage, with recall from memory?

Studies indicate that biases actually occur at every level of cognitive processing of emotion. Studies using a dot-probe paradigm also suggest that there is a deficit in attention in depression. For this task, two faces are briefly presented on a screen, one with a neutral face and one with an emotional face. A probe is then presented in the location of one of the faces, and subjects are asked to respond to the location of the probe. A faster response to the probe following an emotional face indicates a bias towards the emotion. Subjects with depression consistently attended preferentially to the sad faces more than neutral faces, and more than happy faces. This was in contrast to the healthy controls (Gotlib *et al.* 2004). This indicates that there is an attentional bias in depression. There is also bias in memory for emotional information in depression. Patients will recall more negative than positive information. To try and assess whether this relates to the storage and recall of information in memory rather than just a selective attention difficulty, an event-related potential (ERP) study followed the presentation of neutral, happy, and sad stimuli to depressed patients. This showed a lack of attenuation of amplitude in the slow wave component of the ERP in response to sad faces in the depressed group, and a diminished response to happy cues (Shestyuk *et al.* 2005). This indicates that later manipulation and memory processes are affected in depression as well as earlier information attentional processes.

Assessment of mood processing during fMRI studies has used assessment of these affective biases, i.e. the distortion that depressed patients experience towards negative or depressing stimuli. This may be in the form of words, pictures, faces, or sounds. The regions identified form an emotion regulation affective cortico-striato-thalamic loop, including amygdala and ventral striatum. Depressed patients tend to overactivate these areas in response to negative emotional stimuli, and underactivate in response to positive emotional stimuli.

The level of overactivity in the amygdala has been a particular area of focus, and has been associated with severity of depressed mood (Abercrombie *et al.* 1998). This overactivity subsides following treatment with antidepressants (Fu *et al.* 2004; Sheline *et al.* 2001). In trying to separate out the primary abnormality in the prefrontal-amygdala loop, it is suggested that a lack of feedback from anterior cingulate cortex may result in a lack of regulation of amygdala response to emotion. An interesting related finding is the relationship between the polymorphism of the serotonin transporter gene and alteration in the feedback circuitry between amygdala and anterior cingulate in response to fearful emotional faces. This study was in healthy control subjects, but provides a possible mechanism for a susceptibility to depression in those carrying the s allele of serotonin transporter promoter gene (Pezawas *et al.* 2005).

Structural imaging studies of amygdala volumes in depression have been inconsistent, however, with some showing enlarged volumes, and some showing decreased volumes. There is more consistency in the study of children, with small amygdalae being more reliably demonstrated (Campbell and McQueen 2006).

An important associated cortical region in the emotion-processing network is the anterior cingulate cortex, and this region has been consistently identified during functional imaging studies of emotion processing in depression. Further support comes from a structural MRI study of subgenual anterior cingulate cortex that indicated that this area was significantly decreased in a group of depressed patients compared with controls (Drevets *et al.* 1997). A neuropathological study of subgenual cingulate indicated a decrease in glial density and number in patients with a family history of depression.

An interesting avenue of investigation of the functional neural networks implicated in depression is the study of the effects of direct electrical stimulation of some of the areas thought to be pathologically involved in the depressed state. In one study, implantation of deep brain stimulation electrodes in the subgenual anterior cingulate in six patients with treatment-resistant depressive illness produced a remission in four of six subjects. The observation was that the initial response was in melancholic symptoms, with an improvement in sleep in the first week, and increase in psychomotor activity with a concomitant improvement in energy and enjoyment. Following a blinded discontinuation of the stimulation there was a decrease in energy and initiative, concentration, and motivation after a couple of weeks, whilst mood remained euthymic. These symptoms then resolved when the stimulator was turned back on again (Mayberg *et al.* 2005). PET scans in these patients demonstrated a reduced activity in the subgenual cingulate along with other areas, including hypothalamus and mediofrontal and orbitofrontal cortex, as well as increases in other areas, including BA9 and dorsal cingulate and brainstem associated with the deep brain stimulation, supporting the importance of these interconnected regions in the development of cognitive and behavioural aspects of depression. Interestingly, the four who responded had marked melancholic symptoms, whereas the two who did not had more atypical symptoms, as well as a later age of onset.

Deep brain stimulation is also used in the treatment of Parkinson's disease, and the location of the electrodes in these cases is in the subthalamic nucleus area. These studies also report marked effects on mood following treatment, either with acute depression (Berney *et al.* 2002) or transient mania (Kulisevsky *et al.* 2002; Romito *et al.* 2002).

20.6 **Poor motivation, anhedonia, and dorsolateral prefrontal cortex**

Motivation is defined as a drive towards a reward. The lack of motivation seen in depression, which manifests itself in everyday tasks, can be thought of as the lack of pleasure from reward so that, if no pleasure is received from achievement, there is little point in doing the task in the first place.

The lack of motivation experienced when depressed also extends to a lack of motivation in the completion of neuropsychological tests. It has been suggested that a lack of motivation may wholly underlie the other neuropsychological deficits that have been demonstrated. It is difficult to extricate motivation as a factor as it is such a common feature of the disorder. One way to try and address the issue is to compare more effortful with more automatic tasks. If motivation were the only factor underlying neuropsychological deficit then depressed subjects should be less impaired in more automatic processes. A particular example is in memory recall, comparing implicit and explicit memory recall. There is a divergence of opinion with some studies showing impairment on both implicit and explicit tasks and other studies showing no deficit on implicit memory recall in depression (reviewed in Elliott *et al.* 2002)

As a way of demonstrating the lack of motivation seen in depression experimentally, reward-based tasks can be used. In these tasks it would be expected that depressed patients would not respond to positive feedback from a task. Therefore, in tasks where financial rewards are given, depressed patients do not improve their performance on the task following a reward, unlike non-depressed control subjects (Austin *et al.* 2001). Conversely, when negative feedback is given when a task is failed, depressed subjects are more likely to fail subsequent tasks, with the negative comments confirming already held negative views (Elliott *et al.* 1997).

Poor motivation is described in neurological terms as abulia, an impoverishment of volition, and is associated with a frontal lobe syndrome, with particular localization to the dorsolateral region of the frontal cortex. This area is functionally connected to other components of a cortical–subcortical network, and lesions in other parts of this network can also therefore result in a frontal lobe syndrome. Lesions in the caudate(Petty *et al.* 1996), globus pallidus (Strub 1989), and thalamus (Sandson *et al.* 1991) have all been implicated. These regions along with other frontal cortical regions have been regularly identified as having abnormal resting blood flow in depressed patients prior to treatment (reviewed in Mayberg *et al.* 2005).

20.7 **Negative cognitions and prefrontal cortex**

A cognitive concept related to the behavioural manifestation of poor motivation is that of the negative cognitive set. This term, described by Beck (1963), entails the negative views held by a depressed person, and encompasses a global view of the past, present, and the future. This pessimistic standpoint includes the key features of hopelessness and helplessness, so that the depressed person may believe that 'whatever I do, it doesn't make any difference' or 'nothing good will ever happen'. It can be seen that, as a result of these negative beliefs, any positive action or activity seems pointless to the depressed person; this causes a secondary loss of motivation.

Functional imaging studies following cognitive therapy treatment for depression offer an insight into the neural network underlying negative thoughts. Cognitive therapy is effective in depression by helping the patient to challenge these negative beliefs about themselves and the world and to change their behaviour as a result. One study compared a group of patients following treatment with paroxetine with a group following treatment with cognitive behavioural therapy (CBT; Goldapple *et al.* 2004). They demonstrated opposite changes in dorsolateral prefrontal cortex following treatment with CBT and treatment with paroxetine, with a decrease in activity in this region following CBT and an increase following paroxetine. The CBT group also demonstrated increased blood flow in other regions, including the hippocampus and parahippocampal regions, again in contrast with the medicated group. The authors propose that these results could be interpreted as a 'top-down' effect of CBT, altering cortical metabolism, with a downstream effect on ventral and limbic regions, altering the processing of emotional stimuli. In contrast, they propose that antidepressants exert a more 'bottom-up' approach, with an alteration and disengagement of limbic-mediated negative information processing, with the later effect of cognitive remodelling. Support for this study comes from a study administering IV citalopram to healthy volunteers (Harmer *et al.* 2005). Subjects were given rating scales before and after the infusion of citalopram. Patients did not feel any happier after acute administration of the antidepressant, but they did demonstrate an altered perception of emotion, in that they rated faces showing sadness as being less sad. The antidepressant provides a rapid altering of the negative filtering of external information, but the subject does not feel brighter in mood until this information results in a recalibration of negative authomatic thought processes.

20.8 **Do any of these abnormalities persist?**

Whilst it is clearly established that there are neuropsychological and neural network abnormalities in attention, memory, emotion processing, and movement during a depressive episode, it is less clear if any of these deficits persist following treatment of an episode, and can therefore be considered trait markers for the disorder. There are some indications that sustained attention and strategic aspects of working memory continue to be impaired in euthymia following a major depressive episode. There is also some evidence that neuropsychological impairment between episodes is more pronounced in those with more episodes of illness (Paelecke-Haberman *et al.* 2005). This may indicate that the illness is having a progressively toxic effect on brain networks.

Clinically, this would relate to the worse prognosis experienced with increasing numbers of episodes of illness.

It is even less clear if any of these abnormalities can be detected in first-degree relatives to a greater extent than in the general population, both required characteristics for an endophenotypic marker for the disorder (Gottesman and Shields 1973). Large-scale, longitudinal follow-up studies of neurocognitive function are required to fully address this issue, in a well delineated patient population as well as in relatives.

20.9 What is different about bipolar depression?

As a way of demonstrating the limitation of clinical phenotype and the value of neurocognitive evaluation and functional neuroimaging as modalities of investigation, it is worth contrasting the findings in unipolar disorder with emerging findings in bipolar disorder. These disorders have separate aetiologies, with bipolar disorder having a higher genetic heritability, at about 80%, and sharing some genetic linkage with other psychotic disorders, but not with unipolar depression (Badner and Gershon 2002).

In spite of the different nature of the disorder, it is difficult to distinguish unipolar and bipolar depression in a patient presenting with a first presentation of depression. Of those with a diagnosis of unipolar depression, about 30% of patients will in time receive a diagnosis of bipolar disorder. Using clinical phentype is therefore not always sufficient and, if there were therefore a way of distinguishing the diagnosis at presentation using neuropsychological or functional imaging probes, this would have clinical utility as well as providing possible clues as to aetiology.

In studies looking for groupwise differences in clinical presentation, distinguishing features were that depressed patients with a history of bipolar disorder demonstrated more signs of psychomotor retardation, with a non-reactive mood, general slowing of movement, delayed initiation of movement, and facial immobility. However, as these were clinical groups, medication was not controlled for, and bipolar patients tend to be prescribed antipsychotic drugs with extrapyramidal side-effects, indistinguishable from 'psychomotor slowing'. Other features more commonly seen in bipolar depression were of persistent and unvarying low mood and less tearfulness and anxiety. These seem to be the same 'subcortical' features of the depressive syndrome seen in basal ganglia–thalamo-cortical circuit disturbance.

In neuropsychological profiling of bipolar depression, similar abnormalities in attention, memory, and executive functioning have been shown, as well as shared difficulties in problem-solving and decision-making. However, there does appear to be a discrepancy in the bias towards affective information in bipolar depression

In a study using an affective go/no-go task, where subjects have to respond to a happy or sad word shown on a screen, and not respond to a neutral, distractor word, patients showed no difference in their response to sad rather than happy words (Rubinsztein *et al.* 2006). This is in marked contrast to the consistent abnormality in this task shown in unipolar depression. In this study the authors also demonstrated widespread generalized cognitive impairment in patients with bipolar depression, with impairments on tests of attention, visual and spatial recognition, and decision-making. This indicates that there is not a generally improved level of functioning in bipolar depression when compared to unipolar depression, but the converse, with widespread deficits, but a preservation of emotion-processing networks.

Functional imaging studies also demonstrate significant differences between these two depressive disorders. fMRI studies showed enhanced activation by both positive and negative emotional expressions in depressed bipolar patients that was significantly different from the corresponding activation patterns seen in both unipolar depressed patients and healthy controls

(Lawrence *et al.* 2004; Malhi *et al.* 2004). In response to happy faces, depressed bipolar patients significantly overactivated fronto-striato-thalamic regions including superior frontal gyrus, ventral frontal gyrus, precentral gyrus, cingulate, putamen, and thalamus (Fig. 20.1; Chen *et al.* 2006). The particular prefrontal region that appears to be consistently overactive in bipolar disorder is a region of ventromedial prefrontal cortex (Blumberg *et al.* 1999, 2003a; Drevets *et al.* 1997; Elliott *et al.* 2004; Rubinsztein *et al.* 2001; Chen *et al.* 2006). Lesions in this area are associated with symptoms associated with mania including disinhibition and increased risky behaviour (reviewed in Clark *et al.* 2004). It appears that there is a converse overactivity in these ventromedial prefrontal cortical areas, in contrast with decreased dorsolateral prefrontal activity seen in unipolar depression.

In linking the neuropsychological and functional imaging findings together, it is an interesting observation that patients with bipolar depression do not appear to show the dorsolateral prefrontal–limbic functional abnormalities seen in unipolar depression and, in keeping with this, do not appear to have the negative biases in emotion processing on neuropsychological testing. As an extrapolation of these findings it might be hypothesized that those with bipolar depression would also be less amenable to cognitive therapy than those with unipolar depression and,

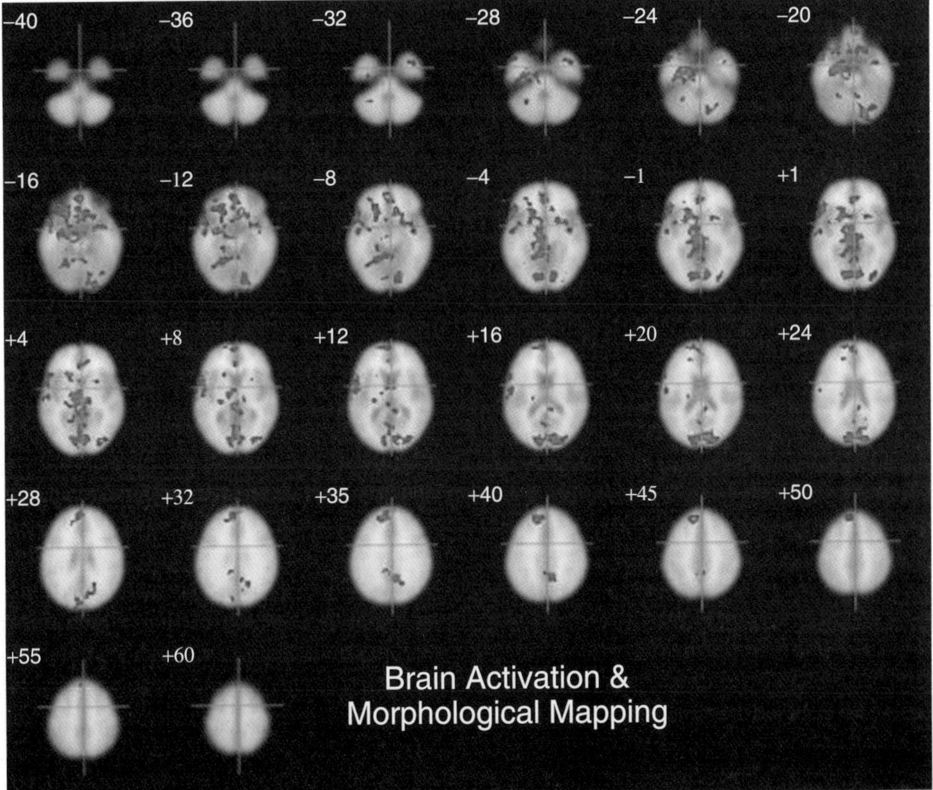

Fig. 20.1 Areas of increased activation in bipolar depressed patients looking at happy faces, relative to matched control subjects. (Data from Chen *et al.* 2006.) Widespread overactivation of fronto-striatal-thalamic regions, including superior frontal gyrus, ventral frontal gyrus, precentral gyrus, cingulate, putamen, and thalamus, in marked contrast to underactivation seen in unipolar depression.

although studies are not consistent, the largest randomized controlled study of CBT in bipolar disorder supports this (Scott *et al.* 2006).

20.10 Conclusions

Depression is an organic brain disorder. It can be viewed as abnormality in different groups of cortico-subcortical neural networks that are often associated, but are to some extent dissociable. Poor memory is associated with abnormality in the hippocampal network, poor motivation and cognitive processing with dorsolateral prefrontal cortical network abnormalities, and psychomotor retardation with abnormalities in basal ganglia and connections. Emotion-processing biases are associated with amygdala–anterior cingulate network abnormality. Bipolar depression appears to be a different type of disorder, with particular abnormalities in the basal ganglia and connections and with a preservation of the amygdala–anterior cingulate network function.

References

Abercrombie, H.C., Schaefer, S.M., Larson, C.L., *et al.* (1998). Metabolic rate in the right amygdala predicts negative affect in depressed patients. *Neuroreport* **9**, 3301–7.

American Psychiatric Association (1994). *Diagnostic and statistical manual of mental disorders*, 4th edn (DSM-IV). APA, Washington DC.

Austin, M.P., Mitchell, P., and Goodwin, G.M. (2001). Cognitive deficits in depression. *Br. J. Psychiatry* **178**, 200–6.

Badner, J.A. and Gershon, E.S. (2002). Meta-analysis of whole-genome linkage scans of bipolar disorder and schizophrenia. *Mol. Psychiatry* **7**, 405–11.

Beck, A.T. (1963). Thinking and depression. *Arch. Gen. Psychiatry* **9**, 324–33.

Bench, C.J., Friston, K.J., Brown, R.G., Frackowiak, R.S., and Dolan, R.J. (1993). Regional cerebral blood flow in depression measured by positron emission tomography: the relationship with clinical dimensions. *Psychol. Med.* **23**, 579–90.

Berney, A., Vingerhoets, F., Perrin, A., *et al.* (2002). Effect on mood of subthalamic DBS for Parkinson's disease: a consecutive series of 24 patients. *Neurology* **59**, 1427–9.

Blumberg, H.P., Stern, E., Ricketts, S., Martinez, D., de Asis, J., White, T. *et al.* (1999). Rostral and orbital prefrontal cortex dysfunction in the manic state of bipolar disorder. *Am. J. Psychiatry* **156**, 1986–8.

Blumberg, H.P., Leung, H.C., Skudlarski, P., Lacadie, C.M., Fredericks, C.A., Harris, B.C. *et al.* (2003). A functional magnetic resonance imaging study of bipolar disorder: state- and trait-related dysfunction in ventral prefrontal cortices. *Arch. Gen. Psychiatry* **60**, 601–9.

Campbell, S. and MacQueen, G. (2006). An update on regional brain volume differences associated with mood disorders. *Curr. Opin. Psychiatry* **19**, 25–33.

Chen, C.H., Lennox, B.R., Jacob, R., Calder, A.J., Lupson, V., Bisbrown-Chippendale, R., Suckling, J., and Bullmore, E.T. (2006). Explicit and implicit facial affect recognition in manic and depressed states of bipolar disorder: an fMRI study. *Biol. Psychiatry* **59** (1), 31–9.

Clark, L., Cools, R., and Robbins, T.W. (2004). The neuropsychology of ventral prefrontal cortex: decision-making and reversal learning. *Brain Cogn.* **55** (1), 41–53.

Drevets, W.C., Price, J.L., Simpson, J.R. Jr, Todd, R.D., Reich, T., Vannier, M., *et al.* (1997). Subgenual prefrontal cortex abnormalities in mood disorders. *Nature* **386**, 824–7.

Elliott, R., Sahakian, B.J., Herrod, J.J., Robbins, T.W., and Paykel, E.S. (1997). Abnormal response to negative feedback in unipolar depression: evidence for a diagnostic specific impairment. *J. Neurol. Neurosurg. Psychiatry* **63**, 74–82.

Elliott, R., Rubinsztein, J.S., Sahakian, B.J., and Dolan, R.J. (2002). The neural basis of mood-congruent processing biases in depression. *Arch. Gen. Psychiatry* **59**, 597–604.

Elliott, R., Ogilvie, A., Rubinsztein, J.S., Calderon, G., Dolan, R.J., and Sahakian, B.J. (2004). Abnormal ventral frontal response during performance of an affective go/no go task in patients with mania. *Biol. Psychiatry* **55**, 1163–70.

Fu, C.H.Y., Williams, S.C.R., Cleare, A.J., Brammer, M.J., Walsh, N.D., Kim, J., *et al.* (2004). Attenuation of the neural response to sad faces in major depression by antidepressant treatment: a prospective, event-related functional magnetic resonance imaging study. *Arch. Gen. Psychiatry* **61**, 877–89.

Goldapple, K., Segal, Z., Garson, C., *et al.* (2004). Modulation of cortical–limbic pathways in major depression. *Arch. Gen. Psychiatry* **61**, 34–41.

Gotlib, I.H., Krasnoperova, E., Neubauer, D., and Joorman, J. (2004). Attentional biases for negative interpersonal stimuli in clinical depression. *J. Abnorm. Psychol.* **113**, 127–35.

Gottesman, I.I. and Gould, T.D. (2003). The endophenotype concept in psychiatry: etymology and strategic intentions. *Am. J. Psychiatry* **160**, 636–45.

Gottesman, I.I. and Shields, J. (1973). Genetic theorising and schizophrenia. *Br. J. Psychiatry* **122**, 15–30.

Harmer, C.J., Shelley, N.C., Cowen, P.J., and Goodwin, G.M. (2004). Increased positive versus negative affective perception and memory in healthy volunteers following selective serotonin and norepinephrine reuptake inhibition. *Am. J. Psychiatry* **161**, 1256–63.

Kendler, K.S., Gatz, M., Gardner, C.O., and Pedersen, N.L. (2006). A Swedish national twin study of lifetime major depression. *Am. J. Psychiatry* **163** (1), 109–14.

Kraepelin, E. (1904). *Lecture on clinical psychiatry*. Republished by Hafner, New York in 1968.

Kulisevsky, J., Berthier, ML., Gironell, A., Pascual-Sedano, B., *et al.* (2002). Mania following deep brain stimulation for Parkinson's disease. *Neurology* **59**, 1421–4.

Lawrence, N.S., Williams, A.M., Surguladze, S., Giampietro, V., Brammer, M.J., Andrew, C., *et al.* (2004). Subcortical and ventral prefrontal cortical neural responses to facial expressions distinguish patients with bipolar disorder and major depression. *Biol. Psychiatry* **55** (6), 578–87.

Lennox, B.R. and Lennox, G.G. (2002). The neuropsychiatry of movement disorders: mind and matter. *J. Neurol. Neurosurg. Psychiatry* **72**, 28–31.

Malhi, G.S., Lagopoulos, J., Ward, P.B., Kumari, V., Mitchell, P.B., Parker, G.B., *et al.* (2004). Cognitive generation of affect in bipolar depression: an fMRI study. *Eur. J. Neurosci.* **19**, 741–54.

Marneros, A. and Goodwin, F.K. (2005). Bipolar disorders beyond major depression and euphoric mania. In *Bipolar disorders: mixed states, rapid cycling, and atypical forms* (ed. A. Marneros and F.K. Goodwin), pp. 1–44. Cambridge University Press, Cambridge.

Mayberg, H.S., Lewis, P.J., Regenold, W., and Wagner, H.N. (1994). Paralimbic hypoperfusion in unipolar depression. *J. Nucl. Med.* **35**, 929–34.

Mayberg, H.S., Lozano, A.M., Voon, V., *et al.* (2005). Deep brain stimulation for treatment-resistant depression. *Neuron* **45**, 651–60.

Paelecke-Habermann, Y., Pohl, J., and Leplow, B. (2005). Attention and executive functions in remitted major depression patients. *J. Affect. Disord.* **89**, 125–35.

Pezawas, L., Meyer-Lindenber, A., Drabant, E.M., *et al.* (2005). 5-HTTLPR polymorphism impacts human cingulate–amygdala interactions: a genetic susceptibility mechanism for depression. *Nat. Neurosci.* **8**, 828–34.

Petty, R.G., Bonner, D., Mouratoglou, V., and Silverman, M. (1996). Acute frontal lobe syndrome and dyscontrol associated with bilateral caudate infarctions. *Br. J. Psychiatry* **168**, 237–40.

Romito, L.M.A., Scerrati, M., Contarino, M.F., Bentivoglio, A.R., Tonali, P., and Albanese, A. (2002). Long-term follow up of subthalamic nucleus stimulation in Parkinson's disease. *Neurology* **58**, 1546–50.

Rubinsztein, J.S., Fletcher, P.C., Rogers, R.D., *et al.* (2001). Decision-making in mania: a PET study. *Brain* **124**, 2550–63.

Rubinsztein, J.S., Michael, A., Underwood, B.R., Tempest, M., and Sahakian, B.J. (2006). Impaired cognition and decision-making in bipolar depression but no 'affective bias' evident. *Psychol. Med.* **36**, 629–39.

Sandson, T.A., Daffner, K.R., Carvalho, P.A., and Mesulam. M.M. (1991). Frontal lobe dysfunction following infarction of the left-sided medial thalamus. *Arch. Neurol.* **48**, 1300–3.

Scott, J., Paykel, E., Morriss, R., Bentall, R., Kinderman, P., Johnson, T., Abbott, R., and Hayhurst, H. (2006). Cognitive-behavioural therapy for severe and recurrent bipolar disorders: randomised controlled trial. *Br. J. Psychiatry* **188**, 313–20.

Sheline, Y.I., Barch, D.M., Donnelly, J.M., Ollinger, J.M., Snyder, A.Z., and Mintun, M.A. (2001). Increased amygdala response to masked emotional faces in depressed subjects resolves with antidepressant treatment: an fMRI study. *Biol. Psychiatry* **50**, 651–8.

Shestyuk, A.Y., Deldin, P.J., Brand, J.E., and Deveney, C.M. (2005). Reduced sustained brain activity during processing of positive emotional stimuli in major depression. *Biol. Psychiatry* **57**, 1089–96.

Sobin, C. and Sackeim, H.A. (1997). Psychomotor symptoms of depression. *Am. J. Psychiatry* **154**, 4–17.

Strub, R.L. (1989). Frontal lobe syndrome in a patient with bilateral globus pallidus lesions. *Arch. Neurol.* **46**, 1024–7.

Videbech, P. and Ravnkilde, B. (2004). Hippocampal volume and depression: a meta-analysis of MRI studies. *Am. J. Psychiatry* **161**, 1957–66.

Chapter 21

'Others' and others: hysteria and the divided self

Sean A. Spence

In hysteria, the incompatible idea is rendered innocuous by its sum of excitation being transformed into something somatic. For this I would like to propose the name of conversion.
[Freud 1894]

21.1 **Introduction**

- In conversion disorder, a key problem lies in understanding how a motor or sensory symptom can be produced in the absence of any known physical cause
- The condition raises a series of uncomfortable questions for the clinician (see Table 21.2):
  - organic or psychogenic?
  - understood in terms of physical or mental processes?
  - feigned or unfeigned?
- One approach to these dilemma is to consider closely the phenomena that comprise hysteria (see Table 21.3):
  - a deficit with no apparent cause;
  - 'unusual features', e.g. improvement when distracted or sedated.
- The observations under distraction may provide a clue that the key cognitive mechanisms in the condition lie at the juncture between automatic and non-automatic behaviour. Under conditions of attentive behaviour (when the executive system is engaged?) the deficit may be clearer. When attention is directed away and the function is automatic, the deficit may ameliorate.
- This interactive model is supported by some data from functional imaging studies suggesting the influence of frontal/attentional systems.
- Any cognitive model of the condition must take into account social factors: the symbolic meaning of the deficit; the setting in which it emerges; the interaction with the clinician and other professionals, culture.

In hysteria, a physical symptom or sign is said to be produced by a psychological mechanism, triggered by a conflict within the patient. Crucially, there is no explanatory physical cause that can be demonstrated.

Hence, the fundamental problem in hysteria is this: 'How can a motor or sensory symptom be produced in the absence of a physical cause?' The man or woman so afflicted reports that they cannot raise their arm, or cannot see; yet physical investigations prove negative and, when sedated or observed unobtrusively over time, symptomatic inconsistencies arise. However, despite these, the diagnostic systems applied (e.g. the DSM-IV; American Psychiatric Association 1994) are quite specific that the patient experiencing and exhibiting such symptoms and signs is not responsible for their production, i.e. they are not 'feigning' (Table 21.1). Hence, the physician is called upon to judge what the patient is thinking and not doing, i.e. to perceive that they are really trying to move or see and are not pretending to be impaired. This is a complex task and, as we shall see (below), the use of language in this area suggests considerable uncertainty among physicians as to what it is they are diagnosing.

21.2 **Terminological ambiguity**

Consider the following comments from the published neurological literature.

1 'I have said to the patient "I know from experience that your pretended [symptom] is the result of some intolerable emotional situation. If you will tell me the whole story I promise absolutely to respect your confidence, will give you all the help I can and will say to your doctor and relatives that I have cured you by hypnotism"' (Sir Charles Symonds 1970, cited in Merskey 1995).

2 'Organic tremor is aggravated by taking the attention away from the area involved and usually improves when attention is directed toward the involved limb ... Functional or psychogenic tremor disappears when attention is withdrawn from the limb or area involved. I will give $25.00 to the first [doctor] who can prove me wrong' (Campbell 1979).

3 'The abductor sign is a useful test to detect non-organic paresis, because (1) it is difficult for a hysterical patient to deceive the examiner ...' (Sanoo 2004).

From these statements one might conclude that, although the neurologists concerned are ostensibly commenting upon 'hysterical', 'conversion', 'functional', or 'psychogenic' disorders (terms that have been used synonymously within the literature), at some level they are acknowledging an element of deception on the part of those whom they diagnose. Hence, the apparent levity at the close of example 2; it is difficult to think of another medical condition where such

Table 21.1 Selected criteria for the diagnosis of conversion disorder (300.11) in the DSM-IV (American Psychiatric Association 1994)

DSM IV criteria A–D for conversion disorder
A One or more symptoms or deficits affecting voluntary motor or sensory function that suggest a neurological or other general medical condition
B Psychological factors are judged to be associated with the symptom or deficit because the initiation or exacerbation of the symptom or deficit is preceded by conflicts or other stressors
C The symptom or deficit is not intentionally produced or feigned
D The symptom or deficit cannot, after appropriate investigation, be fully explained by a general medical condition, or by the effects of a substance, or as a culturally sanctioned behaviour or experience

a challenge might be published. There, is, perhaps, something almost unique about this diagnosis (hysteria), in terms of the difficulties it produces for patients and doctors alike. Does the doctor really believe in the Freudian mechanisms instantiated in the diagnostic systems? Is the doctor acting in good faith if he/she suspects that the patient is feigning? Is there such a condition as 'hysteria' or is it merely a pragmatic label that serves to postpone confrontation? What are the feelings provoked within physicians when they examine and investigate such patients? Some of these difficulties are summarized in Table 21.2.

The problem with hysteria as a diagnosis is that it immediately sets up certain dualisms that may prove to be both inaccurate and unhelpful: is it a disorder of the body (or brain) or mind; one that is organic or psychogenic; conscious (i.e. feigned) or unconscious (the product of conversion); is there a deceiver and their deceived (and which is which); is there villain and victim (and who are they)?

21.3 A phenomenological approach

Perhaps one way through this apparent quagmire is to concentrate, for the time being, upon the objective signs rather than the theories and abstractions that accrue around hysteria. What happens in the clinical encounter? The phenomenology of hysteria has been widely described and revisited recently (see Merskey 1995; Halligan *et al.* 2001; Hallett *et al.* 2006). In the following I will focus upon motor symptoms and signs, largely because they are objectively verifiable and their analysis yields some important clues as to what is going on in hysteria (Table 21.3).

The central finding in the case of motor hysteria is that a movement disorder, either a deficit or an excess of motoric activity, is found to be without demonstrable organic basis. However, in addition, the physical findings on clinical examination do not 'behave' as they should. Hence, the patient may exhibit paralysis in one context but not in another. A tremor may come and go but not in the ways associated with organic disease. Through distraction or sedation the physician may reveal preservation of normal function when the patient's attention is directed elsewhere.

Table 21.2 Some difficulties for patients and doctors when the diagnosis is hysteria

Patient's perspective	Doctor's perspective
Obscure terminology and 'diagnoses'	Various terms are applied: it is not always clear whether illness or malingering is being diagnosed
The cause is unknown	Aetiology is unknown
There are no pathognomonic signs: hence, there is no final 'proof' of illness, no vindication	There are no pathognomonic signs: hence, no 'closure'; the diagnosis is never 'made' but remains conditional
The risks of elaboration: to 'prove' one is 'really' ill	The fear of missing organicity
The question of veracity: knowing one may not be 'believed'	The question of veracity: not wanting to be 'fooled'
The stigma of the psychiatric: the final referral after negative findings	The risk of overinvestigation: repeatedly chasing rare disorders
The implications of litigation, e.g. following a traumatic precipitant: ambivalence, while wishing to recover also wanting to prove harm was done	The implications of litigation: symptoms may not resolve until legal matters have been settled; hence, risk of inferred deception, also therapeutic nihilism
The risk of being 'difficult', diagnostically or personally	'Malignant alienation': failing to help those whom one does not like

Table 21.3 The phenomenology of motor hysteria/conversion (Spence 2006*a*)

Phenomenological characteristics
◆ Relatively acute onset, classically following an emotional precipitant
◆ Biologically implausible: behaves as if 'anatomy did not exist' (Freud)
◆ Variable manifestation: symptomatic inconsistency
◆ Normal movement emerges with distraction (e.g. on the Hoover test) or with sedation (e.g. with benzodiazepines)
◆ If the symptom is a tremor, it reduces during the performance of rhythmic tapping with the contralateral limb
◆ If the symptom is an abnormality of gait, it appears uneconomic: it is more energy-demanding than alternate forms of locomotion, given the implied deficit
◆ Comorbid diagnoses are frequent: commonly depression ±; personality disorder

21.3.1 Distraction and sedation

When performing the Hoover test, the physician examines a patient who is unable to extend his or her affected leg, i.e. cannot press it down on to the couch or bed when requested to do so. Yet, when the patient is asked to flex the contralateral, unaffected leg, bringing it up in the air, the affected limb extends. Now it will press into the surface of the bed. Why did it extend under one condition and not the other?

In the patient presenting with a unilateral tremor, an organic tremor would persist during the performance of rhythmic activity by the contralateral, unaffected limb, yet in hysteria the outcome is different (O'Suilleabhain and Matsumoto 1998). The hysterical tremor reduces when the patient must attend to his or her 'good' limb. Patients do not maintain their abnormal movement.

The implication (as in the quote from Campbell 1979 above) is that the patient's motoric function is more likely to be normal when he or she is not attending to the affected limb, and that when the patient does attend the attending itself somehow interferes with movement, i.e. makes it more likely that the movement will be abnormal.

Similar conclusions may be deduced from the consequences of using benzodiazepines, barbiturates, or general anaesthetics in hysteria: '[I]n the stage of excitement the patient will struggle, cry out...he will often regain consciousness whilst he is in the act of moving the arm which was formerly paralysed or using the voice which was formerly dumb' (Adrian and Yealland 1917).

Hence, whether by distraction or sedation, when the physician interrupts the patient's attentional processes, they can reveal the preservation of normal action (in the previously affected domain). This phenomenology has been elaborated upon elsewhere (Spence 1999, 2001, 2006*a*,*b*). For the present, its principal implications are the following.

- While the patient with hysteria is presenting with manifest physical signs of motor abnormality, there are, latent, within him or her the necessary processes required to carry out physical actions normally.
- The maintenance of the hysterical sign appears to be dependent upon the ability of the patient to attend to its production.
- Distraction or sedation reveals the emergence of normal action.
- Thus, attention is central to the patient's performance of the abnormal act.

21.4 **A cognitive architecture**

The foregoing discussion demonstrates that hysterical phenomena in the motor domain behave like purposeful acts (Spence 1999): the patient must attend in order to produce them; distraction or sedation impairs their performance. Knowing this, can we specify the cognitive neurobiological substrate for such actions?

There is a longstanding, computational distinction that can be drawn between those motor behaviours that organisms perform automatically and those that require conscious attention to action (for a review see Spence 2001). Such a distinction separates those behaviours that have become routine or automated, from those that are difficult, complex, or newly acquired. If we borrow one model, developed by Tim Shallice and colleagues (e.g. Shallice 1988; Shallice and Burgess 1996), we can identify the roles of specific brain regions contributing to the performance of these different kinds of behaviour.

- The engagement of 'lower' brain systems, exemplified by the premotor and motor cortices, and subcortical foci such as basal ganglia and cerebellum, may be sufficient to enable the performance of routine tasks.
- 'Higher' ('executive', 'supervisory attentional system') centres, co-terminus with prefrontal cortices, are implicated in the performance of more novel or complex behaviours.
- In addition, such higher, executive centres may become involved again if an already automated task becomes the focus of renewed attention (see Passingham 1996).

Such a theoretically driven distinction (between the novel and the automated) has its basis in biology. Hence, there is the example of transcortical motor or dynamic aphasia, wherein a patient (often suffering from the effects of a left-sided prefrontal lesion) is unable to generate new speech, spontaneously, but can repeat the speech of others (Lichteim 1885; Freedman *et al.* 1984; Warren *et al.* 2003). Similarly, in many functional neuroimaging experiments involving healthy subjects, patterns of frontal activation elicited by novel behaviours and routines have been shown to differ, for example, during verbal fluency, when the subject's free selection of words beginning with a given letter elicits greater prefrontal, executive activation, than the passive repetition of other people's words (e.g. Frith *et al.* 1991; Spence *et al.* 2000*b*), or during motor skill acquisition, when initial prefrontal activation gives way to posterior and inferior brain activation as the new task becomes automated (e.g., Friston *et al.* 1992; Jenkins *et al.* 1994).

The underlying principle in each of these scenarios is that prefrontal, executive systems appear to be selectively engaged when the task demands attention or the generation of novelty, whereas posterior and inferior systems suffice when the task becomes routine or automated.

Turning once more to hysteria, as we have seen (above) the generation of hysterical motor phenomena seems to require the patient's attention to action. While the physician examines the dysfunctional limb or domain the symptom is present but if the patient is distracted or sedated then the symptom remits. Normal motoric function is more likely to re-emerge under these latter conditions. Therefore, from a cognitive perspective, the latent, preserved, normal behaviour resembles a motor routine that can be performed by subordinate brain systems without the intervention of the prefrontal executive (indeed, it emerges precisely when the latter is impacted by distraction or sedation). In contrast, hysterical motor phenomena appear to be the products of the executive, dependent upon its engagement (see Fig. 21.1).

21.5 **Evidence of the executive**

If the above hypothesis, that executive systems are implicated in the genesis and maintenance of hysterical phenomena, is correct then this should be demonstrable in the domain

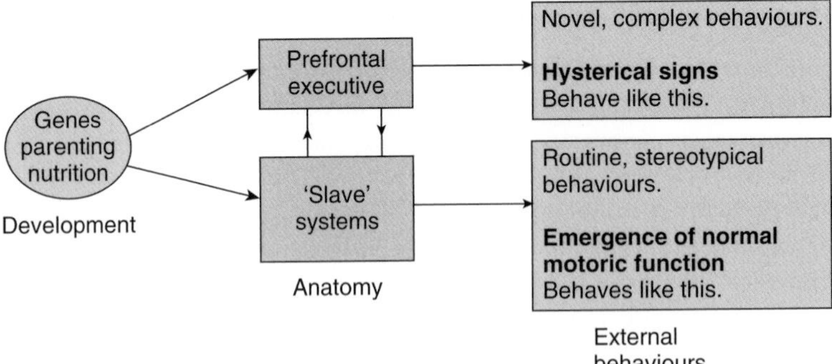

Fig. 21.1 Schematic cartoon demonstrating the relationship between elements of the motor system and emergent motor activity. On the left are developmental factors that might be hypothesized to impact the nascent anatomical structure of the individual (middle column). In terms of current cognitive architecture, the prefrontal executive modulates subordinate, 'slave' systems located in premotor and motor cortices, together with subcortical foci, including the basal ganglia and cerebellum. Simple motor procedures or those that have become routine and automated (right side) require only these lower systems for their enactment. However, novel, complex activities or those that are attended to implicate the prefrontal executive (upper middle and right columns). In the pathological behaviour seen in hysteria (right column), it is clear that the behaviour itself seems to rely for its enactment upon the patient's attention to action (a characteristic of the executive), while preserved, 'normal' action (lower right) behaves like a routine, which emerges during periods of distraction or sedation.

of pathophysiology. Is there evidence from neuroscience that the executive is implicated in the cognitive neurobiology of hysteria? A number of studies of hysterical movement disorders shed some light on this question.

An electromyographic (EMG) study of patients with tremors by O'Suilleabhain and Matsumoto (1998) is informative. They studied patients with Parkinson's disease, essential tremor, and psychogenic tremor. They found that the latter group differed from the former groups in two important ways. First, the tremors exhibited by patients of the first two groups had different frequencies across affected limbs (within the same subject); those in psychogenic disorders did not (i.e. in a given patient with psychogenic tremor all affected limbs oscillated at the same frequency); second, while the former tremors continued while the patients were required to tap out rhythms with their contralateral limbs, those due to psychogenic factors were interrupted. The authors concluded that, while multiple 'oscillator systems' within the central nervous system generated Parkinsonian and essential tremors, psychogenic tremors seemed to rely upon single oscillators. Psychogenic tremors behaved more like voluntary behaviours: 'In psychogenic tremor ... we propose that the motor system *per se* is intact, and that rhythmic contractions are mediated by top-down synchronization involving a common oscillator system, perhaps at a higher cerebral level. The tendency of psychogenic tremor to attenuate when patients are distracted could be explained by a requirement for such high-level involvement' (O'Suilleabhain and Matsumoto 1998).

A somewhat similar conclusion emerges from an electroencephalographic (EEG) study of patients exhibiting psychogenic myoclonus. In the normal state, a spontaneous voluntary action is preceded by an EEG signal over the vertex, termed the readiness potential or *Bereitschaftspotential*, which is thought to emerge from medial premotor cortex. Terada and colleagues (1995) found such potentials in five of the six patients with psychogenic myoclonus whom they studied. 'Therefore, it is most likely that the jerks in these patients were generated through the mechanisms common to those underlying voluntary movement' (Terada *et al.* 1995).

Turning to abnormalities of gait and posture, the available behavioural data suggest that something similar may be happening (i.e. these behaviours are not 'routine'—they seem to require executive control). The postures adopted in the hysterical realm are those that would not be adopted through purely physical expediencies since they are ergonomically 'uneconomic', i.e. they require more energy for their maintenance than alternative strategies for behaving, which subjects would normally be expected to adopt if physically ill (Lempert *et al.* 1991). Also, hysterical postures are improved by distraction.

There is a small literature, mostly comprising case reports and small case series, reporting the application of functional neuroimaging techniques (e.g. positron emission tomography (PET) or functional magnetic resonance imaging (fMRI)) to hysterical disorders. However, it should be noted that frequently there are confounding factors to consider (Table 21.4). So far, most cases described have exhibited comorbid disorders (such as depression and/or personality disorder), and most reports have emerged from tertiary centres, so the patients they describe may be rather atypical of hysteria patients in general. If there is a common theme that emerges it tends to be that where there are sensory deficits (e.g. anaesthesia or blindness) there is hypoactivation of the relevant sensory cortices and evidence of disturbed function in 'higher' frontal regions (Tiihonen *et al.* 1995; Yazici and Kostakoglu 1998; Vuilleumier *et al.* 2001; Mailis-Gagnon *et al.* 2003; Werring *et al.* 2004); when the presenting dysfunction is one of motor disturbance there is evidence in favour of either excessive activation of inhibitory prefrontal (orbitofrontal) cortices (Marshall *et al.* 1997) or hypoactivation in prefrontal (dorsolateral) cortices involved in action generation (Spence *et al.* 2000*a*). A common view has emerged that lower centres are somehow inhibited or suppressed by higher centres. There has been debate as to whether this technology might adequately distinguish hysterical conversion syndromes from feigning or malingering (Marshall *et al.* 1997; Spence 1999; Spence *et al.* 2000*b*). It should also be noted that there is considerable overlap between the functional neuroimaging findings described in these disorders

Table 21.4 Problems for neuroimagers wishing to study hysteria

- A scarcity of cases
- Scarcity of control groups in reported studies
- Symptomatic heterogeneity (thereby making the recruitment of patient groups difficult, and complicating comparisons across studies)
- Frequent comorbidity (especially depression and personality disorder)
- Difficulty in identifying and recruiting suitable control groups (e.g. 'depressed' and 'personality disordered' groups in addition to 'healthy controls')
- Studies tend to emerge from tertiary centres (thus, cases are likely to be atypical)
- May be confounded by reporting bias (those with coherent positive findings more likely to be written up and accepted for publication than negative studies)
- Establishing a suitable protocol for the scanner (whether to choose a task that the patient can perform, and hence risk problems with interpretation, or choose a task they find difficult and risk non-adherence or poor performance as a confounding variable)
- Most studies have not addressed the issue of 'intent' (i.e. how do investigators establish whether or not patients are 'trying' to perform the task)

and those emerging in other literatures describing such conditions as chronic fatigue syndrome, somatization disorder, dysmorphophobia, and other anomalies of bodily experience (for a recent overview see Spence 2006).

21.6 Influence of social context

From the foregoing review, with its emphasis upon both the behaviours and the brains of individual patients, it is possible to overlook the fact that all hysterical phenomena arise within social milieu and that this applies whether one considers their initial appearance in the community or their manipulation in therapeutic encounters (Spence 1999; and see Wenegrat 2001). If this were not the case then the presence or absence of ward staff would not have its effect and unobtrusive observation of patients would not yield evidence of 'symptomatic inconsistencies' in the way that it does at present (for some florid examples, see Baker and Silver 1987).

However, the influence of the social is even more obvious if one considers the emergence of the modern literature on hysteria under quite specific social conditions. At the end of the nineteenth and the beginning of the twentieth centuries there were three settings in which reported case material was particularly abundant and influential: Charcot's practice at the Salpetriere hospital in Paris, Freud's private practice in Vienna, and the battle front of the First World War. When reading the historical accounts, one is struck by the possible contribution of particular personal and social factors to the emergence of some of the more bizarre phenomena described. Consider the impact of Charcot's personality and his milieu upon other people's behaviour.

Example 1: The production of signs

'Strange things were said about [Charcot's] hold on the Salpetriere's hysterical young women and about happenings there ... [D]uring a patient's ball ... a gong was inadvertently sounded, whereupon many hysterical women instantaneously fell into catalepsy and kept [the] plastic poses in which they found themselves when the gong was sounded' (Ellenberger 1994).

Example 2: The resolution of signs

'There was ... a young lady who had been paralysed for years. Charcot bade her stand up and walk, which she did under the astounded eyes of her parents and of the Mother Superior of the convent in which she had been staying. Another ... was brought to Charcot with a paralysis of both legs. [He] found no organic lesions; the consultation was not yet over when the patient stood up and walked back to the door where the cabman, who was waiting for her, took off his hat in amazement and crossed himself.' (Ellenberger 1994).

What is occurring beneath the surface of such spectacular enactments and miraculous recoveries? We seem to witness the manifestation of the force of Charcot's personality and the belief that others had in him, both in manipulating their behaviour and eliciting their recovery. According to Brant Wenegrat (2001), these sorts of concentrations of diagnosis and cure, occurring within very specific clinical settings and involving powerful medical figures, should make us question the veracity of the disease model being expounded. Wenegrat has studied many of our culture's more florid, contemporary, neurotic, and subcultural afflictions (including possession, multiple personality disorder, and alien abduction) and concluded that they involve role enactments, arising under the influence (conscious or otherwise) of powerful people (often doctors). We should be particularly cautious when a new disorder, without demonstrable organic pathology, exhibits incidence rates that fluctuate widely, where certain clinicians diagnose many of the cases (and others do not), and where prestige accrues (to either doctor or patient) through the accordance of 'special' status.

Such considerations are relevant when we consider the emergence of hysteria under particular conditions of inequality and disempowerment. It has been argued that Charcot's patients came from poverty and faced uncertain futures if they did not 'perform' in the clinical setting (for a most graphic demonstration of this thesis, see Didi-Huberman 2003). Similarly, we see in the early psychotherapeutic work of Freud an emphasis upon the plights of women drawn from the bourgeoisie who were subject to the power of men. Then, in the soldiers exhibiting unusual movements in the First World War, we see the explicit application of power, through rank and social class structures, under conditions of very real danger (where the consequences of both failing to fight and recovery itself could be death, by firing squad or returning to action).

Hence, any comprehensive account of hysterical motor phenomena will need to include a role for social influence, for the role of the interpersonal (see Fig. 21.2). One hypothesis might be that the presence of 'superiors' in the prevailing social hierarchy impacts the executive systems of the hysterical patient, such that the emergence of further hysterical motor signs is either facilitated or

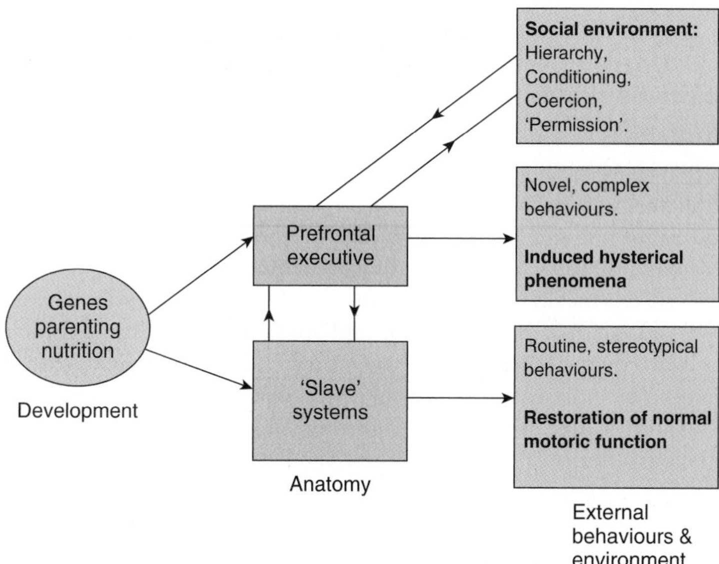

Fig. 21.2 Schematic cartoon demonstrating the relationship between elements of the motor system and emergent motor activity. Figure 21.1 has been modified to demonstrate the impact of social environment upon the emergence of hysterical phenomena. As before, the prefrontal executive is pivotal to the generation of hysterical signs, and it modulates subordinate, 'slave' systems. However, it is clear that the social milieu and, in particular, hierarchical relationships appear to impact the emergence of these phenomena (see the examples from Charcot's Salpetriere cited in the text). The presence of other individuals may either facilitate the performance of hysterical motor phenomena (as in the modern clinical examination or, historically, in the use of Charcot's gong) or lead to their resolution (through withdrawal to unobtrusive observation, in modern accounts, or the more 'miraculous' cures attributed to Charcot).

prevented (as in the Charcot examples above), through either an inhibition of the executive (allowing the emergence, we might say 'escape', of 'normal' motor routines) or its facilitation, through coercion or 'permission', to elaborate new, perhaps even extravagant, motor behaviours (as when the gong sounded at the Salpetriere, above).

The nearest our modern, cognitive literature has come to exploring this feature of hysteria (the role of powerful 'others') is in the modelling of symptoms using hypnosis: where susceptible subjects are influenced to produce physical signs resembling those of hysteria (it is of interest that one such study in the literature reported functional brain images very similar to those of a hysterical patient studied by the same group; see Halligan *et al.* 2000 and Marshall *et al.* 1997, respectively). Clearly, there is a need for further work in this area.

21.7 **Integrating the cognitive and the social**

From this account we may conclude that the motor behaviours exhibited by people with hysteria behave like purposeful actions, although patients deny awareness of their causation. Indeed, our diagnostic systems contain both the stipulation that such motor phenomena be (potentially) subject to voluntary control and the criterion that we conclude that the patient is not consciously controlling them (i.e. the patient is not feigning; Table 21.1). Instead we must believe that hysterical phenomena are generated from within the patient's psyche, while not reflecting their sense of agency (their awareness of their own volition). Hence, it might be concluded that, while the cognitive neurobiological approach taken in this chapter can predict the brain systems that 'should' be involved in the generation of the behaviours described (Fig. 21.1) and that this is consistent with what we know of the empirical literature to date (above), nevertheless, in a sense, we are no nearer to discovering the nature of the underlying pathophysiology and its relation to the contents of consciousness. How do we answer the fundamental question we set ourselves at the very beginning of this chapter:

- 'How can a motor or sensory symptom be produced in the absence of a physical cause?'

To put things another way: Have we really made any advance beyond Freud, who invoked the role of the psychodynamic unconscious? Our response is that we have, for we have demonstrated that consciousness and, more specifically, attention are required for the production of hysterical motor phenomena. It is the diversion of attention away from hysterical symptoms and signs that leads to their resolution. It is the dimming of conscious awareness through sedation or anaesthesia that renders activity normal again. Hence, we may state quite explicitly that attention, not the dynamic unconscious, is what maintains hysterical signs. Therefore, some progress has been made, though no firmer conclusions can be drawn at present.

However, there is a strand of contemporary psychodynamic thought that may be of interest when considering the 'content' of the hysterical symptom. By content we mean the particular manifestation of hysteria exhibited, e.g. a weakness of the right hand. How might we understand these phenomena without recourse to speculative interpretation (e.g. 'the patient cannot move her arm because, unconsciously, she wishes to hit her father')?

In the following, we offer one view that may inform future attempts to reconcile psychodynamic understandings of hysteria with those derived from cognitive neuroscience. To do this we will consider the work of Jacques Lacan (1901–81) and its extension in the current writings of Slavoj Zizek (for an accessible overview see Myers 2003). We must first introduce some Lacanian terms that are pivotal to describing hysteria (below).

Stated simply, Lacan described a distinction between the nature of reality itself, the 'real', which is the true nature of the world, beyond our language and ultimate comprehension, and the 'symbolic', the common language and theoretical constructs that we use to describe what may be put into words. We may not have any choice over the nature of the symbolic universe that we inhabit, for we are brought up to speak a given language by our parents and when we use words we are usually borrowing them, their meanings having been determined by others before us. Hence, we can be said to inhabit the symbolic, yet we have only partial awareness of the real (that which is underpinning our existence and is beyond words). Zizek's contribution has been to extend the Lacanian account into politics and the arts in quite engaging and exciting ways. For instance, he has written much about the films of Alfred Hitchcock and the manifestations of patriarchal authority and power in the work of David Lynch (Zizek 1991, 2000). He has also described how the real may rupture the symbolic order, in circumstances where words will not suffice: hence, in the emergence of violence, or trauma, or even the obscene. If a film comprises a conventional narrative, Zizek argues that it cannot withstand the inclusion of truly obscene, explicit material, for this constitutes the intrusion of the real, and the narrative, the symbolic order, is ruptured. So, for instance, a conventional Hitchcock narrative would be ruptured if he (the director) showed the audience explicit sexual material, rather than resorting to conventional Hollywood signifiers: following the romantic couple's kiss the lights are dimmed; then night becomes morning. For our purposes, it is of interest to consider the tension between the symbolic and the real and what relevance they might have in the clinical case of hysteria.

We have noted previously (Table 21.3) Freud's remark that hysteria behaves as if 'anatomy did not exist', referring to the anatomical and temporal inconsistencies apparent upon physical examination and observation. The symptoms and signs of hysteria do not reflect neurological reality; instead, they reflect the patient's idea of neurology. To borrow the Lacanian terms just mentioned, the patient's symptoms and signs comprise expressions of the symbolic (the lay cultural view of what a given neurological sign comprises) not the real (the 'true' biology constituting our nervous systems). Hence, in hysteria, the symbolic attempts to mask the real.

However, what happens in the clinical examination, if we combine the Lacanian account with a rehearsal of the Hoover Test, is that the patient begins by performing the symbolic (an apparent inability to extend the affected leg) but, when distracted, evinces the real (a non-linguistic sign, which is comprised solely of the physical): the limb extends, pushing into the bed when the contralateral 'good' leg undergoes flexion. The intact motor system has declared itself (non-linguistically). Hence, we may substitute the Lacanian terms for those deployed in our cognitive neurobiological account of hysteria (moving from Fig. 21.2 to Fig. 21.3). The symptom expresses the symbolic; the restored, normal function evinces the real.

But this is not all. The Zizekian account of artistic works also places emphasis upon male power, the dominance of the patriarchal order within and beyond the family, where rules are made (the 'big other'). Such power can be perverse and arbitrary; the 'subject' is literally subject to its will. (One sees this in tyrannical states and abusive homes; those in power may literally 'do as they please' with others.) So this provides another perspective from which to view the conditions prevailing at the outset of modern accounts of hysteria: where the power discrepancy between doctors and patients was most pronounced, the consequences for those patients seen and assessed (particularly at the Salpetriere and the Front) could be most severe indeed. The big other (in the form of the dominant male) might literally make or break symptoms: 'Without any further discussion the motor areas of the cortex were mapped out roughly, the measurements being repeated aloud to impress and mystify the patient. He was told [that] as soon as the shoulder area of the cortex was stimulated by faradism he would be able to raise his shoulder and that the rest of the arm would recover in the same way ... He [moved] at once [after electricity], and in a few minutes the whole of the paralysis had disappeared and he could raise 30 pounds' (Adrian and Yealland 1917).

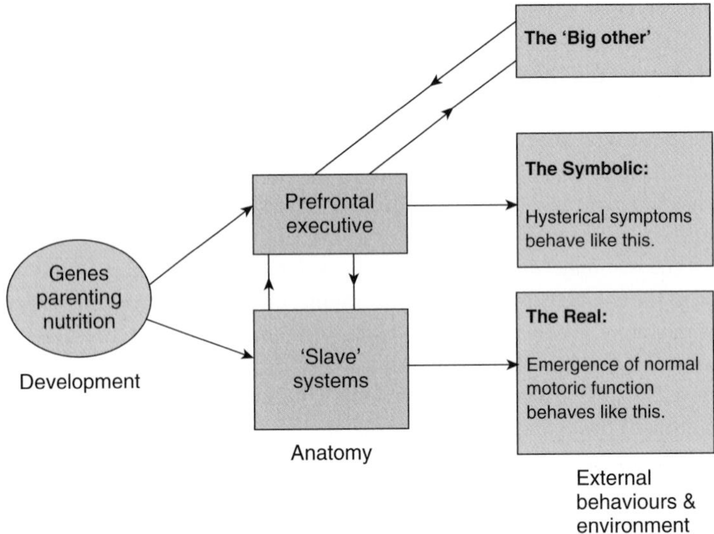

Fig. 21.3 Schematic cartoon demonstrating the relationship between elements of the motor system and emergent motor activity. Here we have substituted the Lacanian terms, the 'big other', the 'symbolic', and the 'real', for aspects of functional influence and behavioural outcome (right side of cartoon). While the symptom represents the patient's (and his/her culture's) understanding of illness (the symbolic) and its enactment implicates the involvement of the prefrontal executive, when the latter is modulated by distraction, sedation, or the impact of powerful social influences (above), the normal motor routine emerges (reflecting the 'real', below).

Thus, to summarize. We may combine our recognition that the cognitive executive is pivotal to the maintenance of hysterical phenomena with an acknowledgement that their symptomatic content reflects the cultural understanding of disease at the time (i.e. it reflects the 'symbolic' order). When the symptom remits, through distraction, sedation, or the influence of the physician, the 'real' emerges, the normal motor routine, which is procedural and beyond words. The influence of specific, sometimes powerful, human beings and of human culture is itself manifest both in the symptom and in the timing of its relapse and resolution. The 'big other' (the dominance culture) and others (our conspecifics) affect the way human beings behave. Any final cognitive neurobiological account of hysteria must find a way of acknowledging and investigating these aspects of the real.

References

Adrian, E.D. and Yealland, L.R. (1917). The treatment of some common war neuroses. *Lancet* **i**, 867–72.

American Psychiatric Association (1994). *Diagnostic criteria from DSM IV*. American Psychiatric Association, Washington DC.

Baker, J.H.E. and Silver, J.R. (1987). Hysterical paraplegia. *J. Neurol. Neurosurg. Psychiatry* **50**, 375–82.

Campbell, J. (1979). The shortest paper. *Neurology* **29**, 1633.

Didi-Huberman, G. (2003). *Invention of hysteria: Charcot and the photographic iconography of the Salpetriere*. [Translated by A. Hartz, first published 1982.] MIT Press, Cambridge, Massachusetts.

Ellenberger, H. (1994). *The discovery of the unconscious*. Fontana, London.

Freedman, M., Alexander, M.P., and Naeser, M.A. (1984). Anatomical basis of transcortical motor aphasia. *Neurology* **34**, 409–17.

Freud, S. (1894). The neuro-psychoses of defence. In *The complete psychological works*, vol. III, standard edn (1962), (ed. J. Strachey), pp. 45–61. Hogarth, London.

Friston, K.J., Frith, C.D., Passingham, R.E., and Liddle, P.F. (1992). Motor practice and neurophysiological adaptation in the cerebellum: a positron emission tomography study. *Proc. R. Soc. Lond. (Biol.)* **248**, 223–28.

Frith, C.D., Friston, K.J., Liddle, P.F., and Frackowiak, R.S.J. (1991). A PET study of word finding. *Neuropsychologia* **29**, 1137–48.

Hallett, M., Fahn, S., Jankovic, J., Lang, A.E., Cloninger, C.R., and Yudofsky, S.C. (eds.) (2006). *Psychogenic movement disorders: neurology and neuropsychiatry*. American Academy of Neurology Press, Lippincott Williams and Wilkins, Philadelphia.

Halligan, P.W., Athwal, B.S., Oakley, D.A., and Frackowiak, R.S.J. (2000). Imaging hypnotic paralysis: implications for conversion hysteria. *Lancet* **355**, 986–7.

Halligan, P.W., Bass, C., and Marshall, J.C. (ed.) (2001). *Contemporary approaches to the study of hysteria*. Oxford University Press, Oxford.

Jenkins, I.H., Brooks, D.J., Nixon, P.D., Frackowiak, R.S.J., and Passingham, R.E. (1994). Motor sequence learning: a study with positron emission tomography. *J. Neurosci.* **14**, 3775–90.

Lempert, T., Brandt, T., Dieterich, M., and Huppert, D. (1991). How to identify psychogenic disorders of stance and gait: a video study in 37 patients. *J. Neurol.* **238**, 140–6.

Lichtheim, L. (1885). On aphasia. *Brain* **7**, 433–84.

Mailis-Gagnon, A., Giannoylis, I., Downar, J., Kwan, C.L., Mikulis, D.J., Crawley, A.P., Nicholson, K., and Davis, K.D. (2003). Altered central somatosensory processing in chronic pain patients with 'hysterical' anaesthesia. *Neurology* **60**, 1501–7.

Marshall, J.C., Halligan, P.W., Fink, G.R., Wade, D.T., and Frackowiak, R.S. (1997). The functional anatomy of a hysterical paralysis. *Cognition* **64**, B1–B8.

Merskey, H. (1995). *The analysis of hysteria: understanding conversion and dissociation*. Gaskell, London.

Myers, T. (2003). *Slavoj Zizek*. Routledge, London.

O'Suilleabhain, P.E. and Matsumoto, J.Y. (1998). Time–frequency analysis of tremors. *Brain* **121**, 2127–34.

Passingham, R.E. (1996). Attention to action. *Phil. Trans. R. Soc. Lond. B* **351**, 1473–9.

Sanoo, M. (2004). Abductor sign: a reliable new sign to detect unilateral non-organic paresis of the lower limb. *J. Neurol. Neurosurg. Psychiatry* **75**, 121–5.

Shallice, T. (1988). *From neuropsychology to mental structure*. Cambridge University Press, Cambridge.

Shallice T. and Burgess, P.W. (1996). The domain of supervisory processes and temporal organisation of behaviour. *Phil. Trans. R. Soc. Lond. B* **351**, 1405–12.

Spence, S.A. (1999). Hysterical paralyses as disorders of action. *Cogn. Neuropsychiatry* **4**, 203–26.

Spence, S.A. (2001). Disorders of willed action. In *Contemporary approaches to the study of hysteria* (ed. P.W. Halligan, C. Bass, and J.C. Marshall), pp. 235–50. Oxford University Press, Oxford.

Spence, S.A. (2006*a*). Hysteria: a new look. *Psychiatry* **5** (2), 56–60.

Spence, S.A. (2006*b*). The cognitive executive is implicated in the maintenance of psychogenic movement disorders. In *Psychogenic movement disorders: neurology and neuropsychiatry* (ed. M. Hallett, S. Fahn, J. Jankovic, A.E. Lang, C.R. Cloninger, and S.C. Yudofsky), pp. 222–9. American Academy of Neurology Press, Lippincott Williams and Wilkins, Philadelphia.

Spence, S.A. (2006). All in the mind? The neural correlates of unexplained physical symptoms. *Adv. Psychiat. Treat.* **12**, 349–58.

Spence, S.A., Liddle, P.F., Stefan, M.D., Hellwell, J.S.E., Sharma, T., Friston, K.J., Hirsch, S.R., Frith, C.D., Murray, R.M., Deakin, J.F.W., and Grasby, P.M. (2000*a*). Functional anatomy of verbal fluency in people with schizophrenia and those at genetic risk. *Br. J. Psychiatry* **176**, 52–60.

Spence, S.A., Crimlisk, H.L., Cope, H., Ron, M.A., and Grasby, P.M. (2000*b*). Discrete neurophysiological correlates in prefrontal cortex during hysterical and feigned disorder of movement. *Lancet* **355**, 1243–4.

Symonds, C. (1970). Hysteria. In *The analysis of hysteria* (2nd edition 1995) (ed. H. Merskey), pp. 407–13. Gaskell, London.

Terada, K., Ikeda, A., Van Ness, P.C., Nagamine, T., Kaji, R., Kimura, J., and Shibasaki, H. (1995). Presence of Bereitschaftspotential preceding psychogenic myoclonus: clinical application of jerk-locked back averaging. *J. Neurol. Neurosurg. Psychiatry* **58**, 745–7.

Tiihonen, J., Kuikka, J., Viinamaki, H., Lehtonen, J., and Partanen, J. (1995). Altered cerebral blood flow during hysterical paraesthesia. *Biol. Psychiatry* **37**, 134–5.

Vuilleumier, P., Chicherio, C., Assal, F., Schwartz, S., Slosmen, D., and Landis, T. (2001). Functional neuroanatomical correlates of hysterical sensorimotor loss. *Brain* **124**, 1077–90.

Warren, J.D., Warren, J.E., Fox, N.C., and Warrington, E.K. (2003). Nothing to say, something to sing: primary progressive dynamic aphasia. *Neurocase* **9**, 140–55.

Wenegrat, B. (2001). *Theatre of disorder: patients, doctors, and the construction of illness.* Oxford University Press, Oxford.

Werring, D.J., Weston, L., Bullmore, E.T., Plant, G.T., and Ron, M.A. (2004). Functional magnetic resonance imaging of the cerebral response to visual stimulation in medically unexplained visual loss. *Psychol. Med.* **34**, 583–9.

Yazici, K.M. and Kostakoglu, L. (1998). Cerebral blood flow changes in patients with conversion disorder. *Psychiatry Res. Neuroimaging* **83**, 163–8.

Zizek, S. (1991). *Looking awry: an introduction to Jacques Lacan through popular culture.* MIT Press, Cambridge, Massachusetts.

Zizek, S. (2000). *The art of the ridiculous sublime: on David Lynch's Lost Highway.* Walter Chapin Simpson Centre for the Humanities, Seattle, Washington.

Part 5

Treatment issues

Chapter 22

Pharmacological treatment

Ulrich Müller

22.1 Introduction

This chapter reviews concepts, available drugs, and indications for pharmacological interventions in cognitive neurology. There is increasing evidence that neuropsychological syndromes like aphasia, unilateral spatial neglect, and memory or executive deficits can be ameliorated by catecholamine-enhancing and cholinergic drugs. The focus of this chapter is on patients with traumatic brain injury (TBI) and stroke, where most controlled studies have been performed. Cognitive rehabilitation will further benefit from discontinuation of medication with cognitive side-effects and psychopharmacological treatment of apathy, depression, involuntary emotional expression, agitation, and sleep disturbances.

Pharmacological manipulation of cognitive processes in healthy volunteers and brain-damaged patients was pioneered by two prominent figures of clinical neuroscience. German psychiatrist Emil Kraepelin (1856–1926) was the first to perform systematic experiments investigating effects of alcohol, sedatives, and stimulant drugs on cognitive processes (Müller *et al.* 2006). Pharmacological interventions in neurorehabilitation were introduced by Russian neuropsychologist Alexander R. Luria (1902–1977), who administered physostigmine to Second World War veterans with brain injury to improve motor and memory deficits (Phillips *et al.* 2003). The underlying model is relatively simple: Some drugs like alcohol and sedatives are bad for cognition and should be avoided in patients with cognitive deficits, whereas other drugs—mainly psychostimulants—can boost impaired cognitive (and motor) functions and their recovery.

The fields of psychopharmacology, clinical neuropsychology, and cognitive neuroscience have flourished in the last decade; however, neurorehabilitation remains a relatively poor cousin of psychiatry and neurology. Despite large numbers of patients with cognitive deficits after acquired brain injury, many of them young adults with many years of handicapped life ahead, pharmacological treatments are surprisingly underinvestigated in cognitive neurology. Cognitive neuropharmacology is one of the few areas in modern medicine where the number of scholarly reviews clearly outweighs the number of randomized placebo-controlled trials (RCTs). The quality of some reviews is not better than the studies that are reviewed, mainly single cases and case series. Some authors have problems in differentiating drug effects from practice effects (e.g. Napolitano *et al.* 2005). Only a few well-controlled studies per indication have been completed and published, but there seems to be an encouraging increase over time (Fig. 22.1).

Uncontrolled studies are often biased towards positive treatment effects (publication bias) and confounded by practice effects (because performance on many cognitive tasks improves with repeated administration). In this chapter the focus is on pharmacological treatments that are based on clear neurobiological models and supported by evidence from RCTs. In order to shorten the list of references most case reports and case series are referenced only indirectly via review articles.

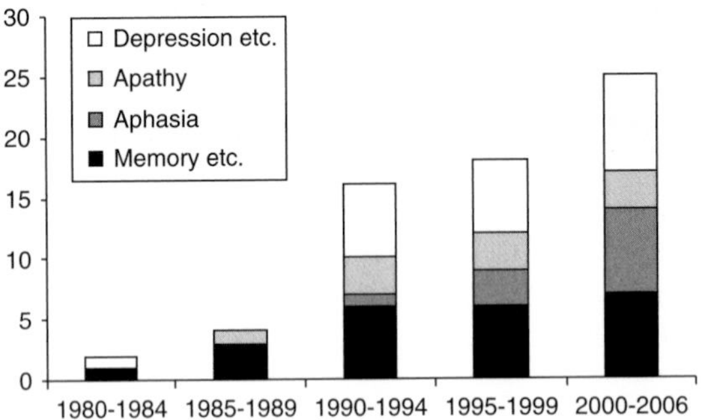

Fig. 22.1 Number of published randomized placebo-controlled clinical trials (RCTs) in cognitive neurology and neuropsychiatry (1982–2006). (Detailed references and data available on request.)

22.2 Neuroplasticity and rehabilitation

Detailed understanding of the neural mechanisms of functional recovery after brain damage is important for targeted pharmacological interventions. The first aim in the *acute phase* is to reduce the extent of a brain lesion, for example, by reducing intracranial pressure. Neurotoxic damage in penumbra zones around necrotic lesions can also be minimized—at least in animal models—by reducing the levels of neurotoxic neurotransmitters with glutamate antagonists, calcium antagonists, or radical scavengers. The time window for early pharmacological interventions is limited because most substances have to be given within the first hour after the brain-damaging event (Goldstein 2006).

In *post-acute and later phases* of neurorehabilitation, redundant neuronal networks can be recruited or existing networks reorganized in order to compensate functional deficits. Pharmacological modulation of neuroplasticity has been demonstrated in animal models with well-defined functional deficits. A good example is the beam-walking paradigm that allows functional testing and training of hemiplegic rats after experimental motor cortex lesions. Motor recovery during the first days can be accelerated by noradrenaline-enhancing drugs (e.g. amfetamine, methylphenidate, yohimbine) and delayed by dopamine antagonists, anticonvulsive, and sedating drugs (Feeney 1997). In an animal model with experimental lesion of the hippocampus, amfetamine facilitated improvement of memory deficits and this was accompanied by higher levels of repair proteins (synaptophysin and GAP-43) in the damaged but not the contralateral hemisphere (Stroemer *et al.* 1998). Using an animal for model TBI, Kline *et al.* (2002) found that chronic treatment with bromocriptine, a dopamine D2 receptor agonist, had positive effects on cognitive deficits.

The *chronic phase* of rehabilitation after acquired brain damage is characterized by persistent sensorimotor and cognitive deficits with minimal spontaneous remission. According to the concept of 'compensatory plasticity', the conditions for effective cognitive training and the use of compensatory aids like memory diaries can be improved by pharmacological treatment of underlying neurological or psychiatric complications like spasticity or apathy.

22.3 Neurotransmitter modulation of cognition and emotion

Pharmacological treatment in cognitive neurology and neuropsychiatry is based on models of neurotransmitter modulation of cognitive and emotional processes. Most available drugs impact on one or more of the major neurotransmitter systems, namely, dopamine, noradrenaline, serotonin, or acetylcholine. These systems consist of neurons ascending from the brainstem and/or basal forebrain into subcortical and cortical regions. Each system has preferential projection areas with different functional specialization. Simple relationships of 'one neurotransmitter = one cognitive function' cannot, however, be expected, because both neuroanatomy and functions overlap considerably (Fig. 22.2). In the last decade substantial progress has been made in fractionating different components of cognition and in elucidating the underlying neural and neurochemical substrates of these processes using a combination of neuropsychological, pharmacological, and neuroimaging methods (Robbins 2005; Cools and Robbins 2004).

Neuropharmacological manipulations in humans have elucidated the neurotransmitter modulation of working memory, attention, and impulsivity. These domains have been classically linked to dopamine, noradrenaline, and serotonin, respectively, and are of particular importance in everyday life and in relation to cognitive deficits manifested across neuropsychiatric disorders. Baseline neurochemical activity can determine not only the magnitude but also the direction of drugs effects on different cognitive domains, according to an 'inverted-U model', where both too little and too much of a neurotransmitter is bad for optimal functioning (Chamberlain *et al.* 2006*c*). Acetylcholine, the fourth major neurotransmitter, plays a modulatory role in early sensory and attentional processing as well as in hippocampal (long-term) and prefrontal (working) memory functions (Thiel 2003).

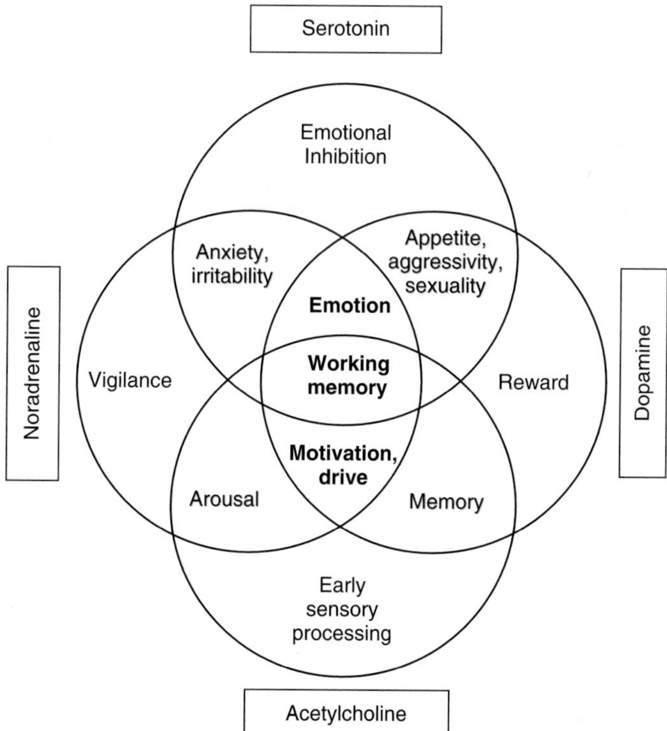

Fig. 22.2 Neurotransmitter modulation of cognitive and emotional processes (modified from Müller 2001).

In order to develop new and targeted pharmacological intervention strategies for patients with acquired brain damage, it is important to understand the biochemical underpinnings of neuroplasticity as well as the neurotransmitter modulation of cognitive and emotional processes.

22.4 Cognitive side-effects

Many drugs that are commonly prescribed in neurorehabilitation have unwanted effects. Cognitive side-effects are especially problematic in patients with acquired brain damage and pre-existing cognitive or behavioural deficits that could be further impaired by some drugs with cholinergic, histaminergic, GABAergic, and dopaminergic mechanism of action. Profiles of cognitive side-effects of general medical, neurological, and psychiatric medicines are summarized in Tables 22.1 and 22.2. Further information on mechanisms of action and side-effects can be found in textbooks (e.g. Stahl 2005) and at various internet resources (e.g. *www.bnf.org* or *www.rote-liste.de*). In most national pharmacopoeias information on available medicinal products is arranged in alphabetical listings of chemical (generic) and products (label) names with detailed information on indication, contraindication, dosing, and side-effects. Data concerning cognitive side-effects are, however, often limited to general statements like 'sedation'.

Sedative drugs should be reduced or withdrawn whenever possible before an attempt at pharmacological stimulation of cognitive deficits. As elsewhere in clinical medicine this may result in a therapeutic dilemma. Brain-damaged patients can suffer from epileptic seizures and need anticonvulsant medication; on the other hand, many anticonvulsants have negative effects on cognition. A trend-setting RCT in 1990 demonstrated that phenytoin was successful in preventing early but not late posttraumatic seizures (Temkin *et al.* 1990). Following that study it became the standard of care to withdraw anticonvulsants within a few weeks of brain injury

Table 22.1 Cognitive side-effects of psychopharmacological drugs

Substance class	Drug(s)	Cognitive side-effects	Comment
Anticholinergics	Biperiden, trihexyphenidyl	(Retrograde) amnesia, sedation, delirium	Budipine more favourable?
Antidepressants (tricyclic)	Amitryptiline, Nortriptyline	(Retrograde) amnesia, sedation, delirium	SSRIs more favourable
Anticonvulsives	Carbamazepine (CBZ), phenytoin (PHE), phenobarbital (PhB)	Psychomotor slowing, sedation	PhB > PHE > CBZ, second-generation anti-epileptic drugs more favourable?
Benzodiazepines	Diazepam, lorazepam, chlorazepate, midazolam	(Anterograde) amnesia, psychomotor slowing, sedation	Avoid long-acting benzodiazepines; buspirone more favourable?
Antipsychotics	Haloperidol	Sedation, psychomotor slowing, apathy	Avoid higher doses, second-generation antipsychotics more favourable
Mood stabilizer	Lithium	Delirium	Risk of overdose

Table 22.2 Cognitive side-effects of medication commonly prescribed in neurorehabilitation

Substance class	Drug(s)	Cognitive side-effect	Comment
Analgesics (centrally active)		Sedation, attention deficits	Duloxetine better for long-term pain relief?
(Some) antibiotics	Aminoglycoside	Ototoxicity (hearing impariment)	
	Sulfonamide	Sedation, focal symptoms	
Beta-blocker	Propranolol	Sedation, cognitive slowing, memory deficits	Calcium antagonists, ACE inhibitors, & peripheral (hydrophilic) beta blocker less problematic
Antispastic drugs	Baclofen	Sedation, delirium, depression	Addictive potential (benzodiazepine)
Glucocorticoids	Dexamethasone, prednisolone	Acute: euphoria; chronic: depression, memory deficits	Dose-related
Virostatics	Aciclovir	Sedation, delirium, psychotic symptoms	

(Chang and Lowenstein 2003; Glenn and Wroblewski 2005). Importantly, it has to be considered that some stimulating psychotropics may lower the seizure threshold (Pisani *et al.* 2002). Profiles of cognitive side-effects should be carefully analysed for individual risk–benefit analyses. Cognitive side-effects are also relevant in the context of recreational drugs like alcohol or cannabis, which are widely used (and abused) in Europe. Behavioural disturbances such as disinhibited or aggressive behaviour and sleep problems require psychopharmacological intervention. Benzodiazepines, neuroleptics, and mood stabilizers can impact negatively on both neuroplasticity and cognition. Atypical antipsychotics, anticonvulsants like lamotrigine, and sedative antidepressants like trazodone may be more favourable alternatives (James and Mendelson 2004).

> The first principle of pharmacological treatment in cognitive neurology is to stop or reduce medication with negative impact on neuroplasticity, cognitive, and motor functions whenever possible.

22.5 **Cognitive enhancing drugs**

In most societies recreational stimulants such as caffeine, nicotine, or cocaine are being used to reduce daytime sleepiness and improve performance at work. There is an increasingly important and complex debate about the neuroethics of cognitive enhancement (Farah *et al.* 2004). Pharmacological agents with positive effects on cognitive processing are increasingly prescribed and investigated in neuropsychiatry. Most psychostimulant medicines boost the function of dopamine or noradrenaline either directly or indirectly. Some cognitive enhancing medicines, such as antidepressants and atypical antipsychotics, are believed to act in part by improving syndromes that are not primarily cognitive. There is an evident overlap of enhancing alertness or cognition and treating apathy or daytime fatigue. Currently available drugs are reviewed in this section with information on mechanism of action, dosing, and licensed indications in Europe (Table 22.3). A few more substances like pemoline or tacrine are still available but not generally recommended due to lack of efficacy or problematic side-effects.

22.5.1 D-Amfetamine

Amphetamines are indirect sympathomimetic drugs that exert their action by stimulating the release of noradrenaline, dopamine, and serotonin. Amfetamine—this is the recommended international non-proprietary name (rINN) spelling that should be used in Europe—was first introduced in the form of 'benzedrine inhaler' and dextroamfetamine (dexamfetamine, D-amfetamine) sulphate tablets in the 1930s. The British Prime Minister Sir Winston Churchill was prescribed D-amfetamine to improve the 'muzzy feelings' he experienced after a first major stroke and he is believed to have taken extra tablets prior to public speaking (Long and Young 2003). Amphetamines are highly addictive and used as recreational psychostimulants. The promising model of enhancing the efficacy of physiotherapy or speech therapy by psychostimulants was first explored in studies with single doses of 10–20 mg of D-amfetamine. Positive results of animal research and pilot

Table 22.3 Overview of stimulating drugs (adapted from Müller 2001)

Substance	Dosage (mg/day)	Mechanism of action	Licensed indication(s)*
Atomoxetine	60–120	NAT inhibitor	ADHD
Amantadine	100–300	NMDA antagonist	PD, antiviral
Dextro-amfetamine[c]		DA/NA releaser, DAT/NAT (SERT) inhibitor	ADHD
Bromocriptine	20–60	DA agonist	PD, hyperprolactinaemia
Bupropion	150–300	DNA	Nicotine withdrawal
Donepezil	5–10	ChEI	AD (mild to moderate)
Galantamine	8–12	ChEI	AD (mild to moderate)
Levodopa/carbidopa	100–300	DA agonist	PD
Memantine	20	NMDA antagonist	AD (moderate to severe)
Methylphenidate[c]	20–40	DAT/NAT (SERT) inhibitor	ADHD, narcolepsy*
Moclobemide	300–600	MAO-A inhibitor	Depression, social phobia
Modafinil[(c)]	200–400	Unclear	Narcolepsy, sleep apnoea syndrome, daytime sleepiness*
Pergolide	3–6	DA agonist	PD
Piracetam	2400–4800	Unclear	Cortical myoclonus
Reboxetine	4–8	NAT inhibitor	Depression
Rivastigmine	6–12	ChEI	AD (mild to moderate)
Venlafaxine	75–150	SNA	Depression, generalized anxiety

ADHD, Attention deficit hyperactivity disorder (children and adolescents); AD, Alzheimer's disease; ChEI, acetylcholine esterase inhibitor; DA, dopamine; D/SNA, dopaminergic/serotonergic–noradrenergic antidepressant; DAT/NAT (SERT), dopamine/noradrenaline/serotonin transporter; MAO-A = monoamine oxidase; PD, Parkinson's disease; * at least in one European country; c/(c) = controlled drug (in some European countries only).

studies with short-term D-amfetamine in patients with hemiplegia or aphasia after stroke could not be replicated in subsequent RCTs (Goldstein 2006). Amphetamines are not available for prescription in most European countries and have to be imported from the US or UK.

22.5.2 Methylphenidate

Methylphenidate is a derivate of amfetamine. Its preferential mechanism of action is inhibition of dopamine (and noradrenaline) reuptake via dopamine transporter (DAT) and noradrenaline transporter (NAT) molecules. In most European countries methylphenidate is the first choice psychostimulant treatment for narcolepsy and attention deficit hyperactivity disorder (ADHD). Due to its addictive potential it is a specially controlled drug in all countries. Methylphenidate can increase blood pressure and pulse; this has to be carefully monitored in patients with cardiovascular disease, but does not seem to be a problem that should prevent its use in cognitive neurology (Burke *et al.* 2003). In elderly people effects of methylphenidate on task-related brain activity during performance of an attentional task were dose-dependent (Müller *et al.* 2005). Slow or dual-release preparations have been developed for the treatment of ADHD symptoms and allow treatment with a single capsule or tablet taken in the morning. There is some evidence from controlled studies that doses of 20–50 mg can improve apathy (Lee *et al.* 2005), executive deficits (Whyte *et al.* 2004; Kim *et al.* 2006), and impulse control (Mooney and Hass 1993) after TBI.

22.5.3 Modafinil

Modafinil is a wakefulness promoting agent that was first licensed for the treatment of narcolepsy in 1994 in France and subsequently around the world. Its mechanism of action is still unclear. However, indirect stimulation of noradrenaline release via orexin-hypocretin as well as enhancement of dopamine and histamine have been shown. Modafinil is a controlled drug in some European countries, but not in all. In the UK it is licensed for the treatment of narcolepsy and daytime sleepiness associated with sleep apnoea and other medical conditions. Despite positive data from RCTs modafinil was not approved by the FDA for the treatment of ADHD in 2006, apparently due to safety concerns after a single case of Stevens–Johnson syndrome, a serious skin disease. In healthy volunteers single doses of 200–400 mg/day of modafinil can improve working memory and attentional and executive functions (Müller *et al.* 2004), especially after sleep deprivation (Wesensten 2006). Modafinil is widely used by the military to remediate sleepiness in combat situations and long distance flights. Its relatively favourable profile of side-effects and low potential of addiction predestines this non-amphetamine psychostimulant as an interesting drug for interventions in cognitive neurology; however, only a few positive case reports have been published so far (DeMarchi *et al.* 2005; Ballon and Feifel 2006) and a high-quality RCT found no effects on fatigue in patients with multiple sclerosis (Stankoff *et al.* 2005). Further research is needed to determine the role of modafinil in cognitive neurology.

22.5.4 Noradrenaline reuptake inhibitors

Two selective noradrenaline reuptake inhibitors (NARIs) with similar pharmacological profiles have been licensed in the last years for the treatment of depression (*reboxetine*) or ADHD in children and adults (*atomoxetine*). Both drugs enhance noreadrenaline levels and possibly dopamine levels in prefrontal cortex, where dopamine is mainly re-uptaken via noradrenaline tranporters (Zhou 2004). There is some evidence for reboxetine 4–8 mg/day to improve cognitive deficits in patients with alcohol Korsakov disease (Reuster *et al.* 2003). In healthy volunteers emotional and memory processes can be facilitated by reboxetine, whereas a single dose of atomoxetine 60 mg improved motor inhibition in a stop signal task (Chamberlain *et al.* 2006*a*, *b*). So far atomoxetine has not been used in patients with acquired brain damage but seems a promising approach to stimulate noradrenaline (and dopamine) dependent cognitive functions. Both dopamine and noradrenaline are involved in the neurotransmitter modulation of prefrontal cognitive processes like working memory and attentional control. Attention deficits and impulsivity in ADHD seem to be related to catecholamine deficits (Frank *et al.* 2007). Similar cognitive and behavioural deficits in patients with acquired brain damage will respond to both noradrenaline- or dopamine-enhancing medication.

22.5.5 Antiparkinsonian drugs

Parkinson's disease is the most comprehensively investigated model of a neuropsychiatric disease caused by neurotransmitter deficits. Degeneration of dopaminergic neurons results in motor, cognitive, and emotional deficits that can be remediated, at least in part, by dopamine-enhancing medication (Brooks 2006). *Levodopa* and dopamine agonists like bromocriptine or pergolide have been used to stimulate motor and cognitive deficits in patients with acquired brain damage (Zafonte *et al.* 2000, 2001). An exemplary RCT in patients with hemiplegia after stroke found significant improvement of motor recovery during 3 weeks of treatment with levodopa 100 mg/day as compared to placebo (Scheidtmann *et al.* 2001). Motor learning in nine patients with chronic stroke was improved after a single dose of levodopa as compared to placebo (Floël *et al.* 2006). *Bromocriptine* is the most widely investigated D2 receptor agonist in cognitive neurology with some positive effects on hemi-spatial neglect, memory deficits, non-fluent aphasia, and apathy (Arciniegas and Silver 2006). Treatment with bromocriptine generally begins with 2.5 mg/day and is gradually titrated to the highest dose tolerated. Dizziness, faintness, orthostatic hypotension, nausea/vomiting, constipation, and diarrhaea are relatively common side-effects that can be minimized by slow titration or co-medication with peripherally active dopamine antagonists like domperidone. Psychotic symptoms during treatment with dopamine agonists are usually dose-dependent and disappear with lower doses. Higher doses of dopamine agonists as often needed in patients with cognitive deficits and apathy can be quite expensive, which is a problem for any longer-term 'off-label' treatment (Müller and von Cramon 1994).

22.5.6 Glutamate antagonists

Amantadine was originally introduced for its antiviral properties in the 1960s and was later found to be effective in treating cognitive deficits and symptoms in Parkinson's disease, multiple sclerosis, and traumatic brain injury. *Memantine* was used for the treatment of apathy in patients with acquired brain damage for many years in several European countries and was formally licensed in 2002 for the treatment of medium to severe dementia in patients with Alzheimer's disease based on evidence from RCTs. Both drugs are moderate-affinity NMDA (glutamate) receptor antagonists and have indirect dopaminergic effects (Arciniegas and Silver 2006). The profile of side-effects is similar to that of dopamine agonists. There are positive RCTs for amantadine 200 mg/day (Krupp *et al.* 1995; Meythaler *et al.* 2002) showing some improvement of apathy in patients with multiple sclerosis and TBI, although practice effects in the later cross-over study are clearly overinterpreted as treatment effects, both in the orginal paper and in most reviews (Napolitano *et al.* 2005; Arciniegas and Silver 2006).

22.5.7 Cholinesterase inhibitors

Physostigmine, the first reversible cholinesterase inhibitor (ChEI), was extracted from the Calabar bean and is still in use for emergency treatment of anticholinergic delirium. Animal and human studies showed cognitive enhancing effects in the scopolamine (i.e. anticholinergic) model of memory deficits and after brain injury (Cardenas *et al.* 1994). Modern ChEIs like *donepezil*, *galantamine*, and *rivastigmine* have a more favourable pharmacokinetics that allows oral administration and single daily dosing. These drugs are generally well tolerated, but some patients experience problems with nausea, diarrhoea, and arrhythmia (Cummings 2003). There is preliminary evidence from small controlled trials that donepezil improves attention and memory deficits after TBI (Griffin *et al.* 2003; Zhang *et al.* 2004) and aphasia after stroke (Berthier 2005; Berthier *et al.* 2006). A large-scale RCT of rivastigmine showed good tolerability and cognitive enhancing effects in a subgroup of TBI patients with more severe memory deficits (Silver *et al.* 2006). Beneficial aspects on apathy and perhaps other aspects of behaviour may result in improved outcome and quality of life for individuals with acquired brain injury (Blount *et al.* 2002). ChEIs are an interesting class of drugs and may become more important for the treatment of TBI sequelae when patents have expired and prices for long-term treatment become more affordable.

22.5.8 **Other stimulating medicines**

The repertoire of pharmacological interventions for patients with cognitive and behavioural deficits after brain injury is not exhausted by the substances portrayed so far. Negative symptoms and apathy in patients with major depression and schizophrenia respond favourably to antidepressants like *bupropion*, *duloxetine*, *moclobemide*, or *venlafaxine* (Fava 2006). Moclobemide is a reversible MAO inhibitor that has shown positive effects in elderly patients with depression and cognitive decline (Roth *et al.* 1996), but not on speech deficits after acute stroke (Laska *et al.* 2005). Another drug that was formally tested in patients with acute and chronic aphasia is *piracetam*, a GABA derivate with multiple mechanisms of action. Piracetam is only available in Europe and licensed for conditions such as dyslexia, cortical myoclonus, and mild cognitive impairment/dementia without supporting evidence from well-performed RCTs. Several RCTs in stroke patients showed positive effects of 4.8 g/day on acute aphasia after stroke (Greener *et al.* 2001). These effects were accompanied by an increase of task-related activation in eloquent areas of the left hemisphere (Kessler *et al.* 2000).

22.5.9 **Herbal stimulants**

Caffeine is worldwide the most frequently consumed psychostimulant drug. It is an adenosine antagonist that indirectly enhances noradrenaline and serotonin in the brain. A typical mug of coffee contains 50–150 mg of caffeine and peak levels are reached within 15–60 min, depending on simultaneous milk and food consumption (Boutrel and Koob 2004). Caffeine has cognitive enhancing properties, especially in sleep-deprived people; any new psychostimulant should be tested against caffeine (Wesensten 2006). *Nicotine* is an acetylcholine agonist widely consumed through cigarette smoking. In patients with schizophrenia deficits, smoking is considered to be a self-medication of cognitive deficits (Kumari and Postma 2005).

Cocaine is a DAT inhibitor, similar to methylphenidate. In most countries it is an illegal (or regulated) street drug. Coca chewing in the Andean regions of South America prevents hypoglycaemia at high-altitude conditions. Nicotine and cocaine are highly addictive. Caffeine, nicotine, and cocaine abuse can result in hypertension, hypervigilance with agitation, and rebound daytime sleepiness. Nicotine abuse is a risk factor for cardio- and cerebrovascular diseases. Nicotine and cocaine are often contributing factors to stroke and traumatic brain injuries in young adults and must be avoided in neurorehabilitation. Caffeine can reduce cerebral blood flow in patients recovering from stroke (Ragab *et al.* 2004). Potential beneficial and detrimental effects of lower doses of caffeine have to be investigated more systematically.

Ginkgo biloba extracts and vitamin E preparations are very popular among people with age-related memory decline. Large-scale epidemiological and placebo-controlled studies showed, however, neither preventive nor therapeutic effects in people with mild cognitive impairment or dementia (Birks *et al.* 2002; Petersen *et al.* 2005). The therapeutic potential of herbal alternative medicines in cognitive neurology has to be further investigated (LaFrance *et al.* 2000).

A variety of stimulating medicines has been used to treat cognitive and motivational deficits in patients with acquired brain injury. So far there is insufficient evidence to support any standards of treatment. The most promising substances are psychostimulants like methylphenidate, which enhance synaptic levels of dopamine and noradrenaline, and cholinesterase inhibitors, which increase acetylcholine.

22.6 Pharmacological treatment of cognitive deficits

Well-defined and measurable cognitive deficits have become a target for pharmacological treatment in cognitive neurology. This is reflected in the publication of Cochrane meta-analyses of interventions for cognitive (Greener *et al.* 2001; Birks *et al.* 2002) and behavioural deficits (Gill and Hatcher 2000; Fleminger *et al.* 2006) and a first multiauthor guideline for the pharmacological treatment of neurobehavioural sequelae of TBI (Warden *et al.* 2006). Pharmacological interventions in cognitive neurology and individual treatment plans must be based on the best available evidence. The number of RCTs in patients with acquired brain injury and cognitive deficits, aphasia, apathy, depression, and emotionalism is slowly increasing over time (Fig. 22.1). Therapeutic strategies and drug regimes that were originally developed for patients with dementia or other neuropsychiatric diseases have been adapted to patients with acquired brain injury. Table 22.4 and the following paragraphs summarize evidence-based knowledge, mainly in patients with stroke and TBI. Most drugs and pharmacological strategies have been or can be applied to treat cognitive and behavioural deficits in patients with other neurological diseases or dementia.

22.6.1 Attentional deficits and neglect

Attentional deficits with cognitive slowing and problems in focusing, dividing, or maintaining attention are common findings in patients with mild to severe TBI (Warden *et al.* 2006) and other brain injury (Cappa *et al.* 2005). Psychostimulants and atomoxetine are well established in the treatment of attention deficit hyperactivity disorder (ADHD), a condition with childhood-onset that is characterized by cognitive deficits, hyperactivity, and impulsivity (Biederman *et al.* 2004). The same cognitive deficits seem to respond to methylphenidate in low performing healthy volunteers, patients with ADHD, and those with TBI. The few controlled trials performed so far used relatively broad and non-specific batteries of cognitive tasks (Zhang *et al.* 2004; Coulthard *et al.* 2006) and only one study focused on attentional functions after cerebrovascular lesions (Lehmann *et al.* 2001).

Unilateral spatial neglect or hemi-inattention is a common and disabling problem after right hemispheric stroke. Patients with neglect fail to explore the left hemispheric field and often bump into obstacles on their left side. Models of disturbed spatial and attentional mechanisms have been proposed to explain this debilitating syndrome (Fink and Heide 2004). Established therapeutic interventions like visual scanning training and visuo-spatio-motor training aim to improve spatial representation deficits (Cappa *et al.* 2005). Pharmacological enhancement of

Table 22.4 Evidence-based pharmacological treatment in cognitive neurology: classification according to EFNS criteria (Brainin *et al.* 2004); last update December 2006

Target symptom	Aetiology	Drug	Evidence class	Level of recommendation*
Attentional deficit, hemi neglect	Stroke(MS, HIV)	Bromocriptine	IV	Unclear
		Guanfacine	IV	Possibly effective (C)
		Imipramine	IV	Possibly effective (C)
		Levodopa	IV	Possibly effective (C)
		Methylphenidate	III	Possibly effective (B)
		Modafinil	IV	Possibly effective (C)
Memory & executive deficits	TBI, stroke (AAD, TBI, brain tumour (post-surgery), encephalitis, MCI)	Bromocriptine	III	Possibly effective (C)
		Clonidine	III	Possibly effective (C)
		Donepezil	III	Possibly effective (C)
		Fluvoxamine	III	Unclear
		Levodopa	II	Possibly effective (B)
		Methylphenidate	II	Unclear
		Physostigmine	III	Possibly effective (C)
		Reboxetine	III	Possibly effective (C)
		Rivastigmine	I	Probably effective (B)
		Vasopressin	IV	Unclear
Aphasia	Stroke	Amphetamine	III	Possibly effective (C)
		Bromocriptine	II	Probably ineffective (C)
		Donepezil	II	Probably effective (B)
		Moclobemide	II	Probably ineffective (B)
		Piracetam	II	Probably effective (B)
Apathy	TBI, stroke (MS, HIV, hypoxia, encephalitis)	Amantadine	II	Probably effective (B)
		Amphetamine	IV	Possibly effective (C)
		Bromocriptine	IV	Possibly effective (C)
		Levodopa	IV	Possibly effective (C)
		Memantine	IV	Possibly effective (C)
		Methylphenidate	II	Probably effective (B)
		Modafinil	I	Unclear
		Pemoline	III	Possibly harmful
		Pergolide	IV	Possibly effective (C)

AAD, Alcohol amnestic disorder; HIV, = HIV encephalopathy; MCI, mild cognitive impairment; MS, multiple sclerosis; TBI, traumatic brain injury; unclear, conflicting findings (and no meta-analysis available).

underlying arousal or attention deficits has been reported in a few promising case series and controlled single-case studies. Improvement of neglect symptoms and normalization of the attentional bias were observed after single doses or short-term treatment with apomorphine, bromocriptine, guanfacine, levodopa, modafinil, and cholinergic substances (Pierce and Buxbaum 2002; Thiel 2003; Parton *et al.* 2005; Luaute *et al.* 2006). The first clinical trials of pharmacological interventions in patients with neglect have been initiated.

22.6.2 Memory and executive deficits

Severe amnesia is common in patients with Alzheimer's disease and after severe TBI and some neurosurgical lesions. Small vascular lesions of memory-relevant brain regions in the basal forebrain, mediotemporal lobe, prefrontal cortex, or basal ganglia can result in more selective *memory deficits*. ChEIs like donepezil are the treatment of choice in mild to medium severe forms of Alzheimer's disease and other dementias: vascular dementia; dementia with Lewy bodies; and dementia in Parkinson's disease (Cummings 2003). Surprisingly, several recent RCTs investigating the therapeutic and prophylactic potential of ChEIs in patients with mild cognitive impairment (MCI) were negative (Jelic *et al.* 2006). Treatment of memory deficits after TBI with ChEIs is based on neuropathological and neuroimaging of lesions affecting the basal forebrain and other cholinergic projections (Salmond *et al.* 2005). A review of published case series concluded that there is sufficient theoretical and preliminary empirical evidence to move beyond pilot studies to large-scale clinical trials (Griffin *et al.* 2003); consequently, a first multicentre RCT of rivastigmine 3–6 mg/day in patients with mild TBI ($n = 157$) has been performed in the USA (Silver *et al.* 2006). This is an exemplary study in terms of overall design, neuropsychological testing battery, and toleration of non-cholinergic concomitant medication (as long as doses remained constant during the trial). Post hoc analysis of the group with more severe memory deficits ($n = 89$) showed positive trends of rivastigmine on memory (Hopkins Verbal Learning Test) and attentional functions (CANTAB Rapid Visual Information Processing). ChEIs may also improve episodic memory functions in patients suffering from basal forebrain lesions and persistent amnesia after rupture and repair of aneurysms of the anterior communicating, the anterior cerebral, or the pericallosal artery casing (Müller and von Cramon 1994). Controlled follow-up studies are necessary to confirm these findings and differentiate drug effects from practice effects and/or spontaneous recovery.

Only a few pharmacological intervention studies focus on *executive deficits*. Executive processes are involved in many memory functions such as encoding, retrieval, or manipulation in working memory. Dopamine (and noradrenaline) enhancement is a theoretically interesting approach to boost executive processing (Knecht 2006). Promising results of improved executive functions after a single dose of bromocriptine 2.5 mg as compared to placebo (McDowell *et al.* 1998) should, however, not warrant guideline recommendation of this intervention (Warden *et al.* 2006). Motor learning in patients with chronic stroke was improved by a single dose of levodopa 100 mg (Floël *et al.* 2006). Studies with single dose application of stimulating medicines are proof of concept experiments that must be followed by clinical trials with longer-term treatment and clinically relevant outcome parameters. The most consistent series of RCTs has been performed with methylphenidate 20–50 mg after TBI with mostly positive (Plenger *et al.* 1996; Whyte *et al.* 1997; Kim *et al.* 2006) but also some unclear (Whyte *et al.* 2004) and negative effects (Mooney and Haas 1993; Tiberti *et al.* 1998) on memory and executive functions (Whyte *et al.* 2002; Siddall 2005).

22.6.3 Aphasia and other language deficits

Language and speech deficits after brain injury are common neurological symptoms that cause considerable disability and handicap. The most frequent aetiology is infarction of the left middle cerebral artery. Currently, the main method of aphasia treatment is speech and language therapy with a pragmatic conversational approach; however, so far the effectiveness of functional treatments over spontaneous recovery has not been shown in properly controlled clinical studies (Cappa *et al.* 2005).

Pharmacological treatment with stimulating and neuroplasticity-enhancing substances is a new approach in aphasia therapy. More than 10 RCTs have been performed during the last decade with some promising results. Among the drugs that have been used to improve *language recovery* after stroke, piracetam 4800 mg/day is a promising candidate with three positive studies. However, the evidence of benefit was weak and there are concerns about its safety. More research is needed into the effects of piracetam before it can be recommended for routine use (Greener *et al.* 2001). Initial positive reports claimed that *non-fluent forms of aphasia* with reduced speech production could be improved by treatment with bromocriptine 10–60 mg; however, all but one (Bragoni *et al.* 2000) of the placebo-controlled trials were negative. In spite of its seemingly sound background, the dopaminergic approach failed to show reliable benefits in controlled studies (Bakheit 2004; De Boissezon *et al.* 2007).

There are apparently no animal models for recovery and treatment of aphasia. Based on models of motor recovery D-amfetamine 10 mg was administered before a series of speech therapy sessions with positive effects on language recovery (Walker-Batson *et al.* 2001). There are, however, still many gaps in our knowledge and the *combination of D-amfetamine and speech therapy* is not ready to become a standard of care. Unanswered questions include the following: How long after stroke can psychostimulants like D-amfetamine be administered and have an effect? What are adequate doses and number of drug administrations needed to provide optimal recovery? What is the amount of use-dependent practice or retraining that must be paired with the pharmacological intervention for optimal recovery? Ongoing trials are exploring the efficacy of D-amfetamine to enhance recovery from stroke (Walker-Batson *et al.* 2002).

Clinical trials in aphasia are relatively difficult to perform due to the heterogeneity of lesions and aphasia syndromes, medical comorbidity, and contraindications, as well as problems with communication and informed consent. The largest RCT published so far found no effects of 6 months of moclobemide 600 mg/day on recovery of aphasia in 89 patients with acute stroke (Laska *et al.* 2005). Another well-designed trial with 26 stroke patients showed greater improvement of aphasia severity and communicative activity after donepezil 10 mg/day as compared to placebo (Berthier *et al.* 2006). ChEIs may well become the only class of drugs that do more good than harm in aphasia treatment. Depression and pain are frequent symptoms and should not be overlooked in patients with aphasia, because pharmacological and psychological interventions are available that may improve preconditions for aphasia treatment (Kehayia *et al.* 1997; Wallesch *et al.* 1997).

Cognitive deficits after acquired brain damage are potentially amenable to pharmacological treatment. The first controlled trials have meanwhile been performed with some positive results for dopamine- or acetylcholine-enhancing drugs on aphasia and memory deficits after TBI and stroke, but there are no recommended standards of treatment at the moment.

22.7 Pharmacological treatment of behavioural deficits

Diagnosis and treatment of psychiatric symptoms in patients with stroke or TBI are often neglected or inadequate because the number of prescribing specialists with expert knowledge in behavioural neurology/neuropsychiatry is limited. Subspecialty training as initiated by the American Neuropsychiatric Association and the Society for Behavioral and Cognitive Neurology (Arciniegas and Kaufer 2006) was approved in the USA (Silver 2006). The new curriculum contains major parts on pharmacological treatment. Similar initiatives should be started to improve the quality of care for patients with acquired brain injury in Europe. The following section reviews pharmacological treatments of behavioural deficits with a focus on recent developments.

22.7.1 Deficits of emotional processing and regulation

Depression is a common complication of many neurological diseases, with frequencies of 30–40% after stroke, the most widely investigated aetiology (Hackett *et al.* 2005). Most authors favour models that combine biological factors like lesion location and psychological factors like maladjustment to neurological deficits or occupational consequences. Two recent meta-analyses found no relationship between the side of a lesion and *post-stroke depression* (Carson *et al.* 2000) but confirmed an inverse correlation between severity of depression and distance of the lesion from the frontal pole (Narushima *et al.* 2003*b*). Depressive comorbidity has a considerable negative impact on psychosocial outcome, quality of life, and even mortality (Robinson 2006). Several RCTs—most of them with relatively small sample sizes—showed positive effects of nortriptyline, trazodone, citalopram, fluoxetine, and sertraline on post-stroke depression. Low to medium doses of selective serotonin re-uptake inhibitors (SSRIs) seem to be relatively safe to use in neurological patients with no increased risk of cerebrovascular events (Bak *et al.* 2002) or epileptic seizures (Kanner *et al.* 2000). A Cochrane meta-analysis concludes that antidepressants may improve mood in stroke patients with depression and that it is unclear how clinically significant such modest effects are in patients other than in those with major depression (Hackett *et al.* 2005). This cautious assessment is supported by some more recent and higher quality studies that could not replicate positive effects of sertraline (Murray *et al.* 2005) or fluoxetine (Almeida *et al.* 2006; Choi-Kwon *et al.* 2006) on post-stroke depression.

There is sufficient evidence from epidemiological and follow-up studies that depression is a risk factor for cognitive decline and dementia (Jorm 2000). Cognitive impairment due to post-stroke depression is reversible and can be quantified separately from cognitive impairment on the basis of the location and extent of ischaemic brain damage. Antidepressant treatment can improve cognitive deficits (Narushima *et al.* 2003*a*). Noradrenergic antidepressants like moclobemide, nortriptyline, or reboxetine and serotonin and noradrenaline re-uptake inhibitors (SNRIs) like duloxetine, milnacipran, or venlafaxine can be used to treat both depression and cognitive deficits (Sato *et al.* 2006). Another clinically relevant issue is the preventive use of antidepressant treatment after stroke. Controlled studies found reduced occurrence of depression in stroke patients treated with mianserin (Palomäki *et al.* 1999), fluoxetine (Robinson 2006), and sertraline (Rasmussen *et al.* 2003; but not Almeida *et al.* 2006).

Depression is not the only deficit of emotional processing and regulation in patients with neurological disease. Involuntary episodes of crying or laughing that are unrelated to or out of proportion to the eliciting stimulus are common among patients with amyotrophic lateral sclerosis (ALS), multiple sclerosis (MS), stroke, and TBI. This emotional disinhibition syndrome has received various names such as pseudobulbar affect, pathological crying, or organic emotionalism and was recently re-branded '*involuntary emotional expression disorder*' (IEED) by a group of leading experts in an attempt to provide a unifying term and operational diagnostic criteria (Schiffer and Pope 2005; Cummings *et al.* 2006). This seems to be part of a marketing campaign funded by Avanir Pharmaceuticals in order to promote dextromethorphan/quinidine (Neurodex®), which may become the first US Food and Drugs Administration (FDA)-approved drug for the treatment of IEED after successful RCTs in ALS and MS (Brooks *et al.* 2004; Panitch *et al.* 2006), but not in other neurological diseases (Pollack 2005). So far, the treatment of choice has been SSRIs, with rapid onset and good tolerability shown in several RCTs (Horrocks *et al.* 2004). Involvement of the serotonin system is supported by a neuroimaging study with beta-CIT SPECT that found lower availability of the serotonin transporter (SERT) in midbrain/raphe regions of patients with post-stroke emotionalism (Murai *et al.* 2003).

22.7.2 Apathy and disorders of diminished motivation

Apathy is characterized by diminished motivation, diminished interest and concern, and diminished emotional responsiveness. It can often have a negative impact on rehabilitation, return to work, and successful reintegration to the community. Apathy is a frequent behavioural symptom in patients with acquired brain damage, neurodegenerative disorders, and psychiatric diseases

(Marin 1996). There is a conceptual overlap between apathy and negative symptoms, fatigue, daytime sleepiness, bradyphrenia, hypobulia, and akinetic mutism. Estimates of frequency of apathy following TBI range from 45% to 70% (van Reekum *et al.* 2005). Apathy can present independently and should be distinguished from depression. Lesion and neuroimaging studies have demonstrated critical involvement of the frontomedial cortex, caudate nucleus, and thalamus in disorders of diminished motivation (Marin and Wilkosz 2005).

Dopamine-enhancing agents and psychostimulants have been used to treat apathy and motivational deficits in patients with acquired brain injury (Müller and von Cramon 1994; Lee *et al.* 2003; Deb and Crownshaw 2004; Keenan *et al.* 2005; Robinson 2006). Activating antidepressants like moclobemide, reboxetine, or venlafaxine are a treatment of choice for patients with mixed apathy and depression. There are, however, only very few controlled studies, most of them in relatively small samples of TBI patients. When patients in the acute stage after moderately to severe TBI ($n = 80$) were treated with methylphenidate, the length of stay at an intensive care unit and at the hospital was shorter when compared to placebo (Moein *et al.* 2006). In another placebo-controlled study of post-acute TBI patients ($n = 30$) both methylphenidate 20 mg/day and sertraline 100 mg/day improved symptoms of depression but methylphenidate seemed to have more beneficial effects on daytime alertness (Lee *et al.* 2005). Two RCTs found no clear effects of amantadine 100–300 mg/day on behavioural deficits after TBI; however, both studies were limited by small sample size and confounded by overall improvement (Schneider *et al.* 1999; Meythaler *et al.* 2002). An appropriately powered RCT ($n = 115$) showed no significant effects of modafinil on fatigue in patients with MS (Stankoff *et al.* 2005). Amantadine, modafinil, and methylphenidate should be further investigated in patients with apathy and prefrontal cognitive deficits.

22.7.3 **Agitation, aggression, and sleep disturbances**

Of the many psychiatric symptoms that may result from brain injury, agitation and aggression are often the most troublesome and require pharmacological interventions. A Cochrane review concludes that beta-blockers have the best evidence for efficacy and deserve more attention (Fleminger *et al.* 2006). Higher doses of beta blockers (propranolol or pindolol) are also recommended for treatment of aggression in USA TBI guidelines (Warden *et al.* 2006). Antipsychotics and benzodiazepines are widely used for sedation in this patient population; however, their negative impact on neuroplasticity and rehabilitative interventions has to be considered carefully. When patients with severe TBI ($n = 26$) were treated with haloperidol they had significantly longer posttraumatic amnesia than untreated patients; agitation and treatment with antipsychotics are indicators of poor outcome (Rao *et al.* 1985).

Disturbed sleep–wake cycles and daytime sleepiness are frequent findings in patients with acquired brain damage. No systematic evaluation of psychotropic interventions is available. Counselling about sleep hygiene should be used as first-line treatment followed by herbal sedatives or sedating antidepressants (e.g. trazodone or trimipramine). Hypnotics with addictive potential should only be prescribed for a short time. Newer substances such as zopiclon or zolpidem are preferable, because they have a better pharmacokinetic profile compared with benzodiazepine hypnotics. Benzodiazepines with long half-life and dopamine antagonist should be generally avoided because of unwanted effects on cognitive and motor functions (Müller 2001).

> The pharmacological treatment of post-stroke depression is well investigated and established. Antidepressants with a favourable profile of cognitive side-effects and sedation are recommended. Psychostimulants and other activating substances should be further investigated for the treatment of apathy.

22.8 General principles of pharmacotherapy

Pharmacological treatment in cognitive neurology should be based on neurobiological models of cognitive (and emotional) deficits and be supported by evidence from clinical trials. A number of general and more specific principles are highlighted in Table 22.5.

At the end of 2006 not a single medication was explicitly licensed for the treatment of cognitive deficits or emotional problems after stroke, TBI, or other forms of acquired brain injury. This has important ethical and legal implications. Off-label prescription of psychotropic medication is possible in most European countries whenever there is good or promising evidence to support an individual indication and after careful risk–benefit analysis (Rummans *et al.* 1999; Fountoulakis *et al.* 2004). The rationale for such a treatment, informed consent, and observed side-effects have to be documented in the patient's notes. Funding of off-label medication can be a big issue in many European countries, especially when expensive drugs like ChEIs, modafinil, or higher doses of dopamine agonists are prescribed. Non-adherence or partial adherence to medication is often a problem in patients with memory deficits and has to be monitored.

22.9 Research perspectives: from bedside to bench – and back

Several approaches have been used to establish the pharmacological treatment of cognitive deficits after acquired brain injury. Experiences and models derived from the treatment of

Table 22.5 Principles of pharmacological treatment of cognitive deficits

General principles

- Take comprehensive history of pharmacological treatment before changing any medication
- Discontinue unnecessary or unclear medication (often more efficient than a new prescription)
- Perform an individual risk–benefit analysis
- Continue successful treatment (never change a winning team)
- Avoid polypragmatics
- Use only a limited number of familiar and well-known pharmaceutical products
- Use 'new' substances only after comprehensive analysis of available literature
- Never chance more than one drug at a time (if possible)
- Consider pharmacokinetics when switching medication and stick to your plan
- Consider and monitor drug interactions (e.g. using Psychopharmacological Drug Interactions Calculator: *www.gjpsy.uni-goettingen.de/interactions_calculator.php*)
- Obtain informed consent and document it
- Monitor side-effects and adherence
- Teach patient and relatives in order to improve adherence

Special principles of pharmacological treatment in neurorehabilitation

- Start with low doses and titrate up quickly in case of good tolerance
- In case of partial response go up to the dose limits
- Perform controlled withdrawal in case of possible spontaneous remission
- Consider dose adaptation in patients with medical comorbidity or leaking blood–brain barrier
- Every patient is different

Alzheimer's and Parkinson's diseases have been used to treat memory and executive deficits. The treatment of aphasia was first introduced in imitation of an animal and clinical model of pharmacological enhancement of functional training after motor cortex lesion and hemiplegia. Treatment of attentional deficits and hemineglect with noradrenaline-, dopamine-, and acetylcholine-enhancing drugs is based on cognitive neuroscience models of neurotransmitter modulation of attentional processes. Better animal models and more translational studies from bench to bedside are necessary (Phillips *et al.* 2003; Floël and Cohen 2006). Single dose studies in healthy volunteers and patients with well-defined brain lesions may help to develop new pharmacological treatment strategies. Pharmacological imaging with fMRI and PET will help to disentangle effects of stimulating and sedating drugs on task-specific or neuroplasticity-related brain activity (Strangman *et al.* 2005; Rijntjes 2006).

Cognitive deficits after TBI have been shown to be influenced by genetic factors like apolipoprotein E (ApoE; Jiang *et al.* 2006). Effects of stimulating drugs on cognition and task-related brain activity may depend on genetic factors, as has been shown in elegant studies with amphetamine and a common catechyl-*O*-methyltransferase (COMT) polymorphism (Mattay *et al.* 2003) or bromocriptine and dopamine receptor (DR2) genotyping (Kirsch *et al.* 2006), where cognitive improvement was only seen in participants with relatively low endogenous dopamine levels. A recent meta-analysis confirmed a small effect of the COMT gene on on executive functioning in healthy volunteers but not in patients with schizophrenia (Barnett *et al.* 2007). Development of post-stroke depression may also be genetically predetermined by factors like the SERT polymorphism (Ramasubbu *et al.* 2006).

There are some promising indications where well-performed RCTs are possible and necessary, such as aphasia after stroke and memory deficits after TBI. Such trials should incorporate methodological considerations including: (1) randomized double-blind placebo-controlled design; (2) sample size selection based on the hypothesized degree of improvement on the primary outcome measure; (3) selection of subjects based on specific cognitive inclusion criteria; and (4) sufficient duration of intervention to allow for measurement of cognitive and functional improvement (Griffin *et al.* 2003). Head-to-head studies of different stimulating drugs are needed to guide clinical decision-making and could be implemented by EU-funded research networks. Future studies will have to investigate the combination and interaction of pharmacological treatment and cognitive training in a more systematic way. Cost-effectiveness studies will have to evaluate comprehensive treatment programmes including different pharmacological strategies (Cardenas *et al.* 2001; Greener and Langhorne 2002). On the one hand, it is good to see that the pharmacotherapy in cognitive neurology and neuropsychiatry has just been discovered as an interesting market by the pharmaceutical industry. On the other hand, independent (publicly) funded research is important in many areas where licences of relevant drugs have already or will soon expire. Comprehensive clinical and research training of cognitive neurologists and neuropsychiatrists is an important strategy to ensure further progress.

The pharmacological treatment of cognitive and emotional deficits after TBI and stroke is a promising area of clinical research. Implementation of evidence- and guideline-based interventions will improve the outcome and quality of life of many patients.

References

Almeida, O.P., Waterreus, A., and Hankey, G.J. (2006). Preventing depression after stroke: results from a randomized placebo-controlled trial. *J. Clin. Psychiatry* **67**, 1104–9.

Arciniegas, D.B., Kaufer, D.I; Joint Advisory Committee on Subspecialty Certification of the American Neuropsychiatric Association; Society for Behavioral and Cognitive Neurology (2006). Core curriculum for training in behavioral neurology and neuropsychiatry. *J. Neuropsychiatry Clin. Neurosci.* **18**, 6–13.

Arciniegas, D.B. and Silver, J.M. (2006). Pharmacotherapy of posttraumatic cognitive impairments. *Behav. Neurol.* **17**, 25–42.

Bak, S., Tsiropoulos, I., Kjaersgaard, J.O., Andersen, M., Mellerup, E., Hallas, J., Garcia Rodriguez, L.A., Christensen, K., and Gaist, D. (2002). Selective serotonin reuptake inhibitors and the risk of stroke: a population-based case-control study. *Stroke* **33**, 1465–73.

Bakheit, A.M. (2004). Drug treatment of poststroke aphasia. *Expert Rev. Neurother.* **4**, 211–17.

Ballon, J.S. and Feifel, D. (2006). A systematic review of modafinil: potential clinical uses and mechanisms of action. *J. Clin. Psychiatry* **67**, 554–66.

Barnett, J.H., Jones, P.B., Robbins, T.W., and Müller, U. (2007). Effects of COMT $Val^{158}Met$ polymorphism on executive function: a meta-analysis of the Wisconsin Card Sorting Test in schizophrenia and healthy controls. *Mol. Psychiatry* **12,** 502–9.

Berthier, M.L. (2005). Poststroke aphasia: epidemiology, pathophysiology and treatment. *Drugs Aging* **22**, 163–82.

Berthier, M.L., Green, C., Higueras, C., Fernandez, I., Hinojosa, J., and Martin, M.C. (2006). A randomized, placebo-controlled study of donepezil in poststroke aphasia. *Neurology* **67**, 1687–9.

Biederman, J., Spencer, T., and Wilens, T. (2004). Evidence-based pharmacotherapy for attention-deficit hyperactivity disorder. *Int. J. Neuropsychopharmacol.* **7**, 77–97.

Birks, J., Grimley, E.V., and Van Dongen, M. (2002). Ginkgo biloba for cognitive impairment and dementia. *Cochrane Database Syst. Rev.* **2002** (4), CD003120.

Blount, P.J., Nguyen, C.D., and McDeavitt, J.T. (2002). Clinical use of cholinomimetic agents: a review. *J. Head Trauma Rehabil.* **17**, 314–21.

Boutrel, B. and Koob, G.F. (2004). What keeps us awake: the neuropharmacology of stimulants and wakefulness-promoting medications. *Sleep* **27**, 1181–94.

Bragoni, M., Altieri, M., Di Piero, V., Padovani, A., Mostardini, C., and Lenzi, G.L. (2000). Bromocriptine and speech therapy in non-fluent chronic aphasia after stroke. *Neurol. Sci.* **21**, 19–22.

Brainin, M., Barnes, M., Baron, J.C., Gilhus, N.E., Hughes, R., Selmaj, K., Waldemar, G; Guideline Standards Subcommittee of the EFNS Scientific Committee (2004). Guidance for the preparation of neurological management guidelines by EFNS scientific task forces, revised recommendations 2004. *Eur. J. Neurol.* **11**, 577–81.

Brooks, B.R., Thisted, R.A., Appel, S.H., Bradley, W.G., Olney, R.K., Berg, J.E., Pope, L.E., Smith, R.A; AVP-923 ALS Study Group (2004). Treatment of pseudobulbar affect in ALS with dextromethorphan/quinidine: a randomized trial. *Neurology* **63**, 1364–70.

Brooks, D.J. (2006). Dopaminergic action beyond its effects on motor function: imaging studies. *J. Neurol.* **253** (Suppl. 4), 8–15.

Burke, D.T., Glenn, M.B., Vesali, F., Schneider, J.C., Burke, J., Ahangar, B., and Goldstein, R. (2003). Effects of methylphenidate on heart rate and blood pressure among inpatients with acquired brain injury. *Am. J. Phys. Med. Rehabil.* **82**, 493–7.

Cappa, S.F., Benke, T., Clarke, S., Rossi, B., Stemmer, B., and van Heugten, C.M. (2005). EFNS guidelines on cognitive rehabilitation: report of an EFNS task force. *Eur. J. Neurol.* **12**, 665–80.

Cardenas, D.D., McLean, A. Jr, Farrell-Roberts, L., Baker, L., Brooke, M., and Haselkorn, J. (1994). Oral physostigmine and impaired memory in adults with brain injury. *Brain Inj.* **8**, 579–87.

Cardenas, D.D., Haselkorn, J.K., McElligott, J.M., and Gnatz, S.M. (2001). A bibliography of cost-effective practices in physical medicine and rehabilitation: American Academy of Physical Medicine and Rehabilitation white paper. *Arch. Phys. Med. Rehabil.* **82**, 711–19.

Carson, A.J., MacHale, S., Allen, K., Lawrie, S.M., Dennis, M., House, A., and Sharpe, M. (2000). Depression after stroke and lesion location: a systematic review. *Lancet* **356**, 122–6.

Chamberlain, S.R., Müller, U., Blackwell, A.D., Clark, L., Robbins, T.W., and Sahakian, B.J. (2006*a*). Neurochemical modulation of response inhibition and probabilistic learning in humans. *Science* **311**, 861–63.

Chamberlain, S.R., Müller, U., Blackwell, A.D., Robbins, T.W., and Sahakian, B.J. (2006*b*). Noradrenergic modulation of working and emotional memory in humans. *Psychopharmacology* **188**, 397–407.

Chamberlain, S.R., Müller, U., Robbins, T.W., and Sahakian, B.J. (2006*c*). Neuropharmacological modulation of cognition. *Curr. Opin. Neurol.* **19**, 607–12.

Chang, B.S. and Lowenstein, D.H. (2003). Practice parameter: antiepileptic drug prophylaxis in severe traumatic brain injury: report of the Quality Standards Subcommittee of the American Academy of Neurology. *Neurology* **60**, 10–16.

Choi-Kwon, S., Han, S.W., Kwon, S.U., Kang, D.W., Choi, J.M., and Kim, J.S. (2006) Fluoxetine treatment in poststroke depression, emotional incontinence, and anger proneness: a double-blind, placebo-controlled study. *Stroke* **37**, 156–61.

Cools, R. and Robbins, T.W. (2004). Chemistry of the adaptive mind. *Philos. Transact. A Math. Phys. Eng. Sci.* **362**, 2871–88.

Coulthard, E., Singh-Curry, V., and Husain, M. (2006). Treatment of attention deficits in neurological disorders. *Curr. Opin. Neurol.* **19**, 613–18.

Cummings, J.L. (2003). Use of cholinesterase inhibitors in clinical practice: evidence-based recommendations. *Am. J. Geriatr. Psychiatry* **11**, 131–45.

Cummings, J.L., Arciniegas, D.B., Brooks, B.R., Herndon, R.M., Lauterbach, E.C., Pioro, E.P., Robinson, R.G., Scharre, D.W., Schiffer, R.B., and Weintraub, D. (2006). Defining and diagnosing involuntary emotional expression disorder. *CNS Spectr.* **11** (6), 1–7.

Deb, S. and Crownshaw, T. (2004). The role of pharmacotherapy in the management of behaviour disorders in traumatic brain injury patients. *Brain Inj.* **18**, 1–31.

De Boissezon, X., Peran, P., de Boysson, C., and Demonet, J.F. (2007). Pharmacotherapy of aphasia: Myth or reality? *Brain Lang.* **102,** 1114–1251.

DeMarchi, R., Bansal, V., Hung, A., Wroblewski, K., Dua, H., Sockalingam, S., and Bhalerao, S. (2005). Review of awakening agents. *Can. J. Neurol. Sci.* **32**, 4–17.

Farah, M.J., Illes, J., Cook-Deegan, R., Gardner, H., Kandel, E., King, P., Parens, E., Sahakian, B., and Wolpe, P.R. (2004). Neurocognitive enhancement: what can we do and what should we do? *Nat. Rev. Neurosci.* **5**, 421–5.

Fava, M. (2006). Pharmacological approaches to the treatment of residual symptoms. *J. Psychopharmacology* **20** (Suppl. 3), 29–34.

Feeney, D.M. (1997). From laboratory to clinic: noradrenergic enhancement of physical therapy for stroke or trauma patients. *Adv. Neurol.* **73**, 383–94.

Fink, G.R. and Heide, W. (2004). Räumlicher Neglect. *Nervenarzt* **75**, 389–408.

Fleminger, S., Greenwood, R.J., and Oliver, D.L. (2006). Pharmacological management for agitation and aggression in people with acquired brain injury. *Cochrane Database Syst. Rev.* **2006** (4), CD003299.

Floël, A. and Cohen, L.G. (2006). Translational studies in neurorehabilitation: from bench to bedside. *Cogn. Behav. Neurol.* **19**, 1–10.

Floël, A., Hummel, F., Breitenstein, C., Knecht, S., and Cohen, L.G. (2006). Dopaminergic effects on encoding of a motor memory in chronic stroke. *Neurology* **65**, 472–4.

Fountoulakis, K.N., Nimatoudis, I., Iacovides, A., and Kaprinis, G. (2004). Off-label indications for atypical antipsychotics: a systematic review. *Ann. Gen. Hosp. Psychiatry* **3** (1), 4.

Frank, MJ., Scheres, A., and Sherman, S.J. (2007). Understanding decision making deficits in neurological conditions: Insights from models of natural action selection. *Phil. Trans. R. Soc. B.* **362,** 1641–54.

Gill, D. and Hatcher, S. (2000). Antidepressants for depression in people with physical illness. *Cochrane Database Syst. Rev.* **2000** (4), CD001312.

Glenn, M.B. and Wroblewski, B. (2005). Twenty years of pharmacology. *J. Head Trauma Rehabil.* **20**, 51–61.

Goldstein, L.B. (2006). Neurotransmitters and motor activity: effects on functional recovery after brain injury. *NeuroRx* **3**, 451–7.

Greener, J. and Langhorne, P. (2002). Systematic reviews in rehabilitation for stroke: issues and approaches to addressing them. *Clin. Rehabil.* **16**, 69–74.

Greener, J., Enderby, P., and Whurr, R. (2001). Pharmacological treatment for aphasia following stroke. *Cochrane Database Syst. Rev.* **2001** (4), CD000424.

Griffin, S.L., van Reekum, R., and Masanic, C. (2003). A review of cholinergic agents in the treatment of neurobehavioral deficits following traumatic brain injury. *J. Neuropsychiatry Clin. Neurosci.* **15**, 17–26.

Hackett, M.L., Yapa, C., Parag, V., and Anderson, C.S. (2005). Frequency of depression after stroke: a systematic review of observational studies. *Stroke* **36**, 1330–40.

Horrocks, J.A., Hackett, M.L., Anderson, C.S., and House, A.O. (2004). Pharmaceutical interventions for emotionalism after stroke. *Stroke* **35**, 2610–11.

James, S.P. and Mendelson, W.B. (2004). The use of trazodone as a hypnotic: a critical review. *J. Clin. Psychiatry* **65**, 752–5.

Jelic, V., Kivipelto, M., and Winblad, B. (2006). Clinical trials in mild cognitive impairment: lessons for the future. *J. Neurol. Neurosurg. Psychiatry* **77**, 429–38.

Jiang, Y., Sun, X., Xia, Y., Tang, W., Cao, Y., and Gu, Y. (2006). Effect of APOE polymorphisms on early responses to traumatic brain injury. *Neurosci. Lett.* **408**: 155–8.

Jorm, A.F. (2000). Is depression a risk factor for dementia or cognitive decline? A review. *Gerontology* **46**, 219–27.

Kanner, A.M., Kozak, A.M., and Frey, M. (2000). The use of sertraline in patients with epilepsy: is it safe? *Epilepsy Behav.* **1**, 100–5.

Keenan, S., Mavaddat, N., Iddon, J., Pickard, J.D., and Sahakian, B.J. (2005). Effects of methylphenidate on cognition and apathy in normal pressure hydrocephalus: a case study and review. *Br. J. Neurosurg.* **19**, 46–50.

Kehayia, E., Korner-Bitensky, N., Singer, F., Becker, R., Lamarche, M., Georges, P., and Retik, S. (1997). Differences in pain medication use in stroke patients with aphasia and without aphasia. *Stroke* **28**, 1867–70.

Kessler, J., Thiel, A., Karbe, H., and Heiss, W.D. (2000). Piracetam improves activated blood flow and facilitates rehabilitation of poststroke aphasic patients. *Stroke* **31**, 2112–16.

Kim, Y.H., Ko, M.H., Na, S.Y., Park, S.H., and Kim, K.W. (2006). Effects of single-dose methylphenidate on cognitive performance in patients with traumatic brain injury: a double-blind placebo-controlled study. *Clin. Rehabil.* **20**, 24–30.

Kirsch, P., Reuter, M., Mier, D., Lonsdorf, T., Stark, R., Gallhofer, B., Vaitl, D., and Hennig, J. (2006). Imaging gene-substance interactions: the effect of the DRD2 TaqIA polymorphism and the dopamine agonist bromocriptine on the brain activation during the anticipation of reward. *Neurosci. Lett.* **405**, 196–201.

Kline, A.E., Massucci, J.L., Marion, D.W., and Dixon, C.E. (2002). Attenuation of working memory and spatial acquisition deficits after a delayed and chronic bromocriptine treatment regimen in rats subjected to traumatic brain injury by controlled cortical impact. *J. Neurotrauma* **19**, 415–25.

Knecht, S. (2006). Optionen der medikamentösen Behandlung kognitiver Störungen. In *Kognitive Neurologie* (*Referenz-Reihe Neurologi—Klinische Neurologie*) (ed. H.O. Karnath, W. Hartje, and W. Ziegler), pp. 230–4. Thieme, Stuttgart.

Krupp, L.B., Coyle, P.K., Doscher, C., Miller, A., Cross, A.H., Jandorf, L., Halper, J., Johnson, B., Morgante, L., and Grimson, R. (1995). Fatigue therapy in multiple sclerosis: results of a double-blind, randomized, parallel trial of amantadine, pemoline, and placebo. *Neurology* **45**, 1956–61.

Kumari, V. and Postma, P. (2005). Nicotine use in schizophrenia: the self medication hypotheses. *Neurosci. Biobehav. Rev.* **29**, 1021–34.

LaFrance, W.C. Jr, Lauterbach, E.C., Coffey, C.E., Salloway, S.P., Kaufer, D.I., Reeve, A., Royall, D.R., Aylward, E., Rummans, T.A., and Lovell, M.R. (2000). The use of herbal alternative medicines in neuropsychiatry: a report of the ANPA Committee on Research. *J. Neuropsychiatry Clin. Neurosci.* **12**, 177–92.

Laska, A.C., von Arbin, M., Kahan, T., Hellblom, A., and Murray, V. (2005). Long-term antidepressant treatment with moclobemide for aphasia in acute stroke patients: a randomised, double-blind, placebo-controlled study. *Cerebrovasc. Dis.* **19**, 125–32.

Lee, H.B., Lyketsos, C.G., and Rao, V. (2003). Pharmacological management of the psychiatric aspects of traumatic brain injury. *Int. Rev. Psychiatry* **15**, 359–70.

Lee, H., Kim, S.W., Kim, J.M., Shin, I.S., Yang, S.J., and Yoon, J.S. (2005). Comparing effects of methylphenidate, sertraline and placebo on neuropsychiatric sequelae in patients with traumatic brain injury. *Hum. Psychopharmacol.* **20**, 97–104.

Lehmann, V., Hildebrandt, H., Olthaus, O., and Sachsenheimer, W. (2001). Medikamentöse Beeinflussung visuo-räumlicher Aufmerksamkeitsstörungen bei rechtshirnigen Media-infarkten. *Aktuelle Neurol.* **28**, 176–81.

Long, D. and Young, J. (2003). Dexamphetamine treatment in stroke. *Q. J. Med.* **96**, 673–85.

Luaute, J., Halligan, P., Rode, G., Rossetti, Y., and Boisson, D. (2006). Visuo-spatial neglect: a systematic review of current interventions and their effectiveness. *Neurosci. Biobehav. Rev.* **30**, 961–82.

Marin, R.S. (1996). Apathy: concept, syndrome, neural mechanisms, and treatment. *Semin. Clin. Neuropsychiatry* **1**, 304–14.

Marin, R.S. and Wilkosz, P.A. (2005). Disorders of diminished motivation. *J. Head Trauma Rehabil.* **20**, 377–88.

Mattay, V.S., Goldberg, T.E., Fera, F., Hariri, A.R., Tessitore, A., Egan, M.F., Kolachana, B., Callicott, J.H., and Weinberger, D.R. (2003) Catechol O-methyltransferase val158-met genotype and individual variation in the brain response to amphetamine. *Proc. Natl. Acad. Sci USA* **100**, 6186–91.

McDowell, S., Whyte, J., and D'Esposito, M. (1998). Differential effect of a dopaminergic agonist on pre-frontal function in traumatic brain injury patients. *Brain* **121**, 1155–64.

Meythaler, J.M., Brunner, R.C., Johnson, A., and Novack, T.A. (2002). Amantadine to improve neurorecovery in traumatic brain injury-associated diffuse axonal injury: a pilot double-blind randomized trial. *J. Head Trauma Rehabil.* **17**, 300–13.

Moein, H., Khalili, H.A., and Keramatian, K. (2006). Effect of methylphenidate on ICU and hospital length of stay in patients with severe and moderate traumatic brain injury. *Clin. Neurol. Neurosurg.* **108**, 539–42.

Mooney, G.F. and Haas, L.J. (1993). Effect of methylphenidate on brain injury-related anger. *Arch. Phys. Med. Rehabil.* **74**, 153–60.

Müller, U. (2001). Pharmacological treatment of emotional disturbances in patients with acquired brain injury [in German]. *Z. Neuropsychol.* **12**, 336–49.

Müller, U. and von Cramon, DY. (1994). The therapeutic potential of bromocriptine in neuropsychological rehabilitation of patients with acquired brain damage. *Prog. Neuropsychopharmacol. Biol. Psychiatry* **18**, 1103–20.

Müller, U., Steffenhagen, N., Regenthal, R., and Bublak, P. (2004). Effects of modafinil on working memory processes in humans. *Psychopharmacology* **177**, 161–9.

Müller, U., Suckling, J., Zelaya, F., Honey, G., Faessel, H., Williams, S.C.R., Routledge, C., Brown, J., Robbins, T.W., and Bullmore, E.T. (2005). Plasma level-dependent effects of methylphenidate on task-related fMRI signal changes. *Psychopharmacology* **180**, 624–33.

Müller, U., Fletcher, P., and Steinberg, H. (2006) The origin of pharmacopsychology: Emil Kraepelin's experiments in Leipzig, Dorpat and Heidelberg (1882–1892). *Psychopharmacology* **184**, 131–8.

Murai, T., Barthel, H., Berrouschot, J., Sorger, D., von Cramon, D.Y., and Müller, U. (2003). Neuroimaging of serotonin transporters in post-stroke pathological crying. *Psychiatry Res. Neuroimaging* **123**, 207–11.

Murray, V., von Arbin, M., Bartfai, A., Berggren, A.L., Landtblom, A.M., Lundmark, J., Nasman, P., Olsson, J.E., Samuelsson, M., Terent, A., Varelius, R., Asberg, M., and Martensson, B. (2005). Double-blind comparison of sertraline and placebo in stroke patients with minor depression and less severe major depression. *J. Clin. Psychiatry* **66**, 708–16.

Napolitano, E., Elovic, E.P., and Qureshi, A.I. (2005). Pharmacological stimulant treatment of neurocognitive and functional deficits after traumatic and non-traumatic brain injury. *Med. Sci. Mon.* **11** (6), RA212–20.

Narushima, K., Chan, K.L., Kosier, J.T., Robinson, R.G. (2003*a*). Does cognitive recovery after treatment of poststroke depression last? A 2-year follow-up of cognitive function associated with poststroke depression. *Am. J. Psychiatry* **160**, 1157–62.

Narushima, K., Kosier, J.T., and Robinson, R.G. (2003*b*). A reappraisal of poststroke depression, intra- and inter-hemispheric lesion location using meta-analysis. *J. Neuropsychiatry Clin. Neurosci.* **15**, 422–30.

Palomäki, H., Kaste, M., Berg, A., Lonnqvist, R., Lonnqvist, J., Lehtihalmes, M., and Hares, J. (1999). Prevention of poststroke depression: 1 year randomised placebo controlled double blind trial of mianserin with 6 month follow up after therapy. *J. Neurol. Neurosurg. Psychiatry* **66**, 490–4.

Panitch, H.S., Thisted, R.A., Smith, R.A., Wynn, D.R., Wymer, J.P., Achiron, A., Vollmer, T.L., Mandler, R.N., Dietrich, D.W., Fletcher, M., Pope, L.E., Berg, J.E., Miller, A.; Psuedobulbar Affect in Multiple Sclerosis Study Group (2006). Randomized, controlled trial of dextromethorphan/quinidine for pseudobulbar affect in multiple sclerosis. *Ann. Neurol.* **59**, 780–7.

Parton, A., Coulthard, E., and Husain, M. (2005). Neuropharmacological modulation of cognitive deficits after brain damage. *Curr. Opin. Neurol.* **18**, 675–80.

Petersen, R.C., Thomas, R.G., Grundman, M., Bennett, D., Doody, R., Ferris, S., Galasko, D., Jin, S., Kaye, J., Levey, A., Pfeiffer, E., Sano, M., van Dyck, C.H., Thal L.J; Alzheimer's Disease Cooperative Study Group (2005). Vitamin E and donepezil for the treatment of mild cognitive impairment. *N. Engl. J. Med.* **352**, 2379–88.

Phillips, J.P., Devier, D.J., and Feeney, D.M. (2003). Rehabilitation pharmacology: bridging laboratory work to clinical application. *J. Head Trauma Rehabil.* **18**, 342–56.

Pierce, S.R. and Buxbaum, L.J. (2002). Treatments of unilateral neglect: a review. *Arch. Phys. Med. Rehabil.* **83**, 256–68.

Pisani, F., Oteri, G., Costa, C., Di Raimondo, G., and Di Perri, R. (2002). Effects of psychotropic drugs on seizure threshold. *Drug Saf.* **25**, 91–110.

Plenger, P.M., Dixon, C.E., Castillo, R.M., Frankowski, R.F., Yablon, S.A., and Levin, H.S. (1996). Subacute methylphenidate treatment for moderate to moderately severe traumatic brain injury: a preliminary double-blind placebo-controlled study. *Arch. Phys. Med. Rehabil.* **77**, 536–40.

Pollack, A. (2005). Marketing a disease, and also a drug to treat it. *The New York Times*, 9 May 2005.

Ragab, S., Lunt, M., Birch, A., Thomas, P., and Jenkinson, D.F. (2004). Caffeine reduces cerebral blood flow in patients recovering from an ischaemic stroke. *Age Ageing* **33**, 299–303.

Ramasubbu, R., Tobias, R., Buchan, A.M., and Bech-Hansen, N.T. (2006). Serotonin transporter gene promoter region polymorphism associated with poststroke major depression. *J. Neuropsychiatry Clin. Neurosci.* **18**, 96–9.

Rao, N., Jellinek, H.M., and Woolston, D.C. (1985). Agitation in closed head injury: haloperidol effects on rehabilitation outcome. *Arch. Phys. Med. Rehabil.* **66**, 30–4.

Rasmussen, A., Lunde, M., Poulsen, D.L., Sorensen, K., Qvitzau, S., and Bech, P. (2003). A double-blind, placebo-controlled study of sertraline in the prevention of depression in stroke patients. *Psychosomatics* **44**, 216–21.

Reuster, T., Buechler, J., Winiecki, P., Oehler, J. (2003). Influence of reboxetine on salivary MHPG concentration and cognitive symptoms among patients with alcohol-related Korsakoff's syndrome. *Neuropsychopharmacology* **28**, 974–8.

Rijntjes, M. (2006). Mechanisms of recovery in stroke patients with hemiparesis or aphasia: new insights, old questions and the meaning of therapies. *Curr. Opin. Neurol.* **19**, 76–83.

Robbins, T.W. (2005). Chemistry of the mind: neurochemical modulation of prefrontal cortical function. *J. Comp. Neurol.* **493**, 140–6.

Robinson, R.G. (2006). *The clinical neuropsychiatry of stroke*, 2nd edn. Cambridge University Press, Cambridge.

Roth, M., Mountjoy, C.Q., and Amrein, R. (1996). Moclobemide in elderly patients with cognitive decline and depression: an international double-blind, placebo-controlled trial. *Br. J. Psychiatry* **168**, 149–57.

Rummans, T.A., Lauterbach, E.C., Coffey, C.E., Royall, D.R., Cummings, J.L., Salloway, S., Duffy, J., and Kaufer, D. (1999). Pharmacologic efficacy in neuropsychiatry: a review of placebo-controlled treatment trials: a report of the ANPA Committee on Research. *J. Neuropsychiatry Clin. Neurosci.* **11**, 176–89.

Salmond, C.H., Chatfield, D.A., Menon, D.K., Pickard, J.D., and Sahakian, B.J. (2005). Cognitive sequelae of head injury: involvement of basal forebrain and associated structures. *Brain* **128**, 189–200.

Sato, S., Yamakawa, Y., Terashima, Y., Ohta, H., and Asada, T. (2006). Efficacy of milnacipran on cognitive dysfunction with post-stroke depression: preliminary open-label study. *Psychiatry Clin. Neurosci.* **60**, 584–9.

Scheidtmann, K., Fries, W., Müller, F., and Koenig, E. (2001). Effect of levodopa in combination with physiotherapy on functional motor recovery after stroke: a prospective, randomised, double-blind study. *Lancet* **358**, 787–90.

Schiffer, R. and Pope, L.E. (2005). Review of pseudobulbar affect including a novel and potential therapy. *J. Neuropsychiatry Clin. Neurosci.* **17**, 447–54.

Schneider, W.N., Drew-Cates, J., Wong, T.M., and Dombovy, M.L. (1999). Cognitive behavioural efficacy of amantadine in acute traumatic brain injury: an initial double-blind placebo-controlled study. *Brain Inj.* **13**, 863–72.

Siddall, O.M. (2005). Use of methylphenidate in traumatic brain injury. *Ann. Pharmacother.* **39**, 1309–13.

Silver, J.M. (2006). Behavioral neurology and neuropsychiatry is a subspecialty. *J. Neuropsychiatry Clin. Neurosci.* **18**, 146–8.

Silver, J.M., Koumaras, B., Chen, M., Mirski, D., Potkin, S.G., Reyes, P., Warden, D., Harvey, P.D., Arciniegas, D., Katz, D.I., and Gunay, I. (2006). Effects of rivastigmine on cognitive function in patients with traumatic brain injury. *Neurology* **67**, 748–55.

Stahl, S.M. (2005). *Essential psychopharmacology*. Cambridge University Press, Cambridge.

Stankoff, B., Waubant, E., Confavreux, C., Edan, G., Debouverie, M., Rumbach, L., Moreau, T., Pelletier, J., Lubetzki, C., Clanet, M.; French Modafinil Study Group (2005). Modafinil for fatigue in MS: a randomized placebo-controlled double-blind study. *Neurology* **64**, 1139–43.

Strangman, G., O'Neil-Pirozzi, T.M., Burke, D., Cristina, D., Goldstein, R., Rauch, S.L., Savage, C.R., and Glenn, M.B. (2005). Functional neuroimaging and cognitive rehabilitation for people with traumatic brain injury. *Am. J. Phys. Med. Rehabil.* **84**, 62–75.

Stroemer, R.P., Kent, T.A., and Hulsebosch, C.E. (1998). Enhanced neocortical neural sprouting, synaptogenesis, and behavioral recovery with D-amphetamine therapy after neocortical infarction in rats. *Stroke* **29**, 2381–93.

Temkin, N.R., Dikmen, S.S., Wilensky, A.J., Keihm, J., Chabal, S., and Winn, H.R. (1990). A randomized, double-blind study of phenytoin for the prevention of post-traumatic seizures. *N. Engl. J. Med.* **323**, 497–502.

Thiel, C.M. (2003). Cholinergic modulation of learning and memory in the human brain as detected with functional neuroimaging. *Neurobiol. Learn. Mem.* **80**, 234–44.

Tiberti, C., Sabe, L., Jason, L., Leiguarda, R., and Starkstein, S. (1998). A randomized, double-blind, placebo-controlled study of methylphenidate in patients with organic amnesia. *Eur. J. Neurol.* **5**, 297–9.

Van Reekum, R., Stuss, D.T., and Ostrander, L. (2005). Apathy: why care? *J. Neuropsychiatry Clin. Neurosci.* **17**, 7–19.

Walker-Batson, D., Curtis, S., Natarajan, R., Ford, J., Dronkers, N., Salmeron, E., Laib, J., and Unwin, D.H. (2001). A double-blind, placebo-controlled study of the use of amphetamine in the treatment of aphasia. *Stroke* **32**, 2093–8.

Walker-Batson, D., Curtis, S., and Unwin, D.H. (2002). Response [to Altieri *et al.* 2002]. *Stroke* **33**, 1170.

Wallesch, C.W., Müller, U., and Herrmann, M. (1997). Aphasia: role of pharmacotherapy in treatment. *CNS Drugs* **7**, 203–13.

Warden, D.L., Gordon, B., McAllister, T.W., Silver, J.M., Barth, J.T., Bruns, J., Drake, A., Gentry, T., Jagoda, A., Katz, D.I., Kraus, J., Labbate, L.A., Ryan, L.M., Sparling, M.B., Walters, B., Whyte, J., Zapata, A., and Zitnay, G. (2006). Guidelines for the pharmacologic treatment of neurobehavioral sequelae of traumatic brain injury. *J. Neurotrauma* **23**, 1468–501.

Wesensten, N.J. (2006). Effects of modafinil on cognitive performance and alertness during sleep deprivation. *Curr. Pharm. Des.* **12**, 2457–71.

Whyte, J., Hart, T., Schuster, K., Fleming, M., Polansky, M., and Coslett, H.B. (1997). Effects of methylphenidate on attentional function after traumatic brain injury. A randomized, placebo-controlled trial. *Am. J. Phys. Med. Rehabil.* **76**, 440–50.

Whyte, J., Vaccaro, M., Grieb-Neff, P., and Hart, T. (2002). Psychostimulant use in the rehabilitation of individuals with traumatic brain injury. *J. Head Trauma Rehabil.* **17**, 284–99.

Whyte, J., Hart, T., Vaccaro, M., Grieb-Neff, P., Risser, A., Polansky, M., and Coslett, H.B. (2004). Effects of methylphenidate on attention deficits after traumatic brain injury: a multidimensional, randomized, controlled trial. *Am. J. Phys. Med. Rehabil.* **83**, 401–20.

Zafonte, R.D., Lexell, J., and Cullen, N. (2000). Possible applications for dopaminergic agents following traumatic brain injury: Part 1. *J. Head Trauma Rehabil.* **15**, 1179–82.

Zafonte, R.D., Lexell, J., and Cullen, N. (2001). Possible applications for dopaminergic agents following traumatic brain injury: Part 2. *J. Head Trauma Rehabil.* **16**: 112–16.

Zhang, L., Plotkin, R.C., Wang, G., Sandel, M.E., and Lee, S. (2004). Cholinergic augmentation with donepezil enhances recovery in short-term memory and sustained attention after traumatic brain injury. *Arch. Phys. Med. Rehabil.* **85**, 1050–5.

Zhou, J. (2004). Norepinephrine transporter inhibitors and their therapeutic potential. *Drugs Future* **29**, 1235–44.

Chapter 23

Rehabilitation of cognitive disorders

Stefano F. Cappa

23.1 Introduction

Many different rehabilitation approaches have been suggested for the treatment of cognitive disorders due to neurological diseases. While the early treatment procedures were developed on a purely empirical basis, in recent years there has been an effort to propose rehabilitation approaches based on what is known about the neurobiology of recovery after brain damage and on explicit models of re-learning.

Two main types of rationale have been applied to the rehabilitation of cognitive disorders. The 'restitution' or 're-teaching' approach consists of the training of lost or damaged abilities by means of extensive practice. On the other hand, the indirect (compensation) approach promotes the use of 'back-up' strategies based on the patient's residual resources. In the latter case, the aim of the treatment is not to restore the function of the impaired cognitive component, but rather to exploit the preserved abilities to compensate for the deficit.

> The two main approaches to cognitive rehabilitation are restitution or re-teaching (training of the affected ability) and compensation (use of residual abilities to circumvent the damaged function).

Unfortunately, the evidence about the effectiveness of cognitive rehabilitation is limited. Only a small number of randomized controlled trials (RCTs) are available, and they are generally of low quality for a number of reasons: small sample size; lack of a control condition; failure to assess the outcome of the treatment at the functional level. This rather discomfiting state of affairs can be attributed to several different reasons.

> The evidence about the effectiveness of rehabilitation of cognitive disorders is limited in the first place because of the low quality of the available investigations.

In the first place, the clinical presentations of cognitive disorders are extremely heterogeneous. To give an example, it is unlikely that the same standardized aphasia treatment may be similarly effective for a patient with a fluent neologistic jargon due to closed head injury and for a patient with agrammatic non-fluent production associated with a fronto-parietal infarction. Research in cognitive neuropsychology has focused on the assessment of specific, theoretically driven treatments on well-defined areas of impairment, usually by means of single-case studies, which are generally considered to provide low-level evidence.

The second difficulty lies in the standardization of the treatment. Several factors, such as dosage, frequency of intervention, etc., are more difficult to standardize for a behavioural treatment than in the case of a pharmacological therapy. Moreover, the interaction between treatment provider and client is laden with interpersonal dynamics factors that cannot be standardized. This has resulted in some enthusiasm for computer-based approaches: however, evidence about their efficacy is not encouraging. Finally, the feasibility of a placebo double-blind controlled intervention is questionable. All these factors indicate that there is the need for methodological improvements in the design of effectiveness studies in cognitive rehabilitation. Here we summarize some of the treatment approaches, organized according to the area of intervention, and briefly comment on the available evidence. (For a detailed summary see Cappa *et al.* 2005; Cicerone *et al.* 2005.)

23.2 **Rehabilitation of focal neuropsychological syndromes**

23.2.1 **Aphasia**

The attempt to rehabilitate speech and language disorders following brain damage dates back to the nineteenth century (Howard and Hatfield 1987). A variety of approaches has been applied to the rehabilitation of aphasia (Basso 2003). The most widely used procedures are based on stimulation-facilitation, i.e. on the assumption that language abilities, rather than lost, become inaccessible after brain damage. The treatment approaches following this model are usually centred on language comprehension, in particular, in the auditory modality. Aphasia is considered as a unitary disorder, with individual patients differing in terms of the severity of impairment, rather than according to the specific features of linguistic breakdown. In contrast, the behavioural modification approaches emphasize the central role of the learning process in rehabilitation, and apply to aphasia the programmed instruction model based on operant conditioning. The techniques include shaping and fading, and other principles of behaviour modification, which are also incorporated in many other treatment approaches. Several specific treatment programmes focus on a detailed psycholinguistic and neurological description of the classic aphasic syndromes. Among the most well-known are the Melodic Intonation Therapy and the Treatment of Aphasic Perseveration programmes (Helm-Eastabrooks and Albert 1991). The neurolinguistic–cognitive approaches attempt to apply linguistic theory to aphasia treatment and have flourished with the development of cognitive neuropsychology. The emphasis is on a detailed assessment of language performance in each aphasic patient and on a precise analysis of the pattern of linguistic dysfunction on the basis of a model of normal processing. The process should lead to a 'functional' diagnosis for each case. The basic assumption of this approach is that a precise identification of the locus of functional damage should provide the ground for a rational intervention (Gainotti *et al.* 2000). A completely different perspective forms the basis of the pragmatic approaches, which aim at improving the patient's ability to communicate, regardless of the linguistic or non-linguistic strategies he or she is using. In the most widely known programme, Promoting Aphasics' Communicative Effectiveness (PACE; Davis and Wilcox 1981), the therapist and the patient are engaged in situations in which the exchange of 'real' information is taking place.

> The single factor that appears to predict the effectiveness of aphasia rehabilitation is the intensity of the treatment programme.

Notwithstanding the long story and the multiplicity of theoretical approaches, the effectiveness of aphasia rehabilitation remains controversial. The conclusion of the Cochrane review is that 'speech and language therapy treatment for people with aphasia after a stroke has not been shown either to be clearly effective or clearly ineffective within an RCT. Decisions about the management of patients must therefore be based on other forms of evidence. Further research is required to find out if speech and language therapy for aphasic patients is effective. If researchers choose to do a trial, this must be large enough to have adequate statistical power, and be clearly reported.' (Greener *et al.* 2000). These rather disappointing conclusions were based on the meta-analysis of a limited number of randomized clinical trials (RCTs), in which the intensity of the therapy was extremely variable. This may be an important issue, since a recent meta-analysis has shown that an intense therapy programme provided over a short period of time can improve outcomes of speech and language therapy for stroke patients with aphasia (Bhogal *et al.* 2003).

23.2.2 Apraxia

Although the incidence of apraxia after acquired brain damage is considerable (Pedersen *et al.* 2001), the literature on its recovery and rehabilitation is very limited. This may be due to the commonly held view that spontaneous recovery from apraxia is usually complete, and that apraxia does not affect the actual organization of purposeful actions in daily life. This traditional concept has been recently challenged by the observation that apraxia has a negative impact on the activities of daily living (ADL; Hanna-Paddy *et al.* 2003).

There is now also evidence that the rehabilitation of apraxia, by means of specific exercises or compensation training, leads to a significant improvement of ADL (Smania *et al.* 2000). If these results are confirmed, a change in attitude towards management of apraxia after acute stroke may be warranted.

22.2.3 Acalculia

Acalculia is frequently observed in patients with left hemispheric stroke, and the functional impact may be considerable in individual patients whose potential for return to work depends on their calculation abilities. The rehabilitation studies in this area have been based on a cognitive neuropsychology approach, focusing on single cases or small groups of patients, studied in great detail. All the main components of number processing and calculation have been the target of intensive training. These include the rehabilitation of transcoding abilites (the ability to translate numerical stimuli between different formats), of arithmetical facts (simple multiplication, addition, subtraction, or division solved directly from memory), and arithmetical problem-solving (the ability to provide a solution for complex, multistep arithmetical text problems) (Deloche *et al.* 1992; Delazer *et al.* 1998; Domahs *et al.* 2003). The results are encouraging as all the studies have indicated the possibility of inducing long-lasting improvements of the trained abilities, with a functional impact on daily life.

22.2.4 Unilateral neglect

As in the case of apraxia, the concept that unilateral neglect (ULN) is characterized by fast spontaneous recovery has led to an underestimation of its potential impact on functional recovery after stroke. However, the considerable evidence that the presence of ULN beyond the acute stage is associated with poor outcome in terms of independence has resulted in considerable interest in its rehabilitation (Denes *et al.* 1982).

> There is now considerable evidence that ULN has a negative impact on functional prognosis, and that ULN rehabilitation may be beneficial.

Many approaches to the treatment of ULN have been proposed in the last decades. These include the training of visual scanning, the use of cueing procedures, and several methods that aim at the modification of the multisensory representation of space, including vestibular stimulation by cold water infusion into the left outer ear canal, galvanic vestibular stimulation, transcutaneous electrical stimulation of the left neck muscles, neck muscle vibration, and changes in trunk orientation (Pierce and Buxbaum 2002). The use of prism goggles deviating by 10 degrees to the right has also recently been shown to significantly improve neglect symptoms (Frassinetti *et al.* 2002).

There is sound evidence of the effectiveness of rehabilitation in reducing ULN manifestations. The Cochrane review concluded that ULN rehabilitation results in significant and persisting improvements in performance on impairment level assessments. There is, however, insufficient evidence to confirm or exclude an effect of cognitive rehabilitation at the level of disability or return to home following discharge from hospital (Bowen *et al.* 2002).

23.3 Cognitive rehabilitation of executive and memory disorders

While executive and memory deficits may follow many types of brain damage, the patients who are most often in need of a treatment of these aspects of cognition are affected by sequelae of traumatic brain injury (TBI). The cognitive–behavioural syndrome of TBI is frequent and has enormous functional impact. While practically any aspect of cognition and behaviour may be affected, the main targets for rehabilitation are attention and memory function.

Attention has been the focus of several training programmes based on different approaches. These include interventions targeting specific attentional mechanisms, often by means of computerized drills. There is considerable evidence for the effectiveness of attentional training only in the post-acute phase after TBI (Gray *et al.* 1992; Sturm *et al.* 1997).

The other crucial area of intervention is memory. As in other areas of cognitive rehabilitation, the main approaches are either targeted to restore or optimize damaged or residual functions, or they are directed towards compensating for lost or deficient functions (Glisky and Glisky 2002).

The use of internal memory aids may have a place in the case of patients with mild memory impairment. An example is visual imagery training on memory functioning in TBI patients (Kaschel *et al.* 2002). Other promising techniques are errorless learning and the spacing-of-repetitions technique. There is evidence that, when patients are prevented from making errors, their memory performance is improved in comparison to errorful (e.g. trial-and-error) learning (Kessels and de Haan 2003). The spacing-of-repetitions procedure is based on the spacing effect, i.e. the improvement of learning when repeated trials are distributed over time (Hillary *et al.* 2003)

External non-electronic memory aids such as calendars, lists, notebooks, and diaries have been used, with good results, in patients with more severe memory disorders (Evans *et al.* 2003). Moreover, assistive electronic technologies, such as computers, paging systems, voice organizers, and virtual environments, have all been used to enhance memory performance. Paging systems and voice organizers have been shown to improve memory and functional status in patients with moderate to severe memory impairments (Cicerone *et al.* 2005).

> The most successful approaches to the rehabilitation of memory disorders are based on the training in the use of external memory aids.

Comprehensive holistic rehabilitation programmes, addressing multiple aspects of dysfunction, not only at the cognitive, but also at the functional, emotional, and interpersonal level, have been considered to be more suitable than cognitive training for TBI survivors, who are often affected at all these levels (Ben-Yishay and Diller 1993). There is some evidence supporting the effectiveness of this approach (Cicerone *et al.* 2005), but further studies are clearly needed.

23.4 Non-pharmacological treatments of dementia

The traditional concept of rehabilitation as restitution or compensation cannot be directly applied to conditions that are not stable, but are characterized by a progressive functional decline. In the case of dementia, the target of any rehabilitation approach is rather the reduction of the functional impact associated with the disease progression. This is a cardinal principle of the rehabilitative treatment of disabling conditions in the elderly (Young 1996). The treatment approach is multidimensional, and involves different professional figures besides the physicians (psychologists, nurses, occupational therapists, physiotherapists) with the aim of improving as much as possible the quality of life of patients with a chronic disease and that of their caregivers.

Cognitive and behavioural interventions may also have a beneficial effect on the rate of progression of dementing conditions. There is adequate evidence for the effectiveness of Reality Orientation Therapy (Spector *et al.* 2000*b*). On the other hand, it is not possible at present to draw conclusions about the efficacy of other rehabilitation techniques, such as validation therapy (Neal and Briggs 1999), music therapy (Koger and Brotons 2000), and reminiscence therapy (Spector *et al.* 2000*a*). There is also some evidence that the cognitive–behavioural rehabilitation and stimulating activities may delay the clinical onset of dementia (Wilson *et al.* 2002).

> Non-pharmacological treatments of dementia may reduce the functional impact of disease progression.

Given the potential impact of effective rehabilitation practices in this patient population, there is no doubt that high-quality studies are urgently needed.

References

Basso, A. (2003). *Aphasia and its therapy*. Oxford University Press, Oxford.

Ben-Yishay, Y. and Diller, L. (1993). Cognitive remediation in traumatic brain injury: update and issues. *Arch. Phys. Med. Rehabil.* **74**, 204–13.

Bhogal, S.K., Teasell, R., and Speechley, M. (2003). Intensity of aphasia therapy, impact on recovery. *Stroke* **34**, 987–93.

Bowen, A., Lincoln, N.B., and Dewey, M. (2002). Cognitive rehabilitation for spatial neglect following stroke. *Cochrane Database Syst. Rev.* 2002 (2), CD003586.

Cappa, S.F., Benke, T., Clarke, S., Rossi, B., Stemmer, B., and Van Heugten, C.M. (2005). Task Force on Cognitive Rehabilitation. EFNS guidelines on cognitive rehabilitation: report of an EFNS task force. *Eur. J. Neurol.* **12**, 665–80

Cicerone, K.D., Dahlberg, C., Malec, J.F., *et al.* (2005). Evidence-based cognitive rehabilitation: updated review of the literature from 1998 through 2002. *Arch. Phys. Med. Rehabil.* **86**, 1681–92.

Davis, G.A. and Wilcox, M.J. (1981). Incorporating parameters of normal conversation in aphasia. In *Language intervention strategies in adult aphasia* (ed. R. Chapey), pp. 169–94. William and Wilkins, Baltimore.

Delazer, M., Bodner, T., and Benke, T. (1998). Rehabilitation of arithmetical text problem solving. *Neuropsychol. Rehabil.* **8**, 401–12.

Deloche, G., Ferrand, I., Naud, E., Baeta, E., Vendrell, J., and Claros-Salinas, D. (1992). Differential effects of covert and overt training of the syntactic component of verbal processing and generalisations to other tasks: a single-case study. *Neuropsychol. Rehabil.* **2**, 257–81.

Denes G., Semenza, C., Stoppa, E., and Lis, A. (1982). Unilateral spatial neglect and recovery from hemiplegia: a follow-up study. *Brain* **105**, 543–52.

Domahs, F., Bartha, L., and Delazer, M. (2003). Rehabilitation of arithmetical abilities: different intervention strategies for multiplication. *Brain Lang.* **87**, 165–6.

Evans, J.J., Wilson, B.A., Needham, P., and Brentnall, S. (2003). Who makes good use of memory aids? Results of a survey of people with acquired brain injury. *J. Int. Neuropsychol. Soc.* **9**, 925–35.

Frassinetti, F., Angeli, V., Meneghello, F., Avanzi, S., and Ladavas, E. (2002). Long-lasting amelioration of visuospatial neglect by prism adaptation. *Brain* **125**, 608–23.

Gainotti, G., Basso, A., and Cappa, S.F. (2000). *Cognitive neuropsychology and language rehabilitation.* Psychology Press, Hove.

Glisky, E.L. and Glisky, M.L. (2002). Learning and memory impairments. In *Neuropsychological interventions: clinical research and practice* (ed. P.J. Eslinger), pp. 137–62. Guilford Press, New York.

Gray, J.M., Robertson, I., Pentland, B., and Anderson, S. (1992). Microcomputer-based attentional retraining after brain damage: a randomised group controlled trial. *Neuropsychol. Rehabil.* **2**, 97–115.

Greener, J., Enderby, P., and Whurr, R. (2000). Speech and language therapy for aphasia following stroke. *Cochrane Database Syst. Rev.* **2000** (2), CD000425.

Hanna-Paddy, B., Heilman, K.M., and Foundas, A.L. (2003). Ecological implications of ideomotor apraxia: evidence from physical activities of daily living. *Neurology* **60**, 487–90.

Helm-Eastabrooks, N. and Albert, M.A. (1991). *Manual of aphasia therapy.* Pro-Ed Publishers, Austin, Texas.

Hillary, F.G., Schultheis, M.T., Challis, B.H., Millis, S.R., and Carnevale, G.J. (2003). Spacing of repetitions improves learning and memory after moderate and severe TBI. *J. Clin. Exp. Neuropsychol.* **25**, 49–58.

Howard, D. and Hatfield, F.M. (1987). Aphasia therapy: historical and contemporary issues. Lawrence Erlbaum Associates, Hove.

Kaschel, R., Della Sala, S., Cantagallo, A., Fahlbock, A., Laaksonen, R., and Kazen, M. (2002). Imagery mnemonics for the rehabilitation of memory: a randomised group controlled trial. *Neuropsychol. Rehabil.* **12**, 127–53.

Kessels, R.P.C. and de Haan, E.H.F. (2003). Implicit learning in memory rehabilitation: a meta-analysis on errorless learning and vanishing cues methods. *J. Clin. Exp. Neuropsychol.* **25**, 805–14.

Koger, S.M. and Brotons, M. (2000). Music therapy for dementia symptoms. *Cochrane Database Syst. Rev.* **2000**, CD001121.

Neal, M. and Briggs, M. (1999). Validation therapy for dementia. *Cochrane Database Syst. Rev.* **1999**, CD001394

Pedersen, P.M., Jorgensen, H.S., Kammersgaard, L.P., Nakayama, H., Raaschou, H.O., and Olsen, T.S. (2001). Manual and oral apraxia in acute stroke, frequency and influence on functional outcome: The Copenhagen Stroke Study. *Am. J. Phys. Med. Rehabil.* **80**, 685–92.

Pierce, S.R. and Buxbaum, L.J. (2002). Treatments of unilateral neglect: a review. *Arch. Phys. Med. Rehabil.* **83**, 256–68.

Smania, N., Girardi, F., Domenciali, C., Lora, E., and Aglioti, S. (2000). The rehabilitation of limb apraxia: a study in left brain damaged patients. *Arch. Phys. Med. Rehabil.* **81**, 379–88.

Spector, A., Orrell, M., Davies, S., and Woods, B. (2000*a*). Reminiscence therapy for dementia. *Cochrane Database Syst. Rev.* **2000** (4), CD001120.

Spector, A., Orrell, M., Davies, S., and Woods, B. (2000*b*). Reality orientation for dementia. *Cochrane Database Syst. Rev.* **2000** (4), CD001119.

Sturm, W., Willmes, K., Orgass, B., and Hartje, W. (1997). Do specific attention deficits need specific training? *Neuropsychol. Rehabil.* **7**, 81–103.

Wilson, R.S., Mendes De Leon, C.F., Barnes, L.L., *et al.* (2002). Participation in cognitively stimulating activities and risk of incident Alzheimer disease. *J. Am. Med. Assoc.* **287**, 742–8.

Young, J. (1996). Rehabilitation and older people. *Br. Med. J.* **313**, 677–81.

Index